The CRC's Guide
to Coordinating Clinical Research

FOURTH EDITION

Sandra "SAM" Sather, MS, CCRC

wcg™ CenterWatch

The CRC's Guide to Coordinating Clinical Research, Fourth Edition

Sandra "SAM" Sather, MS, CCRC

Editor	Susan Salomé
Cover and Interior Design	Paul Gualdoni
Design & Production Associate	Renee Breau

Printed in the United States.

wcg™ CenterWatch

300 N. Washington St., Ste. 200
Falls Church, VA 22046
www.centerwatch.com

Print: 978-1-60430-100-7

TABLE OF CONTENTS

INTRODUCTION

Clinical research is a complex undertaking that involves multiple stakeholders that provide checks and balances to the process of Good Clinical Practice (GCP) to support human subject protections and data integrity.

Sponsors generally plan, initiate and finance the trial and own the compounds or devices being developed. The sponsors commonly have multiple vendors helping to fulfill their responsibilities for a clinical trial. Vendors supplement sponsor resources and/or expertise—often with a contract research organization (CRO). The investigators and their study staff conduct investigations for sponsors. Study participants (also called subjects once they are consented and study procedures begin) range from healthy volunteers to critically ill patients. There are also ethics committees, known as Institutional Review Boards (IRB), that are affiliated with an investigator(s) for a trial where the primary purpose is to ensure human subject protections related to a clinical trial being conducted at a research site. IRBs must approve the studies before an investigator can start enrolling subjects and must review and approve any changes. Last, but not least, are the regulatory bodies (the FDA and the HHS in the U.S.) that regulate the research and make the final decision about whether or not the product is approved for marketing.

The focus of this text is specifically on the role of the study coordinator or clinical research coordinator (CRC) working in the clinical trials setting. This book was written particularly to help and educate CRCs, the people who work in conjunction with clinical investigators at research sites. CRCs are the main liaison between the investigators and the study subjects, and between the site and the sponsor; they also handle a great deal of the study activity at clinical sites.

The book also looks at the many facets of clinical trials, from regulatory matters to the influences of technology.

Whether the reader is a CRC or another stakeholder in clinical trials, or has an interest in learning more about the role, it is hoped you will find the book both informative and useful.

CHAPTER ONE

The Clinical Research Coordinator

A clinical research coordinator (CRC) is a specialized research professional working under the supervision of a clinical research site's principal investigator. Chapter 1 discusses 1) the role of the CRC, 2) the knowledge and skills necessary to be a CRC who performs well across studies and contributes to the protection of those who participate in a clinical trial and the quality of the data generated, 3) the duties and responsibilities of a CRC, 4) the influence of technology upon the role of the CRC and 5) the increased workforce demand for CRCs.

Role and Responsibilities of the CRC

The principal investigator (PI) is legally responsible for the conduct and oversight of a clinical trial at a site. The investigator commonly delegates most of the clinical trial administrative and operational tasks. The CRC plays a critical role in a research site's study conduct and administration. First, it is important to become familiar with the various clinical research roles for the major groups that perform the study tasks within the regulatory framework.

Globally, the three major stakeholders commonly seen within clinical trials include:

1. Sponsor. The organization or individual that funds, designs, collects and analyzes data, and reports updates to regulatory authorities. Sponsors do not conduct their own studies. Sponsors are commonly pharmaceutical, medical device and/or biotechnology companies. Sponsors are required to monitor the quality of the clinical trial. Monitors or clinical research associates (CRAs) perform investigation site monitoring for a sponsor. The sponsor can formally delegate some

of their sponsor responsibilities, such as monitoring sites, to a vendor called a contract research organization (CRO). Commonly, a study has a primary study coordinator that works with the sponsor or CRO monitor for a specific trial.

2. Investigator. The individual who conducts and must oversee the clinical trial at an investigation site. The investigator cannot delegate responsibility of study oversight but is allowed to delegate tasks to appropriately qualified individuals. The CRC works at the research site that is conducting the clinical trial and is who the investigator commonly delegates certain study tasks to.
3. Institutional Review Board (IRB) or Independent Ethics Committee (IEC). The group or company that reviews and approves research for an investigator and the institution where the trial is being conducted also oversees the welfare and safety of study participant at each research study center.

The importance of the CRC in regard to the efficient and effective operation of clinical trials cannot be over-emphasized; in fact, many sponsor companies will not place a trial at a study site that does not assign a CRC to the study. The CRC performs various tasks for the study that involve study participants and some tasks that are more administrative. Examples of study participant-related tasks are scheduling study visits and reviewing the study requirements. Examples of administrative tasks are maintaining the study records and working with sponsor monitors on data verification.

Although not required, many CRCs have been trained as nurses, physician assistants (PAs) or other medical professionals prior to working as a CRC. A CRC who is a medical professional is better prepared to participate and be involved in activities related to the patient visit procedures. Medical personnel are more familiar with the settings in which clinical trials are conducted, and therefore understand medical terminology and the medical facility's systems; this all contributes to a CRC's ability to positively affect the quality of a clinical trial.

Some CRCs are not medical professionals. They may have scientific backgrounds or have worked their way up to their positions through experience-based training in a physician's office or clinic. Many non-medical people have gained the appropriate knowledge to function effectively as CRCs but are more likely working on the administrative tasks for a study. Some studies require a CRC to have specialized medical training due to the complexity of the trial design, the therapeutic area being studied, and how vulnerable the subjects enrolled may be. Some research sites have created an organizational structure that includes both medically experienced professionals and non-medically trained individuals to work as a team.

There are many opportunities for CRCs to obtain training. Ideally, the CRC receives foundational training for Good Clinical Practice (GCP) that includes a practicum component related to the activities performed by the

CRC, e.g., investigational product accountability, obtaining subject informed consent. GCP training provides the regulatory, ethical principles and roles and responsibilities information that a CRC needs to perform the study-specific tasks and make quality decisions from the application of GCP to a specific situation. This requires using critical thinking skills to adapt to different trials and situations to support quality clinical trials to ensure human subjects protection and data integrity.

Most sponsors require CRCs and investigators to complete GCP training prior to working on their studies. Commonly, sponsors provide the GCP training. Therefore, CRCs may take multiple GCP training courses in a year. This has resulted in an administrative recordkeeping burden and unnecessary repeat of GCP basic training. Instead the training needed for the CRC is study-specific application of GCP. Recently, there have been some influential collaborations between various clinical research stakeholders to improve the efficiencies and quality of how clinical trials are conducted, including how clinical researchers are trained on GCP.

One collaboration example is TransCelerate Biopharma[1], a nonprofit organization whose members are large pharmaceutical companies with a mission to promote improved efficiency in running clinical trials. One initiative resulted in their members agreeing to accept past trainings from a certain set of GCP training providers that can be used for a certain period of time to exempt the participant with successful completion from having to sit through yet another generic GCP training.

Another example of a collaboration supporting improving efficiencies for trial conduct is the Clinical Trials Transformation Initiative (CTTI), a private-public partnership between clinical research stakeholders and regulatory authorities. It has various projects ongoing to promote improved quality and efficiencies for clinical trials, including GCP training.

Besides formal GCP training, commonly the CRC receives mentoring by another, more experienced CRC or manager at the same site. If there is no experienced CRC working at the research site, an investigator that delegates to an inexperienced CRC must support the development of the CRC to independently perform core CRC GCP activities, or ensure that more intense oversight activities are in place. For studies with inexperienced CRCs, a sponsor should also recognize this risk and should monitor key data and GCP activities more closely at this site for the study because the inexperience of the CRC can contribute to regulatory noncompliance, challenges with enrollment and subjects' dissatisfaction with their participation in the trial.

Sponsors are required to provide CRC protocol-specific training for their studies. GCP training and study-specific training do not include the basics of how to perform as a CRC. There are various options for training CRCs. Professional clinical research associations can also be a training resource for the CRC; some examples include the Association of Clinical Research Professionals (ACRP) and the Society for Clinical Research Associates (SoCRA).

ACRP and SoCRA offer certification programs for clinical research professionals, including CRCs. There are prerequisites for taking the certification examinations, e.g., minimum years of experience. Becoming certified is an excellent choice for an experienced CRC as it shows a commitment to the position and adds to the CRC's overall credentials. Details of each certification program may be found on each organization's website.

Finally, an increasing number of universities are offering undergraduate and graduate degrees in clinical research management. A formal education in this field enables CRCs to begin their careers with the skills necessary for efficient and ethical management of clinical research and provides them with the knowledge and background needed to advance their careers in clinical research management.

Personality and Skills

The CRC job is multi-faceted, with a mix of administrative, business, medical and patient duties. With such a wide range of responsibilities, CRCs must possess many skills. CRCs must have extremely good organizational skills, including the ability to handle a number of different tasks simultaneously. They must be detail-oriented (being picky and a perfectionist is helpful) in order to handle the paperwork aspects of the job well.

CRCs must be people-oriented, as they interact with patients, sponsor companies and others on a regular basis. CRCs must be self-confident, flexible and adaptable to change. They also must be focused, manage time well and follow through on problems and commitments.

For a CRC, creative and critical thinking skills are very important. For each study, the CRC is using organizational policies and the clinical trial-specific requirements together with their skills to manage trial complexities, change and issues to best support the research participant and comply with the GCP requirements in support of quality data. And finally, a CRC must have a high energy level—they are usually very busy and likely coordinating several trials.

Where Do CRCs Work?

There are many types of investigation sites conducting studies, and CRCs work in all of them. For example, CRCs might work in a medical center, a doctor's office or even perform some activities within study participants' homes.

It is useful for a CRC to have an understanding of these different types of settings when looking for and assessing potential employers. Some of the more common investigative site organizational types are listed below.

Part-Time Sites

Investigators at part-time sites participate in research studies but also maintain their regular medical practices. Sometimes these investigators conduct only one or two studies at a time, while others may participate in research to a greater degree, depending on their interest and their resources for conducting studies. Most sponsors prefer this kind of site because there is greater potential to have study subjects readily available and the site study staff have more experience working on a clinical trial.

A CRC at a part-time site may work only part-time, or likely will have other responsibilities in addition to working on studies. There are other variations of the part-time site; for example, a large clinic may have a separate unit or department that only conducts studies, although the clinic as a whole sees non-study patients also. In this case, a CRC may work full-time as a CRC within the research unit.

Independent Research Sites

These sites are dedicated only to conducting studies; they do not see other patients for managed care or accept private or public health coverage. They generally are more experienced, are very productive and have the advantage of being consistent in their practices. They tend to have organizational structure and processes that support efficient clinical trials. This includes feasibility assessments of potential studies. Therefore, they evaluate which studies they can perform successfully and are less apt to accept studies for which they do not think they can enroll sufficient subjects within the given time period. A CRC at an independent research site will commonly be part of a team of CRCs.

Academic Research Sites

Academic research sites are those located within university teaching hospitals. They tend to do a mix of physician investigator-initiated research and government-sponsored clinical trials, as well as industry-sponsored clinical trials. Often these organizations are headed by thought leaders, the top specialists in their fields. Industry clinical trials may or may not be the academic site's primary interest. But it is sometimes the industry trials that provide added funding to allow these sites to carry on other research.

It is desirable for a sponsor to use some academic sites in its development programs. This allows sponsors to have thought leaders within the list of investigators working on the trial; thought leaders become familiar with the investigational product and, hopefully, become spokespersons in favor of the product once it is marketed. Some research centers have a well-organized quality system for research, some do not. Some have multiple research departments and therapeutic areas. Depending on the amount of research being done, an academic site may have one part-time CRC or several CRCs working within a department.

Site Management Organizations

Site management organizations (SMOs) bring together a group of sites and organize them centrally to conduct studies. They standardize procedures across sites and often provide standardized materials (standard operating procedures, study file procedures, source documents, etc.) to each site in the organization. Many SMOs also provide training for their sites and assist the sites in compiling and submitting the required regulatory documents. They usually provide centralized services for marketing the sites (attracting clinical studies) and for subject recruitment. There are several types of SMOs, from those that own the sites in the group to those with other partnership agreements. Each practice within an SMO may have its own CRC(s) or they may be contracted from the SMO.

A variation of an SMO is the Coordinator Organization. This is usually a group of experienced study coordinators (CRCs) who have formed a business. They recruit investigators to conduct trials and then place an experienced CRC in the investigator's office to manage and help with the trial. These coordinators usually act as the interface with the sponsor/contract research organization (CRO) and manage the operational aspects of the trial; the physician serves as the investigator and is utilized for his or her medical expertise and patient base, as well as providing the regulatory role of investigator. The investigator must still delegate tasks to the CRCs and oversee their performance. The organization of the SMO provides support to the investigator for oversight. But the investigator is still ultimately responsible for the quality of the system. There must be a clear communication mechanism for the investigator to escalate concerns about how a study is being run to higher management of an SMO and have the power to approve CRC assignments.

Regardless of how the physician's research practice is organized, the CRC will have the same general duties and responsibilities.

CRC Responsibilities

The CRC has multiple responsibilities. Although they may vary from site to site, the following list shows the breadth of duties CRCs handle.

The CRC assists in evaluating new protocols for feasibility at the site. This includes:

- Reviewing the protocol and other materials, such as the investigational product's Investigator Brochure and study informed consent form
- Looking at subject eligibility requirements and determining if those subjects would be available in the practice
- Assessing the ability to meet study timelines in light of other site commitments and overall feasibility

- Assessing the resources necessary to conduct the study, including people, physical space, materials, etc. (varies by site—the CRC may or may not be involved in the resourcing aspects of a trial)
- Assessing the financial feasibility of performing the study (varies by site—the CRC may or may not be involved in the financial aspects of a trial).

The CRC prepares the site study team for conducting the study, including:

- Training the people involved or ensuring they receive the training needed
- Setting up and organizing study files
- Creating or reviewing study-specific source documents (i.e., medical records, data case report forms) and other study-related materials and supplies
- Disseminating information about the study to others in the institution and/or the community
- Creating advertising, if appropriate
- Preparing documents for submission to the IRB
- Collecting the documents needed to initiate the study and sending them to the sponsor
- Attending the investigator meeting and sponsor site initiation visits, as appropriate
- Clarifying any study requirements with the sponsor.

The CRC participates in the informed consent process, which may include:

- Assisting in writing or editing consents
- Interacting with the sponsor and/or IRB on informed consent development
- Presenting the informed consent form to potential study participants, discussing the consent and the study with them and answering questions
- Obtaining subjects' signatures on the informed consent forms
- Ensuring that all necessary signatures and dates are on the informed consent forms
- Facilitating that the potential participant's medical questions are answered by the investigator or other qualified individuals
- Documenting, distributing and filing signed informed consent forms appropriately
- Ensuring that all amended consent forms are appropriately IRB approved, implemented and signed.

The CRC manages study conduct throughout the trial. This often includes:

- Contacting and screening potential subjects for the study
- Recruiting subjects
- Scheduling subject and sponsor monitoring visits
- Preparing for each subject visit to ensure that all appropriate study procedures are done
- Assisting the investigator with study subject visits
- Ensuring that all necessary data are gathered and recorded in the appropriate source documents (i.e., subject research charts) and on the sponsor data collection case report forms
- Reviewing case report form entries for completeness, correctness and logical sense and reviewing the source documents for subject changes in baseline health that are adverse events to ensure none have been missed
- Entering subject data into an electronic data capture (EDC) system
- Working with sponsor monitors (CRAs) during monitoring visits
- Making corrections to case report forms, if appropriate
- Resolving data queries
- Ensuring that study documents are complete, current and filed correctly
- Ensuring that the investigational product accountability is done correctly for each subject and overall
- Managing laboratory procedures (drawing samples, processing, packaging and shipping)
- Reordering study supplies as necessary
- Managing payments to study subjects, if applicable
- Completing study closeout activities at the end of the study.

Other duties a CRC may have include:

- Maintaining regular communications with sponsors and/or CROs, IRBs and the institution, if the site is part of a larger institution such as a university or hospital
- Collaborating with other departments performing protocol procedures (e.g., laboratory, pharmacy) as necessary
- Assisting the investigator with financial aspects of the trial, including budgeting and contracts
- Problem-solving and communication to the investigator

- Coordinating sponsor and/or regulatory study audits
- Helping to enlist new studies
- Professionally representing the site to all people/organizations in the best possible light.

On top of all of these responsibilities, the CRC must conduct all trial activities according to the appropriate federal and state regulations. This is considered the strictest enforceable standard of GCP.

The CRC also must be aware of the big picture—how the trial is going overall. With so many duties and so many things to take care of, it can be easy to miss an issue that affects the trial over all subjects and time periods. Most important of all, the CRC helps to ensure the safety and well-being of all study subjects throughout the trial.

As you can see, being a CRC is a challenging position, but one filled with opportunities and rewards with the added benefit of being involved in the process of bringing new treatments to individuals who will benefit from them.

Influence of Technology

As an industry, the adoption of technology is slow for many reasons, aversion to risk, complexity of interpretation of regulations and more. But the use of technology within clinical trials has increased greatly, triggered by a global movement to make running clinical trials more efficient. Technology adoption has been one of the results of the initiatives to do things with a risk mindset and focusing efforts and cost where it matters.

The CRC role includes the use of various technologies to accomplish study site tasks. Some of these are provided by the sponsor for a particular trial, e.g., electronic case report forms (eCRF), and some are part of the quality system of the research site, e.g., clinical trial management system (CTMS) and electronic health records (EHRs).

A CRC needs to learn how to use various types of technology. Sponsors rely on the timeliness and accuracy of the CRC's use of technology to be able to monitor some of the conduct of their clinical trials remotely, like remote study data review.

CHAPTER TWO

Quality Documentation and Data Characteristics

Essential documentation individually and collectively permits evaluation of the conduct of a trial and the quality of the data produced. This documentation serves to demonstrate the compliance of the investigator, sponsor and monitor, and IRB/IEC with the standards of GCP best practice, including all applicable regulatory requirements. Various study documents are grouped in three sections according to the stage of the trial during which they will normally be generated: 1) before the clinical phase of the trial commences, 2) during the clinical conduct of the trial and 3) after completion or termination of the trial. You can find a list of documents for each stage of a clinical trial within International Council for Harmonisation's Integrated Addendum to the Guideline for Good Clinical Practice [ICH E6 (R2)] section 8.2, 8.3 and 8.4.

A description is included of the purpose of each essential document, and whether it is for an investigator/institution's or sponsor's files, or both study files. Study files for clinical trials that are not study participant documentation are commonly called trial master files (TMF). It is acceptable to combine some essential document, as long as the individual elements are readily identifiable. TMFs should be established at the beginning of the trial, both at the investigator/institution's site and at the sponsor.

A final closeout of a trial can only be done when a sponsor has reconciled the essential files of the investigator and sponsor to ensure that all essential documents are there. All essential documents may be subject to, and should be available for, sponsor audit and inspection by regulatory authority(ies). Therefore, good storage systems should be used during the trial and for archiving (irrespective of the type of media used) that supports consistent and efficient document identification, version history, search and retrieval. Essential documents for the trial should be supplemented or may be reduced where justified (in advance of trial initiation) based on the importance and relevance of the specific documents to the trial.

When a copy is used to replace an original essential document, the copy should fulfill the requirements for "certified copies." The investigator/institution should have control of all essential documents and records generated by the investigator/institution before, during and after the trial. Important characteristics of certified copies is covered later in this chapter.

Study documentation is either study participant- or non-study participant-related. This is essential documentation that permits evaluation of the study conduct and the compliance of stakeholders (sponsor/CRO, investigator, IRB) to requirements related to a clinical trial. Study documentation therefore must meet a standard of good documentation practices.

In 2016, there were major updates to the ICH E6 GCP guidelines. One of the updates was related to investigator documentation and reporting when conducting a clinical trial. ICH E6 (R2) section 4.9, Investigator Records and Reports, states, "The investigator/institution should maintain adequate and accurate source documents and trial records that include all pertinent observations on each of the site's trial subjects. Source data should be attributable, legible, contemporaneous, original, accurate and complete. Changes to source data should be traceable, should not obscure the original entry and should be explained if necessary (e.g., via an audit trail)."

The elements mentioned in section 4.9 are referred to as A.L.C.O.A.C. (i.e., attributable, legible, contemporaneous, original, accurate and complete).

- **A**ttributable – Is it obvious who wrote it? Who or what is it about?
- **L**egible – Can it be read? If encrypted, can it be read if printed?
- **C**ontemporaneous – Was the documentation created when the data were observed?
- **O**riginal – Is it a copy? If yes, has it been verified as an exact copy with all the same attributes as the original? Has it been altered?
- **A**ccurate – Are conflicting data recorded elsewhere? If so, has this been satisfactorily explained? Is the information complete?
- **C**omplete – Are the data complete? Are any data missing?

Handwritten and or electronic documentation, and any changes to the documentation, must support these characteristics and answer the associated questions. When document templates or sources are approved for use during a study, for example study-specific source document worksheets, they become "required" and part of the essential documents for a clinical trial.

Quality data must also be made available when needed by those who have permission, which ensures adequate safeguards to protect the participant's privacy but not restrict use for approved research-specific activities over an approved timeframe. For example, a sponsor's monitor requests applicable original source documentation for an enrolled subject, while at the same time complying with the institution's privacy and security restrictions and requirements. A later chapter goes into detail about the privacy regulations applicable in a clinical trial setting. Clinical trial and privacy regulations do not restrict one another and there is no conflict, but knowing both sets of requirements is very important for the CRC.

Knowing the principles of ALCOAC will enable the investigator and CRC to follow good documentation practices even in situations where policy, protocol, etc., do not specifically address the question at hand. A CRC needs to be able to apply the ALCOAC principle when completing or reviewing documentation for a study. This helps prevent documentation issues for a study. This also supports effective issues identification and management. Ultimately, this supports human subjects protection and data integrity.

The following are some core principles of good documentation practices and ALCOAC:

- If it is not written down correctly, it did not happen.
- If you cannot tell who wrote it down, it did not happen.
- If you cannot tell what they meant when they wrote it down, it did not happen.
- If you cannot tell when they wrote it down, it may not matter what they wrote.
- If it is not written legibly, it did not happen.

Handwritten Documentation in Clinical Research

Always follow the policies of the organization you are working for. Here are some generally accepted practices that are related to handwritten documentation in clinical research:

- Keep handwritten notes and signatures legible. In cases when a signature may not be legible, the author should legibly print their full name beneath the signature, but not for someone else.
- Sign and date all entries. Initials are only okay if they can be linked to the individual.
- It must be clear what you are signing and dating. An entry may be one field, one line on a page, one page, or a collection of pages.
- Do not obliterate entries that require correction. Even paper documents have an audit trail, and this trail requires that the previous entries be legible, even though they are marked through.
- Never alter past-dated documentation, even if you wrote it. This includes adding information to an entry you have already signed and dated. If this need arises, handle this as a correction.

- Never alter someone else's recorded documentation. If the individual who wrote the documentation is no longer working for the organization and the data need clarification, there are acceptable practices to be sure the data are up to date. If you are in the same role as the original author, you can correct someone else's documentation as long as it is done in a manner that clearly indicates it is you and not the author that is making the change. But you may never alter documentation even if on the same date without treating this as a correction, no matter how trivial the change may be.
- Record the actual date when you sign the documentation. If this is different from when the data were generated, record that too.
- If you sign a document a day, a month or even a year after the data are recorded, you should still record the actual date you signed it.
- If there is a story to tell, e.g., the original document was lost, and you have re-created this document from other sources, do not hesitate to note that – BUT DATE THE DOCUMENT WITH YOUR ACTUAL SIGNATURE DATE.
- Record data on or about the date when the actual observations occurred. While one or two catch-up documents created a week after an event might be believable, it would be hard to believe that an entire series of documents could be recreated from memory months or years after their occurrence. There are certain late entries that are less likely to be acceptable. These are for things such as medical test measurements like blood pressure, heart rate, etc. If these types of measurements have not been written down, they are considered not to have been done.
- There are a variety of practices related to the color of the ink required to be used and can depend on the context and requirements of the institution. For example, some institutions require blue ink when signing a document to better support copying and recognition of the original. But exercise caution when using certain colored inks since some do not copy well.
- Never use correction fluid because this violates the principle of an audit trail. The appearance of correction fluid on a page will raise questions about what is obscured, and potentially raise questions about the validity of the document.
- Never use pencils or any easily erasable media for the same reasons.
- Maintain records chronologically. This helps to record what actually happened in a way that will best communicate to the future reviewer of the record the clearest picture and supports contemporaneousness.
- Complete all fields in a form. As an example, when completing a checklist with 10 items with columns for date and initials for each

item, if one person completes all the items, it is not sufficient to complete the first one and then draw a line down the page under the initials and date. Each field needs to be addressed.

- All changes or corrections to handwritten materials should be made by:
    - Drawing a single line through the old entry.
    - Writing the correct entry in a space adjacent to the old entry.
    - Dating and signing (or initialing) the new entry and indicating a reason for the correction.
    - If space does not allow for the correct entry, date, signature and reason, then indicate "(OVER)" and record these on the back of the current paper document. This is to be done only when it is NOT possible to make a legible entry on the same side of the page, as there is a greater risk of overlooking entries made this way or losing them entirely when copies or scans of the original document are made.
- Write the date format in such a way as to be completely unambiguous. With various date format standards worldwide, agreement of date format is not so critical as is the unambiguity of that date, unless there is an enforceable standard, like in a Case Report Form (CRF). For example: for the date of March 1st, 2012, various methods can be used, including 01-03-12, 03-01-12, 12-03-01, etc. These are ambiguous as they could also mean January 3, 2012, or December 3, 2001. Unambiguous alternatives would be 01-Mar-2012, March 1st, 2012, 2012-Mar-01.

The following are some additional good documentation practices for creating documents and completing forms. The forms may have been created electronically and then printed for use, e.g., a site worksheet to use for subject source documentation.

- Avoid hand calculations for important study information. Use Excel formulas to show calculations performed. Peer review calculations/formulas for accuracy.
- No blank sections should appear on study templates. If not applicable, explain or remove from the template (where permissible).
- Include appropriate references on every page (e.g., Study # and Document Version or Effective Dates).
- Number all pages (e.g., page x of y).
- Ensure consistent header and footer information (e.g., references to version, date, template).
- Don't leave the final version of documents in a "draft" state.

- Ensure that attachments are clearly identified and easily traceable to their source.
- Don't use sticky notes on documents going to long-term storage.
- Leave blank fields, sections or pages unless the form or procedure indicates they do not need to be completed. No dittos, dashes or arrows in place of information/data. Recent inspection findings at investigation sites have cited incomplete forms.
- Version control and document labeling:
    - Standard document naming convention: location_visit date_document type
    - Location = name of city
    - Visit date = yyyymmdd (dd is the last day if a multi-day visit)
    - Document types = for example quality plans, action plans for deviations

Use of "Memo to Files" (MTF), has increased greatly over the past 10 years of clinical trials. Regulations do not mention memos to the file or explain use or misuse. Sponsor monitors and sites sometimes use memos for many reasons (e.g., to clarify discrepancies between source documents and other study records, to explain specific issues that arise during the course of a study). Although such memos can help with reconstructing practices at a particular site and/or understanding how problems that arose during the study were resolved, there are many cases where the memos did not contribute to the quality of the documentation and serve the purpose intended. Many times, this is because the memos are inaccurate or incomplete. And many times, they are unnecessary (e.g., a deviation is noted in a study subject's research chart and an MTF is created to point out the deviation).

An MTF by itself commonly does not support the corrective and preventive actions agreed upon and completed to address significant deviations. An MTF should not duplicate what is already written or replace what can be written in a study participant's research record. The MTF should also be checked for clarity and accuracy and signed by the appropriate individual related to the content, e.g., if the MTF is indicating clarification of a patient's diagnosis, then the MTF should be attributable to a medically qualified individual. Additionally, this type of MTF may be an example of an unnecessary MTF, since this explanatory note can be written directly in the subject's record to benefit anyone reviewing the information for various purposes. In medical practice, MTFs are not used for updates to a patient's record; the medical record is where the information is updated and the same is true for research.

There are appropriate uses for MTFs, e.g., noting where something is being stored if not currently being filed within the study designated location. This occurs sometimes at research sites for delegation logs since they are used so often. There are some examples of FDA Form 483s and Warning Letters that have cited inaccurate and inadequate documentation at research sites and referenced examples of MTFs at the sites: "Nine months later the subject signed the correct version assent; the coordinator back-dated the signatures as stated in your note to file dated almost a year later." Investigator Warning Letter: CBER-05-020.

Certified Copies of Paper Documents

In a 2007 FDA guidance document, Using Electronic Data and Signatures in Clinical Trials, the agency defines a certified copy as a copy of original information that has been verified, as indicated by a dated signature, as an exact copy having all of the same attributes and information as the original. And more recently, in ICH E6, the definition of certified copies was finally added (section 1.63), expanding the FDA's definition to any media and the concept of validated methods supporting the original as well. So the definition states that a certified copy is "a copy (irrespective of the type of media used) of the original record that has been verified (i.e., by a dated signature or by generation through a validated process) to have the same information, including data that describe the context, content and structure, as the original."

In the process of certification of copies of original documents, a qualified individual producing the copy certifies in writing that the photocopy or printout made is an accurate and complete copy of the original data containing all the attributes of the original. Certification contains: a procedure and training documentation, the signature of the individual making the photocopy, the date the copy was made, and a statement attesting to the accuracy and completeness of the photocopy. The process must be traceable to all pages photocopied or printed.

There are two acceptable methods: 1) each page should be signed, dated and certification statement provided or 2) pages are numbered and a cover page attached to the photo copies stating the document type, the page numbers, and the signed and dated certification statement. The FDA does not require verification of certification process, but some sponsors and auditors may do a quality check. When a site must maintain the original supporting documents and another entity, like a sponsor, must also maintain an original, then copies should be certified. Examples include:

- When original data cannot be monitored directly, and shadow charts are supplied.
- When the subject transfers to another site.
- When original source data is collected, and copies are made for the site.
- Data recorded from automated instruments should be printed and certified if not directly reviewed.

Certification requires a verification process, so creating a scanned copy of an original paper record in itself does not meet the criteria of a certified copy. Having a formal process as described above is needed.

Certified Copies of Electronic Documents

Copies of electronic records are often from printing the electronic record to paper or converting the electronic file to a portable document file (PDF). The act of printing or converting to a PDF by itself does not equal a certified copy. There must be a process that supports the certification. Copies used to replace an original document, no matter whether paper or electronic, should fulfill the requirements for certified copies. The investigator should have control of all essential documents and records generated before, during and after the trial. The CRC should follow those procedures to ensure that quality documentation is maintained. Quality data ultimately supports human subjects protection.

Electronic systems that generate a system-validated copy of the data collected electronically do not require an additional manual certification. An example is a system-generated signed consent where the copy generated comes from the system and that system function has been tested to be consistent and yielding a quality output with all the same attributes. In ICH E6 section 1.63, the definition of Validation of Computerized System was added as "a process of establishing and documenting that the specified requirements of a computerized system can be consistently fulfilled from design until decommissioning of the system or transition to a new system. The approach to validation should be based on a risk assessment that takes into consideration the intended use of the system and the potential of the system to affect human subject protection and reliability of trial results."

A CRC will not be validating electronic systems, but likely using systems during a clinical trial that supports GCP. Some systems produce copies of data. The copies generated from the system should be from a validated process. Another example is central lab reports. An example of a system that does not create validated copies from the system is electronic health records (EHRs). When a CRC prints from an EHR to provide source documentation to the sponsor's monitor, these copies need to be certified as being a complete set as described earlier.

Summary of CRC Duties and Responsibilities

- CRCs perform many critical tasks for a clinical trial.
- The study tasks are delegated to CRCs from investigators.
- Research sites should have clinical trial procedures to support the CRC's good documentation practices.

- The CRC must be trained and educated in the performance of the study responsibilities. The duties include subject and no-subject related activities.
- All GCP activities must be documented or they are considered not done.
- The quality of the documentation must support ALCOAC. A CRC should be able to apply the ALCOAC principle related to documentation and check the adequacy of documentation for audit readiness.
- The research site's clinical trial processes also should support the investigator with the oversight of delegates, like the CRC.
- These oversight activities also should be evident through good documentation.
- A CRC should ensure that the efforts to keep the investigator informed and any escalations to the investigator are documented well within the essential documentation.

CHAPTER THREE

Regulations and Good Clinical Practices

As a CRC, you will want to ensure that you have a thorough understanding of the Good Clinical Practice (GCP) regulations that are applicable for your role. This will help you do a better job of helping the investigators and your workplace perform high-quality studies. In this chapter, we will discuss the GCP requirements that are important for a CRC to understand and apply. This includes pertinent requirements that apply globally and specifically in the U.S. Many of the requirements globally for GCP are results of incidents that significantly compromised human subject protection and led to global recommendations for foundations of ethical principles for clinical trials, for example the Declaration of Helsinki. This declaration has led to regulations and guidances that are important for the protection and well-being of human subjects in clinical trials.

Many clinical researchers think they have a good working knowledge of the regulations and global guidelines when they actually do not. How can this happen? Very easily; instead of reading the regulations for themselves, too many people rely on information by asking someone else, and that someone else actually may not have read them either or misinterpreted the intent or left out important information. This leads to an increasing spiral of misinformation and, thus, misrepresentation of requirements. As a CRC that is well read in the applicable GCPs, you can help prevent this from happening.

The Declaration of Helsinki (first version 1964)

The World Medical Association (WMA) spent more than 10 years working on the statement of ethical principles that became known as the Declaration of Helsinki (DoH). This document defines rules for therapeutic and non-therapeutic clinical research. It repeats the 1947 post World War II Nuremberg Code requirements for consent for non-therapeutic research but emphasizes the importance of consent when enrolling patients in therapeutic research. The Declaration of Helsinki also added that legal guardians need to grant permission to enroll subjects in research, both therapeutic and non-therapeutic, and recommends written consent — an important issue not addressed in the Nuremberg Code. In addition, the declaration requires review and prior approval of a protocol by an ethics committee. Several revisions have been made to the DoH related to the changes or challenges in society and clinical trials. It can be found referenced in many regulations, and the latest version is referenced on the World Health Organization website.

Good Clinical Practice

Good Clinical Practice (GCP) is not a single document that can be referenced, printed or read. GCP describes the responsibilities of the investigator, sponsor, monitor and IRB in the conduct of clinical trials. GCP is the applicable ethical and scientific quality standards for the design, conduct, recording and reporting of a research trial that involve the participation of human subjects.

Applicable GCPs for a clinical trial are made up of the regional regulations and guidance documents, local laws, institutional policy and study-specific protocol requirements. They are recognized as the requirements for the conduct of a clinical trial and encompass pre-study, during the study and post-study activities that ensure human subjects protection and data integrity. This includes such things as staffing qualified individuals, adequate training, the informed consent process, accurate collection of data, maintaining audit trails and permanence of data, adverse event collection and reporting, adequate and accurate records and records retention.

ICH Guideline for Good Clinical Practice

ICH stands for the International Council on Harmonisation of Technical Requirements for Registration of Pharmaceuticals for Human Use. The ICH was organized to provide opportunities for standardized regulatory GCP initiatives to be developed with input from both governmental bodies and industry representatives. ICH regions currently include the European Union, Japan, the United States, Canada and Switzerland.

The ICH releases guidelines within four major categories: 1) quality, 2) safety, 3) efficacy and 4) multi-disciplinary. The category that is directly applicable to the CRC's role is efficacy. These guidelines are concerned with the design, conduct, safety and reporting of clinical trials. The ICH guideline directly related to the role of the CRC is ICH E6 for Good Clinical Practice (GCP).

ICH E6 defines GCP and provides a harmonized standard for designing, conducting, recording and reporting on clinical trials involving human subjects. Compliance with good clinical practice ensures that the rights, well-being and confidentiality of human subjects are protected, and that trial data are credible. The guidelines are pharmaceutical-grounded but have been adopted and adapted by many medical device sponsors for GCP integration along with medical device-specific global requirements. There are some other global GCP guidelines that are more specific to devices and becoming more used, such as ISO 14155: 2011 Clinical Investigation of Medical Devices for Human Subjects, which addresses good clinical practice for the design, conduct, recording and reporting of clinical investigations carried out in human subjects to assess the safety or performance of medical devices.

The latest revision of ICH E6 was released late in 2016, titled Integrated Addendum to ICH E6(R1): Guideline for Good Clinical Practice E6(R2). The revisions are primarily focused on the changes in the industry related to performing trials with a more risk-based approach and provides some clarifications on GCP requirements. Regulatory audit findings of investigators and sponsors were also taken into consideration when the updates were added. Members of the ICH have all adopted the updated standard into their GCPs.

The Belmont Report (1979)

The National Research Act, passed by Congress in 1974, created the National Commission for the Protection of Human Subjects of Biomedical and Behavioral Research. This commission wrote a document entitled Ethical Principles and Guidelines for the Protection of Human Subjects of Research, which became known as the Belmont Report when it was published in 1979. The three basic principles of the Belmont Report are respect for persons, beneficence and justice.

- **Respect for persons** is manifested by the informed consent process, as well as in safeguards for vulnerable populations, such as children, pregnant women, mentally disabled adults and prisoners. Other important concerns of respect for persons are privacy and confidentiality.
- **Beneficence** has two general characteristics: do no harm and maximize benefit while minimizing risk. Beneficence is manifested in the use of good research design, competent investigators and a favorable risk/benefit ratio.
- **Justice** implies fairness and is manifested in the equitable selection of subjects for research, ensuring that no group of people is "selected in"

or "selected out" unfairly based on factors unrelated to the research. This means that there must be appropriate inclusion/exclusion criteria and a fair system of recruitment.

The Belmont Report forms the cornerstone for the ethical treatment of human subjects of clinical research and associated laws in the United States. You can find a copy of it on the Department of Health and Human Services' Office for Human Research Protections' (OHRP) website.

FDA Regulations for Clinical Trials

The primary FDA regulations that the CRC is most impacted by are:

- FDA 21 CFR Part 50 – Protection of Human Subjects
- FDA 21 CFR Part 54 – Financial Disclosure by Clinical Investigators
- FDA 21 CFR Part 56 – Institutional Review Boards (IRB)
- FDA 21 CFR Part 312 – Investigational New Drug Application (IND)
- FDA 21 CFR Part 812 – Investigational Device Exemptions (IDE)

These regulations tell us what is actually required by the FDA when involved in conducting clinical studies under the FDA's jurisdiction. They cover the responsibilities of sponsors, investigators and IRBs for conducting trials involving human subjects.

FDA Guidelines and Information Sheets

The FDA also publishes a number of guidances and information sheets that are very useful in the conduct of clinical trials. These give further explanation of the regulations and often include questions and answers for items of particular interest to assist in interpretation and implementation of the GCP regulations. Although the guidances do not carry the weight of regulations related to enforcement, it is highly recommended that they be followed. In many places throughout guidance documents, specific regulations are cited, and the requirements of the regulations are reiterated. CRCs benefit from reading and referencing regulatory guidance for clinical trial activities frequently performed by the investigator and/or the CRC, e.g., informed consent and adverse event management.

Links to specific FDA guidance documents can be found on the FDA's website under the Office of Good Clinical Practice (OGCP). Some of the more pertinent guidances for the CRC include:

- Information Sheet on Informed Consent
- Information Sheet on Inspections of Clinical Investigators

- Investigator Responsibilities—Protecting the Rights, Safety and Welfare of Study Subjects
- Exception from Informed Consent Requirements for Emergency Research
- Oversight of Clinical Investigations, A Risk-Based Approach to Monitoring

CRCs should familiarize themselves with the various GCP guidances as well as with the FDA clinical trial regulations. Exploring the FDA's website (www.fda.gov) is an excellent way to find all kinds of information about conducting trials. From the main page, look for links under Scientists and Researchers. Here you can visit the OGCP sub-site where you will find GCP resources for drugs, biologics and devices.

FDA BIMO and CPGMs

The FDA requires that the clinical trials it regulates conform to the GCP standards found within the FDA regulations. To help ensure that GCP standards are followed, the FDA inspects those that must comply with the regulations, i.e., sponsors, CROs, investigators and IRBs. The FDA's program of inspections is called the Bioresearch Monitoring (BIMO) program. Each of the FDA's divisions, drug, device and biologics, manages its own BIMO program, which is overseen by OGCP. OGCP ensures the harmonization of policies and best practices across the individual centers and maintains BIMO program manuals for inspecting sponsors, CROs, IRBs and investigators. These are referred to as Compliance Program Guidance Manuals (CPGM).

The CPGMs are used by FDA personnel who perform inspections. Of particular interest to CRCs will be the CPGM for Clinical Investigators, specifically Part III–Inspectional. The investigator's CPGM includes descriptions of what the FDA looks for during inspections of clinical study sites. The CPGM for the investigator was updated in 2008. One of the additions includes a section on the use of electronic data by investigators. (FDA inspections will be discussed in a future chapter.)

Office for Human Research Protections

FDA-regulated trials are often referred to as "industry" studies. But if you are working on government-funded research that is not regulated by the FDA, the set of regulations governing these studies comes from the Office of Human Research Protections (OHRP), for example, studies run through the National Institutes of Health (NIH). The OHRP provides leadership in the protection of the rights, welfare and well-being of subjects involved in research conducted or supported by federal agencies. The OHRP helps ensure this by providing clarification and guidance, developing educational programs and materials, maintaining regulatory oversight and providing advice on ethical and regulatory issues in biomedical and social-behavioral research.

The primary OHRP regulations are found under 45 CFR Part 46, Protection of Human Research Subjects. Subpart A of this set of OHRP regulations is sometimes referred to as "The Common Rule." This set of regulations contains specific sections on working with vulnerable subjects, such as pregnant women and prisoners, which are not found in the FDA regulations. The FDA has also adopted specific sections of 45 CFR Part 46 into the FDA 21 CFR Part 50 regulations: Subpart D for protecting children. The OHRP offers a reference tool online that compares the regulations for the two groups, "Comparison of FDA and HHS Human Subject Protection Regulations."

The Common Rule for Clinical Trials Update

The Common Rule was originally adopted in 1991 by 15 U.S. agencies and departments involved in human clinical research. The rule came from a combination of prior regulations and a number of international bioethics codes and declarations. Some we have already discussed in this chapter, i.e., the Nuremberg Code, the Declaration of Helsinki, the Belmont Report.

The purpose of the Common Rule is to create a uniform body of regulations across various U.S. federal agencies for human subject research.

In 2011, the 15 agencies began work to overhaul the rule to bring it up to date with current research practices and issues. The updated rule was released in January of 2017 and took effect in January 2019.

Clinical trial sites, sponsors and investigators conducting government-funded research have some new rules to follow now that the revision is complete.

The changes in the Common Rule that impact the CRC are the following main topics:

- Addition of "identifiable biospecimens" to the definition of "human subject"
- Update of informed consent requirements to include explanation of what, if anything, will be done in the future with any biospecimens collected during a study
- A new section on "broad consent," which allows study subjects to sign off on future, secondary research that may be conducted with their identifiable information or identifiable biospecimens
- Adding certain types of research to the list that are NOT considered human research and subject to the Common Rule, e.g., scholarly and journalistic activities, public health surveillance and the collection of biospecimens data for criminal justice and law enforcement purposes
- Procedures for limited IRB reviews including:

- New scenarios in which continuing review will no longer be required
- Cooperative research to be overseen by a single IRB
- Independent IRBs can be held directly accountable for certain compliance deficiencies during an institutional study.

HIPAA Privacy Rule

HHS implemented the Health Insurance Portability and Accountability Act (HIPAA) Privacy Rule of 1996 in an effort to protect individuals' rights to have access to, control access to and disclosure of their private health information, and to ensure continuity of coverage between health insurance plans. The HIPAA Privacy Rule encompasses more than clinical trials but has direct impact on clinical research that involves investigators working under a HIPAA healthcare institution, also known as a covered entity.

HIPAA is applicable to FDA- and OHRP-regulated studies. HIPAA regulations can be found in the U.S. Code of Federal Regulations: 45 CFR Parts 160 and 164. Failure to comply with HIPAA can be costly to the covered entity, resulting in significant civil monetary sanctions, or even criminal investigations. The covered entities must have institutional policies that its members, including CRCs, must follow. The regulatory authority that manages the HIPAA Privacy Rule is not the FDA or OHRP but the Office for Civil Rights (OCR). The requirements of HIPAA do not interfere with the FDA and OHRP requirements for a clinical trial and vice versa.

HIPAA Authorization

Under the HIPAA Privacy Rule, a covered entity must obtain HIPAA authorization from an individual before disclosing protected health information (PHI) outside the covered entity. This applies in clinical research as well. A potential study participant must provide authorization to the investigator at the time of informed consent for the investigator to disclose identifiable PHI for the study.

As a member of the covered entity, the CRC can review medical records and share this information freely with other covered entity clinicians who are involved in the subject's care at the site. This is considered part of operations and chart review. In the case of research, this is considered a Review of PHI Preparatory to Research and does not require a patient's authorization. But prior to any release of the information outside the covered entity, e.g., to a sponsor or independent IRB, a HIPAA authorization or an approved waiver of authorization must be obtained.

Since study subjects' pertinent medical records will be reviewed by a sponsor for industry studies and some information collected as well during a trial by the sponsor and/or the FDA, study subjects must be provided with information related to how their PHI may be used and disclosed. HIPAA authorization may be incorporated into the body of the study informed consent form or it may be provided through the use of a separate authorization document. The IRB commonly influences which way the authorization will be presented.

HIPAA regulations cover any patient's information at a site that could be used to identify the person to whom the information pertains. Under the regulation, this PHI includes, but is not limited to, the items or subsets of the following:

- Names (or initials)
- Addresses (any geographic subdivisions smaller than a state)
- Employers' names or addresses
- Relatives' names or addresses
- All elements of dates related to a person except for year
- Telephone numbers
- Fax numbers
- Email addresses
- Social security numbers (or portion of)
- Medical record numbers
- Certificate numbers (including device serial numbers for implants)
- Member or account numbers
- Certification/license numbers
- Voiceprints
- Fingerprints
- Vehicle identifiers
- Device identifiers
- Biometric identifiers
- Full face photographs
- Any other unique identifying number, characteristic or code.

(Appendix D includes an Informed Consent Checklist with HIPAA Authorization elements.)

Use and Disclosure of PHI

There is a difference between the terms "use" and "disclosure" of PHI. HIPAA regulations define these terms in the following way:

> *"Use" happens within a healthcare organization and is under the direct control of the organization. Example: a CRC in a clinic "uses" protected health information when seeing a study subject.*

> *"Disclosure" occurs when the information (PHI) is given to someone who is not part of the organization (not an employee). Example: allowing a sponsor monitor (CRA) to see a study subject's office chart/source document.*

As noted previously, PHI may be accessed for review to screen records for recruitment. It is acceptable to look through the records at your site to locate potential study subjects to contact about a trial. However, if an investigator is screening records that belong to an organization other than his or her own practice, then he or she is not allowed to contact the potential subjects associated with those records. There are ways to recruit subjects for trials that are allowable under HIPAA.

Healthcare providers that also conduct clinical trials commonly list potential enrollment in a clinical trial as one of their services offered to their patients and ask that all practice patients sign an acknowledgement of privacy practices. The privacy practices list how the covered entity manages the patient's PHI. The privacy practices can also include the maintenance of a database that can be used within the practice to identify potential participants. The acknowledgement signed by patients is not an authorization, but documentation that the patient was educated about how their information is protected, used and disclosed as a matter of day-to-day operations that do not require HIPAA authorization.

A physician may discuss a clinical trial with a patient during a regular patient medical visit when the service is listed in the privacy practices. If the patient is interested in the trial, then the physician may refer the patient to the principal investigator, study coordinator or another source of information, such as a website, to learn more about the trial. Sometimes, the study site personnel also are those that see the patient for medical visits and, if the patient is interested, start the consenting process at that same visit. Note that if an individual volunteers information, e.g., completes an online recruitment questionnaire, this act is considered basic authorization or permission to use the information provided.

The Office for Civil Rights (OCR) has issued a guidance document, *Summary of the HIPAA Privacy Rule*, that says that a researcher can look at PHI in medical records to identify potential study subjects, but the information gathered cannot be taken outside the clinic or hospital (covered entity) and the information cannot be used for anything other than research.

However, if the researcher is not an employee or in the workforce of the covered entity, he or she cannot contact the person about the study unless the IRB has granted a waiver of authorization.

Under HIPAA, an investigator or a staff member may communicate directly with patients without patient authorization to discuss the option of enrolling in a clinical trial. This means you can telephone or send letters directly to your patients to tell them about trials and their options for possible enrollment in them.

An investigator may use and disclose PHI for research without an authorization from each individual if the investigator has a waiver from an IRB). However, an IRB can issue a waiver only if the use of the PHI involves no more than minimal risk to the individuals' privacy based on the following:

- There is a plan to protect the PHI from improper use and disclosure.
- There is an adequate plan to destroy the PHI as soon as possible after use.
- There is adequate written assurance that the PHI will not be reused or re-disclosed to any other person or entity (with a few exceptions).
- The research could not be conducted practicably without access to the PHI.
- The research could not be conducted practicably without the waiver.

Always be sure to become familiar with how the institution where you work manages authorizations and review of patient information for consideration for participation in a clinical trial.

Obtaining Informed Consent under HIPAA

As was discussed earlier, under HIPAA, an investigator must obtain permission from patients before disclosing their PHI for most clinical research. Investigators may use a separate authorization for this, or it can be included in the informed consent document that will be used for the study.

The document must list all the types of health information that will be used or disclosed, including such categories as the subject's medical history, physical findings and laboratory test results. If the investigator determines later that he or she needs to use information that was not included in the original authorization, an updated authorization will need to be obtained. The regulation requires the following elements to be included in this authorization:

- The specific information intended to be used
- The people who, or organizations that, may use or disclose the information (usually the investigator and the research team)

- The people who or organizations that will receive the information (usually the sponsor, CRO, central laboratories, IRB, FDA, etc.)
- The purpose of the use and disclosure
- The expiration date or event of the authorization (such as 10 years after the end of the study)
- The right to refuse to sign the authorization
- The right to revoke the authorization.

Even though HIPAA allows the individual the right to refuse the authorization, the investigator cannot allow someone who refuses authorization to participate because the information has to be shared with the sponsor to monitor for safety and effectiveness. If the subject participating in a study revokes authorization, they would not be able to remain in the study. Subjects may withdraw their informed consent and end their participation in a study at any time by most any method, e.g., verbally. Under HIPAA, however, they must revoke the authorization in writing to revoke the subsequent use or disclosure of their PHI. Even after a subject has revoked authorization to use his or her PHI, the investigator may still use enough of the PHI to inform the sponsor of the revocation. Also, if the investigator has already submitted the subject's data to the sponsor, those data do not need to be retrieved. In general, the investigator may not submit any additional data from a subject to the sponsor once a subject has revoked authorization to use his or her PHI; the only exception is for safety information.

In summary, the HIPAA rules and regulations have an impact on the way clinical trials must be conducted. The CRC should understand the institution's policies and procedures regarding HIPAA. (Refer to the Chapter on Informed Consent for more information.)

CHAPTER FOUR

An Overview of Product Development

In this chapter, an overview of the research process for new investigational product development and approval will be presented, to include drug, biologic and device for a particular indication. The main documents that must be filed with the FDA to study an investigational product in humans, and subsequently, for approval, will also be discussed.

It is important that CRCs comprehend the investigational product development process, even though they will not be involved in every step. This will help you to understand why things happen as they do and to participate knowledgeably in the process.

Drug Development and CDER

The Center for Drug Evaluation and Research (CDER) is the organization within the FDA that evaluates and approves new drugs for market release.

CDER's review of new investigational drug (IND) applications is to ensure that drugs are studied enough for safety and effectiveness, and there is enough information to support market approval. CDER makes sure that safe and effective drugs are available to improve the health of consumers. CDER also ensures that prescription and over-the-counter drugs, both brand name and generic, work correctly and that the health benefits outweigh known risks.

CDER requires that various phases of research investigation are performed—preclinical, premarket studies and potentially some post-market studies. The phases are also referred to as Phase I, Phase II, Phase III and

Phase IV. Some of the phases of studies have sub-categories as well, like a Phase IIIb study. The following is a review of the phases of research for drug and biologic clinical trials. Note there may be some exceptions to the rules related to phases of research requirements based on the nature of the product and also the need for treatment for the indication being studied, e.g., ovarian cancer.

Figure 1: Development of a successful new drug

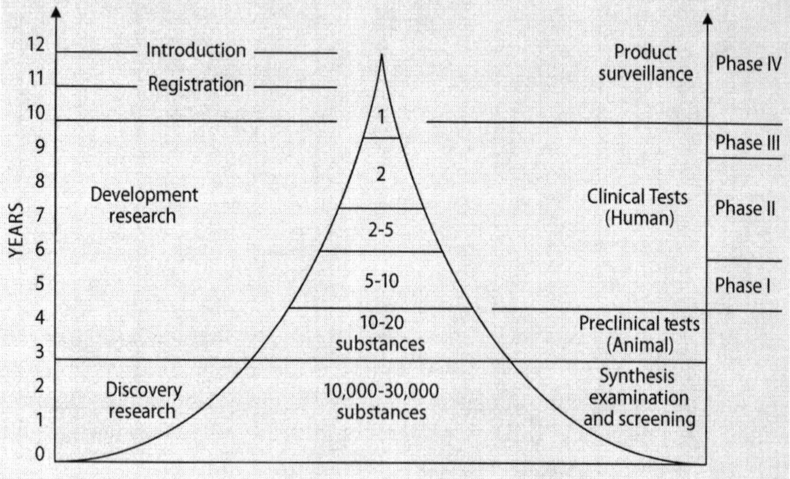

Source: PhRMA

Preclinical Research

In this section, we will look at drug discovery and the preclinical work that must be done before Phase I studies in humans can begin. Preclinical refers to studies that do not involve human subjects. Clinical studies are studies conducted with human subjects. Commonly, the non-human work continues after clinical studies have begun.

Before testing a drug in people, researchers must find out whether there is a potential to cause serious harm or toxicity. The two types of preclinical research are in vitro and in vivo. In vitro is an experiment taking place in a test tube, culture dish, or elsewhere outside a living organism. In vivo is an experiment performed in a living organism, in this case not a human being.

In preclinical research, the FDA requires researchers to use good laboratory practices (GLP). The GLP regulations are found in 21 CFR Part 58.1: Good Laboratory Practice for Nonclinical Laboratory Studies.

Drug Discovery

The discovery of new substances that might eventually become marketed drugs or biologics, occurs in a number of ways. There is direct research, in which chemists create compounds with structures likely to evoke the kind of physiological effect for which they are looking. Another approach is to change the molecular structure of known compounds in the hope of improving safety or efficacy while creating a new chemical entity that is sufficiently different from the parent compound to allow for the filing of a new patent.

In addition to classical chemistry, there are many new laboratory tools for developing viable drug substances. Computer technology provides many methods for molecular structuring. There are also computer-readable chemical libraries, which may contain several hundred thousand molecular structures. Many pharmaceutical companies have contracts with firms that provide these libraries; the companies take these chemical structures from the database and perform structure/function/activity computations and computer modeling to look for a hit on a potential compound. Companies can also perform high-throughput screening and other computer-related inquiries to look for hits. Other methods include gene sequencing, gene vector delivery and recombinant DNA.

In addition to the laboratory synthesis of compounds, naturally occurring compounds are another source of potential pharmaceuticals. A number of drugs have originated from soil samples (antibiotics), plants (digitalis) and other natural materials such as coral (prostaglandins).

Serendipity plays a role in any research program. Some very exciting compounds have been discovered by accident. Many drugs are marketed for an indication that was discovered by accident during studies for a different indication. One example is minoxidil, which was originally developed as an antihypertensive (Loniten®). Its hair-growing capability wasn't known until subjects enrolled in the hypertension studies began exhibiting accelerated hair growth—in all the wrong places. Based on this unwanted side effect, the company eventually developed a topical formulation of minoxidil as a hair growth product; this was approved by the FDA and is marketed as Rogaine®.

Preclinical Studies of Product Candidates

Once a compound appears to be a viable product candidate, it must be determined if it is reasonably safe for initial testing in humans and if it exhibits pharmacological activity that might justify developing it commercially. This preclinical work focuses on collecting data and information to establish that humans will not be exposed to unreasonable risks in early-phase clinical studies. This evidence will be presented to the FDA in an IND application.

The first step is to determine the basic physical, chemical and biological characteristics of a new compound. Once a compound is characterized and satisfactory stability data are in hand, preclinical studies can be initiated. The type of studies and their designs will vary depending on the intended use of the drug or biologic being developed. The purpose of preclinical studies is to characterize the toxic effects of the compound with respect to target organs, dose dependence and relationship to exposure. Many of the studies are in lab animals, sometimes in multiple species with variable durations of dosing.

The preclinical studies will establish a number of different things, including:

- The initial indication to be treated in humans
- The highest dose of the compound that can be tolerated as well as a dose that evokes no overt toxicity, in order to determine initial dosing in humans and to characterize potential organ-specific adverse events
- Proposed dose, route of administration and duration of treatment for Phase I studies
- Whether any adverse effects that are seen are reversible
- Genotoxicity, teratology and reproductive toxicology.

The IND

The FDA IND regulations become applicable in a drug development program when the sponsor has completed enough preclinical work with the compound to determine that it is reasonable to start working with it in humans. This is when the molecule changes in legal status under the Federal Food, Drug and Cosmetic Act. It becomes an "investigational new drug" and is subject to specific regulatory requirements. In order to do this, the sponsor must file an IND application with the FDA.

INDs are not actively approved by the FDA, but during review may be disapproved. After submitting an IND to the FDA, if a company has not received any requests for information, changes or disapprovals, clinical testing of a new compound may begin 30 days after the FDA has received the IND. This allows the FDA time to review the IND for any safety concerns.

An IND contains information in the following areas:

- Animal pharmacology and toxicology studies. These make up the preclinical data that allow the FDA to make an assessment about whether the product is reasonably safe for initial testing in humans.
- Any previous experience with the drug in humans. This might be from foreign studies, especially if the compound is marketed in other countries.
- Manufacturing information.
- Clinical protocols and investigator information. This will include detailed protocols so that the FDA can assess whether the initial phase trials will expose subjects to unnecessary risks, as well as information about the qualifications of clinical investigators.

The IND must be updated on an annual basis. In the update, the sponsor includes any new information about the drug, as well as the results of any studies ongoing or completed during the year. This information includes current enrollment numbers, adverse event information and the overall study status. The update also includes the clinical plan for the next year. This information keeps the FDA abreast of what is happening with the compound over time.

Amendments to the IND may be filed at any time. Amendments are filed for any changes in protocols, dosing, investigators or other changes in the development program.

A CRC will not commonly have involvement with the development and submission of the IND. An exception might be when a CRC is working at an academic medical center and is coordinating an investigator-initiated trial (IIT), called a "sponsor-investigator" trial by the FDA. In this case, the site is serving as the sponsor and the investigator, which requires it to follow both sets of applicable regulations. In these types of studies, a CRC might be managing the IND safety reporting and updates. The IIT study teams tend to be small, so the CRC may have more exposure to the IND management activities.

Additionally, when it is time for the IND annual update, sites working with the compound may be contacted for the necessary current information by the sponsor. Often there are critical timelines involved, so the sponsor will work with the investigator or their delegate to collect the information in a timely manner.

Clinical Trials

In this section we will discuss the clinical development of a compound. The term clinical implies human studies, as opposed to animal studies. Clinical trials are research studies that involve the active participation of at least one human being (trial subject) to test the safety and efficacy of new medical treatments. Clinical trials are not begun until a reasonable amount of preclinical work has been completed and there is evidence that the compound is potentially safe for use in humans.

Clinical trials are divided into phases: I, II, III and IV. Many companies also use the designation of Phase IIa, IIb and IIIb, which will be defined in this chapter. (Note that you also may see the phases numbered using Arabic numerals 1, 2, 3, 3b and 4.) The phases simply serve as markers or milestones in the drug development process and are not necessarily distinct, consecutive periods; for example, in some cases, Phases II and III can be combined, or Phase II may start before Phase I is complete. However, each phase does have distinct characteristics and purposes, and each is important to the development program.

Phase I Clinical Trials

During Phase I, the investigational drug or biologic is given to humans for the first time. The primary goal of Phase I studies is to establish safety—determining if the drug can be given to people without intolerable side effects.

Phase I studies, frequently referred to as safety studies, enroll a small number of subjects. The total number of subjects in Phase I usually is between 20 and 100. Subjects are usually healthy volunteers, although in some cases, patients with the target disease are studied. The type of subject depends on the nature of the disease and the expected toxicity of the investigational drug. It would not be ethical, for example, to give healthy subjects a toxic new drug meant to treat one of the cancers.

The purpose of Phase I studies is to determine the metabolic and pharmacologic action of the drug in humans, assess the adverse effects associated with different doses and perhaps get an indication of whether or not there is any evidence of efficacy. Because this is the first time humans are exposed to the drug, these studies are very closely monitored by medical personnel. Phase I studies often are conducted in special testing facilities designed for this work.

Essentially, Phase I should provide the researcher with sufficient information about the drug's pharmacokinetics and pharmacological effects (safe-dose range and adverse effects) to permit designing safe, well-controlled, scientifically sound Phase II studies. The primary concern of Phase I is subject safety.

Phase II Clinical Trials

When the appropriate Phase I studies have been completed and sufficient safety data are in hand, Phase II studies are initiated. The goal of Phase II studies is to see if the drug has efficacy in the target disease/condition, as well as to determine an appropriate dose.

Phase II studies are rigid, well-controlled studies in a relatively small patient population, usually no more than a few hundred subjects in total. These subjects have the target disease but no other illnesses. Phase II usually consists of double-blind studies using a placebo or comparator drug, or both. Their purpose is to determine whether or not the investigational drug demonstrates efficacy for the proposed indication within the safe-dose range established in Phase I. Short-term adverse effects and risks are also assessed.

While the focus of Phase II studies is primarily efficacy, they also assess safety, as this is always of primary concern. Dose-range finding, e.g., establishing a minimum and maximum effective dose and pharmacokinetic (PK) data correlating blood levels of the drug with pharmacological effect are also studied during Phase II.

Some sponsors also break Phase II trials into two categories.

- Phase IIa: Smaller trials to evaluate efficacy (and safety) in selected populations of patients with the disease or condition. The focus is commonly on dose-response, type of patient, frequency of dosing.

- Phase IIb: Sometimes referred to as pivotal trials to evaluate efficacy (and safety) in patients with the disease or condition. These clinical trials usually represent the most rigorous demonstration of the investigational product's efficacy.

Phase III Clinical Trials

Phase III studies are initiated only if the data generated in Phases I and II show a satisfactory safety profile and there is sufficient evidence of efficacy. The purpose of Phase III studies is to demonstrate the long-term safety and efficacy needed to assess the risk/benefit relationship of the drug and to provide adequate data for the product package insert.

Phase III studies are expanded, controlled studies in large patient populations (often thousands of patients) that represent the types of patients the compound is intended to treat once it is marketed. They may extend over several years. The development plan for the compound usually includes many different studies, including more than one multi-center study using the same or similar protocols. Multi-center studies are those in which multiple investigative sites all follow the same protocol and the data are intended for analysis together in one group.

The FDA requirement for registration of a drug is two "adequate and well-controlled" (primary efficacy) studies. However, under the Food and Drug Administration Modernization Act legislation of 1997, the FDA may allow one study instead of two for a product for which it is determined (by the FDA) that "data from one adequate and well-controlled clinical investigation and confirmatory evidence (obtained prior to or after such investigation) are sufficient to establish effectiveness." This is known as Fast Track designation. A Fast Track product is intended for the treatment of serious or life-threatening conditions and demonstrates the potential to address unmet medical needs for the condition. The decision to do one, rather than two, adequate and well-controlled studies is not one a sponsor will make on its own; this decision will be made after consultation with and support of the FDA.

Phase III trials have two main categories.

- Phase IIIa: Trials conducted after efficacy of the medicine is demonstrated in Phase II, but prior to regulatory submission of a New Drug Application (NDA). These trials commonly provide a lot of the information included in the package insert or labeling of the product.

- Phase IIIb: Clinical trials conducted after the sponsor has filed its application for marketing approval of the product, but prior to FDA approval. These trials may supplement earlier trials, complete earlier trials, or may be directed toward new types of trials (e.g., quality of life, marketing).

The NDA

The NDA is a formal request to be allowed to market a drug. The sponsor submits the NDA to the FDA once the primary efficacy studies (Phase III) are complete. The company is essentially telling the FDA that it has completed the necessary safety and efficacy requirements needed for approval. This signals the end of Phase III, although there are likely to be some studies still in progress.

In the NDA, as in the IND, the sponsor informs the FDA of everything known about the drug to date. This includes copies of all protocols and case report forms from studies. The regulations for NDAs are found in 21 CFR 314. They are very detailed and delineate the particular information that must be included.

CRCs are not involved in putting together the NDA, although there may be a last-minute push to retrieve and/or clean up data needed for the NDA; it seems there are always some outstanding data that must be collected and entered into the database very quickly in order to process material for the NDA. CRCs may also be asked to re-verify information from their study when questions arise during the NDA-writing process.

Part of the NDA is the proposed package insert or labeling that the sponsor would like to use with the drug. This is the information that goes with the drug that tells physicians and patients about the drug and how it should be and not be used.

There is an active approval process for an NDA, as opposed to the passive 30-day wait for an IND. The sponsor must receive a formal approval letter from the FDA before marketing of the drug can begin.

Phase IV Clinical Studies

Phase IV studies are those conducted after the NDA approval, often to determine additional information about the safety or efficacy profile of the compound. They may consist of:

- Studies required as a condition of approval by the FDA
- Long-term safety studies required by the FDA
- Studies conducted to look at the compound in comparison with other marketed products.

If the sponsor were allowed to file the NDA with one, rather than two, adequate and well-controlled studies, the FDA may require that one or more additional confirmatory studies be completed within a certain time period of the approval. This is a condition of the approval; if it is not met, the approval may be withdrawn.

The FDA also may require that a sponsor conduct a long-term safety study as a condition of approval. These studies often are referred to as epidemiologic or post-marketing surveillance studies. These may be required because the FDA has seen problems with similar compounds or because the compound is novel, and the FDA thinks additional safety information will be beneficial.

During the compound's development time, other drugs may have been approved by the FDA and become the new standard of care for the disease or condition. In this case, the sponsor may want to conduct additional studies comparing its drug to these new compounds. The sponsor may also wish to look at different formulations, dosages, durations of treatments or medical interactions with other compounds commonly used by people with the disease targeted by the drug. Note that if the sponsor wants to evaluate the compound for a new indication, these studies will be considered as Phase II studies; a new IND will need to be filed for the new indication(s).

Notes on Studies in Women and Children

Many compounds do not work the same in women or children as they do in men. Consequently, the FDA has determined that studies should include women and children if the compounds would be used to treat them once marketed. The rationale is that it is preferable to determine the effects of the compound under the controlled conditions in clinical trials as opposed to in the uncontrolled use of the drug after marketed.

In 2003, the Pediatric Research Equity Act (PREA) was passed. This act authorizes the FDA to require research in children for drugs that will be used in pediatric patients. Consequently, sponsors must consider pediatric assessment as a routine part of drug development. If children are to be included in clinical trials, repeated-dose toxicity studies and all reproductive toxicity and genotoxicity studies should have been completed. In addition, safety data from previous studies in human adult populations should be available. Sponsors that conduct clinical trials that include children receive some incentives to do so, e.g., 180 days of exclusivity after approval to extend patent protections.

In addition to children, women of child-bearing potential are a major concern in clinical trials because of the possibility of unintentional exposure of an embryo or fetus before data are available relative to potential risk. Some teratology work (Phases I and II) is usually done before entering women of childbearing potential into a clinical trial, although this is not essential. Generally, a woman capable of conceiving a child will not be considered for a clinical trial unless she is not pregnant and agrees to use birth control.

In the U.S., women of child-bearing potential may be included in early studies prior to completion of reproductive toxicology studies, provided the studies are carefully monitored and all precautions are taken to minimize exposure in utero. This generally involves pregnancy testing and establishment of highly effective methods of birth control. Monitoring and testing should continue throughout the trial to ensure compliance with all measures intended to prevent pregnancy.

If women of child-bearing potential are used in a clinical trial prior to completion of the teratology studies, the informed consent process should clearly indicate the possible risk associated with taking the experimental drug, since effects on the embryo or fetus are unknown.

If pregnant women are to be enrolled in clinical trials, all reproductive toxicity studies and genotoxicity tests must be completed. Data from any previous experience in humans also will be needed.

Table 1: Timeline of Pediatric Testing Regulations

1997	**FDA Modernization Act—Pediatric Exclusivity Provision**
	Grants six-month patent extension for pediatric testing of drugs already approved for adult treatments
1998	**Pediatric Rule**
	Requires pediatric testing of all new drugs used by children
2001	**Clinical Investigation of Medicinal Products in Pediatric Populations**
	Sets standards by which IRBs determine if a pediatric trial can be safely and ethically conducted; includes requirement that children give their assent to participate
2002	**Best Pharmaceuticals for Children Act**
	Grants patent extensions to sponsors conducting pediatric trials or offers funding to third parties if sponsors choose not to
2003	**Pediatric Research Equity Act**
	Amends the Food, Drug and Cosmetic Act to authorize the FDA to require research in drugs used in pediatric patients

Biologics and CBER

The Center for Biologics Evaluation and Research (CBER) is the division within the FDA that is responsible for ensuring the safety and efficacy of vaccines, blood and blood products, and cells, tissues and gene therapies designed for the prevention, diagnosis and treatment of human diseases, conditions or injury.

The Biologics License Application (BLA) is a request for permission to introduce a biologic product into interstate commerce (21 CRF 601.2). (This means approval for marketing.) The application, which shows the clinical efficacy and safety of a biologic product in humans and requests marketing approval in the U.S., usually is submitted to the FDA after completion of Phase III trials. The clinical regulations that apply to drugs also apply to biologics.

Vaccine clinical development follows the same general pathway as drugs and other biologics. A sponsor that wishes to begin clinical trials with a vaccine must submit an IND application to the FDA. The IND describes the vaccine, its method of manufacture and quality control tests for release. Also included is information about the vaccine's safety and ability to elicit a protective immune response (immunogenicity) in animal testing, as well as the proposed clinical protocol for studies in humans.

Clinical trials for vaccines are typically conducted in three phases, just like drugs and biologics. Initial human studies, referred to as Phase I, are safety and immunogenicity studies performed in a small number of closely monitored subjects. Phase II studies are dose-ranging studies that may enroll hundreds of subjects. Finally, the vaccine Phase III trials typically enroll thousands of individuals to provide the proof of effectiveness and safety required for licensing treatment.

After the successful completion of all three phases of clinical development, the sponsor can submit a BLA. To be considered, the application must provide the FDA reviewer team (medical officers, microbiologists, chemists, biostatisticians, etc.) with the efficacy and safety information necessary to make a risk/benefit assessment and to recommend or oppose approval of the vaccine.

As with drugs, vaccine approval also requires the provision of adequate product labeling to allow healthcare providers to understand the vaccine's proper use, including its potential benefits and risks, to be able to communicate with patients (and parents if the vaccine is for use in children) and to safely deliver the vaccine to the public. The FDA continues to oversee production of vaccines after the vaccine and the manufacturing processes are approved in order to ensure continuing safety.

Until a vaccine is given to the general population, all potential adverse events cannot be anticipated. Thus, many vaccines are required to undergo Phase IV studies once they are on the market. There is also a Vaccine Adverse Event Reporting System (VAERS) to help identify any problems with a vaccine after marketing begins.

Growth in the vaccine area means that more CRCs will have the opportunity to work on vaccine trials. Although vaccines and drugs fall under the same regulations, there are some significant differences in vaccine trials. One fundamental difference is that many vaccines are typically given to healthy individuals in the hope that the vaccine will keep them from contracting the disease of interest (e.g., flu). Since these trials take healthy people and expose them to an investigational product (the vaccine), there is very little tolerance for risk. There are vaccine studies that are directed at the treatment of disease or a condition and would function more like an experimental drug, starting in healthy volunteers, if ethical, and then to those living with the condition. These types of vaccine trials also might be with multiple doses of the vaccine rather than one or some boosters, e.g., tetanus.

Certain types of vaccine trials tend to be extremely large, and recruiting large numbers of healthy people can be very resource-intensive. There is also the issue of retaining subjects for the duration of the trial because the CRC normally does not see the subjects again after administration of the vaccine until the very end of the trial. There might not be an adequate incentive for subjects to come back for the follow-up since they have received the vaccine.

Also, enrollment time can be very short, especially if you need to "catch the season," as with the flu. When a new strain of flu is expected to become endemic, for example, studies on a vaccine to prevent it must be done before flu season commences.

Medical Devices and CDRH

The precepts of conducting research according to GCP are the same in any clinical trial, but there are some differences in the way they are implemented due to the nature of the investigational product and applicable regulations when working with medical devices. In this section, we will discuss some of these differences. Later in the book we go into more detail about the differences in safety reporting between drugs and devices.

The Center for Devices and Radiological Health (CDRH) within the FDA is responsible for both the premarket and postmarket regulation of medical devices. A medical device is a product used for diagnosis, therapy or surgery purposes in people, and that acts by physical, mechanical or physico-chemical (drug-device combination) means. Medical devices include a wide range of products that vary in complexity from tongue depressors to x-ray machines to artificial hearts.

There are different types of marketing applications a medical device manufacturer may submit to CDRH. Most medical devices reach the market through either the premarket approval (PMA) process or the premarket notification process (510(k)). The great majority are approved through the 510(k) process.

The FDA recognizes different classes of medical devices based on their design complexity, their use characteristics and their potential for harm if misused. "Class" refers to the level of regulatory control attached to the device. The definitions pertaining to the classification of devices are found in 21 CFR 860 (Medical Device Classification Procedures).

Class I devices are lowest risk and are subject only to the general controls authorized under sections 501 (adulteration), 502 (misbranding), 510 (registration), 516 (banned devices), 518 (notification and other remedies), 519 (records and reports) and 520 (general provisions) of 21 CFR 860. A device is in Class I if these general controls are sufficient to provide reasonable assurance of the safety and effectiveness of the device, or if the device is not life-supporting or life-sustaining, or for a use that is of substantial importance in preventing impairment of human health and does not present a potential unreasonable risk of illness or injury. Examples of Class I devices are examination gloves and elastic bandages.

Class II devices are subject to special controls because general controls alone are insufficient to provide reasonable assurance of proper use and to support safety and effectiveness. Special controls can include the need for performance standards, postmarket surveillance, patient registries, the development and dissemination of guidance documents and other appropriate actions the FDA deems necessary to provide this assurance. Examples of Class II devices are powered wheelchairs and infusion pumps. Some Class II devices will require clinical trials if they do not have another device with substantial equivalence that has safety and effectiveness data. Once substantial equivalence is shown, there may not be a need for more trials.

Class III devices require the submission of an Investigational Device Exemption (IDE) application to allow clinical trials to proceed and PMAs to be approved for marketing. These devices tend to have a higher risk or raise new safety and effectiveness questions that must be answered before being approved for marketing. Data in a PMA application must demonstrate a reasonable assurance of safety and effectiveness. Examples of Class III devices include implantable pacemakers and automated external defibrillators.

Manufacturers submit 510(k) applications for devices similar to those already on the market. Data in a 510(k)program are based on non-clinical testing with no clinical data, while the majority of PMA applications do contain clinical data.

Many devices are designed and developed as tools to accomplish a specific task that is already an established practice, so the intended patient population and anticipated effects of the device are known before testing begins. This is different than the drug development process, in which a new molecular entity may be identified before determining any potential clinical applications.

Another major difference between device and drug development is the interpretation of safety events seen in a clinical trial. A control group is commonly necessary to interpret safety information from a drug trial, while a control group may not be needed to identify adverse events related to the use of a device.

Premarket device trials tend to be simpler than drug trials when demonstrating safety with regard to intended use, and compliance is usually easier to measure. But there can be other complexities, e.g., multiple parts to the device or implantable devices that remain in a patient after the study for the life span of the patient. And some clinical trials require that the patient pay for the device. There are a number of other differences between device and drug trials. For example, it may not be possible to "blind" the device, so many device trials are conducted with the investigator and subject both aware of the device being used. It also may not be possible for a direct comparison with a competitor device, either because there is no comparable device or because of the logistics involved.

When studying a drug, the dose may be an issue; with a device, the size of the device may be an issue or the voltage, especially in implantable devices. Implanting a device may carry a greater risk than prescribing a drug, especially in later-phase trials when more is known about a drug. Depending on the device, there may be more precise endpoint determination (especially when there is electronic information storage on the device). Many endpoints in drug trials, on the other hand, are quite subjective (think of a depression rating scale vs. a "hard" measurement such as blood pressure).

Some differences also exist in the collection and reporting of medical events between device and drug trials. (These are discussed in more detail in a future chapter.)

If you will be coordinating device trials, it is recommended that you read the device regulations found in CFR 21 Part 812 (Investigational Device Exemptions) and CFR 21 Part 814 (Pre-market Approval of Medical Devices). 21 CFR Part 860 (Medical Device Classification Procedures) and 21 CFR Part 803 (Medical Device Reporting), which covers adverse event reporting, will also be helpful.

Figure 2: The Research Process

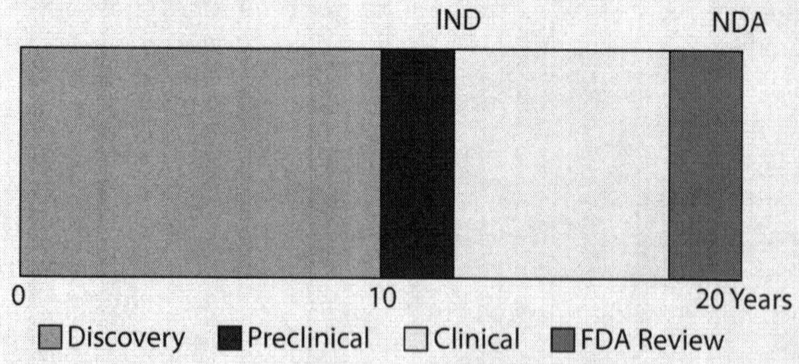

Source: FDA, Tufts CSDD

Summary and Key Points

A CRC may have the opportunity to work on a drug, biologic and/or device study. Having a good understanding of the process for new investigational product development and approval, including drug, biologic and device, for a particular indication is important. Also, knowing the differences overall between drug development and device is essential. The impact of this understanding will allow the CRC to better support the investigator and the subject with documentation, safety and data management.

It is important that CRCs comprehend the investigational product development process, even though they will not be involved in every step. This will help you understand why things happen as they do and to participate knowledgeably in the process.

CHAPTER FIVE

Clinical Site Quality Systems

Performing clinical trials is a complicated business. The conduct of clinical trials is bound by regulations and good clinical practice, with the overriding concern of protecting the safety and welfare of study subjects. Investigators and their study staff must follow each protocol requirement and meet other sponsor study agreements. The best way to ensure that all of these conditions are met, and to decrease the risk of noncompliance, is to have a set of quality systems that support the institution's clinical operations which, in turn, support the investigator to meet his or her obligations.

A quality system includes the following and should be made scalable to the volume and types of research the investigator performs:

- Documented procedures and validated methods being developed, implemented and kept up-to-date
- A documentation system that preserves and allows for the retrieval of any information/documentation (quality records/essential documents) to show actions taken, decisions made and results
- Appropriate training of investigator personnel as well as of the personnel at other service providers contracted by the site to perform any study-specific tasks, e.g., laboratory or pharmacy personnel, if applicable
- Validation of computerized systems used to support clinical trial data or duties
- Quality control, for example overseeing the activities of study staff that have been delegated study tasks, e.g., informed consent
- Quality assurance including internal and external audits performed by independent auditors, as needed

FAQ

If SOPs are not required by regulation, why should we bother with them?

Your site will be better prepared to conduct studies well, your processes will be consistent and you will look much more professional. Most sponsors (and the FDA) will expect a site that consistently conducts clinical trials to have SOPs.

Investigators commonly delegate multiple tasks for a clinical trial; even so, per the regulations, they are responsible for the protection of the subjects and also the data integrity. Oversight of those that perform delegated tasks is challenging and links to most negative site inspection findings. Commonly, an investigator is a very busy person who has responsibilities outside the clinical trials, e.g., running a managed care practice. Therefore, it is essential that the investigator have processes in place to ensure effective oversight. This is accomplished through a quality system that is maintained and updated as changes occur and as instances of site noncompliance are discovered. An investigator should not rely on sponsor monitoring alone to ensure quality. An investigator cannot blame a sponsor for negative inspection findings.

Standard Operating Procedures (SOPs) are just that: the procedures and processes that are used to operate a clinical trial. SOPs have been standardized to ensure that they are followed and enforced as applicable the same way each time. The list of clinical trial SOPs for a site will support the investigator-regulated activities and link the site's way of performing them, e.g., an SOP on obtaining informed consent. SOPs should be clearly written descriptions of how a particular study activity is to be performed, and the SOP should link to the other quality system components, e.g., how to document informed consent, the training on informed consent, the quality control and assurance activities related to informed consent, as well as the validation of the performance of any electronic systems used to support that activity like an electronic trial master file (eTMF).

SOPs should provide critical tools in successful business operations for the investigator and the study staff. CRCs must comply with their SOPs as they may have associated tools, like logs, that can support the GCP activities for the study. Sponsors, CROs and IRBs must also have quality systems that include SOPs for the same reasons investigators do. For example, sponsors must have SOPs for monitoring a clinical trial, which may include a study-specific monitoring plan template.

Global GCP guidelines did not require that investigators have procedures for running a clinical trial until 2016. The update to ICH E6 added the following within the investigator section, 4.2.5 and 4.2.6: *The investigator is responsible for supervising any individual or party to whom the investigator delegates trial-related duties and functions conducted at the trial site. If the investigator/institution retains the services of any individual or party to perform trial-related duties and functions, the investigator/institution should ensure this individual or party is qualified to perform those trial-related duties and functions and should* ***implement procedures*** *to ensure the integrity of the trial-related duties and functions performed and any data generated.*

Ultimately, a clinical quality system should help an investigator be audit-ready and effective in managing issues that risk subject safety and protection of their rights, as well as ensure data integrity, i.e., effective investigator oversight. A quality system should facilitate excellence and should be validated as being complied with and effective, or if there is an issue in the quality system that should be addressed. So, a quality system should have checks and balances components.

Writing SOPs

A CRC might have the opportunity to update or write SOPs. Writing SOPs is not an easy process. It can be time-consuming and involves analysis of your quality system. However, if SOPs are done well, they can be very beneficial in supporting quality and efficiencies. There are many ways to approach the formulation of SOPs. One that has been used successfully by many organizations is described below.

Step 1. Map the Process

Process mapping is a procedure of laying out all the steps in a currently used process and analyzing the process with the goal of making it more efficient and easier to follow. It involves taking each step in the process and mapping it into a process chart. All people involved in carrying out the task should be involved in mapping it into a process chart, and there should be free and open discussion. It is often discovered during this process that all involved people do not do things the same way and have very different ideas about how the current process works and how it should be done in the future.

Consider mapping the steps of your process into a flow diagram, with the primary and secondary steps shown. For example, if mapping the process for making a cup of coffee, the flow chart might look like the diagram on page 52. A convenient way to do mapping is to put a large, long sheet of paper on the wall (tablecloth paper) and write the steps on large (3" by 5") sticky notes to be able to move them around easily when mapping, which is very convenient. This can be done on a computer as well as a whiteboard.

Once you have the process mapped, add the people who are responsible for each step to the map. For this, it's easy to use small sticky notes in several colors with a different color representing each person/position needed. For example, the investigator may be represented by green, the CRC by blue, the receptionist by yellow, etc.

When finished with the mapping, convert the process map to an outline for ease-of-use. The outlines become the building blocks of the SOP. The outline for the process mapped above might look like this:

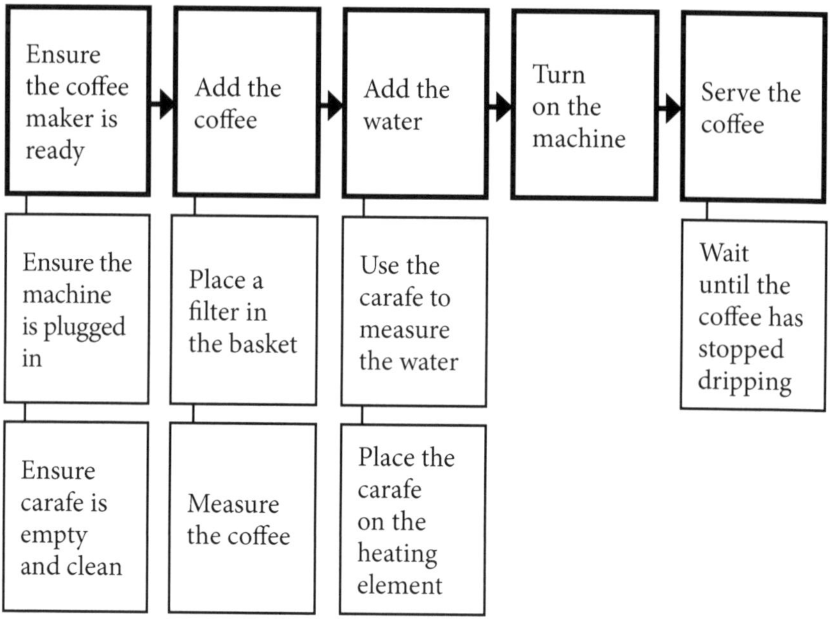

1. Ensure the coffee maker is ready.
    a. Plug in the machine.
    b. Be sure the carafe is clean and empty.
2. Add the coffee.
    a. Place a filter in the receptacle.
    b. Measure the coffee.
3. Add the water.
    a. Use the carafe to measure the water.
    b. Place the carafe on the heating element.
4. Turn on the machine.
5. Serve the coffee.
    a. Wait until the coffee has stopped dripping.

Step 2. Testing the Process

When a procedure has been mapped, it should be tested. Have a person or two involved follow the process to see if it really works. Determine if there are any missing steps or redundant or unnecessary steps that can be eliminated. Does the process meet the requirements? Is it the best way to do the task? Does the SOP map to the other quality system elements? If not, make appropriate changes and retest it.

One approach to SOPs is to have a two-tiered system that includes both SOPs and guidelines. The SOPs give a higher view of the process, and include all the main steps, while the guidelines are significantly more detailed. The guidelines essentially should allow someone to complete the process by following the steps. SOPs are usually approved at a higher level and should not be able to be changed on a whim. One major advantage to a two-tiered system is that the SOPs rarely will need to be changed. The guidelines, on the other hand, may change much more frequently or can be used at a study level, due to changes in organizational structure, equipment or personnel functions. Guidelines are often formulated and updated at a departmental level, rather than at an organization level. A good best practice to support the large differences between projects is to allow more than one guideline linked to an SOP. Some SOPs may not even need guidelines. For example, an SOP on informed consent likely will have a guideline on the process for the department and a guideline for the specific study when there might be multiple consent forms for sub-studies like biospecimens. Another example is an SOP related to managing sponsor monitoring visits that may not have a guideline since there might not be any variance in the process from study to study.

SOP: Making Coffee

SOP #000 Rev #000 Author: Effective date: Page X of X

Purpose

This SOP ensures that any company employee wanting to make coffee does so appropriately and according to company standards, thus ensuring a drinkable brew that satisfies and gives pleasure.

Scope

This SOP applies to all employees of the company and pertains only to use of the approved machine (name of machine) to make coffee. Coffee may be made only by employees who have been trained on the machine and are approved to make coffee (approved coffee makers).

Procedure

1. Ensure coffee maker is plugged in and the carafe is clean and empty.
2. Place a filter in the coffee receptacle and add the appropriate amount of coffee.
3. Fill the carafe with the desired level of water and pour into the water reservoir.
4. Place the carafe on the heating element and turn the machine on.

When the coffee has stopped dripping into the carafe, it is ready to serve.

SOPs often have the following sections: header, scope, purpose and procedure.

Guidelines usually list the tasks necessary to complete the process, as well as the person responsible for completing each task. Here is an example.

Guideline: Making Coffee **Date: February 4, 2019**

Responsible person	Activity
Approved coffee maker	Ensure coffee maker is plugged in. • Plug is located at end of cord attached at back of machine • Outlet is on wall directly to the right of the machine • Insert plug into wall outlet, matching large side of plug to larger hole in outlet • Be sure plug is inserted firmly and completely
Approved coffee maker or custodial staff	Wash out coffee carafe if needed. • Dishwashing soap is located in the cupboard under the sink • Use hot water and a small amount of dishwashing soap • Brush with small brush located on hook under sink • Rinse thoroughly with hot water
Approved coffee maker	Pull out coffee receptacle. • Located in top half of machine • Grasp handle flap firmly and gently pull toward you until receptacle is fully opened Put a filter in the receptacle. • Use a #4 cone filter • Filters are located in the drawer directly under the coffee machine • Be sure the filter is opened correctly • Press the filter firmly against the sides and bottom of the receptacle Prepare to fill the filter with coffee. • Remove can of coffee from the cupboard just left of the coffee machine • Remove the lid from the can • Place the lid on the cupboard top

Guideline: Making Coffee (continued) **Date: February 4, 2019**

Measure and add the coffee to the filter in the pot.

- Use the red scoop found in the drawer next to the filters
- Measure the appropriate number of scoops of coffee and place the coffee in the filter
- For a full pot, use eight scoops
- For a half pot, use four scoops
- Rap the scoop gently on the rim of the filter receptacle to ensure it is completely empty after each scoop
- Rinse and dry the scoop and return to the drawer

Put the lid back on the coffee and return the coffee to the shelf.

Push the filled coffee receptacle firmly back into the pot, ensuring that it is completely in place.

Fill the coffee carafe with water.

- Use cold water
- For a full pot of coffee, fill to the line near the top of the carafe
- For a half pot, fill to the line midway up the carafe

Carefully pour the water from the carafe into the water reservoir at the back of the machine.

- The top of the machine opens up to allow access to the water reservoir
- If any water spills, clean it up with a paper towel (located in dispenser above sink)

Place the carafe on the heating unit at the foot of the machine.

- Be sure it is firmly in place
- Handle should be pointed toward the front of the pot

Turn the machine on by pushing the toggle switch on the left front to the "on" position.

- The red light next to the switch should be glowing
- Pot should start making gurgling noises

Wait until the machine has stopped making noise and coffee is no longer dripping into the carafe.

Pour into cup or mug.

Add cream and sugar to taste, if desired.

Enjoy.

Note that the guideline is much more detailed and may need to be changed even if the SOP is still valid and appropriate. For example, if the brand of coffee maker was changed, some of the steps in the guideline might need to be changed (type of filter, location of switch), but the SOP likely did not need to be changed. Caution: do not make SOPs or guidelines too restrictive when the step does not support quality, e.g., documentation must be completed on the "red" form. What if the form is white but the content is the same? This restriction may cause noncompliance and is not worth the risk.

Step 3. Approval, Training and Implementation

There should be a formal approval process for SOPs and guidelines. To support this, an SOP for developing and maintaining SOPs is needed. In general, SOPs are subject to review by any group or department that is affected by them. This review (and re-review, if changes are made) will help to ensure that they are, in fact, processes that can and should be followed. The final sign-off of SOPs should reside at a senior administrative level in the organization.

Once you have SOPs and guidelines, all involved personnel must be trained on them. SOPs are beneficial only if people know what they are and follow them. Once an SOP is approved, training should take place and then implementation should occur. Note that the approval date usually precedes the implementation date, in order to allow training to be completed for the initial roll-out of the SOP. Each employee also should have easy access to the SOPs and guidelines, either online, in hard copy or both, to refer to when working on studies. Training records should be maintained for audit purposes.

A best practice is that SOPs and guidelines be reviewed at least annually to ensure they are still workable and being followed. If a process changes at any time, the appropriate SOPs and/or guidelines should be revised to reflect the change with clear versioning. The retired version should be archived to prevent following the wrong SOP or guideline. This is why printing an SOP or guideline to refer to during a trial is risky, since it might not be the latest version on file. There should be someone charged with keeping the documents current and maintaining a history of the documents and any revisions. All previous versions of a changed SOP or guideline should be maintained with the history accounted for, so as to see the dates during which it was in effect. This will enable the organization to reconstruct and explain events that may have been done differently in the past and provide a document audit trail for process changes.

SOPs for Investigative Sites

There are a number of SOPs that are useful for an investigative site to have. It is common that some SOPs for studies will need to refer to other institutional policies that are not specific to clinical trials; some examples are listed below in parentheses. The following is a list of common SOP and guideline topic areas for sites:

- Preparing, maintaining and training on SOPs
- Deviations from SOPs
- Pre-study evaluation visits by potential sponsors
- Assessing protocol feasibility
- Contracts and budgets
- Study essential documents/TMF and preparation and maintenance of study files
- Site initiation and investigator meetings
- Informed consent document and process
- IRB submissions and continuing review
- Completion of CRFs
- Managing sponsor monitoring visits
- Correcting CRF and source document errors
- Privacy and confidentiality of study materials (HIPAA policies)
- Adverse event recording and reporting
- Receipt handling and storage of investigational materials, including controlled/scheduled substances (medical center-controlled substance policies)
- Investigational drug accountability (pharmacy policies)
- Preparation and handling of lab samples (lab policies)

FAQ

We have SOPs, but most of our staff are not familiar with them. As long as we don't do anything wrong, does it matter?

Yes. When you are audited by a sponsor or by the FDA, you will be held to your SOPs. It is critical that everyone involved is trained on them and follows them. If an SOP cannot be followed, then it should be rewritten to reflect actual practice (assuming you are adhering to the regulations).

- Shipping of biological specimens
- Internal QC for study documents and case report forms
- Meeting and communications with sponsors/CROs
- Study meetings and minutes
- Study closeout/termination
- Retention and archiving of study documents
- Preparation for sponsor audits or FDA inspections

Sometimes SOPs also have attachments, such as checklists or explanatory documents. To help you get started with SOPs, we are giving you an example of a site clinical trial SOP, guideline and checklist at the end of this chapter. This group of documents covers study closures.

Summary and Key Takeaways

To support busy investigators and ensure efficiencies and quality, clinical research sites' quality systems, including SOPs, are essential. Their primary purpose is to promote consistent quality outcomes and support study teams that work on a variety of diverse projects. They also help to ensure that regulations and good clinical practices are followed.

- An SOP is a clearly written description of how a particular task is to be performed.
- SOPs are essential tools for standardizing processes, ensuring that regulatory and organizational policy requirements are met, training new personnel and managing workload.
- Two of the main keys to a successful research site are good, clearly written, functional SOPs and training on them.
- Process mapping is a procedure of laying out all the steps in a currently used process and analyzing the process with the goal of making it more efficient and easier to follow.
- One approach to SOPs is to have a two-tiered system that includes both SOPs and guidelines.
- There should be an approval and maintenance process for SOPs and guidelines.
- It is critical that all involved personnel are trained on SOPs and guidelines applicable to their role.
- SOPs and guidelines should be reviewed (at least) annually.

- All previous versions of SOPs and guidelines should be retained and archived.
- If the FDA or a sponsor audits an investigator, they will expect to see proof that SOPs have been followed and issues have been prevented and managed effectively based on the systems that support quality.

Study Closeout Checklist

Protocol:________________________________ Sponsor:__________________

Investigator: ______________________________ Date:_____________________

- ☐ Study documents file is complete (refer to Checklist: Study Documents).
- ☐ Final report has been made to the IRB and the sponsor.
    - ☐ All case report forms (CRFs) are complete and have been submitted to the sponsor.
    - ☐ All CRF corrections/queries have been addressed.
- ☐ Any patient diaries, etc., have been submitted as required.
- ☐ All source documentation is in order.
    - ☐ If not with study files, location of materials is noted in the document file.
- ☐ Study personnel form is complete.
- ☐ Subjects' signed informed consent forms are filed.
- ☐ Drug dispensing and disposition forms are complete.
- ☐ Study drug has been returned as per sponsor instructions.
- ☐ All other study materials (extra CRFs, etc.) have been returned to the sponsor.
- ☐ Investigator Brochure is filed with other study materials.
- ☐ All study materials are filed together as per archival procedures.
    - ☐ Location of materials is noted in records.
- ☐ Post-study critique has been held.

Guideline: Study Closure

Revision # 0 **Effective date:**

At the completion of a study, all study documentation and materials must be properly filed or otherwise taken care of. It is important that proper study closeout procedures are done for each completed study.

Responsibility	Action
Investigator, Clinical Research Coordinator	Prepare a final report for the IRB and sponsor, including: • Number of subjects screened, enrolled, completed, dropped • Reasons for dropouts • Listing of all serious adverse events • Listing of any protocol deviations or violations • Other information as requested, or as appropriate Send the report to the IRB and the sponsor.
Clinical Research Coordinator	Prepare the study document file for archiving: • Ensure that all documents are present, including the final report (Refer to the Study Document Checklist) • Include pertinent communications from the sponsor • Ensure that any problems occurring during the study (protocol violations, etc.) have been documented, including the resolution • Include documentation of the final return and/or disposal of unused study materials, including drug, case report forms, etc. • Include the Investigator Brochure in the file.
Clinical Research Coordinator or other designated site personnel	Place all signed consent forms together within the file. • Verify that a signed consent is present for each subject. • Ensure that all case report forms, including Coordinator queries, etc., are present • Ensure that any problems have been addressed and documented • Box these materials for storage.
Study Coordinator or other designated site personnel	Return and/or dispose of unused study materials. • Contact the sponsor for directions.
Designated site personnel	File all documents together according to standard archiving procedures. • Note in central files where these documents are stored.

Guideline: Study Closure (continued)

Investigator and/or Clinical Research Coordinator	Ensure that a post-study critique has been done.

Regulations and Guidances:

21 CFR 312.62 Investigator recordkeeping and record retention

21 CFR 312.64 Investigator reports

ICH Guideline for Good Clinical Practice, Section 4.9. Investigator Records and Reports

ICH Guideline for Good Clinical Practice, Section 4.10. Investigator Progress Reports

References:

SOP: Post-Study Critique

Guideline: Post-Study Critique

Guideline: Study Closeout

Attachments:

Checklist: Study Closeout

Checklist: Study Documents

Keywords:

Closeout, study documents, case report forms, informed consents, study materials, post-study critique, final report, archive

Approved by: ______________________ Date: ________________

SOP: Study Closure

Revision # 0 **Effective date:**

Purpose:

At the end of a study, it is important that all study materials are correctly taken care of and that all necessary documentation is appropriately filed. The purpose of this SOP is to ensure that proper study closeout is done for each clinical trial completed.

Scope:

This SOP applies to all clinical trials.

Responsibilities:

The investigator, clinical research coordinator and other personnel, as appropriate, are responsible for ensuring that proper closeout activities are done.

Procedures:

- A final report will be provided to the IRB and to the sponsor.
- All study documentation will be verified and filed in the study file, including the Investigator Brochure.
- Case report forms and supporting documentation will be filed.
- All signed informed consent documents will be filed with the study documents.
- All unused study materials, including drugs, case report forms, etc., will be disposed of or returned as directed by the sponsor.
- Actions and problem resolutions will be documented in the study file, if not already done.
- All materials will be filed together according to standard archiving procedures.
- A post-study critique will be done.

Regulations and Guidances:

21 CFR 312.62 Investigator recordkeeping and record retention

21 CFR 312.64 Investigator reports

ICH Guideline for Good Clinical Practice, Section 4.9. Investigator Records and Reports

ICH Guideline for Good Clinical Practice, Section 4.10. Investigator Progress Reports

References:

SOP: Post-Study Critique

Guideline: Post-Study Critique

Guideline: Study Closeout

Attachments:

Checklist: Study Closeout

Keywords:

Closeout, post-study critique, final report, archive

Approved by:______________________________ Date: ____________

Case Study: Why do we need SOPs?

I was working with a large study group with seven CRCs and three investigators. They did not have SOPs, and didn't really think they needed to have them. "After all," one of the group said, "as long as we follow the regulations, we're OK." But the reason they asked me to consult with them was that they had a problem.

One of their coordinators had left the group to move to a new state when his wife was transferred by her company. His studies had been divided up among the other CRCs, and this is when the problems started. One problem involved keeping the study documents in order. It turned out that they all kept their study documents in different ways. Some filed them in a binder, some in folders. Some filed by category and others filed by date. Some didn't file them at all—they were just stacked in a box on a shelf. Now the new CRCs for each study had to figure out someone else's system—not an easy task. The CRC who left had his study documents well filed, but his system was his own and wasn't immediately transparent to the other CRCs.

The first thing we did as a group when I joined them was have everyone take a few minutes and write down how to make a grilled cheese sandwich. Should be easy; after all, this is an American classic and everyone knows how to make one. Well, as you can imagine, with 10 people we had 10 very different sandwich recipes. They ranged from:

Put cheese on a piece of bread. Toast in a toaster oven until the cheese melts.

to:

Slice two pieces of San Francisco sourdough bread about half an inch thick. On one slice add a generous handful of shredded sharp cheddar cheese. Spread the cheese out evenly to the edges of the bread. Butter the outside of the top slice of bread, and carefully put the sandwich in a frying pan, butter side down. Gently fry over medium low heat until the bottom of the sandwich is golden brown. Carefully turn the sandwich over. Press down on the sandwich with a spatula. Cook until the bottom side is golden brown and the cheese is melted. Remove from the pan to a plate. Cut in half and serve with a dill pickle spear.

After some heated discussion on the "real" way to make a grilled cheese sandwich, we moved on and everyone wrote down how they kept their study documents in order. Needless to say, there was no agreement on this front, either. What they did recognize, and agree on, was that they needed standard operating procedures in order to have consistency for their study procedures. They realized, thanks to the CRC who left, that workload allocation was one major benefit of SOPs, along with a general ease of knowing how things should be done.

CHAPTER SIX

Institutional Review Boards

When conducting clinical trials, the safety of human subjects is paramount. Two of the main safeguards for individuals participating in clinical trials are institutional review boards (IRBs) and the informed consent process. In this chapter, the roles and responsibilities of IRBs and the interactions between IRBs and investigative sites will be discussed.

The regulatory definition of an IRB (21 CFR Part 56.102(g)) is: "any board, committee or group formally designated by an institution to review, approve the initiation of and conduct periodic review of biomedical research involving human subjects. The primary purpose of such review is to ensure the protection of the rights and welfare of the human subjects." In most cases in clinical research, an IRB must approve a study for each investigator before it can start. Most clinical research conducted involving humans in the U.S. must be approved by an IRB.

IRB Review

Unless the research is exempt from IRB approval and continuing review, like some non-treatment low-risk studies, an investigator planning to conduct a trial must arrange for an IRB to be in place to review the study. An investigator must confirm if the study requires IRB oversight. For investigators working within an institution that has its own IRB, consulting with the IRB is important when determining if IRB review is required. When the study requires IRB review, the investigator must submit the appropriate materials to the IRB, including the proposed study protocol and informed consent form, and wait for formal IRB approval before starting the clinical trial. Initially, interacting with and asking an IRB for the study approval for their site is the responsibility of the clinical investigator, not the sponsor of the research. But the investigator can rely on a third party to arrange the IRB review, e.g., a sponsor arranges a central IRB process through a single independent IRB when an investigator is not already affiliated with a local institutional IRB and/or if the study is multi-center and using a centralized review process where one IRB oversees all the sites in a certain region or country. Here the institutions with a local IRB still need to consult with the IRB to see if they have any additional requirements related to the protections of human subjects for research conducted at the institution.

No matter how the IRB is coordinated for a study, the investigator is responsible for ensuring that the IRB has experience with the type of trial (e.g., drug, device, pediatric, vaccine study) and complies with the applicable IRB regulations (FDA and/or OHRP). For multi-center trials for the FDA and OHRP, an investigator will participate in a centralized, single IRB process to support more efficient and timely IRB review.

Many CRCs work at institutions that conduct FDA- and OHRP-regulated trials, so the CRC needs to be familiar with the institution's policies on IRB review and communication. The CRC should identify the best resources in the IRB to ask questions and get clarifications on requirements. This is also true for specific trial requirements since the IRB can be stricter than the regulations if deemed necessary to protect the individuals being enrolled in a clinical trial. The CRC supports the investigator in ensuring that the IRB approvals, safety reporting and continuing review submissions are carried out per the requirements of the pertinent IRB for the clinical trial.

An IRB separately considers each research project submitted by an investigator for review. It may review a batch of investigators for the same study at one time but review the individual investigator's differences carefully. In order to determine if the research meets all the criteria discussed above, the IRB will review the investigator qualifications, the study protocol and supporting documents, the proposed consent form and any subject compensation or advertising, if applicable.

IRB Membership

An IRB must have at least five members with varied backgrounds. Most IRBs also have alternate members so that they will have a quorum if a regular member is unable to be present. The members must possess appropriate professional competence to review the diverse types of protocols received.

There must be at least one member who is not affiliated with the institution (and who has no immediate family member affiliated with the institution) other than his or her IRB membership. There also must be one member whose interests and background are non-scientific (i.e., a layperson). It's acceptable for one IRB member to fulfill both of these criteria. In addition,

FAQ

Can an investigator sit on an IRB?

Yes, but he or she can participate neither in the discussion leading to the vote nor in the voting for his or her own research. (See the section on conflict of interest.)

an IRB that reviews FDA-regulated products (drugs, biologics and devices) should have at least one member who is a physician.

IRB membership should be selected to ensure appropriate diversity, including representation by multiple professions, multiple ethnic backgrounds and both genders, and must include both scientific and non-scientific members.

Investigators and/or CRCs can present studies to IRBs during the meetings when the clinical trial is being reviewed for approval. This can be very beneficial to the IRB in regard to answering questions about the complexities of a clinical trial and also related to the medical science or technology. This activity is not considered to be voting.

Sponsors review and sometimes collect documentation from investigators that are using an IRB that meets the membership requirements and has no conflict of interest with the membership and the study. Investigators and CRCs can also be members of an IRB. If this is the case, the investigator and CRC must not vote on any study they are conducting. Disclosure of a membership must be present in the study documentation which also must provide confirmation that they did not vote on that study. As noted earlier, the investigator or CRC is allowed to present information about the studies he or she is working on for IRB review.

IRB Operations

Since 2009, IRBs are required by the HHS to be registered. The registration includes key things like whether they review FDA and/or OHRP trials. It also asks about experience with pharmaceutical and medical device products. This requirement came about when inspections revealed some IRBs were reviewing studies without device expertise. Institutions that perform OHRP-regulated trials must also apply, receive and keep updated a Federal Wide Assurance designation (FWA number). This is an institution's commitment to HHS that it will comply with the requirements in the human subject protection regulations at 45 CFR part 46.

IRBs are required by regulation and FWA (when applicable) to follow written procedures. IRBs are audited by regulatory authorities, and they are held responsible for having appropriate written procedures and for following them. IRBs maintain meeting minutes during IRB reviews that document their activities. They must carefully document their decisions and retain this documentation appropriately. IRBs must provide their decisions, regarding study review and approval or disproval, in writing to the investigator. This information is monitored and audited by the sponsor.

IRB Responsibilities

Whether or not the IRB is affiliated with a particular institution, its primary responsibility is to protect the rights and welfare of human subjects participating in research. To fulfill this responsibility, the IRB will answer two basic questions regarding the study it is reviewing for an investigator:

- Should the study be done at all? If yes, are there any areas that need clarification or changes before a human subject is consented?
- What constitutes adequate informed consent for this trial?

The Benefit vs. Risk Assessments

In determining whether the study should be conducted, the IRB must consider several items. The IRB members must have assurance that the study has a valid scientific design, meaning that there is a properly designed protocol. The charge of an IRB is not to judge the scientific merit or worth of the trial. For example, this means that it is not the function of an IRB to decide whether another drug for hypertension is needed, but rather to determine if the research methods being used to study that potential antihypertensive are valid and have protections for the subjects.

Risks to the subjects must be minimized, so the IRB will look for a sound research design without unnecessary exposure to risk. It will also ascertain if the protocol uses procedures that would be performed on these individuals, both diagnostically and for treatment, even if they were not in the study, as far as it is feasible to do so. The idea is to treat people in a study as closely as possible to how they would be treated if they were not in the study, then adding those activities that are required to test the study hypothesis.

The IRB must determine whether the anticipated benefit to subjects and the overall knowledge to be gained from the research compares favorably to the risks. In this evaluation, the IRB considers only those risks and benefits that may result directly from the research, excluding the risks and benefits the subjects would have encountered if they had not been involved in the research (if they just had received the standard treatment for the condition). Remember that there are always risks involved in doing research. The treatments being studied are either experimental and not approved, or newly approved for the treatment of a particular indication; this is why research is conducted to collect information about the treatment's safety and efficaciousness. The IRB looks for a study design that might be coercive, appearing to take something away if they do not participate, like access to care.

The IRB also will want to know the subject selection process in order to ensure the selection is equitable and that no groups of potential subjects are routinely excluded or included based on non-study-related characteristics. The IRB checks for any signs of undue influence (promising something contingent on participation, like a cure, and any coercion, again taking something away they normally would have without participating.) Depending on the particular study, some of these characteristics might include sex, race, ethnic background, weight, smoking, educational background, cognitive ability, etc. In making this assessment, the IRB will consider the particular setting in which the research will be conducted, as well as the purposes of the research.

What Constitutes Adequate Informed Consent?

If the IRB determines that the benefits outweigh the risks and that it is acceptable to do the study, then it will consider the study informed consent form submitted for the investigator. It is a regulatory requirement that informed consent be sought from each subject, or the subject's legally authorized representative, before that person may be enrolled in the research project and before any study protocol procedures are performed. By regulation, informed consent must be documented, usually by having the subject sign the informed consent document. (Consents are discussed in detail in a later chapter.)

Along with the hard copy of the informed consent, the IRB looks for provisions in the research plan for ongoing sponsor safety monitoring of the data, with the goal to ensure the safety of the subjects during the research. It's not sufficient, for example, to have all the adverse event data looked at only at the completion of a trial—it must be regularly reviewed throughout the study period in case problems arise as more is learned about the product under investigation.

The IRB also determines whether or not there are adequate provisions in the research to protect the privacy of the research subjects, as well as to maintain the confidentiality of the data, where appropriate. Regionally there commonly are additional privacy protections of individuals' health information that the IRB reviews to see if they are included in the informed consent or separately, depending on the requirement (e.g., the country-specific privacy law requirements, like HIPAA in the United States, which requires an authorization be obtained for use and disclosure of protected health information in addition to the informed consent.)

Payments to study subjects and advertising are considered by the FDA and IRBs as part of the consent process, as both could encourage a subject to enroll in a trial. If subjects are to be paid for their participation in the research, the IRB will review the planned compensation to ensure that it does not constitute an undue influence that could impact the subject's voluntary decision to participate. Ideally, subjects would not take the risks involved in study participation simply because of the compensation. An exception is in Phase I studies using healthy volunteers; in this case, subjects usually volunteer, at least in part, because of the compensation offered. The IRB's decision will be based not only on the amount subjects may receive for being in the study, but also on the setting in which the study will take place. An amount that may constitute undue influence in one setting may not be in another. Additionally, some institutions do not allow payment to subjects as it is deemed unethical.

The IRB will also review any proposed advertising to ensure it does not make misleading or untruthful claims. Glowing claims of success for a "new" treatment for an unapproved product, for example, can also influence subjects to participate in a trial they otherwise would not want to be involved with.

Vulnerable Subjects

Sometimes special, vulnerable populations are studied in research trials. Vulnerable subjects include children, pregnant women, prisoners, physically or mentally disabled individuals, people with acute or severe mental illness, those who are economically or educationally disadvantaged and people who are vulnerable because they are institutionalized. If any of these categories of people are going to be included in the research, the IRB must determine if there are sufficient additional safeguards to protect them from coercion or undue influence. There are a number of OHRP and FDA regulations regarding research in various vulnerable populations. One such regulation is shared by both for protections of children. Subpart D of the OHRP regulation was adopted by the FDA: *Additional Safeguards for Children in Clinical Investigations*. These regulations must be taken into account when conducting clinical trials that involve children. If an investigator and his or her staff are involved in research with vulnerable populations, they should familiarize themselves with the regulations and guidance. The IRB is a great resource for CRCs as well.

A 2018 guidance from the FDA titled *Pregnant Women: Scientific and Ethical Considerations for Inclusion in Clinical Trials* discusses the ethical and scientific issues when considering the inclusion of pregnant women in clinical trials of drugs and biological products.

State and Local Regulations

The IRB must determine that the research does not violate any existing state or local laws or regulations, or any applicable institutional policies or practices. Some states, notably California and Massachusetts, have regulations that may exceed the federal regulations. People working in these states, and others, should be familiar with their state requirements for doing research. For example, California has an Experimental Research Subject's Bill of Rights that must be provided to every study subject in a trial and commonly is included with the informed consent.

Materials Submitted to the IRB by an Investigator

To ensure an adequate review, the investigator must submit a number of materials to the IRB for review, including the following:

1. A current CV that includes his or her qualifications for conducting the research, including education, training and experience.
2. The study protocol, which includes or addresses the following items, as applicable:
    - Title of the study
    - Purpose of the study, including any expected benefits
    - Sponsor of the study
    - Results from previous related research
    - Subject inclusion/exclusion criteria
    - Study design, including a discussion of the appropriateness of the research methods
    - Description and schedule of the procedures to be performed
    - Provisions for managing adverse events.
3. The Informed Consent document, containing all the appropriate elements, which includes or addresses the following items, as applicable:
    - Payment to subjects for their participation
    - Compensation for injuries to research subjects
    - Provisions for protecting subject privacy
    - Extra costs to subjects for participation in the study
    - Extra costs to third-party payers because of a subject's participation.
4. The investigator brochure or package insert, if applicable.
5. All subject advertisements and recruitment procedures. In general, advertising includes anything that is directed toward potential research subjects and is designed for recruitment.
6. The investigator agreement with the sponsor. For drug studies, Form FDA 1572 (Statement of Investigator) is required for all FDA-regulated

studies conducted under an Investigational New Drug Application. Some IRBs do not require this, but many do. (See form in Appendix D.)

7. Grant application for federally funded research, if applicable.
8. Any other specific forms or materials required by the IRB, such as an application form.

At many, if not most, investigative sites, a CRC is the one who assembles and submits the packet of information to an IRB. It helps to use a checklist so that nothing is forgotten; missing documents cause delays in IRB review. Some IRBs furnish investigators with a checklist that comprises all their particular requirements. If your IRB does not furnish you with one, it is good to make your own and have it ready for each study. There is an example of a checklist in Appendix D.

FAQ

If the IRB disapproves my study, can I take it to another IRB?

No. You should determine why the research was not approved and see if it is possible to modify it to make it acceptable. Note: There could be an exceptional circumstance by which it might be ethical to submit the research to another IRB, but this is extremely rare, and the second IRB should be informed of the first disapproval and the reasons for it.

IRB Deliberations

After the complete documents are received from an investigator, an IRB will schedule the protocol for review. For the initial review of a protocol, the board will meet to decide whether or not to approve the proposed research. In order to make this decision, the board will review all submitted materials and discuss the proposed research, followed by a vote. The IRB may approve the project or request changes or additional information in order to approve or disapprove it.

The IRB must notify the investigator of its decision in writing. If a study is disapproved, the IRB will also notify the investigator in writing of its action and the reasons for disapproval and must allow the investigator to address the IRB concerning the decision, either in writing or in person.

Any planned advertising must be approved before use, although this does not have to be approved before the study begins. Advertising is often started after study initiation, especially when subject recruitment has not been as rapid as anticipated.

Most importantly, IRB approval of the study and the informed consent form must be obtained prior to the investigator enrolling subjects. Most often the investigator delegates who will be in contact with the IRB to check on the status of the approval and the official written notification of approval to the CRC. The CRC should be sure to follow institutional policies on contacting and scheduling potential study subjects and the timing of IRB approval.

Investigator Reporting Responsibilities

Throughout the study, the investigator must report any protocol changes or amendments to the IRB. Any change must be approved by the IRB prior to implementation and may require a change to the informed consent form. The only exception to this is when the change is necessary to eliminate an apparent immediate hazard to the safety and or well-being of a subject, in which case the change should be implemented immediately by the investigator or qualified staff after their discovery, followed by a timely notification and submission to the IRB. For example, if it were determined during a drug trial that taking a particular concomitant medication was unsafe, sites would be notified by the sponsor to immediately stop giving that particular medication to study patients. Investigators would start implementing this immediately, and then notify their IRBs. These exceptions are relatively rare, but it is important to be familiar with what might be an exception if the study is approved at the site.

The investigator must also promptly report "immediately reportable" safety events to the IRB. These usually include deaths and other serious medical events that are unexpected during the study. Occasionally, deaths may be an expected outcome in a study; in this case, the reporting rules may change, and deaths will not be reported as immediately reportable adverse events. This exception must be clearly defined and then approved by the IRB. (Safety reporting will be discussed in more detail in a future chapter.)

The investigator also must promptly report to the IRB any unanticipated problems that arise during the research that involve risk to the study subjects or others. IRBs must have policies that include what is defined as an unanticipated problem. A common example is a serious adverse event related to the study product. Another example is a protocol deviation involving enrolling a subject in the study that does not meet the protocol inclusion criteria or meets an exclusionary criteria.

The investigator is also required to submit periodic reports to the IRB for the IRB's continuing review. This is a detailed report of the progress of the study and many IRBs have a standard template to complete. These reports are submitted at least annually and may be required on a more frequent basis. The exception is for some expedited approved research studies. Continuing review reports are not required, and the trial is exempt from this. Although the investigator is the person responsible for submitting these reports to the IRB, the preparation and submission of these reports is usually delegated to the CRC.

FAQ

The IRB chair notified us in person that our study has been approved. Can we start enrolling subjects now?

No. You must wait for the official written notification. Most sponsors will not send you the investigational drug or device until they have a copy of the IRB approval letter but, even if they have, you may not start until you have the written approval.

Continuing Review of a Research Study

As noted above, the IRB will review each investigator's research project at least annually, although the IRB may require updates on a more frequent basis, such as quarterly, based on the degree of risk to which the subjects are exposed. This is called continuing review, where the IRB will ensure that the: 1) risk-to-benefit relationship remains acceptable, 2) consent and study documents being used are still appropriate and 3) selection of subjects has been equitable.

To help make these determinations, most IRBs will require the investigator to submit an IRB-specific form asking about the progress of the study including enrollment figures and withdrawals, and unanticipated problems, like serious adverse events and significant protocol deviations at each review period. The IRB will ask for any protocol changes during the time period to verify they have been reviewed by the IRB. This information allows the IRB to determine whether or not the research can continue and/or needs any changes. IRBs commonly provide access to the continuing review checklist in advance and the CRC prepares and submits these reports in a timely manner.

The investigator will receive IRB written notification of each formal re-approval. Re-review and re-approval continue throughout the entire research project until such time as all subjects have completed their participation and the IRB has received a request to close the project. If the study is not re-approved prior to the expiration date of the previous approval, the study is out of compliance with the regulations. A lapsed IRB approval is a bad situation for a number of reasons (e.g., it could result in unfavorable audit findings and may affect the treatment of the subjects on the study). If an investigator has not submitted the required study updates to the IRB for review, the IRB has several options. The IRB may send the investigator a reminder that he or she is required to submit the update, with a deadline for receipt of the requested materials. If there is a lapse, the IRB may put enrollment on hold until the updates are received and reviewed. In the worst case, the IRB may withdraw approval of the study. It is important to remember that each approval is good only for a specified time period.

As of 2017, under the revised Common Rule, continuing review will not be required for: research reviewed under expedited review (unless the IRB determines otherwise); research reviewed under limited review; research that has progressed to the point where it involves only one or both of the following as part of an IRB-approved study:

- Data analysis (including the analysis of identifiable private information/identifiable biospecimens); or
- Accessing follow-up clinical data from procedures that subjects would undergo as part of clinical care.

Expedited Review

For the FDA and OHRP, an IRB may use amendment reviews or continuing reviews as part of an expedited review process if they constitute minor changes in previously approved research; this may be done only during the time period for which the approval was authorized. Expedited review may be done by the IRB chairperson or by experienced members who are designated as expedited reviewers. Items may be approved by expedited review, but they cannot be disapproved. If the expedited reviewer(s) thinks something should be disapproved, it must go to the full board. The board also must be made aware of all expedited review decisions, which is usually done at the first regular meeting following the review.

Expedited review is never used in circumstances in which the risk to human subjects would increase. It cannot, in general, be used for the initial review of a research study. There are a few exceptions in which initial review of a project can be done using expedited review; these exceptions may include non-treatment studies. But the IRB can always require more review for any study if they feel it is right.

IRB Registration

As mentioned briefly above, in 2009 the HHS began requiring registration of IRBs that review FDA- and OHRP-regulated studies. Registration gives the regulatory authorities more complete information about the IRBs that review studies and will:

- Facilitate sharing educational and other information with the IRBs
- Assist in scheduling and conducting IRB inspections
- Help prioritize IRB inspections.

Once registered, IRBs are required to review and submit current information every three years, although some information, such as a change in the IRB chairperson, are required to be submitted within a certain amount of time after the change occurs. IRB registration is not accreditation or certification, nor does it address issues of the IRB's competence, expertise or ability to conduct review.

Registering an IRB and obtaining an FWA or accreditation are related but separate processes. An institution working under OHRP must have an FWA in order to receive HHS support for research involving human subjects. Each FWA must designate at least one IRB registered with OHRP. Before obtaining an FWA, an institution must either register its own IRB, (an "internal" IRB) or designate an already-registered IRB operated by another organization (an "external" IRB), after establishing a written agreement with that other organization. The FDA does not require an FWA but permits the use of the FWA as the assurance required by their regulations.

Data Safety Monitoring Boards

Another entity frequently used to enhance safety in clinical trials is a Data Safety Monitoring Board (DSMB). Sometimes known as a Data Safety Monitoring Committee (DSMC) or Data Monitoring Committee (DMC), a DSMB is a group of expert advisors, usually appointed by a sponsor, to periodically review the accumulating data from a clinical trial, primarily to assess the continuing safety of trial subjects. The purpose of this committee is to advise the sponsor, after review of the data to date, whether the trial should continue in its present form, be modified or, perhaps, even be discontinued.

DSMBs were used in some clinical trials as early as the 1960s, mainly in large, randomized, multi-center trials sponsored by NIH and the Department of Veterans Affairs (VA), in which mortality and morbidity were the primary outcome measures. The establishment of these committees was based not only on the premise that monitoring the accumulating study data is essential to ensure the ongoing safety of trial subjects, but also on the premise that sponsor representatives who are closely involved in the design and conduct of a trial might not be fully objective in reviewing the interim data for any emerging concerns. FDA regulations do not require the use of DSMBs in trials except under 21 CFR 50.24(a)(7)(iv) for research studies in emergency settings in which the informed consent requirement is excepted.

A DSMB consists of people who are external to the trial organizers, sponsors and investigators, in order to minimize bias. They need to have the appropriate expertise to evaluate the data, and members usually include one or more medical people, a statistician and others, as appropriate. They may meet on a regular schedule based on time, such as every six months, or they may meet based on enrollment, e.g., after every increment of 50 enrolled subjects or on some other "trigger" appropriate for the trial. The DSMB will receive the data from the study up to the cut-off date for that review.

During their review, they will look at the data, have the DSMB statistician run some appropriate programs for looking at aggregate data, discuss their findings and inform the sponsor of their recommendation. This review usually results in one of three possible recommendations: Continue the trial as is, continue with modifications (or more frequent DSMB review) or stop the trial because of safety concerns. Although the DSMB recommendation is not binding, sponsors take these recommendations very seriously and usually abide by them.

FAQ

If a DSMB is used, will it need to approve our study before it starts?

No. DSMBs do not approve studies. They only review accumulating safety data.

All clinical trials require safety monitoring, but not all trials require monitoring by a DSMB. DSMBs usually have been used for large, randomized, multi-center studies that evaluate treatments intended to prolong life or reduce risk of a major adverse health outcome, such as cancer or cardiovascular events. They are recommended in controlled trials in which mortality or major morbidity is the outcome measured or in trials in which there is a high risk of severe outcomes. They are not usually needed for trials looking at less serious outcomes or for early-stage trials.

Adding a DSMB to a trial adds cost and resources, as well as additional administrative complexity, so the FDA does not recommend using a DSMB unless the trial meets particular criteria related to safety, practicality and scientific validity. The FDA guidance document, *Guidance for Clinical Trial Sponsors: Establishment and Operation of Clinical Trial Data Monitoring Committees,* gives additional information and the FDA's current thinking on the use of DSMBs, as well as practical information relating to the establishment and function of such groups.

A CRC usually will not have any reason to interact with a DSMB; however, there can be situations in which an upcoming DSMB review will necessitate the rapid collection and cleaning of data from study sites. In this case, the sponsor may be expected to retrieve data for the subjects included in the DSMB review without regard to the normal monitoring schedule. The investigator and CRC may need to spend significant time to ensure that the necessary information is available for the DSMB. Also, the decisions of the DSMB that impact the study are communicated to the investigator and filled in the study file at sponsor and each study site, as applicable.

CRC Responsibilities and IRBs

Usually the CRC is the one who puts together the submissions to the IRB, tracks their progress and maintains the appropriate files. This involves gathering together all documents that are required, obtaining signatures from the investigator as needed and ensuring that appropriate copies go to the necessary people by the deadlines. It helps to use checklists, either those furnished by the IRB or ones you have made yourself. It also involves maintaining good, organized files and keeping them current. Ensuring that IRB documentation is done appropriately helps keep your study in compliance and eliminates future problems. Sponsors are increasingly involved in this process and may want to see the documents being submitted to the IRB before they are actually sent or do the submission on behalf of the site. It is important to remember that the investigator is ultimately responsible for working with an IRB for clinical trials. The CRC might access IRB portals for a study to obtain documentation about IRB reviews and new, approved versions of the consent. The CRC needs to stay abreast of what has been approved by the IRB, what is pending and what documentation might be of use to file in the TMF to stay audit ready and also avoid the risk of using outdated study materials with subjects.

Key Takeaways

IRBs

- IRBs are one of the primary safeguards for the protection of human subjects of research.
- 21 CFR Part 56 contains the FDA regulations that pertain to IRBs.
- 45 CFR 46 pertains to human subject protections for OHRP-regulated trials that include requirements for IRBs.
- An IRB must approve a study and the informed consent document before the study can start, unless exempt.
- There are two types of IRBs, those affiliated with an institution and those that are independent.
- The use of a centralized or single IRB review process is becoming more common for multi-center studies.
- When IRB approval is required, no procedures or consenting should be done without consent.
- The IRB must make a risk vs. benefit assessment for each proposed project. The benefits must outweigh the risks for a study to get approved.
- There are special regulations concerning research in vulnerable subjects (children, pregnant women, prisoners, etc.).
- State and local research regulations also must bc followed when applicable.
- IRBs must approve advertising prior to use.
- IRBs must approve any subject compensation.
- An investigator must report unanticipated problems per the IRB reporting requirement timelines and study progress must be reported to the IRB at least annually, unless exempt.
- Continuing review of a study must be done at least annually, unless exempt.

- Expedited review may not be used for the initial review of a project, except in particular instances.
- IRB members may not vote if they have conflicts of interest, but they can present the study to the voting board members.
- The CRC is the primary person who interacts with the IRB at most investigative sites.
- IRBs reviewing FDA-regulated research must register with the FDA.

Case Study: Conflict of Interest

A well-known investigator, Dr. Smith, was in charge of the rheumatology unit at GoodHealth Hospital. During his tenure, he developed a new drug with great potential for helping with rheumatoid arthritis. In conjunction with two other family members, he started a small company to develop, test and market this drug.

The company started clinical trials with the drug, and one study site was at the GoodHealth Hospital Research Group. Dr. Smith was planning to be the clinical investigator for the trial, but the IRB determined this was inappropriate because of the potential conflict of interest.

Think about: Was this an appropriate IRB decision?

The IRB determined that it was acceptable for Dr. Smith to be a sub-investigator, with Dr. Jones acting as the primary investigator. Dr. Jones reports to Dr. Smith in the rheumatology unit.

Think about: Was this an appropriate decision?

The study began, with Dr. Jones as the responsible person. Dr. Smith recommended subjects for the trial and saw subjects for study visits, especially if they were his patients. He recommended the study to other doctors within the hospital and in the community, telling them how beneficial this drug would be for their patients. The study coordinators in the Research Group were concerned that there was still a potential conflict of interest, not only by having Dr. Smith involved, but also by having his company placing a study there, even if Dr. Smith were not involved.

Think about: Do the coordinators have a valid concern?

Discussion:

The IRB was right in not allowing Dr. Smith to be the primary investigator on this trial; even having him as a sub-investigator is a potential conflict, especially as he is Dr. Jones' superior. Added to that, Dr. Smith is recommending the trial not only to his own patients, but also to other doctors within the community. It would be more appropriate if Dr. Smith were not involved in the study at all.

Having his company place a study at GoodHealth Hospital is not ideal, either. There would not be as large a potential conflict if Dr. Smith were not involved in any way, but still it could be a problem, since everyone knows of his involvement and because of his stature at the hospital.

CHAPTER SEVEN

Informed Consent

A potential study participant's decision whether or not to enroll in a clinical trial is not an easy one. A study participant should be provided the information needed to make an informed and voluntary decision. The information provided should be presented at a level of comprehension for the potential study subject, along with opportunity to have questions answered and sufficient time to make an informed decision. One of the main safeguards for the protection of research study subject's rights, safety and well-being is the informed consent process. In this chapter, informed consent and the process of consent, including the regulations governing consent will be discussed.

Informed consent is defined by ICH E6 which states, *"a process by which a subject voluntarily confirms his or her willingness to participate in a particular trial, after having been informed of all aspects of the trial that are relevant to the subject's decision to participate. Informed consent is documented by means of a written, signed and dated informed consent form."*

The terms "voluntarily" and "informed" form the cornerstone of ethical conduct in clinical research and are in place to protect the rights and safety of the research subjects who participate in research. Potential subjects of clinical research must understand what they are getting into and must be free to decline to participate. Overall, the following are standards for any informed consent:

- Consent is legally effective.
- Consent is sought under circumstances that provide sufficient opportunity to discuss and consider whether or not to participate and minimize the possibility of coercion or undue influence.

- The language of consent is understandable to the subject or legally authorized representative.
- The subject or legally authorized representative is provided with information that a reasonable person would want to have in order to make an informed decision about whether to participate and an opportunity to discuss that information.
- The consent form cannot include exculpatory language in which the subject or legally authorized representative waives, or appears to waive, any of their legal rights.

In the 2014 revision of the Informed Consent Information Sheet regulatory guidance for 21 CFR Part 50, the FDA includes in its summary of the informed consent process an important statement: "*To many, the term informed consent is mistakenly viewed as synonymous with obtaining a subject's signature on the consent form. The FDA believes that obtaining a subject's oral or written informed consent is only part of the consent process. Informed consent involves providing a potential subject with adequate information to allow for an informed decision about participation in the clinical investigation, facilitating the potential subject's comprehension of the information, providing adequate opportunity for the potential subject to ask questions and to consider whether to participate, obtaining the potential subject's voluntary agreement to participate, and continuing to provide information as the clinical investigation progresses or as the subject or situation requires.*"

The FDA continues on in this section to say: "*To be effective, the process must provide sufficient opportunity for the subject to consider whether to participate. FDA considers this to include allowing sufficient time for subjects to consider the information and providing time and opportunity for the subjects to ask questions and have those questions answered. The investigator (or other study staff who are conducting the informed consent interview) and the subject should exchange information and discuss the contents of the informed consent document. This process must occur under circumstances that minimize the possibility of coercion or undue influence.*"

Table 1: Tips for an Improved Consent Form

- Provide a summary of highlights, with the details kept separate.
- Provide a glossary; define terms.
- Use layperson language throughout.
- Provide information on clinical trials in general.
- Use larger font for text.
- Emphasize what is important.
- Use graphics and video.

The investigator is responsible to ensure that the research subject is adequately consented prior to study procedures (FDA 21 CFR Part 312.60 and 312.62(b)) and ICH E6 Section 4.8.8). The CRC is commonly delegated various study tasks related to informed consent. This chapter reviews the regulatory requirements of informed consent and the potential role of the CRC in developing, obtaining and/or managing the informed consent for a particular clinical trial for the investigator.

Required Elements of the Informed Consent Document

ICH E6 Section 4.8.10 and FDA 21 CFR Part 50.25 agree on the major elements that any informed consent document should contain. Elements include:

- Statement that the study involves research
- Purpose of the research
- Duration of the subject's participation
- Description of procedures to be followed
- Identification of any procedures that are experimental (e.g., the exposure to the investigational product being studied for a particular indication)
- Description of any reasonably foreseeable risks or discomfort to the subjects (known risks from past trials)
- Description of any benefits to the subjects or others that reasonably can be expected from the research (not potential; must be actually defensible in the data)
- Disclosure of appropriate alternate procedures or courses of treatment, if any, that might be advantageous to the subject
- Statement describing the extent to which confidentiality of records identifying the subject will be maintained and that notes the possibility that the sponsor, IRB and regulatory authority may review pertinent study records
- For research involving more than minimal risk, an explanation as to whether any compensation and whether any medical treatments are available if injury occurs, and, if so, what they consist of, or where further information may be obtained
- Explanation of who to contact for:
    - Answers to questions about the research
    - Emergency contact related to the research

Table 2: Example of an Informed Consent Element Using a Heading

Purpose of the research The purpose of this research study is to find out if the study drug is safe and works for patients with moderately high blood pressure. The study drug has the brand name ANTIACHE Tablets. It is not yet approved for sale, but this is not the first time it has been tested in people. (Grade level is 6.5.)

    - Answers to questions about the research subjects' rights, and who to contact in the event of a research-related injury to the subject.
- Statement that participation is voluntary:
    - That refusal to participate will involve no penalty or loss of benefits to which the subject is otherwise entitled
    - That the subject may discontinue participation at any time without penalty or loss of benefits to which the subject is otherwise entitled.
- The additional elements of consent, which must be included as applicable to the clinical trial (not optional):
    - Statement that the particular treatment or procedure may involve risks to the subject that are currently unforeseeable
    - Or risk to the embryo or fetus, if the subject or subject's sexual partner is or may become pregnant.
- Anticipated circumstances under which the subject's participation may be terminated by the investigator without regard to the subject's consent
- Statement must include one or more examples of such circumstances, e.g., not following protocol instructions
- Any additional costs to the subject that may result from participation in the research (e.g., billable to insurance, expense not covered by the study)
- Consequences of the subject's decision to withdraw from the research and procedures for orderly termination of participation:
    - Participation in the study might impact the subject's ability to have access to treatment (e.g., no primary physician) and might need support to have access to treatment for a chronic disease
    - Termination from the study may also involve the return of supplies and investigational product

    - Protocols commonly include early termination study procedures, and compliance depends on the subject's cooperation.
- Statement that significant new findings developed during the course of the research that may relate to the subject's willingness to continue participation will be provided to the study subject
- Approximate number of subjects involved in the study.

Many states and institutions have additional requirements that may affect the content of the informed consent form. For example, the State of California requires a one-page *Experimental Research Subject's Bill of Rights* that must be attached to all research consent forms (see Table 3). Some states, countries or institutions may have additional consent form document requirements. For example, as of 2011, HHS requires an additional informed consent element to include reference to the website clinicaltrials.gov, and is applicable for drug (including biological products) and device clinical trials. The requirement requires a specific statement that clinical trial information will be entered into a databank. The databank referred to in this final rule is the clinical trial registry databank maintained by the National Institutes of Health/National Library of Medicine. The submission of clinical trial information to this databank by the sponsor of the clinical trial is required. This led to the FDA adding to the required elements in a consent form in 21 CFR Part 50 section 50.25(c) and is designed to promote transparency of clinical research to participants and patients. This requirement is applicable for all U.S. clinical trials, including OHRP-regulated studies. Under FDA 21 CFR 50.25(c), the following statement must be reproduced word-for-word in informed consent documents for applicable clinical trials: *"A description of this clinical trial will be available on http://www.ClinicalTrials.gov, as required by U.S. Law. This Web site will not include information that can identify you. At most, the Web site will include a summary of the results. You can search this Web site at any time."* There is a checklist for reviewing informed consent elements in Appendix D.

Sometimes regional regulation that is not clinical trial-specific also adds to requirements in informed consent documents and processes. An example of a national requirement is the Health Insurance Portability and Accountability Act (HIPAA) privacy requirements to obtain authorization to use and disclose an individual's protected health information (PHI). In this case, it is applicable to clinical trial consent because of the requirement to get permission (authorization) from an individual for an investigator to disclose a person's PHI for a sponsor's use for a clinical trial.

Table 3: Example of a California Patient's Bill of Rights for Study Subjects

Any person who is requested to consent to participate as a subject in a research study involving a medical experiment, or who is requested to consent on behalf of another, has the right to:

- Be informed of the nature and purpose of the experiment.
- Be given an explanation of the procedures to be followed in the medical experiment, and any drug or device to be used.
- Be given a description of any attendant discomforts and risks reasonably to be expected from the experiment, if applicable.
- Be given an explanation of any benefits to the subject reasonably to be expected from the experiment, if applicable.
- Be given a disclosure of any appropriate alternative procedures, drugs or devices that might be advantageous to the subject, and their relative risks and benefits.
- Be informed of the avenues of medical treatment, if any, available to the subject after the experiment or if complications should arise.
- Be given an opportunity to ask any questions concerning the experiment or other procedures involved.
- Be instructed that consent to participate in the medical experiment may be withdrawn at any time, and the subject may discontinue in the medical experiment without prejudice.
- Be given a copy of a signed and dated written informed consent form when one is required.
- Be given the opportunity to decide to consent or not to consent to a medical experiment without the intervention of any element of force, fraud, deceit, duress, coercion or undue influence on the subject's decision.

HIPAA and Informed Consent

The HIPAA privacy rule is enforced by the Office for Civil Rights (OCR), and the HIPAA authorization requirements are found in 45 CFR Part 164.508(c)(1)(2). HIPAA authorizations can be combined with the study informed consent form or may be a stand-alone document. The institution that is conducting the research is responsible for deciding on the format, and for ensuring that the required elements are supported.

HIPAA authorization core elements include:

- Description of PHI to be used or disclosed (identifying the information in a specific and meaningful manner)
- Name(s) or other specific identification of person(s) or class of persons authorized to make the requested use or disclosure (e.g., research site)

- Name(s) or other specific identification of the person(s) or class of persons who may use the PHI or to whom the covered entity may make the requested disclosure (e.g., sponsors of the research)
- Description of each purpose of the requested use or disclosure; this must be research study-specific, but can ask the subject to opt in or opt out for future research related to the purpose of the disclosure
- Authorization expiration date or event that relates to the individual or to the purpose of the use or disclosure (the terms "end of the research study" or "none" may be used for research, including for the creation and maintenance of a research database or repository)
- Signature of the individual and date. If the authorization is signed by an individual's legally authorized representative, a description of the representative's authority to act for the individual.

HIPAA authorization required statements include:

- The individual's right to revoke his or her authorization in writing
    - Note that the right for someone to withdraw his or her consent is similar, except withdrawal of consent is not required in writing.
    - An additional statement is sometimes added to remind the individual that even after revocation, some PHI will still be disclosed if relating to safety and efficacy of a study (e.g., adverse event information about a study subject).
- Notice of the covered entity's ability to condition eligibility for study participation on the authorization (cannot participate without authorization since the data would not be able to be reviewed and shared with the sponsor of the study)
- PHI can be re-disclosed by the recipient (sponsor) for the purposes of the authorization and no longer protected by HIPAA.

A research subject may revoke his or her HIPAA authorization at any time. However, a covered entity may continue to use and disclose PHI that was obtained before the individual revoked authorization to the extent that the entity has taken action in reliance on the authorization. In cases where the research is conducted by the covered entity, this would permit the covered entity to continue using or disclosing the PHI as necessary to maintain the integrity of the research, as, for example, to account for a subject's withdrawal from the research study, to conduct investigations of scientific misconduct or to report adverse events. The Informed Consent Checklist in Appendix D includes HIPAA authorization-required elements.

Related to future use of a subject's PHI, a significant update to HIPAA came from the 21st Century Cures Act of 2016 (Cures Act) mandate to issue "*Guidance Related to Streamlining Authorization*" under HIPAA for uses and disclosures of PHI for research. Specifically, it clarifies that: 1) *the circumstances under which the authorization for use or disclosure of protected health information, with respect to an individual, for* ***future*** *research purposes contains a sufficient description of the purpose of the use or disclosure, such as if the authorization (A) sufficiently describes the purposes such that it would be reasonable for the individual to expect that the protected health information could be used or disclosed for such future research, (B) either (i) states that the authorization will expire on a particular date or on the occurrence of a particular event or (ii) states that the authorization will remain valid unless and until it is revoked by the individual and (C) provides instruction to the individual on how to revoke such authorization at any time; (2) the circumstances under which it is appropriate to provide an individual with an annual notice or reminder that the individual has the right to revoke such authorization; and (3) appropriate mechanisms by which an individual may revoke an authorization for future research purposes, such as described in paragraph (1)(C).*

OHRP Changes to Informed Consent

With the changes in the Common Rule, as discussed in an earlier chapter, the requirements of certain studies and informed consents have changed as well. These changes were primarily triggered by negative inspection findings, but more so to better support the information study participants want to know and currently many times are not provided. The goal of these changes, which took effect on January 20, 2019, is to enhance a prospective subject's understanding of what they are agreeing to. The revision to the Common Rule adds several new required elements to consent forms, primarily related to studies with biospecimens. There are also a few changes to the informed consent process, but the underlying principle of informed consent has remained the same: that informed consent forms must present and organize information with enough detail and in a way that facilitates a potential subject's understanding of why or why not they may want to participate in a clinical trial. During the development of the revisions it was considered to create a standard form template, but it was concluded that the researchers were the ones that were most qualified to do so and there needed to be flexibility due the huge differences between trials.

Section 116(a)(4) of the amended rule states that informed consent must begin with *"a concise and focused presentation of the key information that is most likely to assist a prospective subject or legally authorized representative in understanding why one might or might not want to participate in the research."* This statement must be *"organized and presented in a way that facilitates comprehension."* Informed consent information needs to be written in a way that is patient-centric—taking the needs of the person into account—rather than the highly legalized document currently presented to participants with dozens of text heavy pages. The informed consent document should be readable, engaging and clear. As required by the FDA, the person must be given the chance to ask questions until they understand. So understandability and time to review the document are key.

Another new requirement is contained in Section 116(a)(5)(ii):

"Informed consent as a whole must present information in sufficient detail relating to the research and must be organized and presented in a way that does not merely provide lists of isolated facts, but rather facilitates the prospective subject's or legally authorized representative's understanding of the reasons why one might or might not want to participate."

There's no definition of what the "key information" is or how to balance the need to make that information concise with the need to make it detailed. So IRBs, sponsors and investigators should focus on the type of study participant and what they need and then determine how best to present that information in an easily comprehensible way.

The revised Common Rule requires that the process provides the participant a description of essential "factors" or information at the beginning of the informed consent process and locate said information at the beginning of the informed consent form. These five factors are:

1. Consent is being sought and participation is voluntary
2. The purposes of the research, expected duration of participation and procedures to be followed
3. The reasonably foreseeable risks and discomforts
4. The benefits to the prospective subjects, or others, that may reasonably be expected from the research
5. Appropriate alternative procedures or courses of treatment that may be advantageous to the prospective subject.

The required elements and additional situational elements of informed consent have remained the same in the revised Common Rule, as listed earlier in this chapter for ICH E6 and the FDA.

But four new elements were added, all of them dealing with biospecimens. Some of them also touch on issues around identifiable private information.

1. Section 116(b)(9) requires one of two statements to be given to a prospective research subject:
    a. *That identifiers might be removed from the identifiable private information or identifiable biospecimens and that, after such removal, the information or biospecimens could be used for further research studies or distributed to another investigator for future research studies without additional informed consent from the subject or the subject's legally authorized representative, if this might be a possibility; or*
    b. *That the subject's information or biospecimens collected as part of the research, even if identifiers are removed, will not be used or distributed for future research studies.*

2. Section 116(c)(7) requires a statement "that the subject's biospecimens (even if identifiers are removed) may be used for commercial profit, and whether the subject will or will not share in this commercial profit."

3. Section 116(c)(8) requires a statement "whether clinically relevant research results, including individual research results, will be disclosed to subjects, and if so, under what conditions."

4. Section 116(c)(9) requires a statement "whether the research will (if known) or might include whole genome sequencing (i.e., sequencing of a human genome or somatic specimen with the intent to generate the genome or exome sequence of that specimen)."

The revised Common Rule requires that informed consent forms be published online to a federal website within 60 days of the close of enrollment of the clinical study. This is the informed consent template and not the signed consents. It is not clear who will be posting; it potentially could be the IRB or the sponsor. The website is being developed and will be linked to clinicaltrials.gov. Redaction of commercially sensitive information will be allowed.

Broad Consent for Secondary Research

This part of the revision of the Common Rule has some similarities to the later updates to HIPAA that allowed Authorizations for Future Research. The new element of the Common Rule gives researchers the option of obtaining broad consent from research subjects to store, maintain and use identifiable private information and biospecimens for unspecified future studies.

An identifiable biospecimen is defined by the rule as *"a biospecimen for which the identity of the subject is or may readily be ascertained by the investigator or associated with the biospecimen,"* while identifiable private information is defined as *"private information for which the identity of the subject is or may readily be ascertained by the investigator or associated with the information."* Broad consent should never be required, it's only an available option. If it were required, this would be an example of pressuring someone to give up a right to participate in a study or coercive behavior. So, researchers still have the ability to use non-identified biospecimens or to get specific consent from a subject for a secondary study. If a subject declines to give broad consent, then informed consent is required for every study that would use the subject's identifiable private information or identifiable biospecimens. It's not possible to get a waiver from the consent requirement if the subject declines to give broad consent.

Requirements of Broad Consent

Broad consent generally needs to meet the elements of informed consent described earlier in this chapter.

This means the consent form should contain a description of the information and biospecimens that may be used, as well as the types of institutions and individuals that may perform the research. If the subjects are not going to be told about the specifics of a future study, they need to be told that their specimens may be used for research they haven't actively consented to. If the proposed secondary research is objectionable or controversial—by a *"reasonable person"* standard—the description needs to be more detailed than it would be for non-controversial research.

For instance, how should subjects be advised about future research possibilities if some of those possibilities aren't known?

The Secretary's Advisory Committee on Human Research Protections (SACHRP) has provided a starting point for language that could be included on a consent form. The consent should include broad language about the institutions and individuals that may have access to their biospecimens and information, including: other research, academic and medical institutions; drug and device companies and biotechnology companies; and other types of entities that may be applicable on a case-by-case basis.

The final rule also requires that a broad consent form include a number of elements specific to broad consent (some overlap general requirements of consent noted in FDA and ICH):

1. A description of any reasonably foreseeable risks or discomforts to the subject
2. A description of any benefits to the subject or others that may reasonably be expected from the research
3. A statement describing the extent, if any, to which confidentiality of records identifying the subject will be maintained
4. A statement that participation is voluntary, refusal to participate will involve no penalty or loss of benefits to which the subject is otherwise entitled, and the subject may discontinue participation at any time without penalty or loss of benefits to which the subject is otherwise entitled
5. If applicable, a statement that the subject's biospecimens (even if identifiers are removed) may be used for commercial profit and whether the subject may share in the commercial profit
6. If the research involves biospecimens, whether the research will (if known) or might include whole genome sequencing
7. A general description of the types of research that may be conducted, with sufficient detail to allow a reasonable person to decide whether to consent
8. A description of the identifiable private information or biospecimens that might be used, whether that information or biospecimen may be

shared with other researchers and the types of institutions or investigators who may use the information or biospecimen

9. The length of time the information or biospecimens will be stored, used for research purposes and maintained (which can be indefinite)
10. If it applies, a statement that the subjects will not be informed of specific research studies using the information or biospecimens, including a statement that the subjects may not have chosen to participate had they known of the use
11. To the extent it applies, a statement that clinically relevant results will not be shared with subjects
12. Who to contact concerning questions about the subjects' rights or harms from the research.

There is a template for broad consent available on the OHRP website and a sample list of the kinds of future uses a broad consent form might list, like *"studying the causes and progression of different diseases and conditions."* A clause could also be included that specifies particular types of research that will not be conducted. Once broad consent is obtained, researchers are allowed to conduct secondary research using the identifiable private information or identifiable biospecimens, as long as the IRB determines that the proposed secondary research fits within the scope of the broad consent. The IRB is still involved and will need to approve the conduct of the secondary research.

Developing Study-Specific Informed Consent

Process of Developing Study-Specific Consent

The sponsor of a clinical trial usually develops the study-specific form and then regional-level versions are developed next, e.g., the study-specific U.S. version, the study-specific Canadian form. The sponsor must have a procedure for developing an informed consent document that meets the regulatory requirements for the required elements. The sponsor's procedure commonly includes an informed consent template that is then updated for a specific study. After the regional level, the sponsor facilitates the site or local level. When the sponsor hires investigators to conduct the clinical trial the study consent is updated to include the specific information for each investigator. The CRC commonly is delegated the responsibility by the investigator to verify that the information is correct and adequate for the requirements of the institution where the investigator conducts the trial.

Some clinical trials are sponsored by an institution that is also conducting the trial, e.g., academic medical institutions commonly sponsor a large amount of medical research. In these cases, the study type is called an Investigator-Initiated Trial (IIT). This is also known as a Sponsor-Investigator trial under FDA 21 CFR Part 3(b) definitions: *Sponsor-Investigator means an individual who both initiates and conducts an investigation, and under whose immediate direction the investigational drug is administered or dispensed. The term does not include any person other than an individual. The requirements applicable to a sponsor-investigator under this part include both those applicable to an investigator and a sponsor.* In this case, the CRC is also commonly the delegate that the investigator authorizes to ensure the consent document contains the institution-required content. Ultimately the responsibilities are the investigator's, so his or her oversight is critical and evident in the study essential documentation.

Support for Participant Comprehension

There are many factors that affect the ability of the potential study participant to be able to adequately comprehend an informed consent. The sponsor, investigator and, ultimately, the IRB are responsible to ensure that an informed consent is developed to support the types of research subjects that are to be consented for a study and/or for a particular site's participant demographics.

One factor that impacts a participant's ability to comprehend the consent is the length of the document. Study informed consents today are commonly very long. According to the FDA, the length of the consent has been identified as a contributing factor to the inability for a study participant to comprehend the information presented to support making an informed decision. A consent form may contain a very detailed description of protocol activities and consequences and simply too much information to support the decision-making of the participant. Before approval, the IRB reviewing and approving the study consent for a research site is required to evaluate the length of the consent to ensure that the length would not negatively impact the ability for the participant to be informed. The update to the Common Rule is likely to also affect the development, format and presentation of the consent form, hopefully for the better. A 25-page consent form is not uncommon for some multi-center Phase III clinical trials. A participant's ability to comprehend is questionable.

Another factor that supports the consent comprehension is the complexity of the words. The consent form needs to be technically correct, yet intelligible for nonmedical people. Consent forms should be written at an appropriate reading level for the participants; this is determined by the IRB and is commonly required to be at a 6th to 8th grade level. This is a challenge in an industry filled with research jargon, acronyms and medical terminology. In general, the shorter the sentences and the fewer syllables per word there are in the text, the easier it will be to comprehend and understand. For example, a conscious effort should be made to use common terminology such as "teaspoons" instead of "cubic centimeters or milliliters," or "sick to your stomach" instead of "nauseated." Here is an example of some text from an informed consent document written at different grade levels:

> If any significant new information about the study drug becomes available during your participation in the study, and that information might affect your willingness to continue in the study, the doctor in charge of the study will tell you about it.

The paragraph above is written at the 12th grade level, which is likely too high of a reading level for an informed consent document. This was calculated by using the reading level tool found within most word processing programs being used to develop a consent.

> If we find out anything new about the study drug while you are on the study, we will let you know. This will help you to decide if you would like to continue.

The second example above is written at a 5th grade level.

There are different reading level formulas that can be used. One example is the FOG Index, which is taking the square root of the number of three syllable words in 10 consecutive sentences plus 3. For example, if the number of three-syllable words in 10 consecutive sentences of an informed consent is 16, the square root of 16 = 4, 4 + 3 = 7th grade reading level.

The reading level should initially be determined by the author of the consent, and then approved by the investigator's IRB. In a case where the CRC may be delegated to develop the draft of the study consent in an IIT, checking for reading level should be done and confirmed appropriate by the IRB.

Ensuring that a consent is written in the language that the participant can read and understand is another factor that must be supported in the consent document used for a particular participant, e.g., a Spanish-speaking participant who also reads and speaks English can be consented with a consent in English, but a Spanish-speaking participant who cannot read and understand English cannot be consented using a consent in English even if someone translates it verbally into Spanish during the consenting process. A consent translation must be formally done ahead of time and approved by the IRB. The translation must be confirmed to have the same meaning as the original. Commonly, this is done through the use of a translation company and offers a certificate of translation for the record.

Additionally, it is important to support the special needs of some study participants with decreased mental ability to make an informed decision, e.g., dementia. In this type of case, the study participant must be represented by a legally authorized individual. The investigator must ensure 1) those that have decreased capacity have a legally authorized representative (LAR) that makes the informed decision for that patient, signing for the patient and 2) there is confirmation and documentation of the qualifications of the LAR for a particular subject. The investigator may delegate these responsibilities to the CRC to manage. Adequate documentation is essential.

Another example of supporting the special needs of the potential participant is the circumstance where a subject or their LAR is illiterate or blind, not able to read the consent form. This is not the same as supporting the different language translation needs of the participant or LAR, nor the same as

> **FAQ**
>
> **Sometimes we're caught in the middle between the sponsor and the IRB when it comes to the preferred language for the consent form. Who has the ultimate responsibility for this decision?**
>
> This is always awkward—you can't do the study without IRB approval for the consent and yet, sometimes the sponsor will not budge on the wording it wants, especially when it comes to indemnification language. Sometimes it works best to suggest direct contact between the IRB chairman and the sponsor; having everything go through the site is not very effective. If agreement can not be reached, you may not be able to participate in the study.

supporting a study participant who mentally cannot consent on their own. Consenting individuals who are illiterate require what is termed as "oral" consent, which has additional requirements related to participants for obtaining of consent. There are two ways to perform oral consent.

The standard written consent form described earlier can be used to obtain consent and read aloud. An impartial witness must be present for the consenting process. They are witnessing that the oral consent included the reading of the consent content, adequate time was provided for consent, questions were answered and the participant voluntarily consented. In this case, an LAR is not needed since the subject is competent. To support the other aspects of oral consent, the person obtaining consent must document in the subject's research record the circumstances as to why oral consent was needed and how an impartial witness was obtained.

In some cases, an IRB requires and provides a short form to support the documentation of the process. The short form is discussed in FDA 21 CFR Part 50.27, *Documentation of Informed Consent,* and ICH E6 Section 4.8.9, *Informed Consent of Trial Subjects*. The short form supplements and documents the oral consent process. If this method is used, the form must state that all elements of consent required by regulation have been presented orally to the subject or subject's LAR, and there must be an impartial witness to the oral presentation. The impartial witness is provided a copy of the script being read aloud to the subject. If an additional script is created to perform oral consent and the approved written consent is not used, the IRB must approve the written summary or script of what is to be said to the subject or his or her representative. Only the short form itself is to be signed by the subject or his or her representative. The impartial witness will sign both the short form and a copy of the written summary. The person obtaining the consent will sign a written copy of the summary. A copy of the short form and the summary will be given to the subject or his or her representative. Both short and standard forms must be approved by an IRB before use. Documentation of the approval must be maintained by the site.

Additionally, the industry has seen more efforts toward using electronic consents that use multi-media, but if the length of the content and the readability are not appropriate an eConsent may not improve the process related to comprehension.

Pediatrics and Assent

Some studies include pediatric populations. The IRB decides whether the study requires assent of the child and consent from the child's parent(s) or legal guardian. Assent is the child saying they want to participate, and the consent is completed by the parent or guardian giving permission. Sometimes assents are not used, e.g., the child is too young. Sometimes an assent is combined with a consent into the same form and obtained at the same time. Sometimes they are separate documents. The reading level of the assent is lower than the consent, of course, and may include more pictures or videos. Both the assent and the consent must be approved by an IRB before use. There also may be more than one active version of an assent for different age groups, e.g., 5-7 years old, 8-12 years and 13-17 years old. This is up to the IRB and influenced by state or regional law.

It is important that the CRC know the requirements of a study involving a pediatric population. Additionally, confirm what is legal representation for a legal guardian, e.g., one parent, both parents or the parent with primary custody in divorce situations. It is critical to document this type of confirmation. Children are one of the most vulnerable populations and, at the same time, very underserved in clinical trials.

Obtaining Informed Consent

Who Can Obtain Consent

The investigator is ultimately responsible for obtaining consent. Depending on the study, the investigator may delegate obtaining consent to the CRC working on the study. The person obtaining consent must be trained on the study, be able to explain the action of the investigational product and be able to answer questions about study participation, the study events and medical information. If the CRC is not qualified to answer medical questions the participant may have regarding their medical condition in relation to the study drug, the investigator must ensure that qualified individuals are participating in the consenting process. The CRC should be cautious not to accept the performance of tasks delegated to them if they are not qualified by training, education and experience, as applicable.

Timing of Consent

No person may be enrolled as a research subject unless the person, or the person's LAR, has given informed consent. This informed consent must be obtained before the subject is involved in any study-related activity. The timing of consent is commonly audited by the sponsor or regulatory authority to ensure that this requirement was supported. The reconstruction and evaluation of the events before and after consenting are essential in verifying that the time of consent versus when the subject started the study-specific procedures is appropriate. The negative implications of not obtaining consent prior to initiating study procedures are great to subject safety, usability of data and inspection outcomes.

The Consent Process

As noted earlier, the informed consent process is more than obtaining signatures on a form. The informed consent process includes activities before, during and after consenting: 1) Before the consenting of a subject, e.g., development and approval of a study consent document that supports participant comprehension and assessing if the subject has special needs for consent like translation or oral consent; 2) Supporting the subject during the consenting process, e.g., providing adequate opportunity for the potential subject to ask questions and to consider whether to participate, and ensuring that the right people are present; 3) Obtaining the potential subject's voluntary agreement to participate and continuing to provide information as the clinical investigation progresses or as the subject requires.

FAQ

The consent for our study was changed by the sponsor to reflect new information about adverse events. Nothing else changed—just the addition of two more possible adverse events to the list. Does the IRB need to approve the revised consent?

Yes. Any change in a consent that involves risk should be approved by an IRB before use. Most IRBs will want to approve any change to a consent form. The revised consent form should be dated appropriately to differentiate it from previous versions.

Who must sign the revised consent?

All new subjects enrolled after the revised consent became effective should sign it. Also, all subjects who are still in the trial should sign the revised consent form. Generally it is acceptable for those subjects to read and sign the new consent at their next regularly scheduled visit. Some IRBs allow sites to add the new material as a one-page addendum to the consent and ask their current subjects to review and sign the addendum; new subjects must have the full consent, of course.

Consent Process Documentation and Signature Requirements

The FDA requires the subject or LAR sign and date the consent after agreeing to participate. Under ICH E6, the subject or LAR and the person obtaining the consent must sign the consent. Each person signing the consent must date their own signature. What is commonly seen for studies is the ICH requirement.

The investigator typically delegates the responsibility for confirming the study requirements for each study to the CRC. It is essential that this information be communicated to all study site members working on the clinical trial. Mistakes commonly happen when someone less familiar with the study is covering for the primary CRC coordinating the trial. The CRC is also frequently involved in the actual consent process. During the time of consent and before the subject leaves the site after consent, the CRC should ensure that the consent document was adequately obtained and that all signatures are present; this includes the LAR and impartial witness, if applicable. In addition to the signatures on a form, remember that documenting other aspects of the consenting process is critical and not supported by signatures alone, like including documentation that supports who was present at the consenting, if the consenting was done over several visits, why an LAR or impartial witness was used, and how was it confirmed that these were the appropriate individuals to sign the consent document. All efforts to support the consent process should be documented. If it is not written down, it did not happen. (Refer to the previous chapter on ALCOAC.)

Table 4: Example of a Chart Notation Documenting the Informed Consent Process

June 8, 2019

The informed consent document for the Acme Company protocol 1234/0019 was presented to Bill Smith at 2:15 p.m. This protocol is for an investigational drug (Drug 1234) vs. placebo in moderate hypertension. Details of the protocol procedures were discussed, as well as potential benefits and risks. Alternate therapies were presented. Mr. Smith read the consent (version dated 4/3/2019), asked questions, discussed it with his wife and decided to participate. He signed the consent at 3:25 p.m. 6/8/19. A signed copy of the consent form was given to the patient. His first study visit will take place on Monday, June 10, 2019.

—Cynthia Rodgers, CRC

As mentioned earlier, informed consent can also be obtained through the use of an eConsent (eIC) or hybrid approach between paper and electronic, e.g., video of essential elements and a paper document to sign. The FDA finalized a regulatory guidance on eConsent at the end of 2016. The guidance promotes the use of technology to improve documentation and compliance to the informed consent process, e.g., using the correct IRB-approved version of the consent for a study, and improving efficiencies in consent and the ability to obtain consent remotely from a subject's home. In cases of eIC, a subject might be asked to sign electronically. The electronic system dates and timestamps when the electronic signature is recorded for the consent process. The audit trail created by the electronic system helps support the documentation of the consent process, but also should eliminate the risk of using the wrong version. The regulations for electronic systems and signature, 21 CFR Part 11, apply.

The following are best practices for the CRC to use during the informed consent process:

1. Have the presenter summarize what was read, emphasizing the more important activities.
2. Always ask the subject if there are any questions. Answer them completely and truthfully or obtain someone that can answer them, e.g., the investigator or other medically qualified individual.
3. Never try to convince a subject to participate. Objectively present the study information and answer honestly.
4. Ask the subject some questions about the consent material to determine how well the subject understands what is being presented. This will often generate additional questions from the subject.
5. An IRB-approved video presentation of the consent form can be an effective tool. If the site has a person who is a particularly good presenter, this person could describe the study in the video. Some sponsors have videos to use during the consenting process. In addition to ensuring that all subjects hear the same thing, the video documents what was said by the site staff. The video, however, should never replace the involvement of the site study staff. The investigator or qualified delegate must be available to answer medical questions and/or to make a judgment of subject eligibility. The video must be IRB-approved before use, even if the written consent is already approved earlier.
6. The consent process should not be rushed. Subjects must be given ample time to assess, evaluate and discuss the information they have been given before having to make a decision. A subject may want to take the written form home or to access the electronic consent remotely to discuss with family members.
7. The consent process always should be documented in the patient's chart.

A proper informed consent process should leave the potential study subject the freedom to say "no" without feeling guilty or fear of losing any of their rights or access to care. Many people have a very high esteem for their primary care physician (PCP) and may want to please their physicians, willing to do as their doctor directs. This can carry over into the consenting process; this "need to please" must be avoided by physicians involved in research. Investigators and CRCs must make every effort to help potential study subjects understand that it is entirely acceptable if they choose not to participate, and that they will not lose any benefits of care if they decline. Some research centers choose to have physicians other than the subject's PCP consent the subject to help address the potential influence.

Exceptions from Consent

There are two main situations for FDA trials in which exceptions to consent may be made during a clinical trial. Since the use of consents is usually mandatory in clinical studies, these two situations are unique and must be anticipated in advance through inclusion of protocol components that detail the process to support compliance and help mitigate the risk of improper use of exceptions to consents.

One type of exception is for patients who do not have any other treatment possible. They may not qualify for a current study, to include the disease process being studied, but in the opinion of the investigator, the investigational product may help when no other treatment option has worked or is available. For example, there may be a patient who is near death from a severe infection and all suitable marketed antibiotics have been tried but the infective bacteria are all resistant to these drugs. The patient does not qualify for any ongoing study. Under this exemption, this patient may be treated with an unapproved antibiotic through the clinical trial.

Regulations for this type of emergency research are found in FDA regulations 21 CFR 50.23. Although a physician may treat a patient with an investigational product in a case like this, he or she must meet the following conditions:

- Informed consent is not feasible before the use of the investigational product.
- Both the study investigator and a neutral physician who is not otherwise participating in the clinical investigation certify, in writing, all of the following:
    - The human subject is confronted by a life-threatening situation necessitating the use of the test article.
    - Informed consent cannot be obtained from the subject because of an inability to communicate with, or obtain legally effective consent from, the subject.
    - Time is not sufficient to obtain consent from the subject's legally authorized representative.
    - There is no available alternative method of approved or generally recognized therapy that provides an equal or greater likelihood of saving the life of the subject.

- The exception to this is:
    - Immediate use of the test article is, in the investigator's opinion, required to preserve the life of the subject.
    - Time is not sufficient to obtain the independent determination in advance of using the test article.
        - In this case, the determination of the clinical investigator shall be made and, within five working days after the use of the article, be reviewed and evaluated in writing by a physician who is not participating in the clinical investigation.
- The documentation required must be submitted to the investigator's IRB within five working days after the use of the test article.
- These types of exceptions are rare. If the investigator wants to be able to use the product for this type of patient again in the future, then he or she must submit a protocol to the IRB as for any study.

The second type of emergency research exception involves types of protocols where the subject population enrolled is very sick and without alternative approved treatment. Additionally, there is a chance that a subject might present for the study and qualify but is unable to consent and has no LAR available in time to consent before the subject dies. The protocol design would include the anticipation of the potential recruitment of such subjects and the requirements of consent. The regulations for this type of emergency research are found in 21 CFR 50.24. Examples of these studies are those in which the subject has a life-threatening trauma to the body, such as a head injury or a heart attack. Not only are the subjects in these studies not able to give consent prior to being treated, but there may not be time to identify and locate a subject's LAR before treatment must begin. Frequently, these studies have a relatively short window of opportunity for treatment.

Unlike the first type of exception, waivers of consent must be approved in advance of the study start by the reviewing IRB. It is not the investigator or the sponsor who makes the determination of whether or not the exception is allowed. It must be approved by an IRB, with the agreement from a licensed physician who is not associated with the research project but who may or may not be a member of the IRB. In order for the IRB to make this determination, the following must be documented:

- The subject is in a life-threatening situation, available treatments are unproven or unsatisfactory and the collection of valid scientific evidence is necessary to determine the safety and effectiveness of the particular intervention.
- Obtaining informed consent is not feasible because:
    - The subjects will not be able to give consent because of their

medical condition.

- The intervention under investigation must be administered before consent can be obtained from the subject's LAR.
- There is no way to identify prospectively the individuals likely to become eligible for participation in the study.
- Participation in the research may have direct benefit to the subject because the subject is in a life-threatening situation that necessitates intervention.
- Previous research, both pre-clinical and/or clinical, provides supporting evidence of the potential for the intervention to provide a direct benefit to the subject.
- Risks associated with the intervention are reasonable in relation to what is known about the medical condition of the potential class of subjects, the risks and benefits of standard therapy and what is known, if anything, about the risks and benefits of the experimental treatment or intervention.
- The clinical investigation could not be carried out practically without the waiver.
- The protocol defines the length of the therapeutic window based on scientific evidence and the investigator commits to attempting to contact the subject's LAR or family member within that window of opportunity and asking for consent, if feasible, rather than proceeding without consent. The investigator will summarize efforts to contact LARs and provide this information to the IRB at the time of continuing review.
- The IRB has approved the consent form and process to be used when informing the subject, when possible, or the subject's LAR or a family member.
- Additional protections of the rights and welfare of the subjects will be provided to include:
    - Consultation with the community in which the study will be conducted and the subjects selected
    - Public disclosure (in the community in which the study is to be conducted) prior to initiation of the study, including plans for the study and the risks and benefits associated with it
    - Public disclosure following completion of the study of sufficient information to apprise researchers and the community of the study, including demographics of the

study population and its results

- Establishment of an independent data monitoring committee to exercise oversight of the investigation
- The IRB also has a responsibility to see that the study subject is informed about the nature of the study and his or her involvement in it as soon as that can be done. If the subject remains incapacitated, then the LAR or, if not available, a family member must be updated. The LAR (or family member) also should be told that he or she may request the subject be removed from the study at any time without penalty or loss of benefit.

- A CRC may work on a study that includes emergency research and enrollment of subjects into a trial where there is waiver of consent. All of these requirements are important for the CRC to be familiar with, especially if the CRC is delegated any informed consent tasks. The CRC should be sure that the investigator is adequately involved and that all medical evaluations and decisionmaking is performed by the investigator or a qualified delegate.

Under OHRP-regulated studies there are some additional examples of studies that may qualify for allowing IRBs to waive some or all elements of informed consent when specific conditions have been met. One example is outcomes research at an academic medical facility. To qualify for the waiver, it cannot be practical to obtain the consent—for example, the patient is deceased. This type of research commonly looks at the progression of a disease process related to other circumstances and the data is not gathered on each individual person, but rather as a set of statistics to help better plan standards of care. Note that some studies require consent, but not all the elements of the standard consent. This is common in non-treatment questionnaire studies.

Common Informed Consent Deficiencies & Conclusion

The informed consent deficiencies involve the content of the written consent and/or the process of consent. Common problems are:

- The timing of consent is not correct, e.g., study procedures being done before the consent is signed.
- Proper signatures and dates are not always obtained.
- The consent form does not have all the required and applicable additional elements.
- The person(s) obtaining consent were not adequate.

- The wrong version of the IRB-approved consent was used or an unapproved version was used.
- An additional required element was not included.

The CRC can prevent many informed consent deficiencies, but clear understanding of the regulatory and study-specific requirements is necessary. The IRB is a great resource for questions before a study starts. It is important to proactively anticipate challenges for consent. Even after the consent is approved for a study, identify what things are likely to go wrong and how the investigator and CRC can plan the consenting process for a particular study to prevent issues, e.g., timing of consent, involvement of the investigator, questions to the IRB about the consent process. Directly after consenting subjects on a new study, having a fellow site staff member review the completeness of the consent and the documentation is a good practice to catch errors early in the study and not when the sponsor monitors the study. Early issue identification and documentation of management is essential to maintain audit readiness and, more importantly, human subject protection.

One of the primary safeguards for the rights, safety and well-being of human subjects of research is informed consent. The informed consent process is a complex and important part of conducting clinical research. CRCs must have a working knowledge of consent forms and processes so that deficiencies can be avoided. Ensuring that there is adequate investigator oversight and involvement is essential. It is recommended that CRCs read the regulations governing informed consent (CFR 21 part 50). There is a checklist for reviewing informed consents in Appendix D.

CHAPTER EIGHT

Pre-study: Preparing for a Study

Good Clinical Practice (GCP) includes three main stages with associated activities and essential documents. These stages include: 1) pre-study, before the clinical phase of the trial starts; 2) trial conduct, during the clinical conduct of the trial; and 3) study completion or termination after the clinical trial conduct has been stopped. The investigator or delegate, commonly the CRC, must maintain quality documentation to support the investigational site activities related to each stage. Per ICH E6, "*Essential Documents are those documents, which individually and collectively permit evaluation of the conduct of a trial and the quality of the data produced. These documents serve to demonstrate the compliance of the investigator, sponsor and monitor with the standards of Good Clinical Practice and with all applicable regulatory requirements.*" Timely filing of essential documents can greatly assist in the successful management of a clinical trial.

Essential documents are also routinely reviewed by the sponsor monitors, usually audited by the study sponsor's independent audit function, and inspected by the regulatory authority(ies) as part of the process to confirm the validity of the trial conduct and the integrity of the data collected.

For a study coordinator, becoming familiar with what is the minimum list of essential documents for investigators to maintain is important. ICH E6 Section 8 includes a list of essential documents for investigators and sponsors to maintain during the three stages of GCP. A description of the purpose for each document is included. It is acceptable to combine some of the documents, provided the individual elements are readily identifiable. It is important to remember that the quality of each individual document must meet the ALCOAC standard discussed in an earlier chapter, and collectively the documents map to other essential documents related to their purpose. For example, individually an investigators' CV must be attributable to the investigator, support accurately the investigator's qualifications to perform and oversee the study and link collectively to many other documents to support the investigator's qualifications, such as training records. A study coordinator has to have the ability to review the documents for quality.

Essential documents are filed at sponsors and sites within their TMF. TMFs should be established at the beginning of the trial, both at the investigator/institution's site and at the sponsor's office. The term TMF was derived from ICH E6. The TMF is commonly called a variety of names by sponsors or investigators, i.e., the investigator study file, but no matter mean the same thing. More commonly used are electronic systems for TMF storage and management.

In this chapter, we will discuss a number of activities that take place before a site is selected, as well as activities that must be completed before a study site can start to enroll subjects. Topics include sponsor site qualification, assessing protocol feasibility, budgeting, site preparation for a study, sponsor site initiation, investigator meetings and financial disclosure. Study coordinators usually are involved in all these activities and need to have a thorough understanding of each of them.

Sponsor Site Qualification

Sponsor site qualification is a critical step for both the sponsor and the site. For the investigator, these visits determine whether the site will be selected to participate in the research and provide the site time to determine if the study is right for them. For the sponsor, site qualification activities are the primary method of determining the best sites to conduct their studies and to identify the areas of greatest risk for a site if chosen.

When a sponsor or CRO is looking for investigative sites to conduct a study, the first contact usually is by telephone or email. If it appears there is a high level of interest in the protocol on the part of the potential investigator, and if the sponsor feels there is good potential for placing a study at the site, the sponsor will arrange a time to visit the site in person. This will enable the sponsor to better evaluate the investigator's capability to do the project. Many companies require a signed confidentiality disclosure agreement (CDA) before sharing a protocol summary; in this case, they will email or fax an agreement to the site, and have it completed and returned before sending the materials. Note that some sponsors and CROs send a preliminary questionnaire to sites to assess their suitability for a particular clinical trial. It is a point in the site's favor to return the signed confidentiality agreement and any questionnaires to the sponsor/CRO quickly. If a sponsor or CRO has worked with an investigator within a certain period of time and the investigator performed well with enrollment and compliance with the protocol, the qualification visit might be able to be waived or abbreviated if the sponsor/

FAQ

What are the most important factors in a sponsor's determination of which sites to choose for a study?

Past experience and current capability are probably the most important, but all of the factors mentioned in this section will be taken into account. And many sponsors won't even consider using an investigator who does not have a CRC.

CRO policy supports this. In this case, the sponsor/CRO would verify that conditions at the site have not changed.

When a sponsor representative, often the sponsor site monitor, completes a qualification visit to a potential site, he or she evaluates the investigator's experience in the therapeutic area and research, and interest in the trial, as well as that of the applicable staff and facility. The potential to enroll the sponsor's desired number of subjects is also assessed. The sponsor's monitoring visit report and study-specific requirements guide the CRA in making the site qualification assessment. There is an example of such a checklist in Appendix D.

The sponsor will want a copy of the investigator's CV in order to make a general assessment of the investigator's experience and expertise. The sponsor will want to know if the investigator has conducted trials similar to the one being proposed or has worked with similar compounds. The investigator and the study coordinator should read any materials (protocol synopsis) before the evaluation activities so they are prepared for any discussion or completion of a questionnaire.

The sponsor will also evaluate whether the site has sufficient staff and an appropriate facility to conduct the study. Many sponsors will not place a study at an investigative site that does not have a study coordinator. During the evaluation activities, the sponsor will want to meet and spend some time interviewing the study coordinator. Not only must there be appropriate people available for a study, but those people must have sufficient qualifications and time to do the trial.

During an on-site qualification visit, the sponsor will tour the facilities. The sponsor will want to see that there are appropriate investigational product and study supply storage areas, the equipment necessary for performing the study and a place for the sponsor monitor to work during monitoring visits.

The sponsor will assess the enrollment potential of the site, including whether subjects will come from the investigator's current patient population or if they will be recruited from elsewhere. For investigators that enroll their own patients, access to potential study subjects is easier. But independent research centers usually have good recruiting departments that are efficient in planning and recruitment strategy. In either case, the more thorough the records are concerning access to the study population, the better the enrollment estimates will be.

There are several other items a sponsor monitor will want to discuss during a qualification visit. One is whether or not the site is conducting, or planning to conduct within the same time period, any competing studies. A competing study is usually one in which similar subjects are to be enrolled. In order to meet the enrollment targets, it's important that a study does not have to compete for subjects with another sponsor's study. Competition for subjects can have a great impact on the ability to meet enrollment targets.

Another factor evaluated is the timing for the study related to the investigator and delegate's availability. If the investigator has too many active studies at the same time, a study may not get the attention it needs to be done well.

The sponsor will want to check on the laboratory and pharmacy, if either will be used for the study, to ensure that laboratory accreditations are current, and the facilities are adequate to perform the necessary study activities.

The importance of the site qualification activities cannot be overstated for both the sponsor and the investigator to ensure study conduct quality and success. Site qualifications are done proactively to support identification and risk planning. Consequently, the investigator and the study coordinator should be well prepared for the visit and ready to show their site at its best.

How to Succeed in Getting Studies

Since the study site qualification is so important, here are some things a study coordinator can do to support the process:

- Read the protocol synopsis, and any other sponsor materials before the visit. Be prepared to discuss them knowledgeably.
- Prepare a list of questions for the visit.
- Have all the staff who might be involved with the study available to talk with the sponsor during the visit.
- Allow enough time.
- Be sure confidential materials are filed away.
- Have data on past studies available (maintaining confidentiality, of course). This should include the number and types of studies that have been conducted, number of subjects enrolled and enrollment rates and any other information that might be helpful.
- Provide previous FDA inspection results.

There are many other things besides activities related to the qualification visits that a site can do to find studies, including social media presence, contacting sponsors and CROs, creating brochures and other advertising materials and talking with sponsor sales representatives about whom to contact. Attending industry conferences and speaking at professional meetings are other ways a study coordinator can support public relations for a research site.

All these tasks take time and may not show results immediately. It commonly takes longer than expected. Over time, the site will find what methods are most successful for marketing

Protocol Feasibility

The sponsor is not the only entity that must determine whether a study should be done at a site. It is equally important for the site personnel to make an assessment of whether a proposed study is a good fit for their capabilities. It is always better to turn down a study that is not a good fit than to accept it and fail.

Just as sponsors have checklists and specific items they must assess at a site, the site should have a site study feasibility process that includes a potential study assessment to completed before accepting a study. The study coordinator, the investigator and any other people who will be involved in the study should read the protocol and supporting materials carefully before making a decision. The following is a list of some questions that help uncover the risks of participation and provide valuable insight for decision-making and negotiations:

- Have we worked with this sponsor/CRO before and was it a successful partnership?
- Are the number of subjects to be enrolled and the timeline realistic?
- Will our patients benefit from this study?
- Do we have the necessary resources (staff, time, equipment, space) to do the study within the given time period?
- Are we interested in the objectives of the study?
- Do we have access to the right kinds of patients for this study? How will we recruit and what kind of expenses will need to be included in the study budget?
- How difficult will the protocol be to execute?

FAQ

We've been offered a study, but we don't think we can do it well (enrollment will probably be difficult). We're worried that if we say no to it, the sponsor won't come back.

You will almost always be better off telling a sponsor you cannot do a study when you don't think you can do it well. Most sponsors will come to you again if they have a more suitable protocol. However, if you accept a study and fail, the sponsor can't afford to try your site again.

- Is the budget compensating for time and materials to do the job?

There is a sample site feasibility checklist provided in Appendix D that should be linked to a process. The process should support that after each person involved has made his or her assessment, a group discussion is valuable in reaching a decision. Again, it is much better for a site to pass on a protocol than to take on a project and fail. Most sponsors will respect a decision to not participate when it is based on a thorough analysis and will return to the site with other studies that may be a better fit. However, once a site has failed at a study (not meeting enrollment, not following the protocol), most sponsors will consider that site risky and use caution when considering the site again. Consequently, site study feasibility is one of the most important pre-study tasks to be performed.

Grants, Budgeting and Contracts

Over time, protocols have become more complex and call for more procedures. This means that sites must be careful about whether or not they can actually afford to do a study without losing money, and they need to be very selective about the projects they decide to take on. There are many hidden costs the investigative site has to be aware of, such as time and costs incurred for copying, recruitment, project management, working with sponsor monitors, unscheduled subject visits, amendments to protocols requiring more administrative and study-specific work, re-consenting subjects due to study changes, studies starting later than planned, and so forth.

Most sponsors operate on a fee-for-service basis. This means they will pay for actual work performed, i.e., subjects enrolled and subject visits. Most grants are formulated on a per-subject amount and prorated for the number of visits a subject actually completes. The amount per visit often will vary, as some visits are more labor- and time-intensive than others. Sponsors feel they are buying a service from the investigator and do not expect to pay if the work (subjects and quality data) is not delivered.

There are different ways in which sponsor grant figures are determined. Some companies use commercially available grant management systems that estimate costs for protocol activities. This gives the sponsor a realistic grant range to work from when determining how much it wishes to pay for per-patient grants. Other companies determine grants based on their own actual costs data or on data gathered from other sources. Others rely on information from the investigators they are considering for the study, or a combination of all of the above.

Some sponsors will determine a range or a single per-subject grant figure they will pay and will not budge from this figure. Investigators either accept it or will not be able to do the study. Other sponsors will allow more flexibility, depending on their experience with an investigator or geographic location. Costs do differ in different parts of the world, so it makes sense to allow some flexibility.

Study start-up activities can be quite expensive for a site. These include activities such as feasibility assessment, submissions to IRBs, resource planning, etc. These expenses are not linked specifically by subject. Therefore, a common practice many sites are demanding of sponsors is a non-refundable start-up fee. For sites that have performed well for sponsors in the past, this fee is more acceptable and can be quite large. The amount can vary greatly from site to site. The research institution would need to justify the amount requested. Sometimes the contract and budget negotiations can go on for a long time, so some sites require a separate precontract that covers pre-study activities through actual study contract execution.

Some institutions involve the study coordinator in budget development and some do not. Budgets are typically developed by creating line items for each study activity, attaching a cost to each, including personnel time to perform the activity, and adding an additional amount for overhead and other required activities for study and data management. Then it is tallied. The overhead covers operation costs that are indirectly related to the study activities, like utilities or rent. An example of a grant worksheet is shown in Table 1.

For this hypothetical study, there are eight visits. To determine the amount per visit, add the amounts for each procedure done at that visit from the budget worksheet. This will allow the grant to be prorated for subjects who do not complete the entire study. Items such as IRB fees, advertising or long-term

Table 1: Budget Worksheet—Protocol XXX

Study Activity	Number of visits	Cost	Expanded cost
Phone pre-screen	1	50	50
Medical history	1	50	50
Physical exam	3	150	450
Labs	8	150	1,200
EKG	3	200	600
Treadmill stress test	3	250	750
Office visit—general assessments	8	75	600
Phone assessments	2	50	100
Sub-total for procedures			**$3,800**
Coordinator time	8	50	400
Pharmacy charge	8	35	280
Subtotal			**$680**
Total			**$4,480**
Overhead—15%			672
Grand total per completed subject			**$5,152**

document storage are negotiated and added on as separate amounts, rather than being calculated in the actual per-subject costs.

This is a simple way to calculate grants and prorate visit costs, but it is quite effective if the initial amounts for each procedure and activity are realistic. It is easy to explain and should help negotiate a grant amount that is fair to both the sponsor and the site.

Some sponsor companies utilize their monitor in determining when grant monies should be paid, while others handle all grant payments internally. Companies usually pay either on a timed schedule, such as quarterly, or on the basis of CRF completion and query resolution.

Besides a start-up fee, some sponsors will pay a small amount of the grant up front (maybe two subjects' worth), which will then be applied to the work being done. This allows the investigator to have some cash flow to set up study procedures, pay for initial labs and other tests, etc., without having to use site funds. If subjects are not enrolled for whatever reason, the upfront money will need to be returned. The research site should keep track of the work completed and payments made to be sure that everything balances. Once a study starts, it may be discovered that the budget is not adequate. The contract should support justified renegotiations.

A clinical trial agreement (CTA) between the sponsor and the investigator must be signed before the trial begins at a site. This document usually contains the responsibilities of the investigator, including the number of subjects the site expects to enroll, timelines for enrollment, grant amounts and the regulatory requirements for the investigator. It also contains the responsibilities of the sponsor, including when and how grants will be paid, monitoring of the study and sponsor regulatory requirements. The research site should always ask the sponsor for an indemnification clause for the institution and involved employees. Indemnification is a type of agreement where the investigator asks the sponsor not to hold them liable for things related to the study where the investigator followed the agreement and protocol. This does not cover if the investigator was negligent.

CTAs are commonly signed by the investigator and/or the legally authorized site financial representative. The CTA is not usually filed within the site study TMF. Therefore, a study coordinator may not see the contract or budget for a study. If the study coordinator is involved in grants, he or she must have a good understanding of both the process and the specifics for each protocol, to be able to discuss the grant with the investigator and the sponsor, and to track the figures to ensure that all sums are paid as appropriate.

Investigation Site Trial Master File

Before the study begins, the primary study coordinator ensures that the site study files are set up. Very organized and well-maintained study files will have a significant impact on the quality of a study and, subsequently, the validity and usability of the data.

FAQ

We'd like to work with a particular sponsor, but the grant it is offering us for a study will not cover our costs. Should we do the study anyway, hoping for additional work with the sponsor in the future?

Your first task should be discussing the grant in detail with the sponsor. Show the sponsor your actual figures and see if it can make an adjustment in your grant amount. If not, you have to decide how much money you are willing to lose in the hope of another study. Just remember, the next grant may not be any better.

According to regulations (21CFR 312.62 and 21 CFR 812.140), the investigator must keep records relating to disposition of the investigational product, including dates, quantity and use by study subjects and case histories, including case report forms and all supporting documentation. Supporting documentation includes the signed and dated consent form, pertinent medical records, study progress notes, hospital charts, nursing notes and any other source documents. It also should be documented that informed consent was obtained prior to the subject's participation.

This is the minimum by regulation. In reality, investigator study files contain much more information. One recommendation is to have two major categories for study files: 1) non-subject-related, including regulatory and administrative files and 2) subject-related or clinical files, called source documents or case histories. Sponsors commonly provide a study file binder or an electronic file space for the study coordinator to maintain the associated documents for the first type, regulatory and administrative.

In the regulatory and administrative files there should be:

- Completed and signed Form FDA 1572 (Statement of Investigator)
- Delegation log (Log listing the study activities being conducted by the investigator and to whom they have delegated responsibility for the study tasks)
- Copies of the CVs for the investigator and sub-investigators
- Financial disclosures for the investigator and sub-investigators
- Training records for the investigator and study staff listed on the delegation log
- IRB-approved documents, e.g., the study consent forms
- Written IRB approvals of the study documents, e.g., protocol, consent form and advertising and subject compensation, if applicable
- Investigator protocol signature page(s)
- Copies of the laboratory certification and normal ranges, if applicable

- Investigator's Brochure (IB)
- Sponsor-expedited safety reports, e.g., Suspected Unexpected Serious Adverse Reaction (SUSAR – drug studies) or Unanticipated Adverse Device Effect (UADE – device studies)
- Pertinent correspondence, such as letters, memos, emails including contacts with the sponsor/CRO and IRB, as applicable
- Instructional materials or procedure manuals:
    - CRF completion/correction guidelines
    - Guidelines for handling adverse events
    - Procedures for handling and storing laboratory specimens
    - Investigational product information, including instructions for storing, dispensing and accounting
- Investigational product shipment, dispensing and return records
- Sponsor/CRO contact information
- Various study logs, e.g., screening and enrollment, supplies, investigational product study disposition.
- Records of study meetings and contact with the sponsor and/or CRO
- Monitoring log (a record of CRA monitoring visits)
- Other study-specific files.

The site will also have a research subject record with pertinent information called source documentation. The FDA refers to this as case histories in 21 CFR 312.60 and 21 CFR 812.140. Case histories are the subject's CRFs and supporting source documents, including subject signed consent form(s).

Two items not mentioned in the list above are the grant (CTA/contract) and any reports from sponsor quality assurance (QA) site audits. This information is not routinely made available in the study files. They are not directly reviewed by the FDA or an inspecting regulatory authority. But the regulatory authority can request a review, and the investigator must comply. If these are found in the files supplied to the FDA in an inspection they likely will be reviewed. The investigation site should have procedures for maintaining study files and for managing site audits/inspections.

File retention is discussed in a future chapter. However, investigators and study coordinators must be aware of the study record retention requirements from the start. The CTA will note how long the records must be maintained at the research sites.

The study sponsor monitor or study manager will be valuable in assisting with setting up and maintaining files throughout the study. Sponsors should also check the files regularly throughout the study and again at study closure. If the files are maintained electronically and shared remotely, this can be done off-site.

Being sure the files are complete and in order periodically during the study will ensure that they are in good condition in the event of an audit of the site by the sponsor, the IRB or inspection by the FDA.

During a study, the study subject files need to be kept where they can be easily accessed for sponsor monitor visits. Files can be a combination of paper and electronic. These files usually contain not only the patient medical records, but also any other study source documents and the CRF for the subject. Although these files should be easily accessible during a monitoring visit, sponsor monitors should not have free access to them due to source document control and privacy protections. Rather, the study coordinator organizes access to the needed records per the research site's policies. Depending on the type of records, this may include providing the paper and/or electronic source. Sites frequently conduct studies for different sponsors at the same time, and no monitor should have access to another sponsor's confidential information. In fact, during a site qualification visit, sponsors should check how the confidentiality of materials is maintained at a site and how the sponsor will have access to the records to monitor the study.

For investigators that enroll their own patients, it is important that a subject's medical record indicate they are participating in a study to ensure that practitioners outside the study are aware to prevent protocol deviations, support patient safety and continuation of care. Additionally, many protocols require that a participant not have been on a clinical trial within a certain period of time. For investigators that enroll subjects from outside their institution, obtaining records from the outside may be necessary to confirm the eligibility of the subject before enrollment. The requirements of the study related to medical records should be clear and included in the feasibility assessment and budget development.

A site should have consistent rules for filing all studies. This allows anyone to file and find needed documents easily. Some research institutions also perform managed care where an EHR is maintained. The EHR includes research documentation, but this is separate. Documentation from both the EHR and research chart will need to be used to perform the study and provided access to for the monitor to review.

Some tips for filing regulatory and administrative study documents:

- For paper documents, use binders or hanging files. Separate regulatory documents and correspondence into separate binders, etc.
- Use tabs or file naming conventions to break them into subsections for different categories, such as "1572 Forms," "IRB Approvals," etc.
- Within each section, file in reverse date order (newest documents on top).
- File only one copy of each document in the proper place. Filing multiple copies, especially if they are not in the same place, is very confusing and creates the risk of using the wrong version of a document.

The keys to maintaining good files are to organize them at the start, file things regularly throughout the trial and file everything correctly. Keeping study files organized and current allows for documents to be found quickly and easily. This is critical for audit readiness and for supporting ALCOAC, the quality characteristics of study documentation. It will allow for retrieval and review of any document needed with a minimum of effort. Keeping good, organized, complete study files helps the trial to run more smoothly.

Source Documents and Case Report Forms/Case Histories

A source document is any document on which the data are first recorded. Remember that essential documents are necessary for the reconstruction and evaluation of the study. They must support ALCOA: attributable, legible, contemporaneous, original and accurate. Source documents are the subject-specific records that should be the same as or support the data collected by the sponsor for the trial. The sponsor study monitor will check the source documents throughout the trial per the study monitoring plan; this is known as source document review and source document verification. The purpose of source document review and verification is two-fold: 1) to review the quality of the documentation and compliance to the regulations and protocol; and 2) to check for transcription errors in the data compared to the supporting source. The amount of review and verification is spelled out in the sponsor's monitoring plan for the study.

Other source documents include such things as laboratory reports and electrocardiogram (ECG) and other test readings and reports. If supported by the protocol, the original collection of data may be done directly on the case report form or patient-completed assessments, e.g., paper or electronic diaries; in effect, the CRF and/or diary becomes a source document in this case. This is often seen in rating scales, such as for depression and quality-of-life ranking because it is easier and more accurate to collect the information directly on the CRF as opposed to transcribing it later.

CRFs are data collection tools developed by sponsors of the study. The sponsors provide training to the sites on the completion and management of the study CRF. Each subject enrolled will have a CRF. Within a CRF are many sections. The investigator commonly delegates to the study coordinator the responsibility for CRF completion and updating. The sponsor will query data entered and the study coordinator answers the queries. Once satisfied, the sponsor will close the query. Once the data is "clean" the sponsor will lock the data for analysis. The accuracy of the CRF data is critical; so is the quality of source documentation supporting the CRF.

Certain data that needs to be documented in the source document and transcribed into a CRF requires medical evaluation from a qualified person, for example, a medically licensed practitioner. The study coordinator should only document a source and enter CRF data that is within their qualifications and delegation. An example is safety report evaluations related to causality.

The study coordinator's role in source documentation and CRF management is huge. The study coordinator should always be sure they are working within their scope and ensure that they complete quality documentation of their work.

Storage of Study Materials

Studies often necessitate the use of lots of materials. Not only is there the study drug or other test article to be stored, but there are also CRFs, laboratory kits and miscellaneous other materials. The study coordinator must be prepared to arrange for appropriate storage space for these materials. Adequate supply management is important for protocol compliance. Proactively anticipating the need for study supplies is a key role for study coordinators.

It is critical to discuss the storage criteria for the investigational product with the sponsor before the study begins. If, for example, the study requires an investigator to have a -70° freezer, it is not acceptable to use a -20° freezer instead. The sponsor may be willing to provide a site with the -70° freezer, but only if it is discussed before the study commences and is supported in the CTA. The study coordinator must also be prepared to keep such items as temperature logs to verify that the investigational product has been stored and dispensed properly throughout the study.

Many studies use a central laboratory for all sites. These laboratories will send the site laboratory kits for the collection and shipping of samples for each study subject at each appropriate visit. These kits can take up a lot of space. Most laboratories are able to ship them to the sites in smaller quantities, but they need to know ahead of time.

Good planning and organization in advance of study startup will help ensure that a study runs smoothly and well throughout its course.

Trial Master File

Before a trial can begin, a number of documents must be collected for each site by the sponsor. Most of these are required by regulations, although some sponsors and IRBs may require their own additional documents. Both the sponsor and the investigator must each have copies of certain documents; some documents will only be found at sites; for example, subject source documents are only maintained at the site unless serving both the source and the CRF. Most often, the study coordinator is delegated the responsibility to be in charge of collecting and organizing these documents.

The documents listed below are those a sponsor company must commonly collect from the site before the trial may start:

- Signed, IRB-approved investigator qualifications, protocol and any amendments

- IRB-approved informed consent, preferably containing an IRB-approved stamp or other versioning indication
- IRB approval letter(s), verifying approval of both the protocol and consent document
- IRB approval of advertising and subject recruitment materials, including subject compensation, if applicable (Note: not all research institutions offer payment to subjects for participation.)
- Signed, completed Form FDA 1572 (Statement of Investigator) for drugs or the signed agreement letter for devices
- Financial disclosure forms for the investigator and any other study personnel listed on the 1572
- Appropriate CVs for the investigator and the sub-investigator listed on the 1572
- Current laboratory certification and laboratory normal ranges
- Signed CTA (not required by FDA regulation, but required by most sponsors) especially since some content here maps into the delegation log and also ensures support for controlled trials.

Some sponsor companies have specific people whose primary responsibility is to collect and maintain these documents, while in other companies the sponsor monitors (CRAs) gather the documents for their sites. Since the CRA is the person who visits the site, he or she will probably be involved in the collection and maintenance of documents, even if another internal group has the primary responsibility.

When the IRB reviews the study, it is important that the content of the correspondence related to the review is read carefully. Sometimes IRBs ask for clarifications or additional information to be added. The investigator must not start the study screening and consenting until IRB approval has been granted.

Most sponsors will not ship the study drug until all the documents have been received per their procedure. Note that some companies do ship the CRFs and other non-drug (or device) supplies before receiving all the documents in an effort to speed up the process, while others wait and ship everything only after documentation is complete.

Financial Disclosure

In 1998, the FDA published the regulation for financial disclosure. The requirement became effective a year later and applies to any study of a drug, biologic or device that is used to support a marketing application. The regulation requires sponsors to certify the absence of certain financial interests of investigators, disclose these financial interests or certify that the information was impossible to obtain. If a sponsor does not do this, the FDA may refuse to review the application. A full description of the requirements is found in 21 CFR 54, including the following definitions:

(a) *Compensation affected by the outcome of clinical studies means compensation that could be higher for a favorable outcome than for an unfavorable outcome, such as compensation that is explicitly greater for a favorable result or compensation to the investigator in the form of an equity interest in the sponsor of a covered study or in the form of compensation tied to sales of the product, such as a royalty interest.*

(b) *Significant equity interest in the sponsor of a covered study means any ownership interest, stock options or other financial interest whose value cannot be readily determined through reference to public prices (generally, interests in a non-publicly traded corporation), or any equity interest in a publicly traded corporation that exceeds $50,000 during the time the clinical investigator is carrying out the study and for one year following completion of the study.*

(c) *Proprietary interest in the tested product means property or other financial interest in the product including, but not limited to, a patent, trademark, copyright or licensing agreement.*

...

(f) *Significant payments of other sorts means payments made by the sponsor of a covered study to the investigator or the institution to support activities of the investigator that have a monetary value of more than $25,000, exclusive of the costs of conducting the clinical study or other clinical studies (e.g., a grant to fund ongoing research, compensation in the form of equipment or retainers for ongoing consultation or honoraria), during the time the clinical investigator is carrying out the study and for one year following the completion of the study.*

Having a financial interest in a company or product does not mean an investigator cannot be involved in a trial; it simply means that all parties must be aware of the potential for conflict of interest. The sponsor will want to evaluate the potential for bias based on an investigator's financial interest before deciding whether to use that investigator. The FDA will do the same when reviewing an NDA. The sponsor might have a policy against working with an investigator with financial interest amounts defined within the regulation.

Financial disclosure applies to all the people listed on the Form FDA 1572 for a drug study, in addition to their spouses and dependent children, and those performing significant study activities for a device study. Financial disclosure information must be collected at study start. Any changes that result in exceeding the threshold(s) must be reported by the investigator during the course of the study and for one year following its completion. There is no required form for the collection of this information from the investigator. Consequently, sponsors develop their own forms and ways of collecting and maintaining this information. Financial disclosure information must be reported by the sponsor to the FDA on Form FDA 3454 (certification of absence of financial interest) or Form FDA 3455 (disclosure of financial interest). These forms are submitted as a part of the NDA.

Study coordinators may be involved in the collection of that information or, if they are listed on the 1572 for a study or perform critical study safety and/or data management activities, will need to provide the information for themselves and their families. Because of their potential involvement, it is recommended that study coordinators read the FDA's Guidance for Industry, Financial Disclosure by Clinical Investigators, which is available on the FDA's website.

FAQ

When accumulating the financial disclosure information for a sponsor, do I need to determine whether my mutual funds hold stock in the sponsor company, and how much might be included in my portfolio (in the mutual fund)?

No. It is not necessary to do this.

Investigator Meetings and Site Initiation Visits

For multi-center trials (clinical trials involving several sites performing the same protocol), many sponsors hold an investigator meeting. Although not required by regulation, this meeting, which includes all investigators, their coordinators and appropriate sponsor representatives, is one of the most important activities pertaining to the conduct of a good trial. This meeting is often the first time the investigators and study coordinators meet the sponsor monitor and/or other key study management personnel.

Investigator meetings are scheduled and conducted by the sponsor, sometimes with the help of a CRO or a meeting planning company. The purpose of these meetings is to allow the participants to get to know one another, which facilitates communication throughout the study, and to consistently and efficiently review the entire study and its conduct. The major advantages of holding these meetings are that everyone hears the same thing at the same time and site and sponsor personnel become acquainted with one another; communications during the trial are easier when people have met in person.

Since these meetings are expensive, it is important that most sites are ready to begin the study before the meeting. Sites that start the study more than a month or two after the investigator meeting will have forgotten much of the information by the time they actually begin. Ideally, the study drug is shipped while the meeting is going on. Study coordinators should try very hard to collect and turn in all of their study initiation paperwork before the meeting, so they are ready to immediately enroll the first patients upon their return to the site.

It is important for the investigator and the study coordinator to thoroughly prepare for an investigator meeting and/or site initiation visit. Involved site personnel should carefully read the protocol, the investigator's brochure and any other materials provided by the sponsor before the meeting.

During the meeting, the investigator and study coordinator should be sure that all their questions or clarifications are resolved. Be prepared to take careful notes, especially of any items that have changed or have an interpretation that differs from what was initially presented, to refer to during the study. Also, the investigator meeting and/or site initiation visits (SIV) is a time to get acquainted with each other to support a positive working relationship. This facilitates problem solving throughout the trial. The appropriate site personnel should be sure to attend all training sessions and be an active participant. Documentation of attendance is essential, and the timing should occur before performing study procedures.

Sometimes investigator meetings and SIVs are held by teleconference and videoconference. While this saves tremendously on costs and time, it does not allow people to meet and interact in person, which is a distinct disadvantage. After the meeting, sponsor and site personnel must be sure any necessary follow-up activities are done in a timely manner.

The study SIV is most commonly held at the investigation site just before the study begins. The sponsor monitor, and sometimes additional sponsor personnel, will meet with the investigator, the primary study coordinator and other supporting staff. The purpose of the meeting is to review the study protocol, processes and procedures to ensure that all site personnel understand what is necessary to perform the study.

The study initiation should be held at the point when all regulatory paperwork is complete for the site and the study drug and other supplies have been shipped, but before any subjects have been enrolled. Many sponsors will not allow the site to begin enrollment until after this meeting is held. A good, thorough, informative initiation meeting may take half a day, or even longer for a more complicated study, so the CRC may have to work with the sponsor to find a time when all relevant staff are available for a meeting. Most sponsors are willing to work with sites to find an amenable time.

It is important that all site personnel involved in the study attend the meeting, including the investigator, study coordinator, ancillary personnel such as sub-investigators, other coordinators, the pharmacist, dietician, lab person, etc. If the investigator and coordinator attended an investigator meeting, the initiation visit will serve as a review and a more detailed discussion of the topics covered during that meeting. If there was no investigator meeting, or if it was held a month or more prior to initiating the study, then the entire protocol, processes and procedure should be discussed in detail. Since the investigator and study coordinator usually are the only site people who attend the investigator meeting, other site personnel will not be as familiar with the study. The initiation meeting provides an opportunity for everyone at the site to become familiar with the study and to understand everyone's study roles.

The sponsor prepares an agenda for the SIV. The items to be covered at an initiation meeting usually include:

- Detailed discussion of the protocol, including:
    - Inclusion and exclusion criteria
    - Study procedures
    - Investigational product management (storage, dispensing, return)
    - Randomization and blinding
    - Primary outcome measures
    - Other pertinent details
- Adverse event reporting
- CRF management
- Monitoring visits—approach, how often, what should be ready, what will be covered
- Investigator responsibilities
- IRB interactions
- Any other study-specific or sponsor-specific items of importance
- Regulatory requirements
- Periodic reports of enrollment.

If certain attendees are not able to stay for the entire meeting (investigator, pharmacist), the items critical to their participation should be covered while they are present. Other items, such as completing CRFs, can be covered with the coordinators and others who may be involved in a smaller group.

After the meeting, the monitor will complete an SIV report detailing what was discussed and completed during the visit. Many companies have a special visit report for this meeting. ICH guidelines call for a sponsor initiation monitoring report documenting that trial procedures were covered with the investigator and their staff; this report is to be kept in both the sponsor and investigator study files. The same purpose can be accomplished by the CRA sending the investigator a follow-up letter listing what was covered during the meeting.

If questions arise during the meeting that need further follow up, the sponsor should find the answers and relay them to the site. This meeting can go a long way toward ensuring a successful study. It deserves the full attention of the study coordinator, the investigator and other involved staff.

Working with CRAs

For actual study conduct, the CRC is a pivotal role at the site, and the CRA is one of the most important sponsor representatives. Since they will be spending a lot of time working on the study together, the CRC and the CRA must establish a good working relationship. Each person needs to understand how the other works. The CRA should determine the best times and methods for routine communications and let the CRC know the sponsor expectations.

Other Sponsor Interactions

Study coordinators may need to interact with sponsor personnel other than the CRA on occasion, such as a medical monitor, an in-house CRA, project manager or a data manager. The study coordinator should find the appropriate people and best times to contact the sponsor with questions about the study. Remember that the CRC and CRA are on the same team—both the site and the sponsor have the best interests of the study subjects and the success of the study as top priorities.

Some sponsors will hire a CRO to handle the study monitoring for a project. The dynamics of the working relationships among the study coordinator, the CRA, the sponsor and the CRO can be complex. If not clearly defined during the investigator meeting, the study initiation meeting is a good time to clarify the communication channels for the study. The CRC may be required to communicate regularly with the CRO for some things, such as enrollment updates, and the sponsor for other things, such as serious adverse event reporting. Whatever the situation, being clear on the correct reporting and communication procedures will help the study progress smoothly.

A good relationship with the sponsor throughout a study is one of the major factors in obtaining more studies from the same sponsor in the future. Being able to maintain a good relationship with the CRA, whether a sponsor or CRO employee, plus timely and correct communications about study issues, is not only good for the study, but is also good public relations for the site.

Shipping of Biological Samples

The packaging and shipping of biological samples is often the responsibility of the study coordinator. These activities are highly regulated, and there are significant fines for not complying with the regulations.

The following regulations apply to the packaging and shipment of biological materials:

- U.S. Department of Transportation, 49 CFR Parts 171-180 and amendments

- U.S. Public Health Service, 42 CFR Part 72, Interstate Shipment of Etiologic Agents
- U.S. Department of Labor, Occupational Safety and Health Administration, 29 CFR Part 1910.1030, Bloodborne Pathogens
- International Air Transport Association (IATA), Dangerous Goods Regulations
- U.S. Postal Service, 39 CFR Part 111, Mailability of Etiologic Agents, Mailability of Sharps and Other Medical Devices, and Publication 52, Acceptance of Hazardous, Restricted or Perishable Matter
- International Civil Aviation Organization, Technical Instructions for the Safe Transport of Dangerous Goods by Air
- United Nations, Recommendations of the Committee of Experts on the Transportation of Dangerous Goods

All North American airlines and shipping vendors (e.g., FedEx), use the IATA regulation (also referred to as the Dangerous Goods Regulation or DGR) as their standard. Meeting the conditions of this standard will ensure the provisions of the other U.S. regulations are met.

Most clinics, hospitals, etc., are familiar with the regulations and procedures, but investigators and CRCs have responsibilities for these tasks and if not familiar with them, should read the regulations or get other training. References for this activity can be found by doing a search on Google using the terms "shipping biological samples." Many sponsors require evidence of training in this area when it is relevant to their trial.

Pre-study is a pivotal time for clinical trials to ensure things are set up to support human subjects protection and data integrity for a study. The investigator delegates much of the study start-up tasks to the CRC. At this stage of GCP, the CRC is depended upon to ensure that the regulatory and administrative tasks are done to support the decision to accept a study as a site, budget and contract support the site's requirements and best interests, and that the site is participating in study training before the enrollment of subject begins. This is the beginning of the important CRC and CRA relationship as they move into the second stage of the study, once enrollment commences.

Summary and Key Points

The CRC is usually involved in many of the pre-study activities. The quality of the study relies on the time spent planning and learning. Like sponsors, investigators and their study staff should meet and discuss the things that are risky for the clinical trial. In some cases, this might lead the investigator to reject participating in a study as a site. This can also improve the outcome of the SIV to be sure concerns and questions are discussed with the sponsor/CRO regarding the study to ensure plans and resourcing is put in place to ensure risks are managed to decrease the issues that occur during the study. A CRC should have a risk mindset right from the beginning of the trial.

CHAPTER NINE

Protocols

In this chapter, we will look at protocols, one of the main regulatory documents and tools of clinical trials. Although a study coordinator may never be involved in writing a protocol, one will be used for every study, so it is critical to understand what is in a protocol and what should be expected when a protocol is received from a sponsor.

Protocols

The protocol is the plan for a study and describes how the study will be conducted. If the protocol is well-written and the study design is sound, the study will be able to generate valid data that are acceptable to the scientific community, including the FDA. Even if study coordinators are not involved in writing protocols, it is important for them to have an understanding of protocol elements. The protocol is a basic clinical trial tool and is used in every study the CRC coordinates. Knowing the basics of a protocol makes the study coordinator more effective and the job easier.

A study coordinator should be able to read a protocol and determine whether or not it contains all the elements important to a trial, as well as the critical medical information. A study coordinator should also be able to determine if a protocol is logistically feasible based on what they know.

Contents of a Protocol

No two protocols are the same since the content includes study specifics and regional requirements. Most sponsors start with an SOP for protocols that includes a template. The template is then customized to the specific study and then to the specific regions where the trial will be run, as applicable. So, when a CRC works for the same sponsor in the same therapeutic area, there are some similarities between protocols.

Globally there have been some efforts to standardize a protocol template across the industry. One example was created in 2017—the FDA and NIH launched a protocol template for Phase II and III clinical trials funded by the NIH that are being conducted under an IND or IDE. Investigators for such trials are encouraged to use this template when developing protocols for NIH-funded clinical trials. This template may also be useful to others developing Phase II and III IND/IDE clinical trials.

Another, non-regulatory initiative to develop a globally acceptable common protocol template was initiated by TransCelerate BioPharma. One of the initiatives and workstreams is to develop and promote a Common Protocol Template (CPT). The group released the first version in 2015 and later updated that to coincide with the FDA and NIH efforts described above. The TransCelerate CPT is described by TransCelerate as *"a harmonized and streamlined approach to the format and content of clinical trial protocols. It aims to ease interpretation by the study sites and global regulatory authorities while enabling downstream automation of many clinical processes and aligning to industry data standards."* TransCelerate developed the CPT with input from many stakeholders, from sites to sponsors to regulators and IRBs. The TransCelerate CPT includes common structure, common text and regulator-accepted endpoint definitions that TransCelerate claims can be used *"across protocols with little to no editing at the discretion of the user."*

There are differences in a sponsor's therapeutic protocols depending on the development phase of the drug or the stage of development for a device. For drug and biologic studies, Phase I protocols are more flexible and less detailed than those for Phases II and III, because Phase I studies are early in the development program and less is known about how the investigational drug acts in humans. A Phase I protocol is primarily an outline of the study and should include:

- A description of the number of subjects to be studied
- A description of safety exclusions
- The dosing plan, including duration, dose or method being used to determine dose
- A detailed description of the safety procedures such as vital signs and laboratory evaluations.

Phase II and III protocols are very detailed and describe all aspects of the investigations. The FDA defines some minimal requirements for these protocols, which must contain at least:

- A description of the objectives and purpose
- The name, address and qualifications of each investigator
- The names of all sub-investigators working under the direction of the investigator
- The institution at which the research will be conducted
- The name and address of the IRB
- The inclusion and exclusion criteria for study subjects
- The number of subjects to be evaluated
- The design of the study, including the type of control group being used, if applicable
- The methods employed to minimize bias (usually randomization and blinding)
- The method used to determine dose(s) used, the maximum dose and the duration of administration
- A description of the observations and measurements being used
- A description of the measures (laboratory evaluations, procedures, etc.) being used to monitor the effects of the investigational drug and minimize risks to subjects.

These are minimum requirements; almost all protocols will contain additional elements, as well. The common elements of a protocol, in the order in which they usually appear, are discussed below.

Common Elements of a Protocol

1. **Title Page.** All protocols will have a title page. Essential information for the title page includes:

    - Title: The title should be specific enough to distinguish the protocol from those for similar studies. It should be a concise description of the study that provides the reader with the drug, disease, design and study phase.

      Example: A randomized, double-blind, Phase III trial of (drug under study) in subjects with generalized anxiety disorder. A placebo-controlled, fixed-dose, parallel-group multicenter study of 12 weeks.

- Protocol Number: This should be a unique number that identifies the protocol. Most sponsors have a specific procedure for determining this number that identifies the drug as well as the study.

  Example: 12AB345/0021, where 12AB345 is the drug identifier, and 0021 identifies the protocol within that drug development program.

- IND Number: The IND number of the drug, for studies conducted under an IND.

- Date: All protocols should be dated as part of their identifiers. This also allows various versions to be readily identified.

- Sponsor Medical Monitor: The name and contact information for the sponsor's medical monitor.

- Principal Investigator: The name and address of the investigator conducting the study.

- Some protocol cover pages include the statistician, CRA, sub-investigators, study coordinator and laboratory contact information, but these are optional.

2. **Protocol Summary.** The protocol summary should give a good overview of the study and is highly recommended. The sponsor may send the site the summary when it is interviewing potential investigators, even when the entire protocol is not yet complete. The summary will provide enough information for potential investigators to determine if they are interested in and have the capability to do the study. The summary is usually one to two pages long and typically includes:

   - Protocol Title: Repeated from the title page.

   - Study Objective: A statement of the main objectives and purpose of the study.

     Example: The primary objective is to show that (study drug) is more effective than placebo in the short-term (12 weeks) treatment of generalized anxiety disorder. The secondary objective is to gain information on the short-term safety of (study drug).

   - Study Population: A brief description of the type of subjects to be included.

     Example: Study subjects will be male or female, 18 years or older, with diagnosed generalized anxiety disorder and no clinically relevant co-morbid psychiatric conditions.

   - Study Design: A brief description of design, e.g., single-dose, multiple-dose, pilot, safety, efficacy, randomized or not, single- or double-blind, open-label, parallel, crossover, etc.

Example: The study is a randomized, double-blind, fixed-dose, placebo-controlled, Phase III, multicenter trial.

- Study Medication, including the:
  - Generic name and trade name (if known) of the compound. Example: alprazolam (Xanax®)
  - Dosage form. Example: 0.25 mg tablets
  - Route of administration. Example: Oral
  - Dose and regimen. Example: 0.25 mg three times a day.
- Duration of Treatment: The time period during which the study medication will be administered to the subjects. If the treatment is not continuous, it should be described.
  Example: Subjects will be treated for 10 weeks, followed by a two-week single-blind taper period.
- Methods and Materials: A general description of the procedures, tests, etc., required. Sometimes this is listed in an appendix as well, commonly referred to as a Table of Events. Study visit window requirements are usually found here, e.g., each weekly visit can occur 7 +/-2 days from the date of randomization.
- Duration of Subject Participation: Total duration of subject involvement in the study, including screen and any follow-up.
  Example: Subjects who complete the study will have 12 weeks of study involvement.
- Anticipated Maximum Number of Subjects: Total number of subjects in all treatment groups.
  Example: There will be 440 subjects in each treatment group, for a total of 880 subjects.
- Number of Centers: If known.

3. **Abstract.** An abstract is optional. An abstract should be limited to one or two paragraphs describing the objective, design, population, sample size and major study activities.
4. **Table of Contents.** A detailed table of contents should be included in all protocols.
5. **Introduction.** The introduction should identify the reason for conducting the study and place it in context with previous investigations and with the overall development plan. If the introduction is lengthy, subheadings should be used. Abbreviations and acronyms should be avoided when possible. If they are used, each abbreviation or acronym should be identified in full the first time it is used. Example: Hamilton

Rating Scale for Anxiety (HAM-A). The introduction usually contains:

- A brief discussion of the study medication, including the medical need and rationale for use
- A description of the design and major endpoints, including the rationale for use
- A description of how this protocol differs from other similar protocols for the same treatment
- An identification of the setting in which subjects will be studied (outpatient, hospital, etc.)
- The rationale for the dose and regimen, citing supporting data
- A description of the study control (e.g., placebo) and/or comparator drug, plus the rationale for use
- A general description of procedures and length of the study.

6. **Study Objectives.** These should clearly state the primary and secondary objectives and identify the endpoints that will be used to satisfy them. Primary endpoints usually are the key efficacy parameters to be studied. Secondary endpoints usually consist of efficacy variables that are of lower clinical significance and are also the safety parameters of the trial. State whether the study is intended to show a difference or similarity between treatments (this also could be included under study design).

7. **Study Design.** This section should include a description of the study design, including:

    - Type of study (methodology, pilot, tolerance, efficacy, pharmacokinetics)
    - Controlled or uncontrolled
    - Single- or multiple-dose (fixed or variable)
    - Single site or multi-center
    - Open-label or blinded
    - Randomization scheme
    - Design (parallel, crossover, matched pair, block, sequential).

8. **Randomization.** This section should describe the randomization and blinding procedure, including any stratification. It also should contain instructions for breaking the blind, if it becomes necessary.

9. **Subject Selection.** This section will include a description of the study population, that indicates the number of subjects to be enrolled. If

appropriate, it will differentiate between the maximum number of subjects to be enrolled and the minimum number of subjects required to meet protocol objectives. The subject selection criteria (inclusion and exclusion criteria) should include:

- A description of each requirement for subject eligibility. If there are any exceptions to a criterion, they should be stated.
- Specific disease-related criteria.
- Willingness to sign an informed consent form as an inclusion criterion.
- Allowed and disallowed concomitant medications.
- Criteria that will exclude subjects. Subjects who are taking another investigational medication or who have recently taken an investigational medication within a specified time period (i.e., 30 days) are almost always excluded.
  This section should also include a description of when the entry criteria must be met, e.g., before or following a screening period, after a washout period, etc.
  In some trials, subjects who meet basic study criteria are enrolled in a screening period. During this time, various tests are done (e.g., physical exam, laboratory tests) to determine if the subjects meet the additional criteria for entry into the entire trial. A washout period is a time when subjects are taken off their current (non-study) medications. When the carryover effect from these medications has had time to dissipate, subjects are entered into the main part of the trial.

10. **Subject Enrollment.** This section should identify the point at which a subject is considered enrolled. For randomized studies, this usually is at the time of randomization. Other possibilities might be after the informed consent form is signed or after successful completion of a screening period.

11. **Informed Consent.** The section about informed consent is sometimes located in the body of the protocol and sometimes in an appendix. The protocol section on informed consent should include:

    - A complete description of informed consent requirements, emphasizing the requirement for obtaining consent prior to a subject's involvement in any study-related activity
    - The investigator's responsibility to obtain IRB approval of the consent
    - Specific instructions if vulnerable populations, such as minors, will be included in the study.

12. **Screening Procedures.** This section should contain the following:
    - A description of all activities and tests related to the screening of subjects for study enrollment
    - The specific timing relative to tests, meals or the start of treatment
    - Results of any screening tests that will be used as baseline for within-group comparisons
    - A description of discontinuation of any concomitant medications, if required.
13. **Replacement of Subjects.** This section should specify whether subjects who drop out will be replaced and any conditions associated with replacement. If replacement is allowed, the protocol should specify how replacement subjects would be assigned to treatment groups.
14. **Treatment.** This section should provide the following information about the investigational medication and any comparator medication, including a placebo:
    - Generic, chemical and trade name (if known).
    - Formulation of the placebo.
    - Dosage forms and formulation, in general terms. If any medication contains excipients to which some subjects may be sensitive, such as lactose, this should be indicated.
    - Packaging (e.g., bottles, blister packs).
    - Special storage procedures and stability considerations. If the medication requires reconstitution, the stability in the reconstituted form should be specified.
    - Route of administration; include any special instructions for reconstituting medication or preparing individual doses. If it is administered intravenously (IV), specify the infusion rate.
    - The dosage regimen and time schedule for each dose. Clarify the duration of administration, including any medication-free periods or washout periods. As appropriate, specify the timing of dosing in relation to meals.
    - Rationale for the dose and regimen.
    - Procedures for dosage adjustments, if applicable.
    - Compliance parameters, e.g., the number of allowable missed doses, etc.

15. **Concomitant Medication**, as appropriate. This section should include the policy on the use of concomitant medications, including over-the-counter (OTC) medications, herbals and vitamin supplements. Indicate that all concomitant medication must be recorded. If concomitant medications are allowed, there should be information about how they may be used and why the use will not confound the treatment effect. Interaction data should be cited, as appropriate:

    - If the analyses will be stratified based on concomitant medication, this should be stated, with reference to the analysis plan.
    - If smoking, alcohol, caffeine or illicit drugs are prohibited or restricted, this should be mentioned in this section.

16. **Study Activities and Observations.** This section will give all the activities that are to be done at each study visit. It also should include an overall activity schedule that shows at a glance each event, procedure, observation and evaluation that will be done for each visit. Other considerations to keep in mind for this section are:

    - Each time period should be clearly defined.
    - All study activities, observations and evaluations to be made during each period should be listed and defined.
    - If any non-study medications are to be discontinued during a period (usually a screening period), the procedure should be described.
    - The acceptable leeway or "treatment window" for each visit should be specified.
    - If there is a tapered discontinuation of the investigational medication, the exact procedures, including the specific dose adjustments and time schedule to be followed, should be described.
    - Clinical assessments also need to be described in this section, including:
        - Specific criteria (as appropriate) for the various observations and assessments at each study period
        - The rationale for the selection of specific endpoints or assessment tools, unless discussed elsewhere
        - Any special conditions under which assessments are to be made, or specific equipment that should be used

- The rules or criteria for changing the management of the subject if there is either marked improvement or worsening of the subject's condition.

17. **Adverse Events.** There should be a very explicit section covering adverse events definitions, documentation and adverse event reporting.
18. **Data Recording Instructions.** This section should:
    - Indicate how data will be collected, if detailed instructions have been prepared, specify their location (e.g., study manual, appendix, etc.)
    - Discuss the use and management of source documents
    - Discuss the procedure for correcting errors.
19. **Data Quality Assurance.** This section should:
    - Describe procedures for assessing subject compliance
    - Describe any special training or other measures for site personnel to ensure valid data
    - Discuss source document review
    - Provide GCP references.
20. **Analysis Plan.** Items that may be included are:
    - Discussion of the general study design issues
    - A statement of the planned sample size, reasons for choosing it and power calculations
    - Classification of study variables (e.g., primary versus secondary)
    - Identification of statistical model(s) to be used
    - Description of specific analyses, including any subgroup analyses
    - Information about the timing and purpose of any planned interim analyses
    - Handling of missing or non-evaluatable data.
21. **Risks and Benefits.** This section should briefly summarize the risks and potential benefits associated with the use of the test compound or procedure. This section should be consistent with the consent form.
22. **References.** All references for the protocol should be in this section.
23. **Appendices.** Appendices may be used to detail information that might be confusing if placed in the body of the protocol.

For device studies, the stages commonly are divided in early stage pilot studies, pivotal studies and post-approval studies. Protocols are written based on the stage and become more complicated at the pivotal stage. Another significant influencer of protocol content for a device is whether the study is for a significant risk vs. non-significant risk device. The sections of a protocol are similar to the ones listed above for drug and biologic studies, but in areas of adverse event requirements are significantly different. Safety reporting requirements are specifically detailed in a different chapter.

Protocol Complexity

Over the past several years, protocols have become more complex and more demanding in their requirements. In looking at over more than 10,000 protocols covering all phases and all therapeutic areas, the Tufts University Center for the Study of Drug Development (CSDD) found that all measures of complexity have risen considerably. The median number of procedures per protocol has risen by almost half and the total number of eligibility criteria has risen by more than half. This places an increasing burden on study sites, and the study coordinator bears the brunt of this extra work.

More complex protocols also require larger and more complex CRFs, at a great expense to both the sponsor and the sites. Not only does it take more time to develop, review and approve more complex protocols, but the time from protocol readiness until the first subject is enrolled commonly increases, as does the time until the final subject visit takes place. Simplifying a protocol while still making it adequate to meet the study goals will pay dividends to the sponsor, the site and the study subjects.

Protocol Amendments

In 2016, CSDD conducted a study on protocol amendments. It looked at 3,413 protocols and found that 3,596 amendments had been made, encompassing 19,345 changes. This study found that 69% of all protocols have at least one amendment, and that almost half of the amendments (46%) occur before any study subjects even have been dosed. Not only that, they determined 37% of the amendments could be considered either "somewhat" or "completely" avoidable (see Figure 1).

In fact, the CSDD study found that it takes an average of 61 days and costs more than $450.000 to implement each amendment. So, let's break down this amendment cost—for just the amendments in this study (3,596 of them), that's about 601 years of implementation time and a cost of more than $1.618 billion. And these are only from the protocols included in the study, which came from just 24 companies.

Constant protocol amendments are difficult for sites to manage. They are often confusing, especially when it comes to determining the changes and

Figure 1: Prevalence and avoidability of amendments

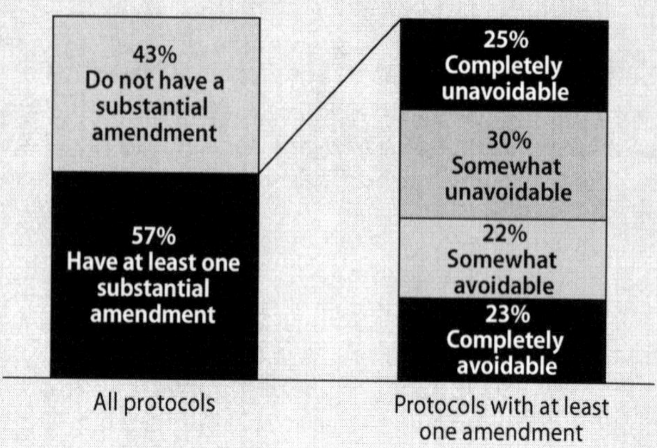

Source: Tufts CSDD, 2016

when they are to be implemented, which can make compliance with study procedures difficult. Amendments also cause sites a great deal of extra time, especially if subjects need to be re-consented. Unfortunately, study coordinators undoubtedly will still have to contend with multiple protocol amendments in the future, but if the site is asked up front to provide input on a protocol, think carefully about what can be done to eliminate changes later. CRCs must be sure that they are following the latest approved protocol and not implement any protocol changes unless approved by the IRB first. The only exception is if the investigator must deviate the protocol to save a life of a study subject. Luckily this is rare and is not included in a standard amendment procedure.

During the Study

Just before the site begins enrolling subjects in the trial, a good practice is to reread the protocol carefully. The investigator and the study coordinator, and any other involved site personnel, must be very familiar with the protocol and all of its ramifications. Remember, it is the study plan and must be followed exactly. Also remember that the initial protocol training might have happened a long time before the start of enrollment. Sites are likely conducting many protocols all at once, so implementing tools to help support compliance is common. Some sites create worksheet tools to help comply with the protocol. The study staff must also be clear on what is required.

Reading the protocol again after enrolling the first subject is a good practice. If there was anything in the protocol that didn't work or caused a problem, discuss it with the sponsor before enrolling subsequent subjects. Occasionally things that seem straightforward when reading the protocol aren't quite as

Figure 2: Top areas addressed by amendments

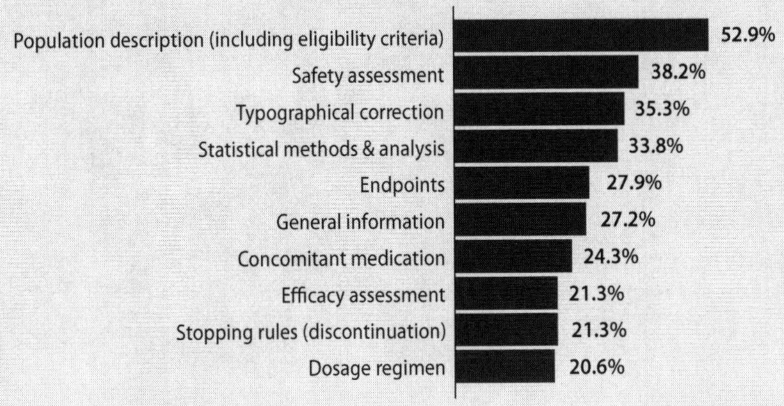

Source: Tufts CSDD, 2016

simple when executing it.

If the protocol is amended during the study, there are a number of things to think about and do:

- The amendment will need to be submitted to the IRB, and usually will need approval before the changes can be implemented.
- Do these protocol changes require changes to the informed consent form? If so, that also must be approved by the IRB. If it is necessary to re-consent subjects still in the trial, check to see if it may be done at their next regular study visit. Sometimes the IRB approval will include instructions indicating who needs to be consented (active and/or new subjects).
- Do these protocol changes necessitate any changes in the CRFs? If so, the sponsor will need to update the CRFs and make the changes as instructed. This might also require some changes to the site's source documents.
- Be sure that all relevant people are trained regarding the changes.
- Check the implementation date(s) and start using the new materials at that time. Also, check to see if the subjects need to be contacted or trained.
- Be sure to add the appropriate documentation to the study files.

Remember that the protocol is a guide/instruction book for conducting the study. Be very familiar with it and use it throughout the trial.

Summary and Key Points

The protocol is a pivotal document for CRCs to use for planning and performing GCP tasks that are subject and non-subject related. Proactively look for things in the protocol that are unclear or can be interpreted differently that might impact the compliance of the subject and audit readiness. How can the CRC help prevent protocol deviations? Some CRCs use tools to support compliance with the protocol procedures since a CRC is commonly working on multiple studies and protocols. Be sure any tools meet the ALCOAC standard.

Case Study: Protocols

A CRC recently told me about a protocol she had received to review for a potential study. It was a comparatively easy study, as it was just an "add-on" to a standard procedure. Subjects who qualified had their regularly scheduled procedure and then were to wear a Holter monitor at home for a few days. At the end of the Holter monitoring period, they detached the monitor and sent it back to the sponsor, where their data were downloaded.

The study actually required very little effort on the part of the site. Once the subjects were identified, they were given some Holter monitor training, it was attached and they were sent home.

When the CRC read the protocol, she had some concerns. Her primary concerns were that there was no mention of safety or adverse event collection in the protocol, nor were there any follow-up visits with the subjects after they left the hospital.

What should she do?

The CRC was right to have these concerns. Safety assessments and final evaluations are standard elements in protocols and omitting them seems to be a safety issue.

The first thing she probably should do is discuss the protocol and her concerns with the clinical investigator at the site who would be responsible for the study. Then the investigator can contact the sponsor with their concerns. It would be reasonable to expect the subject to come back in for a final visit, at which time the Holter monitor could be collected and there could be a discussion of any adverse events or other subject concerns. At a minimum, there should be a follow-up phone call to the subjects asking them how things had gone with the Holter, if they experienced any adverse events and so forth.

As a side note, even if the investigator had decided to do the study as written, it is doubtful an IRB would approve it in its original state.

CHAPTER TEN

Case Report Forms and Electronic Data Capture

Whether using paper forms or electronic forms, recording the data collected during a clinical study is one of the major tasks of the study coordinator. With advances to technology, it is likely that those CRFs a CRC works with will be electronic (eCRF). Technology has influenced an increase in other forms of electronic data capture (EDC) that link to data collection, such as randomization and investigational product assignment platforms, such as interactive voice or electronic registration systems (IVRS/EVRS), and electronic patient-reported outcomes (ePRO) for study patient diaries, and eConsent. A study coordinator is likely to have multiple electronic systems to work with and some not merged with another. The ability to coordinate the multiple computerized systems used for a clinical trial is one important skill set that is needed more and more by CRCs.

CRFs

CRFs are used during a clinical trial to record the protocol-required data for each study subject. CRFs standardize the collection of study data and help to ensure that the medical, statistical, regulatory and data management needs of the study are met. It is the "deliverable" data of the study and forms the basis for all analysis of the drug/device. Working with CRFs is a significant part of the workload of many CRCs and is a major factor in the performance of a clinical trial. Some research sites divide the responsibilities of the coordinator into two or three types, 1) patient, 2) regulatory and/or 3) data coordinating. Some CRCs might work more with CRFs than others depending on the study operations structure.

Paper CRFs are being used less and less for studies but are unlikely to be phased out completely. Some small studies sponsored by startups in early phases and/or some investigator-initiated studies are among types of studies that are likely to continue to use paper due to cost and operation complexity. This chapter discusses the collection of data on paper CRFs first, and then electronic data entry. In both situations, it is critical to properly record the data from the trial. Remember that decisions regarding the investigational product are based on the observations from study sites, so it is essential that the data recorded are valid and accurate. Additionally, many of the topics discussed for paper CRFs also hold true for electronic forms.

CRF Completion

After or during a study subject visit, the required data need to be recorded for the sponsor.

When completing the CRFs for a subject, the CRC must keep a number of things in mind. The study coordinator must be sure that the data entered on the forms are accurate, complete and legible. The data must be derived from original source data that is linkable to the subject and the author, thus meeting ALCOAC, as covered in Chapter 2.

The CRC should ensure that each item has been completed and each blank filled in. Check that the answers are within range, the form is signed, if appropriate, and by the correct person, and the header is complete and correct. (The header is the top part of each paper form that lists the subject and study identifiers.)

Next, check all the pages for a single visit. Also, check for completeness, correct dates and that the visit was within the allowed window. Check to be sure that the timing of procedures was appropriate. If, for example, there was to be a blood draw followed by another activity, then the blood draw should have been done first, and the times should reflect this. Any time there is a specific order to be followed for activities, that order must be followed. If the source data reveals that the protocol was not followed, the data should be entered into the CRF as-is in the source, and the CRC should complete a protocol deviation report or documentation as required by the study sponsor. It is critical that any deviations are documented within the subject's source document with any actions performed in relation to the issuc. For example, if it was discovered that a test was not performed at a visit and the subject was called and asked to come in for an unscheduled study visit, this should be documented. The interventions needed due to the deviation might also require additional CRF forms to be completed (e.g., the unscheduled visit CRF page). The CRC will find they are working between the source documents and CRF quite a bit.

The CRC should ensure that there is consistency across forms. If the subject is getting better according to various ratings, then the overall rating should reflect an improvement. If a form says there was a concomitant medication administered for an adverse event, then the medication should

FAQ

One sponsor insists that we have a source document for every entry on the case report form. Is this in the regulations?

No. However, the sponsor may not agree to let you conduct the study if you cannot meet its internal requirement.

be listed on the concomitant medication form and the adverse event entered on the adverse event CRF. In addition, the CRC should think about what appears on the forms, and whether it makes sense given the subject's condition and the study activities. Sometimes it's easy to see individual data but miss the view of the overall data trend.

The CRC should also check the current visit against previous visits. Are the data consistent from visit to visit? Was the timing of procedures appropriate? Do the data match where necessary? Are the visit windows for all of the visits specified by the protocol? Visit windows should be clearly defined in the protocol, but this is not always the case. The CRC should ask for clarification if they are not clear. Within a protocol, there is commonly a Table of Events where the study windows are commonly found.

Lastly, the CRC should be sure to have correctly identified the same subject at each visit, with the same initials, numbers and/or other study identifiers. It is always better to straighten out any problems the CRC may find when completing the CRFs before the study monitor comes to review them. Remember that CRAs are on the same team with the same objective—clean, accurate data.

Subject Source Document Review

Source document review (SDR) is when the sponsor monitor reviews the quality of data. This includes the compliance with the protocol and ALCOAC and the accuracy and completeness of the data recorded. Sometimes a part of SDR is source data verification (looking for transcription errors or finding that what is in the source does not meet the CRF). Source data verification (SDV) by itself would not support quality data. For certain critical data points, a high accuracy rate is necessary in the data entered in the CRF (e.g., information about endpoint data procedures and AEs), but the quality of the source that the data came from is critical. So, the focus of monitoring is SDR with some SDV. Study coordinators also perform SDR when completing the CRF and working with the monitor.

A source document is any document on which the data are first recorded. Remember that the investigator is required to maintain adequate and accurate case histories (21 CFR 312.62 and CFR 812.140). All observations pertinent to the study should be documented; however, not all of them will be requested in the CRF. The source will have more information than the CRF. The source allows reviewers to be sure the study subject was alive and

FAQ

We have a new CRA, and she wants us to enter some of the information in the CRFs differently than the way the previous CRA told us to do it—plus, she wants us to go back and change all the previous entries so they match her instructions. For example, she wants all weights recorded in kilograms, not pounds. Do we have to do this?

It's an enormous amount of work. This can be a real problem. Your best bet is to contact the sponsor's medical monitor, explain the problem and ask for advice. Chances are that the difference can be resolved internally, not at the site. If you do need to go back and change all previous entries, you might ask for some additional financial compensation to pay for this "unbudgeted" time.

available during the time on the study. To accomplish all the documentation and to remember what is required by one study versus another, some sites use source document worksheets. These worksheets should not be a copy of the CRF because that encourages under-documentation. The source worksheets are a job aid to help the user remember what is next on a study visit. Pre-printed statements on the worksheets should be avoided since they are not contemporaneous. Take, for example, a pre-printed section that says, "the study subject was consented prior to any study procedures, and all questions were answered and the subject was provided a copy of their consent." Just because it is written does not mean that it happened. Describing who was at the consenting, how long it took, what questions there were, etc., is more supportive of the reconstruction of what actually occurred.

Some sponsors provide study source worksheets, but this is not a common practice as much as in past decades. The reason the sponsors stopped providing the worksheets is primarily due to the liability—if there are errors in the forms this can be risky for the sponsor to be contributing to noncompliance. Ultimately the investigator is responsible for the accuracy of any study-specific tool. Additionally, initially study coordinators created the worksheets to help conduct a visit but also to learn the protocol when creating them. If worksheets are used, they should not be designed to discourage documentation of what occurred at the visit and also should not solicit or pre-document a source that is documented somewhere else, like a medical chart. Duplication of documentation is risky and commonly leads to incompleteness or inaccuracies in one of the sources. The CRC should follow good documentation practices and ensure that all study documentation supports ALCOAC. An investigator is ultimately responsible for the quality of the case histories. They delegate a good deal of managing source to the CRC.

It takes a lot of time and effort to construct source document worksheets and a great deal of attention to detail and understanding the protocol. It is very easy to miss things that should be on the form or to misinterpret what is actually called for by the protocol. There are some things the CRC can do to help ensure the accuracy of these forms when used. First, have another coordinator, or the investigator, carefully review the forms to see if they are clear and complete. This is a good practice for any critical source documentation. Second, ask the study CRA to review the forms, before they are used. The CRC should also check the forms against the study activity chart in the protocol to ensure that all activities are captured. As an aside, if the sponsor is asking the site to prepare the source documents for the study, the site should be sure to include this activity in the study budget.

Purpose of Source Documentation

The purpose of source documentation is threefold: 1) to confirm that the subjects exist, 2) to be sure that what has been accomplished is documented and 3) when applicable, to verify that data in the CRF are consistent with the information found in the source documents, which validates the integrity of the data.

For example, one would expect to see basic demographic information in a medical practice chart for a patient, including name, address, phone number, insurance information and a social security number. When monitoring, the CRA is not interested in the particulars of this information, but only that it exists, and that the patient appears to be unique. The usual medical record will also contain lab reports or reports of other tests. The name and identifying information should match the other information in the chart. This information is indicative that the person entered in the trial actually exists.

When the data in the CRFs are in agreement with data contained in source documents, it is an indicator of the quality and veracity of the information being gathered for the study. It is not necessary for every entry in a CRF to have a matching entry in a source document, but where the data do appear in both, they should agree. Not every data point in the CRF will be checked by the CRA; it depends on the sponsor monitoring plan requirements. Sponsors are less inclined to require monitors to verify every data point, but rather SDR, looking for the quality of the data and compliance to the protocol. SDV does not look at compliance.

Under 21 CFR 312.62(b), *"An investigator is required to prepare and maintain adequate and accurate case histories that record all observations and other data pertinent to the investigation... Case histories include the case report forms and supporting data including, for example, signed and dated consent forms, progress notes of the physician..., hospital chart(s) and nurse's notes."*

ICH E6 says only that the study monitor shall verify that *"the data required by the protocol are reported accurately on the CRFs and are consistent with the source data/documents."*

As mentioned previously, upon occasion, the original collection of data may be done directly on the CRFs; in effect, the CRFs become source documents. This is frequently seen in rating scales, because it is easier to collect the information directly on the CRF as opposed to transcribing it later. The protocol must support what data can be entered directly. With EDC this is happening much more, for example ePRO diaries.

If a discrepancy is found between the CRF and the source document during monitoring, the CRA will query the investigator or study coordinator to determine what is correct. This also enables the study coordinator to make the appropriate corrections. Usually the source document takes precedence. If the source document is corrected, the original must not be obliterated, and the audit trail must be maintained. Additionally, the author of the source must update his or her own documentation noting the date of the correction and why. If the author is no longer working at the site, someone in that same role may update the source following proper error correction, never impersonating the original author. The CRC should not change an investigator's source document note. Any change must be signed and dated in real time with an explanation as to why there is an update. Remember the source is the original and that must be upheld.

Sponsor CRAs should not make changes on either the source documents or the CRFs; this is the responsibility of the investigator or appropriate delegate. As noted, there are significant differences among sponsors with respect to the amount of SDV a CRA must do, and there are no guidelines in the regulations. This must be included in a monitoring plan with the rationale for the monitoring approach. The rationale is based on many factors that revolve around the risks of the study and the sites. Some companies still require "100% source document review," but the definition of 100% source document review may require a percentage of the patients' charts to be reviewed and/or a focus on the endpoint data monitored only for each subject. Whatever the scheme, subjects' CRFs are normally reviewed for critical information, such as inclusion and exclusion criteria, a signed informed consent form, adverse events and critical study-specific parameters.

Errors, Queries and Corrections

Some of the most critical errors made during a clinical trial are those that result in protocol deviations. These include such things as a subject not meeting the inclusion criteria or meeting exclusion criteria. Other examples include a wrong diagnosis or a subject taking disallowed medications. When a CRC is completing the CRF, discrepancies and or deviations are frequently identified. These should be addressed because so much of what could be identified by the CRA with SDR and SDV has been identified and even addressed. Waiting for and depending on the CRA to identify errors is risky. More and more, sponsors are also doing monitoring through data analytics.

For paper CRFs, when potential errors are found during a monitoring visit, the CRA should note them in the corrections/questions log and discuss them with the CRC. Some monitors use sticky notes as well, but it is not a good practice for sticky notes to be used because they may be left on documents between visits. Once the discrepancies are resolved, the CRC should make the necessary corrections to the CRFs; CRAs do not make the corrections. Corrections are made by drawing a line through the incorrect entry, making the correct entry and dating and initialing it. If the reason for the change is not clear, a reason should also be added to the form. It is never acceptable to use correction fluid or erase an incorrect entry before correcting it; anyone reviewing the forms must be able to see what was changed, when and why. Write-overs are also unacceptable. See the example below for a correctly made change.

Date 01/16/~~08~~ 09 JAK 2/5/09

Be sure that the changes made are legible. Sometimes there isn't much space to record the change, initials and date, but if it's not legible it will generate a query. If the space is crowded near the query, the CRC can circle the correct answer.

Paper CRFs are commonly three-part carbon paper; all copies must be legible. It is in the CRC's best interest to correct errors at the site before sending the CRFs to the sponsor. However, despite everyone's best efforts, additional errors often are found when the CRFs are sent to data entry at the sponsor. The data must be manually entered in the sponsor database by their data management team. Data management can generate computer-generated error reports that can be sent back to the site and/or to the CRA. These are usually called queries. Queries are questions about the data. These can be about the logic or the compliance to the protocol. Different sponsors have different query methods, but usually there is a query form sent to the site; it lists the errors and where they are located on the CRF, and asks for a correction or explanation to be made and sent in. Sometimes the CRA is involved in the correction process; sometimes it is solely between the site and data management. The sponsor personnel never answer queries. The site should be responsible for that task. When paper CRFs are involved, the investigator may have to sign off on queries. The answered queries are sent back to the sponsor and a copy is maintained at the site with the applicable CRF, so the latest data is present at both the site and the sponsor.

Whether errors are found by the CRA or come in the form of queries, the CRC should think of them as training tools. If it is not clear, the CRC should ask the CRA to explain why each one is an error and how it can be avoided in the future. It is important to have the CRA review and submit the forms for the first few subjects as early as possible, in order to give timely feedback so that similar errors can be eliminated in the future. This is especially important in the case of repeated errors, which usually are due to misunderstanding. Error rates should decrease as the study progresses, due to feedback and training by the CRA and data management, as well as experience on the part of the CRC and other site personnel. Errors are very costly, both in terms of money and people hours to correct. Although most of the cost is borne by the sponsor, about one-third of the cost of correcting errors is borne by the site.

Electronic Data Capture

Although it has taken many years to become accepted, EDC is now being used for most studies.

The advantages of EDC applications over paper-based clinical trials are numerous. First, as data are entered (for example, into a CRF or medical record), automated programmed data edit checks alert the site to possible errors in data entry. The site can check while the source document is readily available, rather than months later in a typical paper-based process. This immediate feedback not only can help the site correct the initial issue, but also can help educate the site to avoid similar errors in the future. Since there is no delay as is typical in the paper process, costly errors can be avoided much earlier in the process.

Some EDC is web-based, and the site can sign on to a secure website. For some studies, the EDC is programed on a sponsor's laptop and a computer is supplied to the site. When sponsors provide a laptop to a site, a workstation and storage space must also be provided.

Sites should also provide the resources necessary so that data entry can be done. EDC entry timelines per subject is commonly included in the clinical trial agreement (CTA) and is something like three days after the subject's visit. The CRC is commonly the delegate and needs to have time to enter CRF data. Occasionally a site, especially larger sites, may have a data-entry coordinator for this task, but if this person is not medically trained and is not familiar with the study, this can be problematic. Sometimes the sheer number of trials at one site, with different EDC systems for each, makes it difficult to keep everything straight and organized.

Subject confidentiality also can be an issue. Good EDC systems will have strict security measures in place that limit access and use of the system, as well as secure ways to transfer data between the site and the sponsor. EDC represents a huge paradigm shift, with changing roles and redefinitions of jobs and responsibilities. CRAs, data managers and study coordinators at the site all share responsibility for data quality when EDC is used. As these roles evolve, there probably will be further blending of the critical responsibilities of these positions. For example, at sponsors, the role of data analyst is becoming more common. This is usually not the monitor. Identifying trends and data outliers is more commonly becoming the trigger for site monitoring visits instead of routinely scheduled periodic site visits. An example of a common outlier is a site study subject with no AEs or a site where the blood pressure of each subject does not deviate over several visits.

At its best, EDC can significantly affect the time necessary to finish a project, which can have a favorable impact on the time needed to bring a new product to the market. EDC can also decrease the time and money spent on CRA travel to sites. CRCs need to remain vigilant to changes in the industry and be prepared to adapt as new technologies come along. There is no question that sites and CRCs will see and be involved more with EDC in the future. EDC is here to stay.

Query resolution in EDC is done either automatically or as the CRC is entering data. These are pre-programmed edit checks. So, the CRC would receive a query as they enter data. They answer the queries as they go along and learn as they go. Additionally, monitors, data managers and other sponsor personnel can create queries to sites for a specific subject from on-site and remote review. If source documents are available remotely and they are needed to SDV and/or SDR, monitoring can happen remotely if the sponsor procedures to support confidentiality are followed. Currently the data source documents are primarily not available remotely, so onsite monitoring of critical data with SDV is still on-site. But the industry is moving toward finding solutions to support remote review. This will likely be the next change on the horizon; one example is eIC support remote review. The FDA released a guidance document in 2015 on eIC.

Internal Data Quality Control vs. Quality Assurance

Sites that are dedicated to conducting clinical studies often have their own quality systems that include procedures to support quality clinical trials that with quality control (QC) checks and/or QA audit plans. In both cases there is likely to be some SDV and SDR depending on the situation and resources available.

One example is when the site has a procedure that requires a QC check after each subject consents. Another CRC completes SDR by looking at a consent for a subject still at site that was obtained by a co-worker to be sure it has been completed appropriately and to catch common errors at the time of consent before the subject leaves the site.

One example of QA at the site level is at the time of accepting a study, the site identifies if the study is high-risk for regulatory audit. If so, an internal audit plan could be created. Audits must be performed by independent function, so they are not the same as the QC of the informed consent as described above. The audit function must be separate from the clinical research study group within the site. The identification of a high-risk study might be triggered by enrollment, the risk of the study product and/or the vulnerability of the patients to be enrolled. It is more common for sites to have some QC and less likely to have QA programs. QC is integrated within the day-to-day operations, but QA is a larger integration and financial commitment. Regulations do not require formally either for investigation sites, but the investigator must have systems in place to support their oversight. We are seeing more sites have formal research processes than ever before.

Summary and Key Points

The CRC commonly is managing multiple studies. Ensuring clarity on protocol requirements is key to supporting data integrity and to prevent issues. A CRC can use tools but should ensure that they support ALCOAC and have a clear understanding of the protocol(s). CRCs rely on other team members commonly for QC checks related to compliance and documentation. Timely completion of CRFs is essential for sponsor oversight and the site should be compliant with the timeline in the CTA. If there are barriers to meet the timelines, the CRC should work with the investigator, sponsor and internal team to address the root cause of the issue.

Key Points:

- Quality source documentation meeting the ALCOAC standard must support the data in the CRF.
- Technology continues to advance and support data collection and management.
- Source document worksheets are still used by many sites to support protocol compliance, but less supplied by sponsors/CROs.
- Timely data entry and QC is essential.

Case Study: The Cost of Errors

"Everybody talks about the cost of errors, and how expensive it is to correct them," said Susan, a CRC. "I don't see what the big deal is—all you have to do it draw a line through, put the right thing in, then initial and date it. That doesn't take more than a few seconds."

Does she have a point? Maybe it isn't such a big deal after all.

Unfortunately, Susan is wrong, but it's not quite as straightforward as that. After all, there are different kinds of errors to think about. Let's look at the simplest case first—a simple error discovered by the CRC before the study monitor visit. A very typical one is putting the wrong year in a date when the new year arrives.

Date 01/16/~~10~~ 11 SSC 2/5/11

She's right about this one. She found it herself before the monitor came and it didn't take very long to correct.

Now let's look at another error, one missed by Susan and also not noticed by the CRA during a monitoring visit. A subject was given a new concomitant medication, an anti-hypertensive, a type of medication not taken by the subject before. When the data were entered into the computer at the sponsor, the program noted the new med didn't have an adverse event (AE) to go along with it. The program recognized that if the subject was given an anti-hypertensive, there must have been an increase in blood pressure (the adverse event) associated with it.

This caused the computer to kick out a query, which was then reviewed by the data manager and sent to the CRA, who sent it on to the site. The CRC had to pull the CFR and the chart for the subject, look at the blood pressures, check to see if an AE of hypertension was recorded and maybe even had to contact the subject for more information. She had to change the case report form, check other forms for consistency and complete the query form. She had to discuss it with the CRA at the next monitoring visit and point out all the changes that were made. The CRA had to review the changes, send in the corrected forms, ensure the query form was correct and complete and that appropriate documentation of the changes was filed correctly at the site. The query form was sent in and reviewed by the data manager, and the data was updated appropriately in the computer.

How long did all of this take? Remember that it involved the CRA, the data manager, the CRC and possibly even the investigator, who must review and sign off on adverse events. Also, there is an actual cost associate with the time, based on the salaries of the employees involved.

A study was conducted at a large pharmaceutical company to look at the cost of errors. It used 45 minutes as the average time for correction of an error, at a cost of $50 each. Looking at all of its major programs over a year, the error rate was less than 1%, about the industry average. And it was a large company, so it conducted a lot of studies in a year's time. What do think this error rate cost?

It took 6.5 years to correct these errors, at a cost of over $11 million. It also determined that about one-third of this cost was borne by its study sites. Pretty costly to correct errors, isn't it?

CHAPTER ELEVEN

Investigational Product Accountability

The investigational product is the drug, device or biologic being studied in the clinical trial. Sometimes, the IP is already marketed but may be studied for a new indication or other reasons. Even if the IP is an approved product, if it is being studied in a clinical trial it is considered an investigational product and needs to be handled and accounted for correctly.

Responsibilities

The regulations describe what the sponsor and the investigator are responsible for doing, but not how it must be done. It is important for both sponsors and investigators to have systems in place to adequately meet the regulatory requirements. Guidance documents such as ICH E6 list certain activities for IP control and management. ICH E6 has a drug focus. We mentioned earlier in the book that in 2011, a global standard for device GCP was released, ISO 14155. It is not a regulatory guidance but a quality standard document available from the International Organization for Standardization (ISO). The FDA does not mandate use of the standard but has said the standard has value. If a sponsor adopts this standard into its quality system, then it becomes required and sites that are working on their trials will need training for ISO 14155 related to their role. ISO 14155:2011 is required to be used for device clinical trials in the European Union (EU).

Drugs and Biologics

Drugs and biological products are governed under the same FDA regulations. For these products, under 21 CFR 312.57, 312.58 and 321.59, the sponsor must:

- Maintain adequate records showing the receipt, shipment or other disposition of the investigational drug, including:
    - The name of the investigator to whom the drug is shipped
    - The date, quantity and batch or code mark of each shipment.
- Follow the special rules for controlled substances, which include that the drug is kept in a securely locked, substantially constructed enclosure at the investigative site.
- Ensure the return of all unused supplies from each investigator.
- Maintain written records of the drug disposition.
- Discontinue shipments to investigators who fail to maintain records or make them available.

It is also the sponsor's responsibility to retain drug samples and reference standards.

Regulations 21 CFR 312.61 and 312.62 give the responsibilities of investigators with respect to drug accountability. The investigator must:

- Administer the drug only to subjects under his personal supervision or under the supervision of a sub-investigator responsible to the investigator
- Not supply the investigational drug to any person not authorized to receive it
- Maintain adequate records of the disposition of the drug, including dates, quantity and use by subjects
- Return unused supplies of the drug to the sponsor.

The sponsor may authorize alternative disposition of the unused drug by the investigator, as long as it does not expose anyone to risks from the drug (21 CFR 312.59). However, it is much more common for the sponsor to require the site to return the unused drug. Disposing of these supplies usually is not a simple task, and many sites are not equipped to do this properly.

Most sponsors cover investigational drug management quite specifically in their SOPs and for the study specifically in the protocol. Drug disposition records should be part of the site study file and should be retained according the record retention requirements of the sponsor. Developing user-friendly forms is a real asset to completing this requirement; there are samples of both a drug dispensing form and a return of drug form in Appendix D.

Devices

Under device regulations, a sponsor shall ship investigational devices only to qualified investigators participating in the investigation (21 CFR 812.43(b)).

The investigator will permit the investigational device to be used only with subjects under his personal supervision and will not supply the device to anyone not authorized to receive it (21 CFR 812.110(c)). It is essential that the delegation log supports the investigator's oversight of anyone using the device in relation to study subjects. The investigator commits to this in the investigator agreement (similar to the drug 1572 form). The device division under the FDA does not have a standard form, but the sponsor uses a standard template supported by their policies to ensure that the investigator signs an agreement to follow the regulations. In device trials, any sub-investigator also using the device with a subject without the principal investigator present must also sign and commit to an Investigator Agreement. It is not uncommon in implantable device trials to have more than one investigator agreement.

ISO 14155: 2011 Clinical Investigation of Medical Devices for Human Subjects — Good Clinical Practice

The international standard ISO 14155 was first released in the late 1990s and updated in 2011. *ISO 14155 section 6.9 Investigational Device Accountability* supports the following investigational device management requirements for GCP:

- *Access to investigational devices shall be controlled and the investigational devices shall be used only in the clinical investigation and according to the Clinical Investigation Plan (CIP, another name for protocol).*
- *The sponsor shall keep records to document the physical location of all investigational devices from shipment of investigational devices to the investigation sites until return or disposal.*
- *The principal investigator or an authorized designee shall keep records documenting the receipt, use, return and disposal of the investigational devices, which shall include:*
    - *a) the date of receipt,*
    - *b) identification of each investigational device (batch number/serial number or unique code),*
    - *c) the expiry date, if applicable,*
    - *d) the date or dates of use,*
    - *e) subject identification,*
    - *f) date on which the investigational device was returned/explanted from subject, if applicable, and*
    - *g) the date of return of unused, expired or malfunctioning investigational devices, if applicable.*

During a Clinical Trial

The investigational product must be available at the site before subjects can be enrolled. For some studies this means that a supply of the product is shipped to the site. For a medical device, it is common to do "just in time" delivery to the site right before use. Usually, the site is alerted to how the product will be shipped before the investigational product is released, so that the correct storage is ready upon arrival and the product is not left unattended, e.g., refrigerated product left on a loading dock in hot weather.

Investigational product is shipped with a shipping invoice that must be reconciled with the actual product when received. The shipping invoice should be checked against the contents of the boxes for accuracy, dated and signed by the receiver, and filed in the study documents. The content should be assessed for any damage or obvious quality issues. Any issues should be escalated to the sponsor as soon as possible. The investigator or delegate should document the process and maintain this in the essential documentation for IP receipt. For some sites and studies, it may be a pharmacist that receives the shipment.

The CRC is usually responsible for managing the investigational product accountability at the site. One exception is with medical devices. With just-in-time delivery, the sponsor's device engineer may be the one bringing the device to the site for the procedure. Unlike drug studies, medical device studies are set up where the sponsor is allowed to place a device engineer at the site during device implantation to support the investigator and set-up of the device. The placement of sponsor personnel at the site, as described under device trials, is not allowed in drug trials. For device studies the medical device engineer should be listed in the site's study delegation log. The investigator must oversee that the sponsor representative is performing well. The sponsor representative commonly maintains some of the documentation of the investigational device accountability. The investigator needs to be sure that the sponsor engineer documentation gets to the study file.

For both drug and device, careful accounting must be done as the IP is either distributed to study subjects or placed in contact with the subject, like for a medical device. This is normally recorded in the source documents and/or logs, then in the CRFs at each appropriate time frame, an example of which is subject site visit or surgery, as noted in the above table.

For drug and device, there is also commonly an overall drug distribution form to record the dispensing and usage for all study subjects throughout the study (sample forms are in Appendix D). A simplistic way to look at drug accountability is what is received is recorded, what is dispensed to and returned by study subjects and the amount returned to the sponsor or destroyed at site, when applicable. But somehow, drug accountability does not always go smoothly.

Drug reconciliation should be done throughout the study, rather than left to the end. As soon as a discrepancy is identified, actions should be taken to reconcile the discrepancy. When the subject is still at the site is ideal, so

Number of pills returned at this visit: ______

Did the subject miss any doses: Yes No

If so, how many doses were missed: ______

Number of pills dispensed: ______

the issues can be resolved before the subject leaves the site. The longer a discrepancy is unresolved, the more difficult it is to close it. Sometimes sponsor monitors may not be at the site for some time and/or do not conduct an IP accountability often, so a site should not rely on the monitor for IP compliance. For medical devices, there may be a device that is a single device used for a subject but might have many parts that are interchangeable or sized, or just for the procedure. Conducting inventory to be certain all the supplies and components are accounted for is critical.

Sometimes, unused investigational product and/or supplies are returned to the sponsor periodically throughout the study, and it is certainly returned at the end of the study. Drug return is usually done by the CRA, according to company policy, but can be done by the research site if supported by sponsor and protocol. A copy of each IP return inventory form should be kept in the site's study file. Commonly, at the end of the study a copy of the accountability records are copied for the sponsor's TMF.

Keeping good, accurate drug accountability records, including shipping, disposition and returns, is important for ensuring overall compliance and the validity of the study. The study coordinator commonly plays a major role in investigational product accountability and documentation.

Summary and Key Points

CRCs support IP control and commonly are involved with receipt, storage, dispensing, accountability and return and subject teaching, as applicable for the clinical trial and appropriate investigator delegation. Detailed and timely documentation is critical to ensure audit readiness and subject safety.

Key Points:

- Good documentation and compliance with the ALCOAC principles are necessary.
- Teaching of the subject is essential.
- Studies vary greatly on accountability requirements and documentation.

Case Study: Investigational Product Accountability

I was recently reviewing a device study for a research group. As part of this review, I wanted to check the device accountability logs. This device had three component parts, which were manufactured by different suppliers, so they were not necessarily shipped to the site at the same time. Each study subject usually had only one of each of the three parts assigned; however, there were occasionally some malfunctions, which necessitated extra parts being used.

The accountability records were not well-organized. Some records were in with subject case report forms, some were found throughout the regulatory binder and others were scattered throughout the correspondence binder and the study documents binder. Shipping invoices, distribution sheets, hospital use records and return lists were found here and there. Device serial numbers also were recorded in the case report forms. There were multiple recordings of the same data. Items were not recorded in chronological order or serial number order.

Components actually used for subjects were implanted, and thus not returned unless they malfunctioned and had to be removed.

Most items had both a part number and a serial number, and there was no consistency about which had been used on the distribution sheets. Unfortunately, the part number was not a unique identifier; only the serial number was. There were different part numbers for the same component, with serial numbers "nested" under each.

Does it sound like a mess? It was.

To straighten things out, we really had to start from scratch. We started from the shipping records and made a list for each component part by date and by serial number. We made another list, by subject (in numeric order) of the parts used by type and serial number. We also verified that hospital records of serial numbers matched those in the CRFs for each subject. The third list was for those device components that had been returned to the sponsor, either due to expiration dates, malfunctioning or because they had not been used by the end of the study.

We also inventoried the parts on hand, in order to cross-check the information.

Once this information was complete, we could make a "master" device disposition list. We actually made three lists, one for each separate component device, since this seemed to be the most straightforward presentation. The final lists were formatted like this:

Device Accountability – Protocol 12345 – Sponsor Name

Device part: Component A

Part Number	Serial Number	Received	Subject	Returned	Comment
A243	1267-429	1/16/2011	7-001 (DFC)		In use
A243	1267-435	1/16/2011		5/2/2011	Expired
A243	1267-506	3/22/2011	7-002 (JAK)		In use

And so forth…

Case Study: Investigational Product Accountability (continued)

When the lists were done, they allowed us to easily find the information for any part or any subject. They were filed together under a Device Accountability tab in the Study Documents binder.

It took hours and a lot of effort to straighten this out. Just think what it would have been like if it were a drug, with dispensing and return by subjects at multiple visits!

The site also developed a standard operating procedure for investigational product accountability and requires all CRCs to follow this procedure. Among other things, this procedure requires that accountability be done regularly throughout the study and that standard forms and a standard method of filing be used.

CHAPTER TWELVE

Working with Study Participants

In this chapter, we will cover some of the most difficult aspects of conducting clinical trials overall: recruitment of subjects into the trial, scheduling of study subject visits, retention of subjects after they have been entered, and subject compliance with the protocol throughout the study.

Recruitment of Study Subjects

Given enormous development costs, it is obvious that companies want to speed up the process as much as possible, allowing for more marketing time before their patent protection for the product expires. The timely enrollment of appropriate subjects into trials is critical to managing the timelines for a development program. Finding, enrolling and retaining study subjects are some of the largest and costliest challenges facing clinical research professionals today.

The majority (approximately two-thirds) of clinical trials fail to enroll the desired number of subjects within the specified enrollment period. Enrollment delays result in significant direct development costs for the study sponsor. Extended enrollment periods also can cause delays in new product introductions—a substantially higher cost due to missed market opportunity. The following chart shows the probability of successful enrollment for drugs in Phases II through IV.

Knowing the patient population and being able to accurately estimate the number of subjects that can be enrolled are critical to completing a trial in a given time period. Before a study actually starts at an investigative site, there always seem to be more than enough potential subjects waiting in the wings. For some reason, however, it frequently happens that as soon as the trial starts, these potential subjects disappear.

Estimating Enrollment Potential at Sites

One of the most important pre-study activities a CRC performs is helping to accurately estimate the number of subjects the site reasonably can expect to enroll in each trial. Investigators frequently overestimate the number of potential subjects they have. Often, this is due to the fact that they are looking only at the number of potential subjects who match the overall diagnosis, for example, depression. However, there are a number of other factors that must be weighed and taken into account, including the protocol and the subjects themselves.

Protocol considerations include the inclusion and exclusion criteria, activities and logistics. The largest constraints on enrollment usually are the inclusion and exclusion criteria for study entry. These criteria delineate the specific characteristics of the population to be enrolled. They will include demographic parameters, such as age and sex, disease and diagnostic criteria and study-specific requirements. In a study of depression, for example, the following (simplified) inclusion/exclusion criteria might be found:

- Age 18 to 65 years
- Men, and women who are post-menopausal, surgically sterile or using acceptable birth control
- Depression lasting at least six months, but no longer than one year
- No previous depressive episodes
- Not taking any other medications that might interfere with the study medication (list provided)
- Able to read and comprehend the informed consent document
- Willing to sign the informed consent
- Able to take pills
- Able to make weekly visits to the clinic site for three months.

Let's look at how these criteria might affect the ability of a site to enroll subjects.

The upper age limit of 65 may limit enrollment from sites that treat a large geriatric population. Depression is a disease that tends to recur in people over time, so the criterion that does not allow previous depressive episodes may be a problem. Willingness and ability to make weekly clinic visits is apt to interfere with a potential subject's life situation, especially when working. On top of these problems, many people just are not willing to participate in research, especially if the protocol requirements are burdensome and they do not see much potential value to themselves for participation.

How can these factors influence the ability to enroll? As a rough estimate, take the number of subjects in the practice who meet the diagnosis for the study (depression), then halve that number for each major inclusion/exclusion criterion, the number that remains is apt to be close to the number of subjects that will be enrolled. If we assume in our example that the site does not see many geriatric patients, then the three main criteria we need to be concerned with are: no previous episodes, the ability to make weekly visits and the willingness to sign a consent form. Note that if most patients in the practice are under 65, then most probably work, so weekly visits to the clinic may be a problem. Let us also assume that the investigator says there are about 300 patients in the practice who suffer from depression. Take 300 and divide it in half for each of three major inclusion/exclusion criteria.

$$300 \rightarrow 150 \rightarrow 75 \rightarrow 37$$

It can be assumed the site probably will be able to enroll about 37 subjects into the study, in total. This number may be acceptable, but the rate of enrollment needs to be factored in as well. (Note that if a site regularly does research similar to the protocol in question, it may be able to estimate enrollment much more exactly based on recent experience. In this case, there should be hard data about recent past trials, including the inclusion/exclusion criteria, number of subjects enrolled and rates of enrollment to back up the estimate.)

Remember, too, that it is necessary to attract a much higher number of patients through recruitment than are needed to finish the trial in order to yield the required number of subject completions, as some subjects will not complete the study for one reason or another.

The CRC must help the investigator analyze the requirements for the rate of enrollment. The sponsor may expect, for example, two patients to be enrolled every week, for a total of 25. Two patients a week does not seem too onerous, but remember that we have a three-month study, and that subjects are seen on a weekly basis. Let's look at what happens as the site begins enrolling. At week one, the site enrolls two subjects. During the second week, it enrolls two more, for a total of four subjects on study. By week six, the site is up to 12 subjects, and by week 10 it has 20 subjects on study. Since this is a three-month study, all of these subjects still are being seen on a weekly basis and there are still five more to enroll. (We will assume no dropouts for the purpose of this example.) The site personnel must determine if they are able to see and manage that many study subjects within a given week. Assessments must be made that include the available staff and space, as well as the ancillary help needed for such things as scheduling visits and calling subjects to remind them of their visits and other study responsibilities.

Unfortunately, most sponsors and investigators do not look at the cumulative workload as the study progresses. This is an area in which a good CRC can make a significant difference in accurate assessments of enrollment and study load capacities. Before beginning a study, the investigator and the CRC should feel confident that their site can manage the enrollment rate and numbers of subjects appropriately. Understanding what will be required in terms of time, staff and space throughout the trial will add to the overall chance of success.

Figure 2: Total subjects enrolled

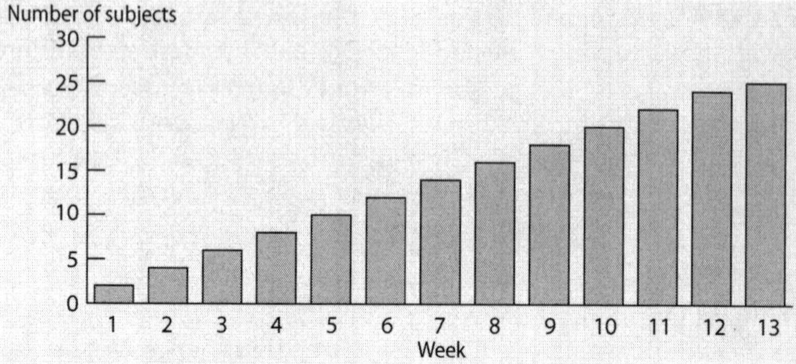

Note: Bars represent cumulative number of subjects enrolled over time.

Other Factors That Influence Enrollment

Another major factor influencing enrollment is competing studies. CRCs need to be aware of the enrollment problems that can result from having a competing study at the investigative site. Competing studies automatically reduce the resources available to each study, including the pool of available subjects. Even if the study is not competing for the same subject population, too many studies at a site can be a problem; study subjects will compete for other resources, including coordinator and investigator time and space.

General interest in the trial, on the part of both the potential subjects and the investigator and staff, can have a major impact on enrollment. The more interesting the trial and the compound being studied the faster enrollment will be. It is human nature to want to spend the most time on the most interesting projects; CRCs and investigators should carefully assess their interest in a trial before agreeing to participate. It is also important to thoroughly consider the available staff and space at a site, even if there are no competing studies. If the CRC and other involved personnel do not have sufficient time to conduct study activities, or if there is no room to put study supplies and perform study activities, they will be more hesitant to enroll additional subjects.

Advertising for Study Subjects

Sometimes advertising for study subjects is planned right from the start of a study. In general, advertising planned from the start is used when it is expected that subjects will be difficult to find and enroll, when the timeline for enrollment is extremely ambitious or when a site routinely advertises for all of its studies. In other cases, it becomes necessary to advertise for study subjects when enrollment targets are not being met as the study progresses; i.e., there already is an enrollment problem. The goal of advertising—to find and enroll suitable subjects into a trial—is the same no matter when it begins.

FAQ

Can we advertise our site as a study site—doing studies in many different areas—instead of advertising for only one specific study?

Yes. These are often referred to as "generic" ads. They still must be approved by an IRB.

The FDA has deemed that advertising for potential study subjects is not objectionable. In general, advertising is anything that is directed toward potential study subjects with the goal of recruiting them into the study. It may consist of radio or television spots, newspaper ads, posters on bulletin boards, flyers or any other items intended to directly reach prospective subjects. For example, one large general practice that conducts studies has multiple copies of a notebook in its waiting room. Each study it is conducting has a brief explanatory page in the notebook that gives basic details and who to contact for further information. The explanatory pages in these notebooks count as advertising.

The FDA considers advertising for study subjects to be the start of the informed consent process. Consequently, all advertising should be reviewed and approved by the IRB before use. Note that advertising may not be needed until later in the study, when it is apparent that enrollment goals are not being met. It does not matter that advertising materials were not submitted to the IRB when the study was first reviewed and approved; they simply must be approved before they may be used.

There are some items that do not count as advertising under FDA rules. Not included as advertising are:

> *"(1) communications intended to be seen or heard by health professionals, such as "dear doctor" letters and doctor-to-doctor letters (even when soliciting for study subjects), (2) news stories and (3) publicity intended for other audiences, such as financial page advertisements directed toward prospective investors."*

However, some sponsors require that doctor-to-doctor letters have IRB approval.

Submitting all advertising to the IRB for review and approval is probably the best course of action, as this eliminates the doubt and the need to make a determination of what is and is not appropriate material for the general public. Most sponsors also require that sites submit advertising for their approval before it goes to the IRB; some IRBs also want to see the approval from the sponsor when the advertising is submitted for review.

Advertising is reviewed by the IRB to ensure that it is not coercive and does not make promises about a cure or favorable outcome or promise things other than what appears in the protocol or the consent. This is especially important if the study involves subjects who are considered vulnerable according to the regulations—children, prisoners and economically or educationally disadvantaged people.

For written advertisements, such as those designed for use in newspapers, the IRB may want to see a finished copy, so it can evaluate the whole ad, including type size and any visual effects. For advertising with an audio component (radio, television, web, video), the IRB may review both the written text script and the audio version. Most IRBs will advise the investigator to submit the text first to be sure it is acceptable before the actual audio- or videotaping is done.

Advertising must not make any explicit or implicit claims that the drug, biologic or device is safe and effective, or that it is equivalent or superior to any other product. Remember that the reason the clinical trial is being conducted is to determine these things; they are not yet known. The ads must explain that the test article is investigational (experimental). Using a term such as "new treatment" implies it is a proven and approved product and is not appropriate. Advertisements may say subjects will be paid for participating in the study, but the payments should not be emphasized by big, bold type or other methods.

Below is an example of an unacceptable advertisement. Note that it says "new treatment," promises to cut the time of the cold in half and emphasizes the overly high payment amount.

New Treatment For
The Common Cold!!!

Cut your sniffle time in half!!!
Get paid $1,000 after only 7 days

Study subjects needed. Three shots a day for 4 days.
Call Success Clinical at 1-800-999-9999

What information should go into an advertisement? In general, the information should be limited to what prospective subjects need to know to determine if they might be interested in and eligible for the study. These may include the following items, although the FDA does not require that they all be included:

- Name and address of the investigator or research facility

- Condition under study and/or purpose of the research
- Brief summary of the primary criteria for study eligibility
- Brief list of benefits (e.g., no-cost health examination)
- Time or other subject commitment
- Contact information.

A more appropriate advertisement might look like this:

> **Research Study**
>
> **Subjects needed for a study to investigate the effects of an experimental medicine on lessening the symptoms of the common cold.**
>
> Subjects must be seen by the second day of the cold and must be at least 18 years old.
>
> For details, contact Shirley Williams at Eastside Clinic. (222) 222-2000

CRCs should be familiar with the information about advertising in the FDA's guidance for IRBs and clinical investigators, so they may better assist investigators in the proper development and use of advertising materials.

New Strategies for Subject Recruitment

Google

Today, it is common for potential study subjects to do Google searches on their medical conditions or even search for possible clinical trials in which they might participate. If the site wants their web page to be available to potential trial subjects, there are two ways this might happen. The first is in the unpaid section, called the "organic search" section. The other is in the paid section, "sponsored links." The sponsored links section is the list that shows up on the right-hand side of the page, or in the top section. Sponsored links are paid for on a "cost-per-click" basis.

If a site is planning to advertise this way, it is important that their web page is carefully and professionally designed for each trial, with the appropriate keywords and information to both attract potential subjects and aid in achieving a higher level in the organic search section. Remember, all advertising, including Internet advertising, must be approved by an IRB before use.

Social Networks

There has been an explosion in the growth and use of social networks such as Facebook and Twitter, and this has created new opportunities for the recruitment of subjects into clinical trials. Used correctly, social networking can be an effective method for generating pre-qualified patient referrals.

Ads can be run on social networks, as well as on Google. Since people have chosen to belong to these networks, they are more inclined to accept and act on messages received on these sites than they are to unsolicited advertising. Messages also are shared exponentially, without huge cost to the messenger.

Social networking sites have the ability to target ads to individual user pages based on information in the user profile, including location. Because these networks are global in scope, geo-targeting can be used for specifying areas for desired recruitment of study subjects.

YouTube videos also might be used to disseminate information about a trial. A YouTube video can also have a link to a web page, so it could connect a viewer directly to the site's web page with additional information about a clinical trial.

Other Recruitment Methods

Although advertising immediately comes to mind when discussing recruitment for study subjects, there are several other methods of finding subjects. The starting place for most sites is their own records. Many sites have their patients in a computer database that allows them to search based on diagnostic criteria. After they have found patients with an appropriate diagnosis, they are able to contact them to ascertain their interest and suitability

Figure 3: Do you have a profile on a social network?

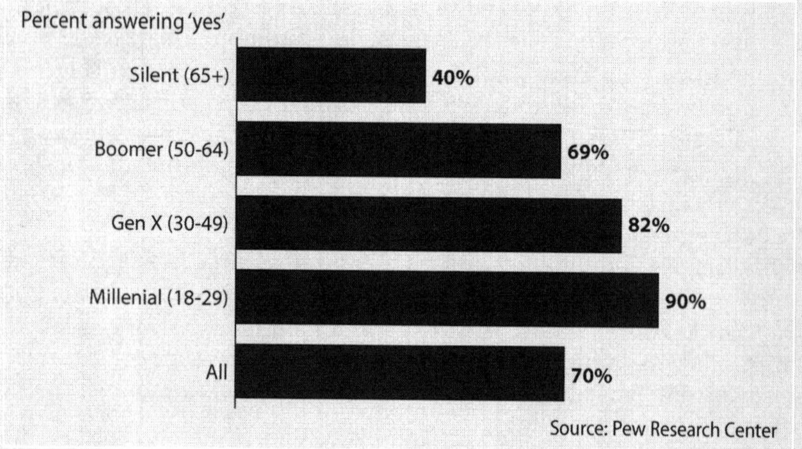

for the trial. In the case of studies in chronic diseases, such as diabetes or hypertension, most subjects probably will come from the investigator's own practice. In the case of acute diseases, such as pneumonia and other infectious diseases, searching the records from the investigative site may not be particularly useful.

Many potential subjects hear about a trial by word of mouth, perhaps from a friend who is in the trial. Sites that do a number of trials often have "free advertising" from current or past study subjects spreading the word. Subjects also find clinical trials by talking to people, contacting organizations, including disease-related groups and pharmaceutical companies, and doing web searches.

There are many websites available to potential study subjects that list trials in process or that are about to start. CenterWatch, for example, has an online database listing of clinical trials that is easily accessible (centerwatch.com).

There are sites, particularly through the NIH, that list active trials with information for potential subjects. The most comprehensive government database is www.clinicaltrials.gov.

Advocacy groups for various diseases, are sources of information about trials; sites may receive interested subjects from these groups or from people who have been in contact with these groups.

Frequently, other physicians or healthcare professionals will refer potential subjects to a trial. Investigators often contact other physicians in the community to inform them of the trial and ask that it be mentioned to suitable subjects. The investigator may make these contacts by phone or send letters to other healthcare professionals in the community. CRCs often help make these contacts.

Usually finding subjects for a trial is accomplished by a combination of methods. The more difficult it is to enroll, the more variety there will be in the methods used to attract potential subjects. It is important for a CRC to monitor enrollment and enrollment rates from the start of each study and to think about ways to enhance enrollment before it becomes a major problem. It usually is much easier to make changes when trouble is just starting than to wait until there is no doubt a major problem has occurred. For enrollment problems, the way to fix things often is by implementing several small ideas and suggestions; not everything works in each case and one change frequently is not sufficient.

Information for Potential Study Subjects

Potential study subjects may not be very knowledgeable about clinical trials and the clinical trial process. Some tend to think that receiving treatment in a clinical trial is the same as receiving treatment as a regular patient in a medical practice. This is not true. Clinical trials are designed to answer scientific questions, not to provide medical treatment. Anyone who is thinking about participating in a clinical trial needs to understand the difference between participating in a clinical trial and receiving treatment at a doctor's private practice. It is the responsibility of investigators and CRCs to help educate their potential subjects about the differences in these activities.

There are, of course, many benefits to participating in clinical trials. Many subjects receive treatment with new compounds that may be much more efficacious in treating their disease or condition than standard treatments. Individuals with severe and life-threatening illnesses may receive treatments that offer them hope. Some subjects receive treatment they otherwise would be unable to pay for and some, especially in Phase I trials with normal healthy volunteers, participate to earn extra money. People often participate out of a desire to help others with similar afflictions. No matter what a person's reason for participating in a clinical trial, however, it is important that the person know and understand that clinical trials are not a substitute for other regular medical care, but rather an enlargement of his or her regular care team and support.

Compensation to Research Subjects

It is quite common for subjects to be compensated for participating in clinical trials, especially in the early phases of development. When subjects are compensated, however, it is viewed by the FDA as a recruitment incentive, not as a study benefit. All compensation schedules must be approved by the IRB in advance of the study, or in advance of being used. The IRB will look at both the compensation amount and the timing of the compensation, to be sure it is not coercive and would not present an undue influence on the subject's trial-related decisions.

Subjects are usually compensated on a regular basis throughout the trial, based most commonly for each completed visit, although they do not have to be compensated at each visit. It is rarely appropriate to compensate subjects only if they complete the entire trial; this might encourage them to continue with the trial even if they otherwise would have discontinued due to side effects or other reasons.

The amount of compensation to subjects varies with respect to the complexity of the study and the involvement of the subjects. Compensation is usually designed to cover any costs the subjects might incur by participating, such as transportation, parking, lunch and child care. Compensation must not be so large as to be coercive; that is, the subjects should not be entering a trial only because of the compensation. Before approving subject's compensation, the IRB also will take into account where the study is being conducted and the patient population. Compensation of $25 per visit may be no enticement at all to people in some neighborhoods, but it may constitute a great deal of money and enticement to subjects in another.

Some sites routinely compensate subjects for participating in trials while others never compensate study subjects. Either is acceptable. The important things to remember about compensation to study subjects are that it must not be coercive or present undue influence and that it must be pre-approved by the IRB.

Incentive Payments to Healthcare Professionals

There are two types of incentive payments: those paid by the investigator to other professionals to encourage them to find study subjects, and bonus payments by study sponsors to investigators and their staff to enhance enrollment. Incentive payments to healthcare professionals by an investigator for the referral of study subjects are known as referral fees or finder's fees. Some examples include payments made to a coordinator or nurse, resident or intern physicians, or other local physicians for each subject referred and entered into a study. These payments usually are not acceptable and may compromise the integrity of a trial. They also may be in violation of regulations or institutional policies.

Some states have laws that prohibit referral fees. For example, the California Health and Safety Code § 445 clearly prohibits referral fees. It states:

> *"No person, firm, partnership, association or corporation, or agent or employee thereof shall for profit refer or recommend a person to a physician, hospital, health-related facility or dispensary for any form of medical care or treatment of any ailment or medical condition."*

Also, the American Medical Association (AMA) has stated in its Code of Medical Ethics that referral fees for research studies are unethical. Section 6.03 of the code, Fee Splitting: Referrals to Health Care Facilities, states:

> *"Offering or accepting payment for referring patients to research studies (finder's fees) are also unethical."*

Incentive payments to healthcare professionals also include bonus payments by the study sponsor to investigators and CRCs for enhanced (faster or more) enrollment. True bonus payments usually are not acceptable because they may encourage the enrollment of "borderline" subjects or subjects the investigator otherwise would not recruit. This creates a conflict of interest and should be avoided.

There is no problem, however, with a sponsor covering true extra costs for enrollment procedures. These payments might be for additional people to help with the screening of potential subjects, advertising costs or other direct costs borne by the investigative site. This is frequently decided upon before the study starts, even though not implemented unless necessary to increase enrollment or speed the rate of enrollment. For example, a sponsor may be willing to pay a per screen amount for the pre-screening of study candidates. In this case, there usually is a limit to the number of screen failures it will pay for in relation to the number of subjects actually entered into the trial. This ensures that the site is actually looking for and pre-screening suitable candidates. If site personnel are not sure whether a payment plan is appropriate, they should contact their IRB for an opinion before implementation.

Summary: Recruitment

Timely and appropriate recruitment and enrollment of subjects into clinical trials is essential for a drug, biologic or device development program. CRCs must be aware of the regulations and institutional policy regarding recruitment and have an understanding of the potential problems and solutions for enrollment. It is important to remember that at each step, from initial recruitment to actual study enrollment, the number of potential subjects decreases. The Venn diagram patterned after one developed by Bert Spilker shows this in graphic form in Figure 4.

Scheduling Subjects

Scheduling subjects for their study visits is more difficult than scheduling normal office visits, because study visits must be in accordance with the protocol and there is not much flexibility around the required visit dates. Since it is not always possible for subjects to come in for study visits on the exact dates, most protocols allow a few days prior or after the calendar date; this is known as the visit window. If a subject is not seen during the visit window, that visit is usually regarded as a missed visit; this is a problem for the analysis of the data and some sponsors will not pay for these visits. The investigator can, however, call the sponsor to discuss a specific case when it occurs; the sponsor may make an exemption on the visit window in certain circumstances.

Figure 4: Venn diagram showing stages of enrollment for a clinical trial

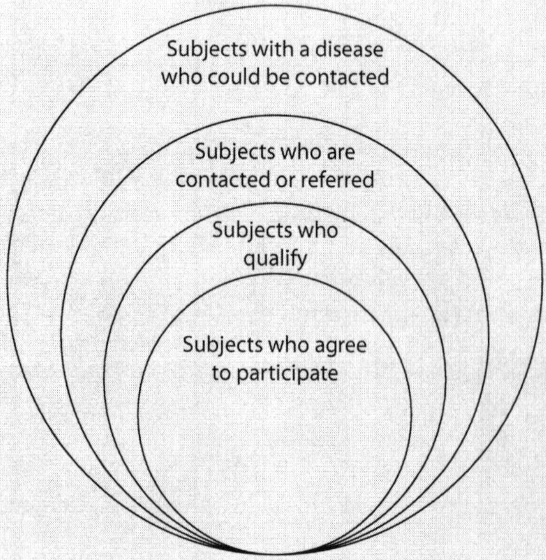

For example, let's assume a subject is to come in every week for a visit. If a subject starts on Tuesday, ideally he or she would come in every week on Tuesday. The visit window might be plus or minus one day, which means that it would be acceptable for the subject to come in on Monday, Tuesday or Wednesday for the visit. This allows some flexibility in case there is a reason the subject cannot come in on the usual Tuesday. Generally, each visit window is calculated by going back to the starting or baseline date, rather than from the previous visit. The reason is that if a subject is always two days late, and if the window is calculated from the last visit, there is always going to be the addition of two days and two more days and two more days and so forth. Because the subject must take the drug every day, after a certain time there will not be enough study drug for the subject to finish all the visits specified by the protocol.

If the study sponsor does not give a reference sheet with dates and study windows, the CRC might find it useful to make one on their own, as it is a very valuable tool to use when scheduling subject visits. Table 1 is an example of how a visit schedule sheet might look.

Notice that in this visit window schedule, the baseline dates are when the subjects actually came in for their baseline visits. At each other visit, the top date is the projected visit date, starting from baseline at each time period, and the bottom dates are the potential dates that the subject is allowed to come in based on the acceptable visit windows. Dates other than those in parentheses would be outside the window for each visit. There are other ways to make visit window schedules, but no matter which format is used it is a useful tool for the CRC.

It also helps, in relatively short studies, to schedule all the subject visits when each subject comes in for the baseline visit. This allows everyone to plan ahead and will help to eliminate scheduling problems. In longer-term studies, the CRC should schedule at least the next few visits in advance. Scheduling in advance does not eliminate the need for visit reminders for study subjects. Some sites send postcard visit reminders, and most sites find that telephone reminders a day ahead are very good aids in helping study subjects keep their appointments. Coming in on the appropriate days for study appointments is very important for study compliance, which will be discussed later in this chapter. A good CRC will do everything possible to maximize compliance with study visit dates.

Table 1: Visit Schedule and Visit Windows

Patient Number	Baseline (+/- 1 day)	Week 1 Visit (+/- 1 day)	Week 2 Visit (+/- 1 day)	Week 4 Visit (Final visit) (+/- 1 day)
001	April 4 (Actual)	April 11 (April 10, 11, 12)	April 18 (April 17, 18, 19)	May 2 (May 1, 2, 3)
002	April 8 (Actual)	April 15 (April 14, 15, 16)	April 22 (April 21, 22, 23)	May 6 (May 5, 6, 7)

Retention of Study Subjects

Once subjects are enrolled into a trial, it is important that they stay in the trial until it is completed, if at all possible. It would be ideal if every subject enrolled would complete the entire study, but this does not usually happen. There are valid reasons for a subject to discontinue his or her study participation, such as intolerable side effects, but there are other reasons that do not have anything to do with subject safety or well-being. When a subject drops out before the study is complete, he or she usually is counted as a "failure" in the statistical analysis; hence, too many dropouts can bias the results of the trial. This is one reason CRCs should be familiar both with why subjects drop out and how retention can be enhanced. In this section, we will explore why subjects leave trials and what can be done to increase retention.

Reasons Investigators and/or Sponsors Discontinue Subjects

Before discussing the reasons subjects choose to discontinue their participation in clinical trials, it is important to differentiate between subjects who choose to drop out on their own and subjects who are discontinued by the investigator and/or the sponsor.

Investigators may discontinue a subject for a number of reasons. Some are medical, some are based on the patient's compliance and cooperation and some are trial-related. Some of the more common reasons for discontinuing a subject are listed below.

Medical reasons for potential discontinuation:

- Lack of efficacy of the drug
- Intolerable adverse events
- Serious adverse events (SAEs)
- Patient's condition deteriorates
- Patient develops an intercurrent illness (an illness other than the one under study, but which occurs during the course of the trial)
- Pregnancy
- Abnormal laboratory values
- Did not meet original entry criteria (discovered after study entry)
- Died.

Patient compliance and cooperation reasons:

- Unacceptable compliance with protocol activities
- Unacceptable compliance in taking the study medication
- Not keeping appointments
- Not cooperating with study staff and/or study procedures

- Use of non-approved concomitant medications
- Moved out of the area.

Trial-related reasons:

- Trial was terminated by the sponsor due to:
    - Safety concerns
    - Benefit so great trial is no longer ethical because some subjects are not receiving active treatment
    - Business reasons.
- Investigator no longer able to continue the trial (retired, died, moved)
- Investigator did not meet enrollment targets or did not comply with the protocol or the regulations.

Since it was either the investigator or the sponsor who decided to discontinue patients for these reasons, we will not discuss them further. The main concern for CRCs is helping to retain subjects who would have decided to drop out of the study on their own.

Other Reasons Subjects Drop Out of Trials

There are many reasons study subjects decide to stop participating in a trial. The most common are valid medical reasons such as intolerable adverse events or a lack of efficacy of the treatment. These cases are usually discussed with and agreed to by the investigator.

There are, however, other reasons subjects drop out, which are not so compelling and could perhaps be avoided. This is when the CRC must understand what causes some of the problems and how they might be prevented from occurring. The key for the CRC is catching problems, or patterns of problems, early so they can be fixed. After all, once subjects are lost from a study, they are lost forever. The CRC wants to ensure that losses do not become the standard and that they do not exceed what normally would be expected during a study. Some reasons subjects drop out are:

- The subject does not understand the importance of remaining in the trial even when the disease condition has improved.
- The study requirements are too burdensome.
- The subject loses interest in the trial.
- The medication is unpleasant to take.
- The subject does not like some of the study staff.
- People at the site are unfriendly (could be anyone, including the receptionist).

- The subject has to spend too much time at the clinic.
- The subject has difficulties with transportation, childcare or time off from work.
- The subject is upset about some aspect of the trial.
- Friends or family are unhappy about the subject's participation.
- The subject has a change in his or her personal situation.

Many sponsors will want the site to keep a list of all subjects who drop out with the reasons categorized by general headings such as adverse events, lack of efficacy, lost to follow-up, withdrawal of consent, etc.

When a patient does not return for study visits, a diligent effort should be made to contact the patient and either have him or her return or find out why he or she is unwilling to return. Most sites will try to call the person at least three times, followed by a registered letter with a stamped return envelope included so the patient can reply easily. Proof of each contact should be kept in the patient's records. After several documented unsuccessful contact attempts, the patient can be classified as "lost to follow-up."

FAQ

Our sponsor wants us to drop a subject from our study because he does not come in during the specified visit windows. He is a busy professional and is often out of town during the visit times. Do we have to drop him?

Remember that compliance is ultimately a safety issue, as well as a statistical issue. You may discuss this with the sponsor, but the subject probably will need to be discontinued if he cannot adhere to the protocol requirements.

Maximizing Retention in Clinical Trials

The secret to subject retention in clinical trials is easy. It is not really a secret at all but is just plain common sense (although sometimes sense is not so common). All site staff have to do is be nice, treat subjects well, spend time with them, listen carefully to what they are saying and communicate openly and often.

Investigators and study coordinators are very busy people. They get rushed and behind on things, have good and bad days and experience the same problems as the rest of us. Nevertheless, if a study is to go well, they must be able to set aside their concerns and problems when study subjects walk in the door. Study subjects want to feel that their contribution is important, and they want to be the sole focus of attention during their time with the investigator and/or coordinator.

When a study subject comes in for a clinic visit, he or she wants to be able to discuss what has happened since the last visit, to have any study concerns allayed, to be praised for doing well, to have questions answered and to be treated like an important partner in the study venture. In short, a study subject wants to be appreciated. After all, there are risks to becoming part of a study, there is no guaranteed outcome and it is voluntary—no one has to participate. People who volunteer for studies are special, and they should be treated as such.

Given the premise of wanting to be treated well, there are many things, frequently small things, that can make a subject decide that trial participation may not be worth the effort. Some of these things are:

- Having to wait when coming in for an appointment
- Not being treated kindly and with respect
- Not being seen by the investigator or the coordinator but being seen by a "substitute" that he or she doesn't know
- Not seeing the same person at most visits (developing a one-on-one relationship)
- Being rushed and hurried through the appointment
- Feeling that the investigator/coordinator doesn't really want to see him or her
- Not being asked about how he or she feels and how the study is going
- Not having the opportunity to ask questions
- Being afraid to ask study-related questions
- Being made to feel dumb or silly when asking questions
- Being berated for doing something wrong
- Having the investigator or coordinator disparage the study.

There are also situations in which the subject does not return and is lost to follow-up, or in which the subject drops out but refuses to give a reason, other than personal choice. These situations are difficult to combat, and the study site cannot do much about them. If there are many of these cases at a site, however, they should serve as a wake-up call. Chances are the real reasons are in the list above, but the subject just doesn't want to tell the site personnel.

These problems can be remedied, but they first need to be recognized and acknowledged. It's critical to catch them early. Some problems are easy to fix. For example, if a subject has a logistical problem, such as transportation to the site, one solution may be to pay for a taxi to transport the subject back and forth. If childcare is a problem, perhaps the visit time can be adjusted to an evening or weekend time so the subject can come in while is there is someone home to stay with children. Questioning the subject about problems and being willing to help with arrangements or adjustments may allow the subject to continue participation.

In addition to treating study subjects well, some successful sites have very clever ways to make their study subjects feel happy, important and wanted. Some of the ideas and little steps that have added to retention success for sites are:

- Reminder calls the day before each visit
- Giving each volunteer a special study T-shirt ("I'm a research volunteer," "Volunteer for XXXXX (study acronym)," big smiley face)
- Mugs, tote bags, gym bags for a study in which there is exercise testing
- Separate waiting room with coffee, tea and doughnuts—and current magazines and newspapers
- Sending a cab to pick up someone if transportation is a problem
- Thank you notes from the coordinator after a few weeks on a study
- Thank you notes at the end of the subject's participation (leads to repeat volunteering)
- Balloons
- Birthday cards
- Bonus gift certificates.

When site personnel would like to incorporate ideas, check with the sponsor and IRB regarding the need for prior IRB approval; it's better to check than to assume it is okay without approval.

It helps if the CRC and the investigator plan out a strategy at the beginning of the trial to help retain subjects. Many sponsors are willing to foot the bill for little extras, such as mugs or T-shirts, that may encourage subjects to feel good about their participation and remain in the trial through completion. But some sponsors are bound by state gift laws that prohibit or limit any gifting between sponsors and sites. It is also important to check with institutional policy on all sides.

Any time there is a pattern of more than expected dropouts due to nonmedical issues, the sponsor monitor should meet with the investigator and coordinator to discuss the situation. Each case should be analyzed. Perhaps the reasons are clear-cut and recognizable, or perhaps they are not. It may be time to reflect on the atmosphere at the site and take a hard look at how subjects are being treated. The site might even want to talk with subjects about their perceptions of how the study is going, how they feel when they come in for visits and if they feel there are ways in which the site could improve the study process. Difficult as it is, site personnel must take an honest look at their interactions with study subjects. Sometimes it helps to think about how one would feel if they were in the study, or how they would feel about having one of their loved ones participate.

There is also a movement within clinical trials related to patient centricity. Including what study patients want to see in studies and including patients in some of the decision-making are some examples of how this works. Informed consent is another area that is a focus of some global initiatives to improve and make more patient-centric and not mainly a legal document protecting sponsors and investigators.

Summary: Retention

Retention of subjects in clinical trials is critical to the completion of an informative, sound clinical trial. Sites should help subjects understand that a successful trial is a partnership between the subjects and the investigative staff. Respect, courtesy, honesty and open communication on the part of both subjects and investigators will increase the chances of successfully completing a study.

Subject Compliance

Clinical trials are conducted to assess the safety and efficacy of a new investigational products and procedures. To be able to accurately assess safety and efficacy, study subjects must take the medication as it is prescribed. Unfortunately, subjects do not always do this. In this section, we will look at compliance, what can go wrong and how to increase the probability of good compliance.

Undetected poor compliance can lead to invalid study results. Lack of compliance in one subject may have an impact only on that particular subject. If several subjects are non-compliant, however, it can invalidate the entire study. Non-compliance can have the following results:

- An effective medication may look ineffective. This can mean a medication that would be effective, and that would be of benefit to patients, never makes it to the marketplace. This is an unfortunate result for the company that has made the development investment in the investigational product and even more unfortunate for those people who would have benefitted from it.
- An ineffective medication looks effective. This result is worse than the one above because, once marketed, the medication will be relied on to effect a cure and will not be effective in doing so.
- Failure to detect an investigational product-related safety issue.
- Inappropriate dosage recommendations. Depending on the type of non-compliance, the investigational product labeling could recommend either too high or too low a dose. This is not good in either direction—patients could be taking too little to be an effective treatment or more than they need, which could lead to an excess of adverse reactions.

The effects of the investigational product in non-compliant subjects cannot be extrapolated to compliant subjects. It is very important that all study subjects are as compliant as possible during their involvement in clinical trials.

Negative Study Results

There are a number of reasons for negative study results. They may be due to the failure of the medication; that is, the investigational product just might not work. Remember that the reason clinical trials are conducted is to find out if the investigational product is safe and effective. Although it would be nice if every investigational product under development worked as expected, they do not always do so. Sometimes they are not safe, and sometimes they are not effective. In these cases, it is better if they are never marketed.

Negative results also can be due to poor subject compliance, although it usually takes more than just a few non-compliant subjects to affect the entire study. We will explore subject compliance in detail as we go along.

Reasons for Non-Compliance

Sometimes study subjects are non-compliant for disease-related reasons. One reason is a lack of symptoms, or what can be called the "antibiotic effect." As many of us know from personal experience, it is hard to remember to take medications when you are feeling better and have very few or no remaining disease symptoms. A prime example of this is the standard 10-day course of treatment with many antibiotics. After five or six days, when the patient appears to be over the disease, it is very common to stop taking the pills. The subject has become non-compliant with the medication schedule; this happens in trials as well as in general practice.

There are also compliance problems with people suffering from terminal diseases. When people know they are going to die soon, they do not have the same incentive for taking a course of medications that they might have otherwise.

There are many other reasons subjects are not compliant when it comes to taking medication. Sometimes they just forget to take their pills. Sometimes there is a lack of belief in the treatment—"It isn't going to work anyway, so why bother?" If the medication is unpleasant to take, such as having a bad taste, or pills so big they are hard to swallow, compliance may be poor.

Non-compliance can result from how the investigational product is packaged. Think about using safety containers (childproof lids) in an arthritis study, for example. The subjects may not be able to open the containers without help, which will surely affect compliance. Sometimes the investigational product is packaged in large blister packs containing several days' worth of IP, with each day's investigational product clearly marked as to when it should be taken. At first glance, it appears this would help compliance, but think about it a bit more. What happens when a subject has to go to work? Most people do not want to carry a large blister pack to work with them and have others ask about it. Consequently, subjects might take the day's investigational product out of the package and just carry it in a pocket, not knowing that the ordering of the pills for the day is important—they become non-compliant.

Sometimes subjects just do not understand the dosing scheme, especially if it is complicated. "Oh... it's two white ones and one pink one? I thought it was two pink ones and one white one. That's why I ran out of pink ones last week." Sometimes it is the regimen that is confusing, with too many pills or too many different times per day to take them, or confusion about the times and/or doses. It also may be the duration of the study, as subjects can lose interest over time.

Subjects also may become non-compliant because of adverse reactions. If a subject becomes nauseous after taking the medication or thinks it is causing headaches, he or she may not take it as often as required, if at all. A subject may not take medication appropriately because of mistrust, either in the medication or in the physician. A subject may be influenced by family or friends in ways that affect compliance also; if people important to the subject do not want him or her to take the pills, or be in the study, this may affect compliance. "I'm not sure you should be taking anything not approved by the government, dear..."

Other ways in which subjects may be non-compliant related to the study medication are by not filling their prescriptions, by prematurely discontinuing the investigational product or by sharing the investigational product with other people. Other examples of noncompliance include:

- Taking other medications at the same time, when the other medications are not allowed by the protocol
- Using alcohol or other disallowed substances such as marijuana while in the study
- Changes in their living situations that influence when and how the investigational product is taken
- Their mental conditions have a negative impact on their ability to follow protocol instructions.

There also are compliance issues not related directly to the medication. Subjects may be non-compliant by missing visits or not coming in for visits within the visit windows. They may not adhere to other study requirements such as special tests (eye exams, for example), dietary requirements or keeping diaries.

Sometimes compliance problems stem from investigator-related reasons. Subjects will be less compliant if it is difficult to schedule study visits or if they are kept waiting when they come in for a visit. If study staff do not keep appointments, subjects are apt to do the same. Worst of all is a poor physician-patient relationship. In general, subjects want to please the physician and do things correctly, but if the relationship is poor the subject is not as likely to care about complying with study requirements.

Unfortunately, there are many ways to be non-compliant, both on purpose and by mistake. The key is discovering and fixing the problem before it has a negative impact on the entire study.

Managing Compliance

Study protocols should be designed to enhance compliance as much as possible. They also should make it possible to monitor compliance.

CRCs and investigators must understand why compliance is important and how they can help to ensure compliance during the study. They need to work with their patients, both before and during the trial, in order to assure compliance. There are certain things study patients must be aware of and do during the study. Just as clinical trials are different than clinical practice for investigators, they are different for study subjects. The investigator and the CRC must ensure that potential study subjects are aware that if they are in the study, they must:

- Come in for all study visits on time and within the visit windows.
- Answer the questions truthfully, especially with respect to their medical histories and disease histories.
- Cooperate fully with study procedures. This is one reason it is critical that the investigator fully explains the study to potential subjects.
- Allow tests to be done as appropriate, and on time.
- Take study medications as prescribed.
- Follow all study directions.
- Ask if something is not clear and inform the site of any problems or snags.

The CRC should tell the study subjects how important it is to answer questions truthfully, especially about their compliance during the study. Subjects need to know that it is better to let the investigator and coordinator know they missed some doses than to not say anything at all, and that they will hurt the study if they are not forthcoming with this information. The CRC or the investigator must thoroughly question each subject about compliance at each visit. They should let subjects know they should call if they are having any problems complying with study activities or are confused about what needs to be done.

There are a variety of ways to test for compliance in studies. Every study will have some way of asking about and maintaining investigational product accountability. Usually a record is kept for each subject of the amounts and dates the investigational product is dispensed, and the amounts and dates of the investigational product returned. Subjects are told to bring back any unused medications at each visit. The returned investigational product is counted and recorded by the coordinator. This is a reasonable way to assess compliance but, unless the subject admits a problem, there is no way to know about the pill that fell down the drain or was swallowed by the dog. The person seeing the subject should also question him or her about whether or not all doses were taken.

Watching subjects take the pills in person would encourage good compliance, but studies usually are not set up in such a way that the subject is at the site each time a dose needs to be taken. This would work only if there is a single dose of medication given, an IV drug is administered or the drug is given in an in-patient hospital setting, etc.

Subjects sometimes are asked to keep diaries and record when each medication dose is taken. This is probably valid with very compliant subjects, but for the others it is as easy to forget writing in the diary as it is to forget to take the medication.

The "gold standard" for testing for compliance is to check blood levels. This is done in some studies, but mostly only in the very early (Phase I and II) studies. It is expensive and is not feasible to do most of the time.

What can site personnel do to maximize compliance? First, it helps to know the subjects enrolled. If an investigator and a CRC have worked with a subject before, they should have an idea of whether or not the person will be compliant. They should question subjects before entering the study as to their willingness to comply with study activities, if they can swallow the pills, if they can come in for visits, etc.

The investigator and coordinator must pay attention to the signs of potential non-compliance. Does the patient show up for visits? On time? Did the subject complete any necessary pre-study activities? Is the person really interested in the study and aware of the requirements?

The CRC should ask the subject about anything that may interfere with completing the study. Does the subject have a vacation planned during the time of the study? Does he or she understand what is involved in participating? Does the patient's lifestyle allow for complying with the study rules and activities?

In short, if the CRC or the investigator knows or thinks a subject will not be a good, compliant patient, he or she should not be enrolled in the study at all. This is a safety issue—if a subject is not compliant with the study protocol, he or she could be putting himself or herself at a greater than acceptable risk.

When Non-compliance Happens

If the CRC is aware that a subject has been non-compliant, either in taking the medication or in other study activities, he or she should inform the sponsor of the non-compliance issue. Details of any non-compliance situations should be documented both in the site's source documents and in the case report form. The CRC or the investigator should discuss the situation with the subject and do some retraining in study procedures. If the subject continues to be non-compliant, he or she may need to be dropped from the trial. Keeping subjects who are not compliant in a trial is not good for the subject (safety concerns) or the trial. When subjects are dropped from a study for non-compliance, the relevant information must be recorded both in the source documents and in the case report form.

By working closely with each potential subject before enrollment into a trial, and by working closely with the subjects throughout the trial, compliance can be maximized, and study results will be more reliable than if there had been major compliance problems.

Good study designs and protocols will anticipate non-compliance and give instructions for minimizing it and handling it if it occurs. If the CRC and the investigator do their jobs, both to minimize noncompliance and to detect and report it, the study should remain valid.

Summary and Key Points

A CRC has a significant role in these key activities that are commonly linked to the most challenging areas of clinical trials: recruitment of subjects into the trial, scheduling of study subject visits, retention of subjects after they have been entered and subject compliance with the protocol throughout the study. A CRC can make a big difference for the success of the trial with the insights they have and obtain regarding what supports the subjects the most. No matter the technology the site team members' relationship with the subject is very impacting on the positive success of the study. Balancing time communicating with subjects and other activities that a CRC performs is very important for recruitment and retention of trial subjects.

Key Points:

- Recruitment of subjects can be supported by social media and other online systems.
- Clear and often communication to the study subjects is essential.
- Patient centric focus is an evolving focus of trials that will hopefully lead to better recruitment and retention.
- Subject compliance is an important focus and knowing why there are deviations is important to be sure actions matter.

CHAPTER THIRTEEN

Study Closure or Termination

When a study is over at an investigation site, it must be officially closed. When a study has been concluded at the site, it means one of four things: 1) that the site enrolled subjects and they have finished, the data has been monitored and queries resolved, 2) the sponsor stopped the study sooner than expected, maybe for a safety issue or the lack of efficacy of the product overall, 3) the investigator has not performed well and is being closed early by the sponsor or IRB or 4) less common, the investigator decides to withdraw participation, maybe retiring, for example, or because of a poor relationship between the site and sponsor/CRO.

Study closing duties are usually shared by the site and sponsor, with the CRC and the CRA performing a large amount of the activities. In this chapter we will look at the what must be done to close a study. We also will discuss site post-study critique.

Orderly Study Closure

A sponsor may discontinue a trial at all sites at the same time or at individual sites at different times. Whatever the timing, the activity is essentially a single site activity, that is, it must be done at each site regardless of the activity at any other sites. ICH E6 requires sponsor reconciliation of essential documentation before study closure at a site (section 8). One cautionary note: If the study is stopped abruptly while subjects are still taking the study medications, the sponsor should have an orderly plan for discontinuing each subject. This plan will be communicated to each investigator. The investigator and the CRC, when delegated, should be prepared to explain the plan to subjects. The site must also be prepared to notify subjects promptly and assure them of appropriate therapy and follow-up outside of the trial.

Closing a study because it is finished and complete at a site is the most common situation. It is also the easiest to handle. The data and the TMF have been monitored and things should be in good shape for closing. If the monitoring has been thorough sometimes the site closure can be done remotely by teleconference. In this case everyone is usually pleased that it was finished and hopeful of a favorable outcome. If a study is closed for a compliance reason, the study closure may not be as easy at a site. No matter the reason for closing a study, much of the same procedures must be followed.

Closure Procedures

A CRA commonly will visit the site to do a closure visit, but as mentioned earlier if all monitoring activities that require the CRA to be on-site have been accomplished at other visits, the site can be closed through remote activities. The main items the CRA will address during a close-out visit are: data query closure and CRF cleaning, investigational product accountability and disposition, the investigator's study file and administrative items, and lastly, being sure the investigator is aware of his or her responsibilities after closure. The CRC should coordinate the preparation for the closeout visit by having everything completed and ready before the CRA arrives.

Data Query Closure and Case Report Forms Clean

If all CRFs have not been entered/submitted, monitored and queries closed, this must be done during the closeout or a period of time with data management, but the site cannot be considered closed without all queries resolved. If the study has come to its natural end, this activity probably has been done already before closeout. If the study has had poor monitoring or has been stopped abruptly or early, data monitoring may not be complete. It is always better to have the CRF data submitted and reviewed before the closeout visit, in case final corrections need to be made that include the need to see original source documentation to verify data accuracy. The CRC should make sure all case report forms, as well as any corrections or queries, are complete before the visit. It is beneficial to have a call before the on-site visit to discuss the action items before closeout. The CRA and the CRC should both review the subjects' CRFs before the visit to understand the amount of data cleaning needed before the visit. Even though this is close to the end, the CRC should be sure to not compromise quality for speed.

Investigational Product Accountability and Disposition

If there are still investigational product and/or supplies at the site, the CRA will complete a final inventory at the closeout visit. These materials should then be packaged for return to the sponsor, according to protocol, federal and state shipping regulations and sponsor and site company policy, if applicable. A copy of the return inventory form should be placed in the investigator's study file and a copy retrieved by the CRA for the sponsor file. There are some cases where supplies or IP can be disposed of at the site, but it must meet the requirements of the protocol, site and sponsor requirements, as well as local biohazard laws, if applicable.

Hopefully, investigational product reconciliation has been done throughout the study, rather than left to the end. In this case, it should be relatively easy for the CRA and the CRC to finish the reconciliation quickly.

Investigator's Study File

The sponsor is required to do one last reconciliation of the investigator site file in-house compared to the study file at the site. There are some studies that have electronic trial master files (eTMF) which makes it easier to reconcile remotely. But many studies still have paper trial master files at sites and require a CRA to inventory what is at the sponsor versus at the site, and to collect copies of any documents not at the sponsor from the site file or vise versa. The CRC should check the study file before the closeout visit to ensure that nothing is overlooked. This is a good time to use a study document checklist (see Appendix D). All documents must be present, including appropriate IRB re-approvals and IRB correspondence. If there were protocol amendments during the study, or amendments to the informed consent form, all versions should be in the file.

Informed consent forms for each subject must be present. The CRA will double check to be sure they were all signed and dated appropriately. There should also be documentation for any protocol deviations. The investigator's brochure should be available in or with the site study file.

If any documents are missing from this file, the CRA can help the site obtain copies. When the file is complete and in order, it is ready for storage. The storage address, if different than the investigation site address must be obtained by the monitor and documented in the closeout visit report.

Reminding the Investigator of Study Responsibilities After Closure

The investigator must be reminded of responsibilities post-closeout visit. This at minimum, includes:

- Retaining study records for the timeframe agreed upon in the contract

- The investigator must inform the sponsor if they are contacted by the FDA for a notice of inspection
- The investigator must notify the IRB of study closure, submit a final report and send a copy to the sponsor (unless done during the closeout visit). The IRB notification of study closure should not occur before study site termination.

The investigator is required to make two final study reports at the end of the study: one to the sponsor and one to the IRB. As noted above, many times the report sent to the IRB is also used to send to the sponsor. The IRB commonly supplies a template to complete. The report typically includes:

- Enrollment summary, including the number of subjects entered, those who completed and those who dropped, including the reasons for dropping
- Serious adverse events and any other safety information relative to the trial at that site
- List of major deviations and actions taken and outcomes.

Frequently, it is the CRC who will draft these final reports for the investigator. At the closing visit, the CRA will verify that these reports were done, collect copies for the sponsor, if appropriate, and ensure that the reports are in the investigator study file.

Since this is probably the last visit the CRA will make to the site for the trial, any outstanding action items should be resolved as much as possible before leaving the site. If there are action items pending, they can be addressed after the visit as long as they do not require a site visit. It is important that the CRC work with the monitor to get all items resolved as soon as possible after the visit.

The investigator and/or the CRC will want to verify that all appropriate grant monies have been paid, requested or are in process.

If there are unused study materials at the site (case report forms, unused laboratory kits, etc.), they should be returned or disposed of according to the sponsor's direction.

Any outstanding issues from previous visits, or issues that arose during sponsor review, should be resolved before the site is closed. If not documented elsewhere, a note detailing the resolution should be put in the investigator's study file.

Of course, the study sponsor may require other documentation or requirements that are study specific.

Record Retention

The CRC should discuss record retention with the CRA. The record retention requirements should have been established and agreed upon at the

FAQ

We have some boxes of old study papers that have been sitting in our storage room for years. Can we get rid of them? We need the space.

Contact the sponsor first. You should not dispose of study records without the concurrence of the sponsor; this is usually in the written contract. If you no longer have room for the materials and the sponsor does not want them destroyed, the sponsor may assist by arranging for off-site storage.

SIV. Not only do the records need to be stored and maintained, but there also must be a record of where they are stored. So the CRA usually collects the location of where the documents will be stored and documents this in their monitoring visit report. According to the regulations, records must be kept for two years after the NDA is approved for marketing or, if an NDA is not filed or is disapproved, for two years after the investigation is discontinued and the FDA notified. However, most sponsors expect the investigator to retain all study records until notified by the sponsor that they may be disposed of; this will usually be in the contract the investigator signed before starting the study.

The site may want to bill the sponsor an annual storage fee; this can be negotiated with the overall study grant or it might be negotiated at the end of the study. If the site is going to move documents, the CTA requires them to notify the sponsor of the new location. ICH E6 (R2) requires the investigator to carefully store records and communicate with the sponsor. Sites do not always keep study records as long as they should. Years go by and circumstances change—they run short of storage space, move to a new facility or just don't think they need to "keep all that old stuff" around any longer. Unfortunately, these records may be needed years after the study has ended for inspection or audit. For example, the sponsor may decide to file a new application based in part on old studies. When the FDA visits investigative sites as part of the NDA review process, it will expect to see all the documents in place, even if the study was conducted many years earlier. It would be an embarrassment to the investigator if he or she has thrown them away, and it may have a negative impact on the sponsor's NDA.

It is recommended that the boxes in which study information is filed be labeled on the outside "DO NOT DESTROY," with the names of both the investigator and the sponsor as contacts for questions about them. Sometimes sites scan all records and store them electronically. This must be supported by a procedure to ensure compliance and protection of the documentation. If there is some reason a site can no longer maintain the records, the site should contact the sponsor. In most cases, the sponsor will arrange storage for these materials so that they are not destroyed.

Post-Study Lessons Learned

After a clinical trial has been completed, it is beneficial for an investigator to have a post-study evaluation meeting that includes all site personnel who were involved in the study. The study coordinator may be the one to organize and facilitate the meeting. During the meeting, the study should be critically evaluated in terms of enrollment, procedures, successful completion and financial viability. What went well, what did not? What are some opportunities for improvement?

Before the evaluation, the investigator and/or the CRC should compile a summary of pertinent data from the study. The summary should include:

- Number of subjects
    - Screened
    - Enrolled
    - Completing
- Timeframe for enrollment, completion
- Serious adverse events
- Summary of problems encountered, protocol violation, changes to the research, etc.
- Any other pertinent information.

A copy of the summary, plus the pre-study assessment sheets, should be sent to all of the people on the site's study team, including the investigator, sub-investigator, CRC(s) and other involved personnel. Everyone should be requested to review the material before meeting for the actual post-study evaluation and critique.

The investigator or delegate will also want to review the grant and costs associated with the study to determine if it actually was economically feasible to do the project. If not, perhaps budget assumptions will need to be adjusted for future work.

During the meeting, the group should discuss and determine what went well during the study and what did not. They also should check the validity of the initial assessments that were made before agreeing to do the study (from the Protocol Feasibility Assessment Checklist in Appendix D). Finally, the group will want to determine where consistent improvements can be made in the future. The Post-Study Critique Worksheet found in Appendix D is a useful tool for this review. Once it is completed, it can be filed for future reference.

By the end of the post-study evaluation session, the group should have a good handle on how the study went, whether or not it was a good fit for the site, if it was beneficial for the subjects involved, if the workload was manageable and appropriate and if the study was financially beneficial. The last determinations to be made should be:

- Was the overall study experience favorable?
- Would we like to work with this sponsor again?

By completing a post-study evaluation after each clinical trial, the investigator and CRC will be more adept at picking those projects that are best suited to the site in the future. This evaluation will also show where to make needed changes or adjustments in site procedures for increased efficiencies in conducting clinical trials.

A post-study critique should be done at the completion of each study conducted by a site.

Summary and Key Points

The study closeout is usually a welcome event. The sponsor and site are moving on to other projects. The skill set of the CRC (organization, communication and attention to detail) can positively contribute to a smooth closeout. Timely answering of queries and filing of study documents are essential. Closing the study with the source data and the essential documents supporting the ALCOAC principles means a smoother closeout, which leaves the CRC's site audit ready and without the need to spend precious time on old and unresolved issues.

Key Points:

- Conducting lessons learned sessions are very beneficial for quality system improvements.
- Record retention must be clear and followed.
- Changes in document storage needs to be reported to the sponsor.
- Closeout of a study can be for several reasons.
- Study closeout might not need to happen on-site if there has been monitoring of essential documents and data.

CHAPTER FOURTEEN

Adverse Events and Safety Monitoring

In this chapter, we will discuss adverse events (AEs) and safety monitoring. It is critical that adverse events are collected during clinical trials, for the accuracy of the study results, protection of the subjects enrolled in the trial and proper use of the drug once it is marketed.

Reporting on safety during a clinical trial is one of the most important tasks the investigator and the CRC perform. At the same time, safety reporting is one of the most difficult things for the site study team to do adequately. There often are misunderstandings about what is necessary for documenting and reporting on safety issues in clinical trials, stemming at least in part from the differences in clinical studies as compared to clinical practice. Also, although the regulations charge the investigator with protecting the rights, safety and well-being of subjects in trials, they don't give much information about actual safety reporting. We will look at the regulations and some helpful guidance in detail.

Drug Regulations and Definitions

21 CFR 312.64 (Investigator Reports) requires investigators to report AEs during clinical trials. It states:

> ***Safety reports***. *An investigator must immediately report to the sponsor any serious adverse event, whether or not considered drug related, including those listed in the protocol or investigator brochure and must include an assessment of whether there is a reasonable possibility that the drug caused the event. Study endpoints that are serious adverse events (e.g., allcause mortality) must be reported in accordance*

with the protocol unless there is evidence suggesting a causal relationship between the drug and the event (e.g., death from anaphylaxis). In that case, the investigator must immediately report the event to the sponsor. The investigator must record nonserious adverse events and report them to the sponsor according to the timetable for reporting specified in the protocol.

By signing Form FDA 1572, the Statement of Investigator, the investigator commits to reporting to the sponsor study subject AEs that occur during the course of a trial, in accordance with 21 CFR 312.64.

ICH E6 has more detailed information. In the glossary there are many helpful definitions. The following are some of those definitions and associated key concepts that are important for a CRC to be familiar with and apply when working on any clinical trial. Remember that GCP requirements can vary from one study to the next regarding study-specific and local requirements. The following definitions and concepts are a baseline. There can be additional requirements for a study as long as they are less strict as the regulation.

Adverse Drug Reaction (ADR) Section 1.1

In the pre-approval clinical experience with a new medicinal product or its new usages, particularly as the therapeutic dose(s) may not be established: all noxious and unintended responses to a medicinal product related to any dose should be considered adverse drug reactions. The phrase responses to a medicinal product means that a causal relationship between a medicinal product and an adverse event is at least a reasonable possibility, i.e., the relationship cannot be ruled out.

Regarding marketed medicinal products: a response to a drug which is noxious and unintended and which occurs at doses normally used in man for prophylaxis, diagnosis, or therapy of diseases or for modification of physiological function (see the ICH Guideline for Clinical Safety Data Management: Definitions and Standards for Expedited Reporting).

Adverse Event (AE) Section 1.2

Any untoward medical occurrence in a patient or clinical investigation subject administered a pharmaceutical product and which does not necessarily have a causal relationship with this treatment. An adverse event (AE) can therefore be any unfavourable and unintended sign (including an abnormal laboratory finding), symptom, or disease temporally associated with the use of a medicinal (investigational) product, whether or not related to the medicinal (investigational) product (see the ICH Guideline for Clinical Safety Data Management: Definitions and Standards for Expedited Reporting).

Serious Adverse Event (SAE) or Serious Adverse Drug Reaction (Serious ADR) Section 1.50

Any untoward medical occurrence that at any dose:

- *Results in death,*
- *Is life-threatening,*
- *Requires inpatient hospitalization or prolongation of existing hospitalization,*
- *Results in persistent or significant disability/incapacity*
- *Is a congenital anomaly/birth defect.*

It is important to distinguish between the terms "serious" and "severe." The term "serious" is used with the definition above and categorizes events (i.e., either they meet the definition for serious or they don't). The term "severe" refers to the intensity of the event and can be used with any event, without regard to whether or not it meets the criteria for being classified as "serious." For example, a subject can have a severe headache, but it is not a serious event.

Other Terminology Related to Safety Reporting

Related to or Associated with the Drug: This is defined to mean that there is a reasonable possibility that the event could have been caused by the investigational product.

Expected/Unexpected: An expected event is one for which the specificity and severity of the event are consistent with the information in the investigator brochure or labeling for the product. Unexpected events are all others.

Life Threatening: A life-threatening event is one in which the patient is in immediate danger of death unless intervention is done. It does not mean the patient may die at some time in the future from the event or may have died if the event had been more serious or specific.

Significant Disability: A significant disability is one that causes substantial disruption to the person's normal life and activity.

ICH E6 also contains section (4.11.1) on investigator safety reporting. In this section, it states that:

> *All serious adverse events (SAEs) should be reported immediately to the sponsor except for those SAEs that the protocol or other document (e.g., Investigator's Brochure) identifies as not needing immediate reporting. The immediate reports should be followed promptly by detailed, written reports. The immediate and follow-up reports should identify subjects by unique code numbers assigned to the trial subjects rather than by the subjects' names, personal identification numbers, and/or*

addresses. The investigator should also comply with the applicable regulatory requirement(s) related to the reporting of unexpected serious adverse drug reactions to the regulatory authority(ies) and the IRB/IEC.

The investigator must report SAEs to the sponsor immediately per the protocol and at minimum report SAEs not described as expected in the Investigator's Brochure (IB). It is common that some sponsors will want all SAEs, expected or not, reported to them. The investigator and the CRC must comply with the strictest requirements. Additionally, the investigator should comply with regulatory requirements for reporting SAEs to regulatory authorities and the IRB.

In clinical studies, sponsors are required to report to the FDA suspected unexpected, serious, adverse reactions (SUSARs) (related to the study drug) that are fatal or life threatening by telephone and/or facsimile within seven calendar days. For all other types of events, the reporting time frame is 15 calendar days. The timeline for reporting starts at the time the sponsor becomes aware of the event, including the study sponsor or CRO monitor. Once the investigator has notified the sponsor of an SAE, the sponsor's reporting clock starts. The sponsor must make the expectedness determination that is not part of the investigator's responsibility even though it has access to the IB, but the sponsor has much more recent information about any events globally, so it is in a better position to make that judgment.

A written report detailing all of the information the sponsor has about the SUSAR event is sent to the FDA within a 15-day time period. The sponsor also must send out IND Safety Reports (SUSAR reports), which will be covered later in this chapter.

Besides ICH E6, refer to ICH E2A, *Clinical Safety Data Management: Definitions and Standards for Expedited Reporting*. Additionally, refer to the FDA 2012 guideline: *Safety Reporting Requirements for INDs and BA/BE Studies* for additional definitions and examples.

Adverse Events in Clinical Trials

The adverse events with which CRCs will be involved with most are those collected during clinical trials of drugs not yet marketed, but still in the development process. In these types of studies, all AEs that occur during studies are documented in the subjects' source documents and then transcribed into the sponsor's study CRF. Some protocols, especially in postmarketing studies, may require that only certain AEs are placed into the CRF, but the investigator is required to document all observations and changes related the subject's time on the clinical trial. The CRC should be familiar with the study-specific requirements for a trial. Events that are documented need to be further classified by the definitions for serious, related and severity, as described earlier.

Most of the AEs seen during clinical trials will not be serious, as defined in the regulations. For some studies we can anticipate more frequent SAEs,

Table 1: Differences between clinical trials and marketed use of a product

Clinical Trials	Marketed Use
• Relatively small number of patients	• Millions of patients
• Tight control	• No control
• Extra care	• Standard care
• Highly-trained physicians	• Any physicians
• Narrow patient population	• Anyone prescribed the drug

an example of which is a study with a seriously ill study population that is commonly in and out of the hospital. In general, non-serious adverse events will be recorded by the CRC in the CRF and transmitted to the sponsor for review and analysis. Additionally, CRAs commonly review AEs during regular monitoring visits or remotely through the eCRF. Remember that non-serious events can be severe in intensity but still not meet the definition of serious. Also, monitoring visits can be triggered by a lack of or an abundance of AEs at a site. There is an expectation per-study around AEs per subject based on what is known, so when a site performs significantly differently than the rest of the majority of the sites, it usually means an assessment needs to occur, root cause needs to be determined and interventions to address any gaps in safety reporting need to be considered. This is an example of sponsor safety surveillance which is a combination on-site and remote with automation.

In most cases, sponsors want all SAEs that occur during a trial to be reported by the investigator per the protocol. The timing of the reporting requirements starts when the investigator has determined that the event is serious. This is for two reasons: first, to ensure the continued safety of subjects in the trial; and second, to help the sponsor meet the reporting requirements for the FDA.

There are some instances where a sponsor does not require all SAEs be reported. The regulations note that related SAEs be immediately reported. Many sponsors are on the conservative side and require that all be expedited to them, as noted above, but there are certain studies where the amount of SAEs expected is high and the criteria of expedited SAEs is more specific, e.g., related to the study drug or not related to the disease exacerbation. This will be detailed in the protocol. The investigator and the CRC must be very familiar with the requirements. If there are any questions in regard to the reporting criteria, these should be clarified and documented for the whole site study team. If the sponsor does not provide documentation, then the CRC can facilitate that documentation and the investigator signs off.

The investigator must ensure that all AEs are documented and then reported, as required by the sponsor.

Safety Reporting Sections in Protocols

Every protocol for a clinical trial should contain a detailed plan for the collection and reporting of all AEs, both serious and non-serious. There are several key items that should be included.

Definitions

The protocol should include the regulatory definitions for an adverse event and a serious adverse event, as well as the definitions for related/associated and for expected/unexpected events.

Sources of AEs

In general, the standard sources of all AEs will be the investigator reporting:

- All directly observed events. [I see you have a rash on your arm...]
- Events elicited from the subject by means of a general non-directive question. [Have you had any problems with your health since you were here the last time?] The use of a specific question allows the sponsor to standardize procedures across all sites. A non-directive question does not prompt a subject to answer in a specific way. Asking subjects about specific events [Have you had any headaches?], although appropriate in some studies, will lead to a higher reporting rate for the specific event than a non-directive question.
- Events spontaneously volunteered by the study subject. [You know, Doc, ever since I started taking these pills, I have had an upset stomach.]
- Laboratory, EKG or other test results that meet protocol requirements for classification as adverse events. [Example: laboratory values more than 10% outside the normal range.]
- Events that led to a healthcare provider visit and medical records are requested. [Example: post-hospitalization or surgery.]

Event Collection Periods

The study periods during which AEs will be collected should be specified. Some protocols require AEs to be collected during a pre-treatment period as baseline data, while others require collection only during active treatment. It also is quite common to collect AEs during a post-treatment follow-up period. Adverse events are always collected during the entire period that a subject is on or could be on (in the case of blinded trials), the investigational product or study drug.

Diaries and Other Data Collection Instruments

Whenever data collection instruments are used that may elicit information about AEs (e.g., quality of life questionnaires, patient diaries), the methods for handling these events should be specified in the protocol. Some data collection devices are linked directly to the CRF but may lack any evaluation or other important information about the AE that needs to be in the source and later transcribed or verified in the CRF. Paper diaries may offer a subject a place to write comments; sometimes those comments link to an adverse event. This needs to be assessed by the CRC and evaluated by the investigator for relationship to the study drug or not.

Notice that the patient in the example in Table 2 was filling in the times she took her investigational medication, but she also added some additional information—the migraine headache. Certainly, the study site personnel would want to know about the migraine, but this is not the place for it to be recorded. The CRC will need to ensure that this event is recorded on the appropriate AE CRFs and not missed.

Table 2: Example: Patient Diary

ACMEPHARMA STUDY 1234 — Patient Diary—Week 4

Name: ____________________ Betsy Smith______

Each day, please enter the time you took your study medication. Remember, you should always take one pill just before breakfast (about 8:00 am) and two pills before dinner (about 6:00 pm).

Sunday	Date:	2/2/10		
	Morning dose time		am	
	Evening dose time		pm	
Monday	Date:			
	Morning dose time		am	
	Evening dose time		pm	
Tuesday	Date:			
	Morning dose time	8	am	
	Evening dose time	6	pm	migraine—felt dizzy

Unresolved Adverse Events

Sometimes AEs that occur during a study are unresolved at the time the subject's study participation ends. The protocol should state what is to be done in this case. Usually serious AEs are followed to resolution, that is, until they resolve, disappear or become stable. There is often a time period during which any events that are ongoing at the end of the study are followed. Thirty days is a frequently used time period, but it varies depending on the compound, its half-life, the length of time the subject was in the trial and the complexity of the diagnosis and protocol.

Exposure in Utero

If women of child-bearing potential are allowed entry into the trial, the protocol should include instructions for reporting exposure *in utero* and the subsequent outcome of the pregnancy. In general, the investigator will be required to follow up on any cases of pregnancy that occur during the study until the child is born or the pregnancy is terminated. There is usually no requirement for interim visits throughout the pregnancy, just an assurance that the subject will be contacted periodically to determine the outcome. Each sponsor has a procedure to manage such a scenario. A pregnancy itself is not an AE or SAE unless described as such in the protocol.

Timely Notification

The sponsor will want to be notified of serious events by the investigator in a timely manner, usually within 24 hours. It is extremely important that the investigator notify the sponsor per protocol of a serious adverse event as soon as possible, even if all details are not yet available. Additional details can be reported as they become available; the initial report never should be delayed while awaiting more information.

An investigator may not know about an event for some time after it has occurred, especially if he or she is not the subject's primary physician. The study site may not know about the event until the subject comes in for his or her next appointment or fails to show up for the appointment because of the event. However, the investigator should inform the sponsor of the event as soon as he or she becomes aware of it. Non-serious AEs also are reported to the sponsor. This reporting is done by way of the case report form and the regular data collection process per protocol.

Devices

In device trials, unanticipated adverse device effects (UADEs) are expedited reports from the investigator. A UADE is defined as any serious adverse device effect on the health or safety or any life-threatening problem or death caused by, or associated with, a device, if that effect, problem or death was not previously identified in nature, severity or degree of incidence in the investigational plan or application. If a UADE occurs, the investigator is required to report the event to the sponsor within 10 working days. Note that in device, commonly not all AEs are reported to the sponsor. Neither are SAEs (related or not). Also, the investigator is required to assess whether the event was anticipated or not. Remember that in drug expectedness, an assessment is done by the sponsor and not the investigator. In devices, it is in the regulations that the investigator do the initial evaluation to determine UADE.

Once reported, the sponsor must make an assessment whether it agrees, but they must investigate and report the UADE to the FDA within 10 working days of receipt and to all participating investigators and all reviewing IRBs. Notice the difference from drug trials, in which the investigator notifies the IRB, and for device, in which the sponsor notifies the IRB.

If the sponsor determines that the device UADE presents an unreasonable risk to subjects, it must terminate all of its investigations, or at least the ones that present the risk, as soon as possible, but at least within five days after making the determination.

Investigator Reporting Responsibilities

Investigators are required to collect, assess and report all adverse events that occur during a trial. The following information is usually gathered for each event: onset (date/time), duration, severity (mild, moderate, severe), relationship to the study drug and whether or not it is serious. All events are to be recorded on the CRF. In addition, if an event is serious, the investigator usually is expected to report it to the sponsor quickly (e.g., within 24 hours).

Not only must the investigator report AEs to the sponsor, but he or she also has a requirement to report these events to the IRB in the manner in which the IRB has requested. As with sponsors, some IRBs will want notification of all serious events while others will want to hear only about events that are serious and related, or only those that are serious, related and unexpected. For example, many IRBs do not want each individual IND safety report. The IRB will tell the investigator what is expected and the report timing and mechanisms. It is important that the investigator notify the IRB according to the rules the IRB has established.

The study coordinator supports the investigator on many of these activities. It is essential that the investigator has delegated the responsibility to the CRC when appropriate, prior to the CRC performing the activities. The CRC must also have the training and experience to conduct the safety evaluation tasks. Delegation must be documented in the study file and all activities must be documented in the subject source documents.

Evaluation of an AE's causality must be done by a medically qualified individual, commonly the investigator, but CRC who has the qualifications, would be able to evaluate an AE's relationship to the study product. The investigator and CRC should always follow the protocol.

Differences Between Clinical Studies and Clinical Practice

One reason AE reporting is fraught with problems stems from the fact that clinical practice and clinical research are not the same thing, and it is easy to get the two confused when it comes to safety reporting. It often is confusing for investigators and CRCs to realize that the definitions used for adverse event reporting in trials are regulatory definitions, not clinical definitions. An investigator and a CRC must understand the definitions and reporting requirements before subjects are enrolled.

In studies, the investigator has a dual role as a medical expert and investigator. It is the investigator's duty to act in the best interest of the subject while on the study and at the same time, to perform good research. These duties are not necessarily in conflict, but there are differences in the roles that must be understood.

Some examples of these differences are the following:

- Concomitant medications that normally might be prescribed for a patient may not be allowed under the protocol.

- Treatment periods may be longer or shorter under the protocol than are usual in general practice.
- AEs that are "normal" for the disease usually must be reported under study rules.

A worsening or progression of the disease may or may not be reported as an adverse event. For example, a worsening of anxiety in an anxiety trial usually would require reporting, while a progression of Alzheimer's disease in an Alzheimer's trial might not be reported, as this is a progressive disease.

The investigator must remember his or her regulatory responsibilities with respect to conducting trials, which include proper reporting of adverse events. He or she also is bound by the contract with the sponsor, and most contracts require the investigator to report adverse events as mandated by the regulations. Additionally, the well-being of the subject is paramount, and the investigator must ensure adequate medical care, even when adverse events that occur are not related to the disease being studied (intercurrent illnesses). If the investigator is not qualified to treat the events, then the investigator must refer the subject outside the study to support continuation of care. Therefore, the awareness of both study requirements and ensuring quality care must be met and balanced.

Assessing the Relationship of an AE to the Study Drug

Investigators usually are asked to assess the relationship between an adverse event and the investigational product by picking the term that best characterizes the relationship of the adverse event to the investigational product. The choices are commonly in the order of not related, probably not related, possibly related, probably related, definitely related. Clear documentation of this assessment is important to support the data collected. The following are some of the characteristics of the events and situations pre and post that can support the investigator's decision related to causality.

Temporal Relationship

Does the timing of taking the investigational drug make sense in relationship to the timing of the event? For example, assume the subject takes the drug, comes in two days later and is diagnosed with cancer. The cancer is probably not related because it occurred too soon after taking the study drug. Or, assume a subject has been taking the study drug without a problem but develops an AE just after the dose was titrated upward; in this case, the event might well be related to the drug.

Known Patterns of Reaction

Assume the study drug causes a distinctive rash, and a study subject develops that type of rash. Chances are good that the rash is related to the study drug. Is there something else that would explain the occurrence of the event? For example, assume the subject is allergic to chocolate, but couldn't resist that piece of devil's food chocolate birthday cake last night. He ate some and ended up with hives. The hives are probably not related to the study drug, but to the chocolate.

Does it Make Sense?

Assume a study subject suffers from regular migraines, takes the study drug and has a migraine. It's probably not related. However, assume the subject usually has one or two migraines a month, but ever since starting the study drug has them every two or three days. They are probably related to the study drug. This might, in fact, be reported as an exacerbation of a previously existing medical condition, e.g., a change in severity. Is this logical?

Dechallenge/Rechallenge

In this scenario, the subject has an AE. The study drug is stopped (the dechallenge), and the event stops. The study drug is restarted (rechallenge), and the event occurs again. It is probably related to the drug under study. This is a very definitive test, but it may not be done unless allowed in the protocol. Although an investigator may stop a study drug (dechallenge) at any time it is deemed appropriate, he or she may not restart it (rechallenge) unless allowed by the protocol or after discussion with, and agreement by, the sponsor.

Common Reporting Problems

There are a number of common misunderstandings that result in incorrect adverse event reporting. Many of these errors can be avoided if the sponsor takes time to clarify them to site personnel in advance. One of these misunderstandings involves symptoms vs. a syndrome. Usually, sponsors want a syndrome reported rather than the individual symptoms when possible; for example, flu versus cough, sniffles and sore throat all reported separately. But a syndrome is a diagnosis and must be assessed and documented by someone that is medically qualified, e.g., M.D.

Another common error is the reporting of a procedure, as opposed to reporting the disease/condition that resulted in the procedure. An example of this is reporting a coronary bypass as the event, instead of reporting the heart condition (e.g., myocardial infarction) that necessitated the bypass.

Changes in severity are frequently reported incorrectly, or not at all. The general convention is that if an event worsens in severity, it is reported as a new event, even if the event is in the pre-study history for the subject. Some protocols also require the reporting of changes in events when the change is for the better.

It is critical for the investigator and the CRC to understand the distinction between the terms "serious" and "severe," as "severe" refers to the intensity of an event, without regard to whether or not it meets the criteria for being classified as "serious."

The CRC significantly impacts the safety reporting for a study conducted at the site. The investigator must oversee the CRC to be sure the solicitation and documentation of AEs is done correctly. A CRC must be sure he or she is delegated these tasks appropriately. Clarity of the protocol requirements is critical. Quality documentation of safety reporting management is essential.

Summary and Key Points

The CRC has an important role in AE solicitation, documentation, training, follow-up and more. A CRC must be clear on what appropriate delegated activities are. Depending on the CRC credentials, he or she may or may not be able to evaluate AEs for causality for the relationship to the study product. This activity takes a medically qualified individual that can diagnose, many times a medical doctor but may be a physician's assistant or nurse practitioner. Clarity of roles and responsibility should be defined at the beginning of the study and the CRC should escalate to the investigator any time the requirements seem to be followed or monitored inconsistently. Subject safety and quality data are at stake and, again, the CRC's role is pivotal.

Key Points:

- Safety reporting requires quality documentation by the appropriate site personnel, adverse event name, relationship, causality, start and stop and follow-up.
- The protocol needs to be specific on the definitions of reporting requirements and what needs to be reported in an expedited fashion.
- Timely reporting is critical to the sponsor from the site.
- Device has some differences from drug in reporting timelines, 10 working days versus 7 or 15 calendars days for drugs for events that are serious, related and unexpected/unanticipated.

Case Study: Caught in the Middle with Adverse Events

"Help," the CRC said to the CRA during a monitoring visit for a study looking at a potential new drug for osteoarthritis. "You and my investigator are telling me different things about what adverse events need to be reported. I'm caught in the middle, and I don't like it."

The CRC explained that she understood from the investigator's meeting that all events needed to be reported during the trial, but the investigator told her this was silly and that they certainly wouldn't do that. He told her that it was too time-consuming to report things that weren't related to the trial or things they would see in their patients even if they weren't in the trial (e.g., increased knee pain in a patient with osteoarthritis). "Why would we report colds in an arthritis study?" he told the coordinator. "That just doesn't make sense, and I'm not going to do it."

What to do?

First, the CRA told the CRC she would be happy to talk with the investigator and the CRC together about the requirements for adverse event reporting in clinical trials. Here are the points she covered during this discussion:

- Clinical trials and clinical practice are not the same. In clinical trials, we know very little about the substances we are putting into people, so we need to collect data on everything that happens to them. There might be a particular event that each involved investigator has seen, and no one thought it was related to the drug, but when the sponsor looked at events over all sites and did an analysis, it was related.
- Adverse event collection is required by regulation and ICH GCPs.
- The protocol is very specific about the procedures for collecting events and specifies that all events occurring during the trial must be collected. When the investigator agreed to do the study, and to follow the protocol, he agreed to do this.
- When the investigator signed the 1572 form, he agreed to "report to the sponsor adverse experiences that occur in the course of the investigation in accordance with 21 CFR312.64." He also agreed to "conduct the study in accordance with the relevant, current protocol."

Usually, when this kind of situation occurs, the investigator just isn't fully aware of the relevant responsibilities and will make the necessary changes after these things are pointed out. If this doesn't happen, what are the next steps to secure compliance?

The next step is for the CRA to alert management. Probably, the sponsor's medical monitor, and perhaps a regulatory associate, will call the investigator for further discussion. If the investigator still will not agree to the appropriate reporting of AEs, the site may have to be closed.

CHAPTER FIFTEEN

Audits and Inspections

During the clinical development process, the FDA may conduct inspections of investigators, sponsors and IRBs clinical trial activities associated with their regulatory obligations. Inspection programs are a regulatory authority's process for ensuring that the regulations they enforce are followed. The FDA inspection program is called the Bioresearch Monitoring Program (BIMO) and includes regulatory audits of sponsors, IRBs, investigators and other group types not applicable to this book. These inspections can be study-focused and/or compliance-focused. Sponsors, IRBs and investigators should remain audit ready to decrease the risk of regulatory sanctions. The ultimate goal of the BIMO program is to support human subject protection and quality data.

Since part of the responsibilities of sponsors and IRBs is to oversee the investigator's performance related to quality data and human subjects protections, the sponsor and IRB may audit investigative sites to support their regulatory responsibilities and support audit readiness. In this chapter we will discuss investigator inspections and audits, including the role of the CRC.

Sponsor Audits of Investigative Sites

There are two main purposes for a sponsor to audit a study site. The most common reason is to ensure that the investigator is complying with the regulations while conducting a study and that everything is in order in case of an FDA inspection. The second reason is that there is evidence the site is out of GCP compliance, and the sponsor wants to ensure that the investigator has an adequate corrective and preventive action plan in place, is following it and it is effective.

A sponsor's right to audit a site is based on both the regulations and the contractual agreement between the investigator and the sponsor. Most contracts will state that the investigator agrees the sponsor may conduct audits of the site. The regulations under which sponsor audits are loosely covered are found in 21 CFR 312.56(a)(b), which states:

> *"(a) The sponsor shall monitor the progress of all clinical investigations being conducted under its IND," and "(b) A sponsor who discovers that an investigator is not complying with the signed agreement (Form FDA 1572), the general investigational plan or the requirements of this part or other applicable parts shall promptly either secure compliance or discontinue shipments of the investigational new drug to the investigator and end the investigator's participation in the investigation."*

If the sponsor knows or suspects that a site will be audited by the FDA, a routine audit may be conducted, either while the study is in process or after it has been completed and during the NDA/PMA review period. The sponsor knows the FDA will inspect some sites during its review of the NDA, so the sponsor will focus on the sites that are logical for the FDA to pick, such as high enrollers. When an investigator has contributed a significant number of subjects for a sponsor's primary registration study, the chances of an audit by the FDA are relatively high.

For a sponsor audit, the sponsor will send in an audit team that will follow the same inspection plan used by the FDA. This inspection plan can be found in the FDA *Compliance Program Guidance Manual for Clinical Investigators* (Program 7348.811).

A written report of sponsor audit results is not often given to the investigator. Instead the sponsor monitor completes a follow-up of any audit findings and facilitates any action items for sites. This ensures that the FDA inspectors do not have access to sponsor audit findings as the site and any issues are addressed and documented between the sponsor monitor and investigator.

IRB Audits of Investigative Sites

IRBs also may audit affiliated sites for a particular trial. There are many reasons why an IRB might audit an investigator, e.g., the IRB is not located nearby and want to be assured that the site is managing studies correctly or visit if there is reason to think the site has ethics or compliance deviations. IRBs are required to report to the FDA any instances of unanticipated problems with investigators involving risks to human subjects, serious or continuing noncompliance with the regulations or IRB requirements, or any suspension or termination of IRB approval.

FDA Inspections of Investigative Sites

The FDA conducts two main types of inspections of investigators: study-related and investigator-related. For either study or investigator-related audits, the purpose is threefold:

1. To determine the validity and integrity of the data
2. To assess adherence to regulations and guidelines
3. To determine that the rights and safety of the human subjects were properly protected.

> **FAQ**
>
> **What are our chances of being inspected by the FDA?**
>
> Not very high, as it inspects only a few hundred sites each year. However, if your study is a primary efficacy study for an NDA and you were among the top enrolling sites, your chances are much higher. They are also higher if there is a suspicion of regulatory non-compliance or other major problems at your site. Remember—if you do everything correctly during a study and follow all of the regulations, you do not have to worry about an inspection.

Study-Related Audits

Study-related inspections are almost always conducted on the studies that are important to an NDA/PMA that has been submitted to the FDA. These studies are the primary efficacy studies on which a sponsor relies to show that the product works and should be approved for marketing.

The sites selected for inspection are usually those that contributed the most data to the application, either by high enrollment or by conducting multiple studies. Because of this, sponsors usually have a reasonable idea of which sites have a high probability of being audited. The sponsor also knows that studies will be inspected during the NDA/PMA review time, which, for an NDA, is now six months or less for a Fast Track product and one year or less for all others from the date the FDA receives the application. The primary efficacy studies are closed at this point, as the trials are complete and analyzed before being submitted; in fact, they may have been closed for quite some time.

The sponsor usually will alert those sites that are most likely to be inspected. Often, CRAs are sent to the sites with high probability of being audited to ensure that all study materials are available and organized for FDA review. Also, a site should inform the sponsor when it is contacted by the FDA to schedule an audit, in which case the sponsor may send the CRA in to help the site prepare. If missing documents or other problems are found during this review, the situation may be able to be remedied before an FDA audit occurs.

Investigator-Related Inspections

Investigator-related inspections are initiated for a variety of reasons, many of which are listed below:

- Investigators have done a large number of studies or have done work outside their specialty areas.
- An investigator has done a pivotal study that is critical to a new product application and it merits extra attention.
- The safety or efficacy findings of an investigator are inconsistent with the results from other investigators working with the same test product.
- The sponsor or IRB has notified the FDA about serious problems or concerns at the site.
- A subject has complained about the protocol or subject rights violations at the site.
- There were an unexpected number of subjects with the diagnosis under study, given the location of the study.
- Enrollment at the site was much more rapid than expected.
- The study and investigator were highly publicized in the media.
- Any other reason that piques the curiosity of the agency.

Site Audit Preparation

The best preparation for an audit is for the site to have done things correctly to begin with, in which case an audit will reveal no significant problems. However, once an audit is scheduled, the site should prepare by amassing all study documents in one easy-to-get-to place and by reviewing them to be sure everything is accounted for, complete and well organized. The study documents that should be available for review include all informed consent forms, subject source documents, CRFs and the study regulatory file. When an inspector asks to see a document, the site should be able to retrieve it easily and quickly.

A site's audit readiness is also accomplished by identifying and managing issues throughout the study. This involves focusing on activities that are essential for subject safety and data integrity that we have discussed in all the chapters. When there are issues in these areas, e.g., documentation, IP accountability, AE reporting, source documentation, informed consent and IRB communications, the effective management is critical to audit readiness. Issues need to be found early. When the issue is significant as defined by the protocol, sponsor, IRB and GCP, the investigator is expected to identify the root cause of the issue and develop an action plan to correct and prevent the recurrence. Additionally, the investigator needs to oversee that the action plan was effective. Some of the issues in that management process may be delegated to other study team members, like the CRC. The study works with the sponsor monitor to ensure he or she is informed and kept up-to-date on the progress of the action plan. A monitor may find issues that were not discovered by the site study team. It is better if the site is aware of issues as soon as possible. The site works with the sponsor as a team to ensure compliance and good documentation of the efforts. Significant issues must be reported by the investigator to the reviewing IRB for the study. The IRB may have additional actions that the investigator may have to do related to subject safety. Ultimately, the investigator wants to show improvement and not repeating issues. So during an audit, the FDA would confirm the issue and the adequacy of the action plan. There are significant negative consequences for not effectively managing issues that matter.

The Inspection Process

The first step in the inspection process is notification to the site. The FDA field investigator usually contacts the site by telephone to arrange a mutually acceptable time for the visit within a specific period of time. Sites are usually given 72 hours to five days notice; it is acceptable to negotiate a delay in the visit date, as long as the investigator has a good reason and the time is not lengthened too much.

If the inspection is investigator-related, and if the FDA has concerns about subject safety or compliance, the time between the notification and the visit probably will be very short and delays will not be acceptable. The FDA will reveal the study(ies) being inspected and, if asked, may provide more details about the inspection and how long the inspection is expected to last. If there are serious concerns, the FDA may appear at the site without advance notice. Most sponsors stipulate in the investigator contract that they notify the sponsor immediately of an impending inspection.

The site should have an inspection policy and perform some mock inspection drills. When the FDA arrives, the receptionist should ask for identification (photo ID) and contact the appropriate people, per policy. The FDA field investigator will present credentials (a photo ID) and a Notice of Inspections (Form FDA-482).

The role of the investigator and the CRC in the audit is to be present and provide the FDA representative with a space to work. The site should not leave the FDA representative unattended. Any copies requested should be made for the representative and someone should take notes of everything requested by and provided to the FDA representative.

The investigator and CRC should be polite, courteous, cooperative and reasonable when interacting with the FDA inspector; antagonism is inappropriate and will undoubtedly be regretted later. The investigator should provide all the materials/documents the FDA inspector requests but should never give the inspector free access to the files. All questions should be answered, but extra information should not be volunteered. The inspector knows what

FAQ

Can FDA auditors ask to see anything they want to see?

Yes. But give the auditor only what he or she requests. Do not give the auditor free rein to look at any and all of your files.

he or she is asking for. Although the responsibility for the audit remains with the investigator, it usually is the CRC or the site's QA staff who prepares the materials for the inspection. Both the investigator and the CRC usually will interact with the FDA.

Site personnel should not offer the inspector any gifts or food. The FDA representative should be escorted everywhere. Study information should not be left on desks or computers left on unattended; study binders and supplies should be securely and appropriately stored. There should be a way for the site to announce to the staff that the FDA is on-site so there is an awareness to be on alert and be cautious about conversations and potential for the FDA to ask questions.

During the inspection, the FDA will meet with the investigator, the CRC and any other appropriate study staff, and will review study documents. If people who played substantial roles in the study are no longer working at the site, the investigator should be able to contact them if he or she wishes to talk with them. Two main aspects of the study will be looked at during the inspection: study conduct and study data. According to the FDA guidance, the conduct of the study will be considered by reviewing the following items:

- Who did what study tasks and the degree of delegation of authority
- Where specific aspects of the study were performed
- How and where data were recorded
- How test article accountability was maintained
- How the study was monitored by the sponsor
- How the monitor evaluated the study's progress.

Notice that the monitor (CRA) is mentioned in two of these items. At the very least, you should have the monitor sign a study visit log at each monitoring visit to verify that the site was actually visited. There is an example of a study visit log in Appendix D.

When the inspector audits the study data, he or she will compare a sample of the data that were submitted to the agency with the site records that support the data, i.e., the CRFs and all pertinent source documents, including patient charts, study research records, laboratory reports, other test reports and any other study-specific documentation. Sometimes the FDA will also have copies of the study data from the sponsor. The inspector will pay close attention to:

FAQ

If an FDA auditor is at our site for several days, are we expected to provide lunches and/or dinners?

No. In fact, you should not offer an FDA auditor anything beyond a cup of coffee, etc. An offer of anything beyond this could be misconstrued.

- The diagnosis
- Whether the subjects were properly diagnosed based on their past history
- Subject consenting
- Whether or not the subjects met the protocol inclusion/not the exclusion criteria
- Concomitant medications, especially those that were not allowed
- Appropriate evaluation and follow-up of adverse events.

The FDA may look at data for only a sampling of subjects or, if there appear to be problems, it may look at the data from all subjects. All informed consents and re-consents are usually reviewed.

The length of an FDA inspection depends on the amount of data to review, the findings and the amount of time the FDA inspector has available. As mentioned earlier, the FDA inspector should be asked how long the audit may take, but the investigator or CRC can also ask at the end of each day what the expected duration of the inspection will be and if there were any new findings or questions. The days of the inspection may not be consecutive for the entire period, but rather a day or two at the site at a time until the review is complete.

At the end of the inspection, the FDA will conduct a meeting with the investigator and other appropriate site members, like the CRC, to review the findings. During this meeting, the investigator may ask questions about anything that is not understood and may clarify things that may have been interpreted incorrectly. Sometimes a misunderstanding or negative finding can be explained satisfactorily at this point and will not be included in the follow-up correspondence. If there are failures to fulfill the regulatory responsibilities, the FDA may issue a Form FDA 483 (Notice of Observations) to the investigator. This form will detail the findings that may constitute regulatory compliance violations.

Most sponsors ask that an investigator call them after the FDA finishes and send a summary and/or a copy of the results of the inspections. If the investigator has received a Form FDA 483, the sponsor usually will offer to help the investigator formulate a reply. A reply is not always mandatory. The investigator should also seek legal counsel before sending the FDA any response to violations.

After the Inspection

After the audit is completed, the FDA prepares an Establishment Inspection Report (EIR). This report goes through FDA compliance channels, includes the pre-, during and post-trial documentation, including any investigator response. A classification is assigned to the inspection and noted in the EIR. The investigator will receive a copy of the EIR report usually only if requested through the Freedom of Information Act; most sponsors will request copies for their files as well.

The results of the inspection may take some time to compile depending on the follow-up.

The EIR classifications are:

- **No Action Indicated (NAI).** This is the best outcome and means that no significant deviations from the regulations were found. The clinical investigator is not required to respond to this report (72% of investigator inspections in 2018).
- **Voluntary Action Indicated (VAI).** This report will provide information about findings of deviations from the regulations and GCP. The letter may or may not require a response from the investigator. If a response is required, the letter will specify what is necessary. A contact person also will be listed for any questions. Even if not required, a response can be sent. If a response is promised during the inspection, this has been noted in the EIR and should be done (27% of investigator inspections in 2018).
- **Official Action Indicated (OAI).** This is the most severe inspection result to receive. This report identifies serious deviations from the regulations that require prompt action from the investigator. The FDA also may choose to link a sponsor inspection if it concludes monitoring of the study was deficient. In many cases, this leads to a warning letter, depending on how the investigator responded related to corrective actions taken and planned. In addition, the FDA may take other action, such as regulatory and/or administrative sanctions against the investigator, including restrictions related to performing clinical trials (1% of investigator inspections in 2018).

Results from FDA Inspections

Inspections are conducted by different divisions of the FDA: the Center for Drug Evaluation and Research (CDER), the Center for Device and Radiologic Health (CDRH) and the Center for Biologic Evaluation and Research (CBER). Each of these divisions inspects investigators, sponsors, CROs and IRBs.

Figure 1: FY2018 Clinical Investigator Inspections Classified

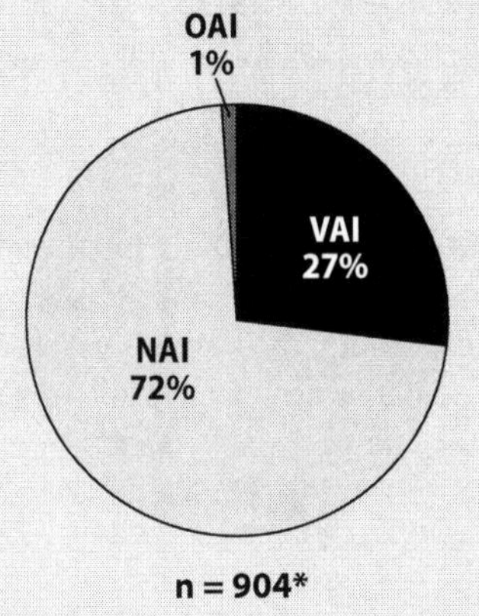

NAI=No Action Indicated; VAI=Voluntary Action Indicated; OAI=Official Action Indicated

***Data includes domestic and international inspections classified in fiscal year 2018**

*Inspections classified in FY18 by CBER, CDER, CDRH and CVM. Some inspections may have occurred in a different FY.

Source: FDA Bioresearch Monitoring Program

CDER, CDHR and CBER conducted 701 investigator inspections in 2017, down from 822 in 2015. The most common inspection findings have not changed in 10 or more years. Common inspection findings of clinical investigations are:

- Failure to follow the regulations and investigational plan
- Failure to follow the protocol
- Inadequate recordkeeping
- Inadequate subject protection, including adverse event and informed consent issues
- Inadequate accountability for the investigational product
- Inadequate communications with the IRB.

To give you an example of the kinds of problems found during inspections, here are two citations from an investigator warning letter from 2016. These quoted paragraphs are excerpted from an actual warning letter, which is posted on the FDA website.

1. You failed to maintain adequate and accurate case histories that record all observations and other data pertinent to the investigation on each individual administered the investigational drug or employed as a control in the investigation [21 CFR 312.62(b)].

As a clinical investigator, you are required to prepare and maintain adequate and accurate case histories that record all observations and other data pertinent to the investigation on each individual administered the investigational drug or employed as a control in the investigation. Case histories include the case report forms and supporting data including, for example, signed and dated consent forms and medical records, including, for example, progress notes of the physician, the individual's hospital chart(s) and the nurse's notes. For Protocol [redacted], case histories include study records of required procedures such as medical history, psychiatric evaluations, physical and neurological examinations and suicide risk assessments. You failed to maintain adequate and accurate case histories when your sub-investigator's name was recorded as having conducted certain required study procedures that, in fact, you or another study employee conducted.

2. You failed to ensure that the investigation was conducted according to the investigational plan [21 CFR 312.60].

   As a clinical investigator, you are required to ensure that your clinical studies are conducted in accordance with the investigational plan. The investigational plan for Protocol [redacted] required you to ensure that study subjects met the protocol inclusion and exclusion criteria before their enrollment. The investigational plan for Protocol [redacted] required that you perform the [redacted] approximately 24 hours after dosing. You failed to adhere to these requirements.

Sponsors also are inspected by the FDA. There were 106 sponsor inspections conducted in 2017. The most common findings in sponsor audits during the year were inadequate monitoring, failure to bring investigators into compliance and inadequate accountability for the investigational product. Note that these are all things that also involve study sites.

Figure 2: OSI warning and NIDPOE letters

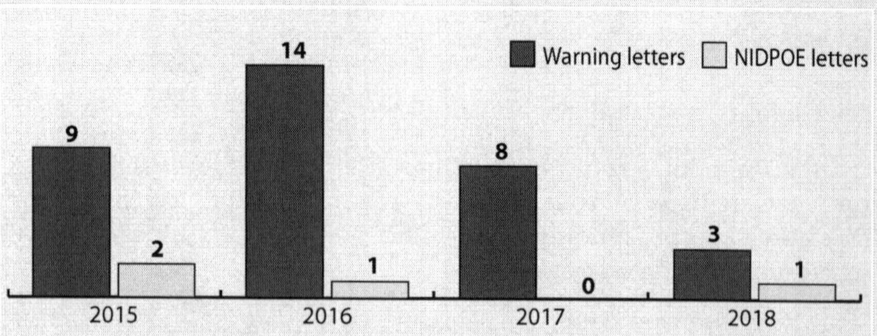

Note: NIDPOE = Notice of Initiation of Disqualification Proceeding and Opportunity to Explain

Source: FDA Office of Scientific Investigations

Consequences

The consequences of finding problems during inspections can be significant, especially when they affect a large amount of the data for a pivotal trial. The study at a particular site may be invalidated, especially if sufficient source documents were not available, if there were significant unreported concomitant therapies or if there was a failure to follow the protocol. If the site was a high enroller and generated a significant amount of data in support of the sponsor's NDA/PMA, these problems could delay the NDA/PMA or result in a disapproved application. A sponsor may even have to repeat a study, which could add years to the drug development cycle.

There also are significant consequences for the investigator in these cases. An investigator may be disqualified or restricted from conducting clinical trials. This puts him or her on the infamous "black list," known more formally as the List of Disqualified and Restricted Investigators. Investigators can be added to the list through a court hearing or through a consent agreement; they can be totally disqualified from ever conducting clinical studies or may have other restrictions placed on them, such as conducting studies only as a sub-investigator or conducting not more than one study every two years, etc. Once on the list, an investigator stays on the list forever, even if corrective action has been taken. It does not happen often, but in the worst cases, an investigator can be fined and/or sentenced to prison.

Remember that documenting study activities in compliance with the ALCOAC principles will support audit readiness for the research institution, but also compliance with the protocol and GCP regulations. A site that has an established quality system to support the investigator and their study team will have what it takes to prevent issues and manage issues well, when there are issues, to ensure audit readiness.

Summary and Key Points

A conscientious, knowledgeable CRC is key to a good, valid study and favorable audit results. The CRC is part of the investigator's team that fulfills the study requirements. When preparing for an inspection or audit, the team follows an inspection procedure to ensure that the quality system has supported audit readiness. Anything found that is a risk should be addressed as much as possible before the audit. Communicating to the sponsor and IRB is very important. Documentation is critical.

Key Points:

- Investigators are audited more than sponsors and IRBs.
- Sites should be audit ready and should have a quality system that supports this as an ongoing effort and not just in preparation for an audit.

- Documentation is key to show compliance and effective issues management.
- Effective issues management is key and includes issues identification, root cause, corrective and preventive actions, monitoring for effectiveness and proof of improvement.

Case Study: Audit Attitude

When the FDA inspector called in late March to set up an appointment at the site, the investigator stalled and tried to put it off as long as possible, asking the inspector to wait until late May. The inspector did not want to wait that long and finally arranged to come in late April. After the call, the investigator told the CRC that she just didn't have time "for any FDA nonsense. ... It's just a lot of busy work, anyway. We certainly aren't going to put in any extra time for this."

When the FDA inspector arrived on the specified day, he was told by the receptionist that the investigator was in meetings all day but that he could work with the study coordinator and the investigator would try to stop by later. The CRC was called and came out to meet the inspector. Telling him she had study subjects scheduled for most of the day, she took him into the study file room, pointed out the shelf that held the documents for the study he was reviewing and said she would check back with him before lunch.

Was this appropriate behavior?

No. First, although FDA inspectors realize that sites are busy, they also expect that an inspection can be scheduled within a reasonable amount of time, say two to three weeks. The investigator certainly should have been there to greet him when he arrived and should have kept herself and the CRC available to meet with him initially and at least periodically throughout the day.

Second, you should never leave an inspector alone with all of your files to look through at will. Take the inspector to a conference room. Ask him what he would like to see and provide him with only the requested material. Spend some time with him to answer any initial questions. If an inspector requests additional material, give it to him; otherwise, keep your other studies and materials in a different location.

By the time the CRC finally checked in again before lunch, the inspector had numerous questions for her. She said she was sorry but she didn't have time to look into them. After all, she needed to have lunch before her afternoon study subjects came in.

The investigator stopped in briefly (only because the receptionist reminded her the inspector was there) about 5:30 p.m. Again, the inspector said he had several things he needed to discuss with her, but she put him off saying she had to leave because she had a dinner engagement. The inspector said he would be back every day until he was satisfied that he had all the materials, information and answers he needed.

Was this inspection going well?

Absolutely not. The investigator and the CRC were not cooperative, and the inspector was getting extremely annoyed. In fact, this inspection ended up taking three weeks to complete. The inspector looked at everything in great detail and finally insisted on reviewing every aspect of the study with both the investigator and the CRC. He issued a 483 when he left, and it detailed every single thing he found, even if it had been corrected.

Both the investigator and the CRC learned the hard way that it doesn't pay to be uncooperative with the FDA.

AFTERWORD

This book has covered a great deal of information, and I hope you found it useful and helpful for your position as a CRC. Remember, it's the little things that often make a big difference, both in how your job progresses and in the success of clinical trials at your site. There is no doubt about it—the job of the CRC is not for the faint-hearted. It carries a lot of responsibility and an enormous amount of work. It requires multiple skills and the ability to stay organized under pressure. It's also fun and challenging, with constant opportunities to learn new things and meet new people. I hope you enjoy both the job and the chance to make a difference in the lives of everyone who will benefit from new drugs and devices, once they are marketed. I'll leave you with a few last thoughts to help you as a CRC.

- The safety and well-being of your study subjects always comes first.
- Establish a good, collegial working relationship with your investigator.
- Know your protocols and case report forms thoroughly.
- Keep all study documents up to date and properly filed.
- Stay organized.
- Read the regulations.
- Monitor the progress of all of your study sites regularly.
- Think of your sponsor monitors (CRAs) as the other half of the team.
- Don't be afraid to admit you don't know something—find out.
- Don't burn bridges. It's a small world.

- Don't be afraid to admit mistakes.
- Remember, you are making a difference in people's lives.
- Be nice.
- Smile.

APPENDIX A

Abbreviations & Acronyms

ACRP	Association of Clinical Research Professionals
ADR	Adverse Drug Reaction
AE	Adverse Event
ALCOAC	Attributable, Legible, Contemporaneous, Original, Accurate, Complete
AMA	American Medical Association
BIMO	Bioresearch Monitoring Program
BLA	Biologics License Application
CBER	Center for Biologics Evaluation and Research
CCRC	Certified Clinical Research Coordinator
CCRP	Certified Clinical Research Professional
CDER	Center for Drug Evaluation and Research
CDRH	Center for Devices and Radiological Health
CFR	Code of Federal Regulations
CI	Clinical Investigator
CPI	Certified Principal Investigator
CPGM	Compliance Program Guidance Manual
CRA	Clinical Research Associate
CRC	Clinical Research Coordinator
CRF	Case Report Form
CRO	Contract Research Organization
CTA	Clinical Trial Agreement
CTMS	Clinical Trial Management System
DGR	Dangerous Goods Regulation
DMC	Data-Monitoring Committee
DSMB	Data Safety Monitoring Board
DSMC	Data Safety Monitoring Committee

ECG	Electrocardiogram
eCRF	Electronic Case Report Form
EDC	Electronic Data Capture
EHR	Electronic Health Record
eIC	Electronic Informed Consent
EIR	Establishment Inspection Report
eTMF	Electronic Trial Master File
FDA	Food and Drug Administration
FDAMA	FDA Modernization Act
GCP	Good Clinical Practice
GLP	Good Laboratory Practice
GMP	Good Manufacturing Practice
HAM-A	Hamilton Rating Scale for Anxiety
HHS	Health and Human Services
HIPAA	Health Insurance Portability and Accountability Act
IATA	International Air Transport Association
IC	Informed Consent
ICH	International Council on Harmonisation
IEC	Independent Ethics Committee
IND	Investigational New Drug
IRB	Institutional Review Board, Independent Review Board
ISO	International Organization for Standardization
IVRS	Interactive Voice Response System
NAI	No Action Indicated
NCI	National Cancer Institute
NDA	New Drug Application
NIH	National Institutes of Health
OAI	Official Action Indicated
OCR	Office for Civil Rights
OHRP	Office for Human Research Protections
OTC	Over-the-counter
PA	Physician Assistant
PDUFA	Prescription Drug User Fee Act
PhRMA	Pharmaceutical Research and Manufacturers of America
PHI	Protected Health Information
PI	Principal Investigator
PM	Project Manager
PMA	Pre-Market Approval
PMS	Post Marketing Surveillance
QA	Quality Assurance
QC	Quality Control
RDE	Remote Data Entry
SAE	Serious Adverse Event
SC	Study Coordinator
SMO	Site Management Organization
SoCRA	Society of Clinical Research Associates

SOP	Standard Operating Procedure
Sub-I	Sub-investigator
SUSAR	Suspected Unexpected Serious Adverse Reaction
TMF	Trial Master File
UADE	Unanticipated Adverse Device Effect
VA	Department of Veterans Affairs
VAI	Voluntary Action Indicated
WMA	World Medical Association

APPENDIX B

Glossary

510(k) Pre-Market Application

A 510(K) is a premarket submission made to the FDA to demonstrate that the device to be marketed is at least as safe and effective, that is, substantially equivalent, to a legally marketed device (21 CFR Part 807.92(a)(3)) that is not subject to premarket approval.

Adverse Drug Reaction

An unintended reaction to a drug taken at normal doses.

Adverse Event (AE)

Any untoward medical occurrence in a study subject administered a pharmaceutical product; it does not necessarily have to have a causal relationship with this treatment.

Beneficence

Doing no harm. Maximizing benefits while minimizing risks.

Bioresearch Monitoring Programs (BIMO)

These are used to inspect study facilities, clinical investigators, or sponsors/monitors/contract research organizations. The BIMO compliance programs help to assure the integrity of scientific testing and the reliability of test data submitted to the FDA. BIMO inspections allow the agency to assess, through audit procedures and real-time inspections, whether data submitted to the FDA will permit sound judgment regarding the safety and effectiveness of regulated products.

Biologic
A virus, vaccine, toxin, antitoxin, blood product, therapeutic serum or similar material for the prevention, treatment or cure of disease or injury in humans.

Biotechnology
Any technique that uses living organisms or substances from living organisms, biological systems or processes to make or modify a product or process, to change plants or animals, or to develop microorganisms for specific uses.

Blinding
The process through which study subjects, the investigator and/or other involved parties in a clinical trial are kept unaware of the treatment assignments of study subjects.

Case History
The investigator's subject source documents and case report forms for a trial.

Case Report Form (CRF)
A record of pertinent information collected on each subject during a clinical trial, based on the protocol.

Certified Copy
A paper or electronic copy of the original record that has been verified (e.g., by a dated signature) or has been generated through a validated process to produce an exact copy having all of the same attributes and information as the original.

Certified Principal Investigator (CPI)
A clinical investigator who meets the required experience and educational levels and has earned certification by passing an exam offered by organizations such as ACRP.

Certified Clinical Research Coordinator (CCRC)
CRC with more than two years of experience and certification earned by passing an exam.

Clinical Trial (Clinical Study, Clinical Investigation)
Any experiment that involves a test article (drug, device, biologic) and one or more human subjects.

Clinical Research Associate (CRA)
The sponsor monitor who visits sites periodically during a study to monitor data and assess progress.

Clinical Research Coordinator (CRC) (Study coordinator)
The person at an investigational site who manages the daily operations of a clinical investigation, and who reports to the investigator.

Compliance Program Guidance Manuals (CPGM)
The FDA uses CPGMs to direct its field personnel on the conduct of inspectional and investigational activities. The purpose of each program is to ensure the protection of research subjects and the integrity of data submitted to the agency in support of a marketing application.

Contract Research Organization (CRO)
A person or organization contracted by the sponsor to perform one or more of a sponsor's trial-related duties and functions.

Double-Blind
The design of a study in which neither the investigator nor the subject knows which treatment the subject is receiving.

Essential Documents
Documents which individually and collectively permit evaluation of the conduct of a study and the quality of the data produced.

Good Clinical Practice (GCP)
The regulations and guidelines that specify the responsibilities of sponsors, investigators, monitors and IRBs involved in clinical trials. They are meant to protect the safety, rights and welfare of the subjects in addition to ensuring the accuracy of the data collected during the trial.

Human Subject (study subject, study participant)
An individual who participates in research, either as a recipient of the test article or as a control. A subject may be either a healthy subject or a patient.

Inclusion and Exclusion Criteria
The characteristics that must be present (inclusion) or absent (exclusion) in order for a subject to qualify for a clinical trial, as per the protocol for the trial.

Informed Consent
The process by which a subject voluntarily confirms after reviewing and then by signing his or her willingness to participate in a clinical trial.

Institutional Review Board (IRB) (Independent Review Board (IRB) Independent Ethics Committee (IEC)
Any board, committee, or group formally designated to review biomedical research involving humans as subjects, to approve the initiation of and conduct periodic review of such research.

Investigator (Clinical Investigator [CI], Principal Investigator [PI])
An individual who actually conducts a clinical investigation, i.e., under whose immediate direction the test article is dispensed, or, in the case of an investigation conducted by a team of individuals, is the responsible leader of that team.

Investigator Brochure (IB)
A compilation of all information known to date about the test product, including chemistry and formulation information and preclinical and clinical data. It is updated at least annually. Once the product is marketed, it is replaced by the labeling (package insert) for the product.

Investigational Device Exemption (IDE)
An exemption that allows the investigational device to be used in a clinical study in order to collect safety and effectiveness data. Clinical studies are most often conducted to support a PMA. Only a small percentage of 510(k) s require clinical data to support the application. Investigational use also includes the clinical evaluation of certain modifications or new intended uses of legally marketed devices. All clinical evaluations of investigational devices, unless exempt, must have an approved IDE before the study is initiated.

Investigational Product (IP)
A new drug, biologic or device that is used in a clinical investigation.

Investigational New Drug (IND) Application
The application submitted to the FDA per regulations within 21 CFR Part 312 to start clinical testing of a new drug or biologic in humans.

***In Vitro* Testing**
Non-clinical testing conducted in an artificial environment such as a test tube or culture medium.

***In Vivo* Testing**
Testing conducted in living animal and human systems.

IRB Approval
The determination of the IRB that the clinical investigation has been reviewed and may be conducted within the constraints set by the IRB and applicable regulations.

Minimal Risk
The probability and magnitude of harm or discomfort anticipated in the research are not greater than those ordinarily encountered in daily life or in the performance of routine physical or psychological examinations or tests.

New Drug Application (NDA)
The marketing application for a new drug submitted to the FDA under the requirements of 21 CFR Part 314. The NDA contains all the nonclinical, clinical, pharmacological, pharmacokinetic and stability data required by the FDA.

Open Label Study
A study in which the subjects and the investigator are aware of the drug that is being administered.

Preclinical Testing
Studies conducted on animals to determine that the drug is safe to use in studies on humans.

Protocol
The formal plan for carrying out a clinical investigation.

Quality Assurance
Systems and procedures designed to ensure that a study is being performed in accordance with Good Clinical Practice (GCP) guidelines and that the data being generated are accurate.

Randomization
A method in which study subjects are randomly assigned to treatment groups. It helps to reduce bias in a trial by ensuring that there is no pattern in the way subjects are assigned to treatment groups.

Serious Adverse Event (SAE)
Any untoward medical occurrence at any dose that results in death, is life-threatening, requires hospitalization (or a prolongation of hospitalization in a patient who is already hospitalized), results in persistent or significant disability or incapacity, or is a congenital anomaly/birth defect.

Site Management Organization (SMO)
A group of investigational sites that have banded together and organized centrally to conduct studies.

Source Documents
Original documents and records including, but not limited to, hospital records, clinical and office charts, laboratory notes, memoranda, subjects' diaries or evaluation checklists, pharmacy dispensing records, recorded data from automated instruments, copies or transcriptions certified after verification as being accurate and complete, microfiches, photographic negatives, microfilm or magnetic media, x-rays, subject files, as well as records kept at the pharmacy, laboratories and medico-technical departments involved in a clinical trial.

Sponsor
The person or entity who initiates a clinical investigation, but who does not actually conduct the investigation.

Standard Operating Procedures (SOPs)
Official written instructions for the management and conduct of clinical trial processes. SOPs ensure that processes are carried out in a consistent and efficient manner.

Study Coordinator (Clinical Research Coordinator)
The person at an investigational site who manages the daily operations of a clinical investigation and who reports to the investigator.

Sub-Investigator
Any member of an investigational team other than the investigator.

Serious Unexpected Suspected Adverse Reaction (SUSAR)
A serious adverse drug reaction (SAR) that is unexpected or for which the development is uncommon (unexpected issue) observed during a clinical trial and for which there is a relationship with the experimental drug, whatever the tested drug or its comparator.

Unanticipated Event
Problem involving risks to human subjects or others participating in a clinical research study (e.g., breach of confidentiality, incarceration of subject, suicide attempt or incorrect labeling of study drug). These, too, need to be collected and reported.

Unanticipated Adverse Device Effect (UADE)
Any serious adverse effect on health or safety or any life-threatening problem or death caused by, or associated with, a device, if that effect, problem, or death was not previously identified in nature, severity, or degree of incidence in the investigational plan or application (including a supplementary plan or application), or any other unanticipated serious problem associated with a device that relates to the rights, safety, or welfare of subjects.

APPENDIX C

Resources

Food and Drug Administration

www.fda.gov

- Bioresearch Monitoring Program (BIMO)
https://www.fda.gov/inspections-compliance-enforcement-and-criminal-investigations/compliance-actions-and-activities/fda-bioresearch-monitoring-information
- Center for Biologics Evaluation and Research (CBER) Guidance, Compliance and Regulatory Information
https://www.fda.gov/vaccines-blood-biologics/guidance-compliance-regulatory-information-biologics
- Center for Drug Evaluation and Research (CDER) Guidance, Compliance and Regulatory Information
https://www.fda.gov/drugs/guidance-compliance-regulatory-information
- Center for Devices and Radiologic Health (CDRH) Resources for Industry
https://www.fda.gov/medical-devices/resources-you-medical-devices/industry-medical-devices
- Clinical Trials and Human Subject Protection
https://www.fda.gov/science-research/science-and-research-special-topics/clinical-trials-and-human-subject-protection
- Clinical Trials Guidance Documents
https://www.fda.gov/regulatory-information/search-fda-guidance-documents/clinical-trials-guidance-documents

- Office of Good Clinical Practice
https://www.fda.gov/about-fda/office-special-medical-programs/office-good-clinical-practice

Health and Human Services Department – Office of Human Research Protections
www.hhs.gov/ohrp

- Belmont Report
https://www.hhs.gov/ohrp/regulations-and-policy/belmont-report/index.html

International Council on Harmonisation
www.ich.org

National Institutes of Health
https://grants.nih.gov/policy/humansubjects.htm

- ClinicalTrials.gov
www.clinicaltrials.gov
- Department of Bioethics
https://bioethics.nih.gov/publications/index.shtml
- Nuremberg Code
https://history.nih.gov/research/downloads/nuremberg.pdf

Declaration of Helsinki – World Medical Association
https://www.wma.net/policies-post/wma-declaration-of-helsinki-ethical-principles-for-medical-research-involving-human-subjects/

APPENDIX D

Sample Forms, Checklists and Logs

- Audit Preparation Checklist
- Budget Worksheet
- Documents Submitted to the IRB
- Elements of Consent
- Enrollment Tracking Form
- Error Query/Correction
- HIPAA Authorization Checklist
- Informed Consent Checklist: Required Elements
- Inventory of Returned Investigational Material
- Investigational Drug Dispensing Record
- Meeting Communication Record
- Post-Study Critique Worksheet
- Protocol Feasibility Assessment Checklist
- Protocol Deviation Report
- Report: Medication Blind Broken for a Study Subject
- Request for Study Supplies
- Sample SOP Format
- Site Evaluation
- Study Closeout
- Study Documents
- Study Document File Verification Log
- Study Monitor Visit Log
- Study Personnel Log
- Study Subject/Chart Master List
- Study Subject Visit Tracking Log
- Subject Identification Code List
- Telephone Communication Record
- Training Verification Form
- Training Verification Master List
- Study Subject Visit Tracking Log

Audit Preparation Checklist

1. Ensure that arrangements have been made for the audit
   - ☐ Conference room is arranged/reserved
   - ☐ Appropriate personnel have been notified and are available
   - ☐ All requested materials are available
   - ☐ The investigator will be available to meet with the auditors

2. Ensure that the following materials have been checked and are ready for the audit:
   - ☐ Copies of signed informed consent forms for all subjects entered in the study
   - ☐ Copies of all case report forms for all subjects
     - ☐ Copies of any corrections made, queries, etc.
   - ☐ Source documents for all subjects (office charts, test results, etc.)
   - ☐ Study document file
     - ☐ All study initiation records
     - ☐ List of involved study personnel and dates of involvement
     - ☐ All IRB communications
     - ☐ Sponsor communications
     - ☐ Study notes, etc.
     - ☐ Grant information should **not** be present
   - ☐ Drug dispensing records for all subjects
   - ☐ Overall drug accountability forms
   - ☐ Other materials, as requested or as appropriate

Budget Worksheet

Date:

Number of subjects to be enrolled: **Number of visits:**

Activity	Cost per procedure	Number of times procedure is done	Total cost per subject
Labor costs:			
Recruitment **			
Screening **			
Administering informed consent			
Per visit activities			
Vital signs			
Laboratory			
Interview, instructions, scheduling			
Study medication/material dispensing and accounting			
CRF completion			
Serious Adverse Event forms			
Total labor costs per subject			
Direct costs:			
Safety laboratory panel			
Urinalysis			
Diagnostic procedures			
Other laboratory tests (list):			
Total direct costs per subject			
Salary/fees:			
Investigator **			
Subinvestigator			
Study coordinator/nurse **			
Secretarial support			
Phlebotomist/lab technician			
Other			
Pharmacy fee			
Subject compensation			
Total salary/fee cost per subject			

** These figures plus labor cost for one visit of investigator and coordinator comprise screening costs.

Budget Worksheet (continued)

Administrative costs	Total cost
Advertising and recruitment	
Data archiving	
IRB fees	
Miscellaneous study activities and overhead	
Total administrative costs	

Total Study Budget Calculations

1. Cost per enrolled subject:
   Labor: ______________________________
   Direct: ______________________________
   Salary/fees: ______________________________
   Total: ______________________________

2. Cost per screened, not enrolled, subject (screen failure):
   Labor: ______________________________
   Salary/fees: ______________________________
   Total:______________________________

3. Subjects to be enrolled
   Cost per subject______ x No. of subjects ______ = Total (A)________

   Screen failures (estimate)
   Cost per subject______ x No. of subjects ______ = Total (B)________

4. Total administrative costs (Total C) = ______________________

5. Total study cost (A + B + C) = ______________________

6. Grant per subject
   Cost per subject______ x No. of subjects to be enrolled ______ = Grant per subject ______

Note: If the sponsor wants a per patient grant figure, divide the total cost per study (A+B+C) by the number of subjects to be enrolled. This will give a per subject grant figure that will cover the total study expenses.

Note: The number of screen failures will need to be estimated based on previous experience, the diagnosis and the number allowed by the sponsor.

Note: Overhead may need to be listed as a percentage of the overall grant per subject.

Documents Submitted to the IRB

Protocol ______________________________

Sponsor ______________________________

Investigator ______________________________

The following documents were submitted to the IRB on ____/ ____/ ____

- ☐ Protocol and amendments (if any)
- ☐ Draft informed consent form
- ☐ Investigator brochure (or package insert, if marketed drug)
- ☐ Proposed advertising or recruitment materials, if applicable
- ☐ Proposed payments to study subjects, if applicable
- ☐ Completed, signed 1572 form
- ☐ CV for the investigator and copy of current license
- ☐ IRB submission form, if applicable
- ☐ Other (list)

If any items are not applicable for this study, write "NA" next to the item.

When all relevant items have been sent, sign below.

Name ______________________ Date ____/ ____/ ____

Elements of Consent

Required elements

- ☐ Statement that the study involves research.
  - ☐ Explanation of the purpose of the research.
  - ☐ Expected duration of subject's participation.
  - ☐ Description of procedures to be followed.
  - ☐ Identification of any procedures that are experimental.

- ☐ Description of reasonably foreseeable risks and discomforts to subject.
- ☐ Description of benefits which may be reasonably expected.
- ☐ Disclosure of alternate procedures or treatment.
- ☐ Statement re confidentiality of records.
  - ☐ Statement that FDA may inspect the records.

- ☐ Statement re compensation for any research-related injury.
- ☐ Contact person for questions about the research and subject rights.
- ☐ Contact person in the event of research-related injury.
- ☐ Statement that participation is voluntary.
- ☐ Statement that refusal to participate will not result in the penalty or loss of any benefits to which the subject is otherwise entitled.
- ☐ Statement that the subject may discontinue at any time without penalty or loss of any benefits to which the subject is otherwise entitled.

Additional elements (include as appropriate)

- ☐ Statement that the treatment may involve risks to the subject (or embryo or fetus) that are currently unforeseeable.
- ☐ Circumstances under the subject's participation may be terminated by the investigator without regard to the subject's consent.
- ☐ Any additional costs to the subject.
- ☐ Consequences for withdrawal and procedures for orderly termination.
- ☐ Statement that significant new findings will be provided to the subject.
- ☐ Approximate number of subjects involved in the study.

Enrollment Tracking Form

Protocol:________________________ **Sponsor:**________________________

Investigator: ____

Date	Screened	Enrolled	Completed the study	Dropouts (due to AEs)	Currently in the study
MM/DD/YY (example)	30	19	4	4 (1)	11

Error Query/Correction

Protocol ______________________ **Protocol date** __________ **Sponsor** __________________________

Patient	Visit	Page	Field	Problem	Correction	Initials

HIPAA Authorization Checklist

- ☐ 1. A description explaining that medical record information may be accessed for research purposes.
- ☐ 2. Identification of individuals or entities who may use/access or disclose the information.
- ☐ 3. Identification of individuals or entities who may receive the information.
- ☐ 4. A description explaining the purpose of the use or disclosure of the information.
- ☐ 5. Illustration of an expiration date of authorization. If not present then waiver must be obtained.
- ☐ 6. Illustrations of how long identifiable data will be retained.
- ☐ 7. Individual's signature and date (if authorization is on addendum sepa rate from informed consent).
- ☐ 8. Explanation regarding the subject's right to revoke authorization.
- ☐ 9. Explanation illustrating the subject has the right to refuse to sign authorization.
- ☐ 10. Explanation that the research subject's rights to access study related information are to be suspended while the clinical trial is in progress. The subject's rights will be reinstated at the conclusion of the trial.
- ☐ 11. Explanation that information disclosed by the researcher to another entity may no longer be protected by the privacy rule.

Other: (e.g., Project Specific, signature requirements)

____

____

____

____

____

____

Informed Consent Checklist: Required Elements

- ☐ 1. A statement that the study involves research.
- ☐ 2. An explanation of the purposes of the research.
- ☐ 3. The expected duration of the subject's participation.
- ☐ 4. A description of the procedures to be followed.
- ☐ 5. Identification of any procedures that are experimental.
- ☐ 6. A description of any reasonably foreseeable risk or discomfort to the subject.
- ☐ 7. A description of any benefits to the subject or to others.
- ☐ 8. A disclosure of appropriate alternative procedures or courses of treatment.
- ☐ 9. Degree to which confidentiality of records identifying the subject will be maintained.
- ☐ 10. Statement noting the possibility that the Food and Drug Administration may inspect the records.
- ☐ 11. An explanation as to whether any compensation is available.
- ☐ 12. An explanation as to whether any medical treatments are available if injury occurs and, if so, what they consist of, or where further information may be obtained.
  - No exculpatory language may be included in which the subject or the representative is made to
    - waive or appear to waive any of the subject's legal rights or
    - releases or appears to release the investigator, the sponsor, the institution or its agents from liability for negligence.
- ☐ 13. Contact person for answers to pertinent questions about the research (and phone number/address).
- ☐ 14. Contact person for questions about research subject's rights (and phone number/address).
- ☐ 15. Contact person in the event of a research-related injury to the subject (and phone number/address).
- ☐ 16. A statement that participation is voluntary, that refusal to participate will involve no penalty or loss of benefits to which the subject is otherwise entitled, and that the subject may discontinue participation at any time without penalty or loss of benefits to which the subject is otherwise entitled.
- ☐ 17. A statement that the particular treatment or procedure may involve risks to the subject (or to the embryo or fetus, if the subject is or may become pregnant) which are currently unforeseeable.
- ☐ 18. Anticipated circumstances under which the subject's participation may be terminated by the Investigator without regard to the subject's consent.

☐ 19. Any additional costs to the subject that may result from participation in the research.
☐ 20. The consequences of a subject's decision to withdraw from the research and procedures for orderly termination of participation by the subject.
☐ 21. A statement that significant new findings developed during the / course of the research which may relate to the subject's willingness to continue participation will be provided to the subject.
☐ 22. The approximate number of subjects involved in the study.
☐ 23. Includes the statement for www.clinicaltrails.gov

Other: (e.g., Project Specific, signature requirements)

____

____

____

____

____

____

Inventory of Returned Investigational Material

Sponsor/Address ____

____

Protocol Number ____

Protocol Title ____

Investigator/Address ____

____

Contact Person/Telephone Number ____

The following investigational material is being returned.

Drug	Lot Number	Code Number	Full Containers	Partial Containers	Empty Containers	Total Containers

Comments ____

____

Inventory of Returned Investigational Material (Example)

Sponsor/Address Acme Pharma

Returned Goods Department, 1234 Main Street, Pharma City, CC 23456

Protocol Number XYZ-1234-001

Protocol Title Study of Drug A vs. Placebo in Moderate Hypertension

Investigator/Address John Smith, M.D.

BCCCR, Kalamazoo, MI 49001

Contact Person/Telephone Number Robert Doe, R.Ph. (616) 555-5555

The following investigational material is being returned.

Drug	Lot Number	Code Number	Full Containers	Partial Containers	Empty Containers	Total Containers
Blinded	12345	101	0	4	4	8
Blinded	12345	102	0	0	8	8
Blinded	12345	103	2	3	2	7-see note

Comments Patient #103 – missing one bottle – patient did not return – threw out.

Investigational Drug Dispensing Record

Protocol Number ______________________________

Protocol Title ______________________________

Investigator ______________________________

Subject Number/Initials ______________________________

Treatment Code (if applicable) ______________________________

Complete the following information using a new line each time medication is dispensed or returned. Use a separate sheet for each subject.

Date Medication Dispensed or Returned	Lot Number and Identification Code	Quantity Dispensed (Number of Tablets)	Quantity Returned (Number of Tablets)	Initials	Comments

Investigational Drug Dispensing Record (Example)

Protocol Number XYZ-1234-001

Protocol Title Study of Drug A vs. Placebo in Moderate Hypertension

Sponsor Acme Pharma

Investigator John Smith, M.D.

Subject Number/Initials BBC – #101

Treatment Code (if applicable) Blinded – #101

Complete the following information using a new line each time medication is dispensed or returned. Use a separate sheet for each subject.

Date Medication Dispensed or Returned	Lot Number and Identification Code	Quantity Dispensed (Number of Tablets)	Quantity Returned (Number of Tablets)	Initials	Comments
2/20/00	Lot 12345 #101	60		KW	
3/06/00	Lot 12345 #101		4	KW	
3/06/00	Lot 12345 #101	60		KW	
2/20/00	Lot 12345 #101		0	KW	Patient forgot extra pills. Will bring next visit.

Meeting Communication Record

Protocol number____

Investigator ____

Date:

People present, including organization:

Purpose of meeting:

Synopsis of meeting discussion:

Actions taken and/or required:

Completed reports are to be filed in the study file.

Post-Study Critique Worksheet

Protocol title ______________________________

Study articles ______________________________

Phase or study type ______________________________

1. General

How many subjects were enrolled? ______________________________

Was the goal met? ☐ Yes ☐ No

How long did it take to enroll? ______________________________

Was the enrollment time goal met? ☐ Yes ☐ No

If enrollment goals were not met, please comment: ______________________________

____

____

____

2. Procedures/clinical assessments

Were procedures/clinical assessments difficult? ☐ Yes ☐ No

If so, describe why below.

Was sufficient staff available? ☐ Yes ☐ No

Were there other factors that make this protocol difficult to perform? If so, describe below.

Comments: ______________________________

____

____

____

3. Workload

Was the workload reasonable? ☐ Yes ☐ No

Were adequate staff available? ☐ Yes ☐ No

Were the facilities adequate? ☐ Yes ☐ No

Were problems encountered in dispensing study material? ☐ Yes ☐ No

Was the study article dispensing/accountability complicated? ☐ Yes ☐ No

Comments: ______________________________

____

____

____

4. **Case report forms (CRFs)**

Were the CRFs appropriate for the study? ☐ Yes ☐ No
Was enough time allowed for completing CRFs? ☐ Yes ☐ No
Were the forms "user-friendly"? ☐ Yes ☐ No
Comments: ______________________________________

5. **Sponsor interactions**

Were communications with the sponsor acceptable? ☐ Yes ☐ No
Was the CRA capable and easy to work with? ☐ Yes ☐ No
Comments: ______________________________________

6. **Other considerations**

Did our patient population benefit from the study? ☐ Yes ☐ No
Was this study desirable to do from a scientific standpoint? ☐ Yes ☐ No
What can we do to improve things the next time we do a similar study?

Was the overall study experience favorable? ☐ Yes ☐ No
Would you recommend working with this sponsor again? ☐ Yes ☐ No
Comments: ______________________________________

Signature Date

Protocol Feasibility Assessment Checklist

Please assess each item as realistically as possible in terms of our ability and capacity to do this study. All assessment forms are to be completed by:

____

Protocol title ____

Sponsor ____

Study material (drug/device/other) ____

Phase or study type ____

Investigator/Coordinator ____

1. General Considerations

Have we worked with this sponsor before?	☐ Yes	☐ No
If so, was the partnership successful?	☐ Yes	☐ No
Is the number of subjects to be enrolled realistic? (N = ______)	☐ Yes	☐ No
Is the enrollment rate realistic? (Rate = ____________)	☐ Yes	☐ No
Is the enrollment period realistic? (Time = ____________)	☐ Yes	☐ No
Will our patients benefit from this study?	☐ Yes	☐ No
Is the IRB apt to have problems with any aspects of this protocol?	☐ Yes	☐ No
Is this study scientifically sound?	☐ Yes	☐ No
Do we have any competing studies?	☐ Yes	☐ No
Are there any competing studies in the community?	☐ Yes	☐ No
Can we make the necessary time commitment?	☐ Yes	☐ No
Is sufficient staff available?	☐ Yes	☐ No
Is this study interesting?	☐ Yes	☐ No

Comments: ____

____

____

____

2. Study Population

Diagnosis ______________________________

Acute	☐ Yes	☐ No
Chronic	☐ Yes	☐ No
Life-threatening	☐ Yes	☐ No
Healthy volunteers	☐ Yes	☐ No
Adults capable of giving consent	☐ Yes	☐ No
Impaired adults	☐ Yes	☐ No
Minors	☐ Yes	☐ No

Comments: ______________________________

____

____

____

3. Study Procedures

How many visits per subject are required?______________________________

What is the visit window (e.g., visit ± 3 days)?______________________________

Are procedures complicated or difficult? If so, describe below.	☐ Yes	☐ No
Are there invasive procedures (other than blood draws)? If so, describe below.	☐ Yes	☐ No
Are any outside specialists needed? If so, list:	☐ Yes	☐ No

Are there other factors that make this protocol difficult to perform? If so, describe below.

Comments: ______________________________

____

____

____

4. Case Report Forms (if available)

Number of pages per subject?______________________________

Time period for completing forms after each visit?______________________________

Are the forms "user-friendly"?	☐ Yes	☐ No
Do laboratory values need to be transcribed?	☐ Yes	☐ No
Are patient diaries to be used?	☐ Yes	☐ No
Do the diaries need to be transcribed?	☐ Yes	☐ No
Is the study drug/other material dispensing/ accountability complicated?	☐ Yes	☐ No

Comments: ______________________________

____

____

____

5. **Overall Assessment**

Do you recommend that the study be conducted at this site? ☐ Yes ☐ No

Comments: ______________________________________

____

____

____

____

Signature Date

____

Protocol Deviation Report

Protocol ______________________________

Investigator ______________________________

Subject number/identifier______________________________

Sponsor______________________________

Date of report ______________________________

The protocol deviation was:

Reason for the deviation:

The protocol variation was approved in advance by the sponsor: ☐ Yes ☐ No

Comments:

Signature Date

This report should be placed in the subject's study file records.

Report: Medication Blind Broken for a Study Subject

Protocol ____________________

Sponsor ____________________

Investigator ____________________

Subject number/identifier ____________________

Medication ____________________

Reason the medication blind was broken:

Did sponsor agree to the unblinding before it was done? If yes, give name, title and contact information for sponsor representative: ☐ Yes ☐ No

---

Comments:

File completed report in study file and in subject's chart.

Request for Study Supplies

Protocol ____

Sponsor____

Investigator____

City and State _______________________________________

Supplies needed, and number requested:

Example: Case report form books – 6
Randomized study drug – 6
Lab kits – 6

Date needed:

By April 23, 2009

Comments:

Two new subjects scheduled to start the study on April 26, 2004.
All other study drug has been allocated to current subjects.
No more case report forms available.

For more information, please contact:

CRC
Telephone number

Sample SOP Format

Name of Organization

SOP #000	Revision #	Dept. or Proces owner:	Effective date:	Page x of y

Purpose
The purpose of this SOP is to...

Scope
This SOP applies to...

The (appropriate person /title) has responsibility for...

Procedure
1. Steps listed in order
2.
3.
Etc.

Regulations
21 CFR and ICH Guideline for Good Clinical Practice details, etc.

References
To other SOPs and guidelines that are related

Attachments
If applicable

Keywords
Significant words and phrases from the SOP

Approved by	Date

Site Evaluation

CRA should evaluate each item below, making notes.

Investigator

- ☐ Qualifications
- ☐ Licensure
- ☐ Specialty
- ☐ Clinical trial experience
  - ☐ Number of previous trials
  - ☐ Number of similar trials
  - ☐ Enrollment in previous trials (numbers, time to enroll)
- ☐ FDA audits
- ☐ Number of trials assigned and status

Staff

- ☐ Study coordinator
- ☐ Other specialized personnel
- ☐ Training and licensure
- ☐ Experience
- ☐ Turnover
- ☐ General interest and attitude
- ☐ Number of trials assigned and status

Facility

- ☐ Appropriate for trials
- ☐ Ample storage for study supplies
- ☐ Appropriate drug storage
- ☐ Special storage equipment available (freezer, centrifuge, refrigerator, etc.)
- ☐ Special equipment available
- ☐ Active practice
- ☐ Facilities tour taken
- ☐ Study records storage, study records format (electronic or paper based), study records access
- ☐ Staff working areas
- ☐ Monitoring area
- ☐ Patient treatment areas

IRB

- ☐ Local IRB available
  - ☐ Frequency and timing of meetings
  - ☐ Average time to approval
  - ☐ Responsiveness
- ☐ Use central IRB

Laboratory/Tests

- ☐ Local lab available
- ☐ Necessary tests can be done
- ☐ Timeliness
- ☐ Certification
- ☐ Have experience with central lab

Protocol feasibility

- ☐ Experience with similar studies
- ☐ Interest level
- ☐ Availability of potential subjects
- ☐ Competing studies (in practice and in community)
- ☐ Timing appropriate
- ☐ Study coordinator availability
- ☐ Can attend investigator meeting

Study Closeout

Protocol ______________________________

Sponsor ______________________________

Investigator ______________________________

Date ______________________________

- ☐ Study documents file is complete (refer to Checklist: Study Documents).
- ☐ Final report has been made to the IRB and the sponsor.
- ☐ All case report forms (CRFs) are complete and have been submitted to the sponsor.
  - ☐ All CRF corrections/queries have been addressed.
  - ☐ Any patient diaries, etc., have been submitted, as required.
- ☐ All source documentation is in order.
  - ☐ If not with study files, location of materials is noted in the document file.
- ☐ Study personnel form is complete.
- ☐ Subjects' signed informed consent forms are filed.
- ☐ Drug dispensing and disposition forms are complete.
- ☐ Study drug has been returned as per sponsor instructions.
- ☐ All other study materials (extra CRFs, etc.) have been returned to the sponsor.
- ☐ Investigator Brochure is filed with other study materials.
- ☐ All study materials are filed together as per archival procedures.
  - ☐ Location of materials is noted in site records.
- ☐ Post-study critique has been held.

Study Documents
(based on ICH GCPs)

Protocol ______________________________

Investigator ______________________________

Pre-Study

- ☐ Investigator Brochure
- ☐ Signed protocol and amendments (if any)
- ☐ Informed consent form
    - ☐ Any other information to be given to subjects
    - ☐ Any advertising materials for recruitment
- ☐ Dated, written IRB approvals for:
    - ☐ Protocol [Date:]
    - ☐ Amendments, if any [Date:]
    - ☐ Consent and any other material to be given to subjects [Date:]
    - ☐ Advertising, if any [Date:]
    - ☐ Subject compensation, if any [Date:]
- ☐ CVs for investigator, subinvestigators
- ☐ Laboratory certification and normal ranges
- ☐ Study manual, if available
- ☐ Shipping records
- ☐ Decoding procedures for blinded trials
- ☐ Financial disclosure sheets
- ☐ Contract
- ☐ Sponsor-specific documents

During the conduct of the trial

- ☐ Investigator Brochure updates
- ☐ Protocol amendments and/or revisions
- ☐ Consent revisions
- ☐ Dated, written IRB approvals of:
    - ☐ Protocol amendments [Dates:]
    - ☐ Revised consents [Dates:]
    - ☐ New or revised subject materials [Dates:]
    - ☐ New or revised advertising [Dates:]
- ☐ CVs for new investigators and/or subinvestigators
- ☐ Laboratory updates of certification and/or normal ranges
- ☐ Shipping documentation (receipt of trial materials)
- ☐ Monitoring visit log
- ☐ Communications with sponsor (letters, telephone reports, etc.)
- ☐ Signed consent forms
- ☐ Source documents

- ☐ Signed, dated, completed case report forms (CRFs)
- ☐ Documentation of CRF corrections
- ☐ Notification to sponsors and IRB of serious adverse events and related reports
- ☐ IND safety reports received from the sponsor
- ☐ Interim and/or annual reports to the IRB
- ☐ Subject screening log
- ☐ Subject identification code list
- ☐ Subject enrollment log
- ☐ Investigational product accountability
- ☐ Signature sheet (all persons making CRF entries or corrections)
- ☐ Record of retained body fluids and/or tissue samples, if any

After study completion or termination

- ☐ Drug (device) accountability
- ☐ Documentation of drug/device return or disposal
- ☐ Completed subject identification code list
- ☐ Final report to the IRB [Date:]

Comments ____

____

____

Checklist should be kept in front of study file and updated as appropriate.

Study Document File Verification Log

Study Document File Review	**Initial / /**	**Initial / /**	**Initial / /**	**Initial / /**
Signed, IRB-approved protocol or cover sheet				
Signed, IRB-approved amendments ■ Amendment #, date ■ Amendment #, date ■ Amendment #, date				
IRB-approved informed consent document				
Signed, completed FDA 1572 form (Statement of Investigator)				
IRB approval letter, verifying approval of both the protocol and consent document				
IRB approval of advertising and subject recruitment materials, including any subject compensation				
Investigator Brochure (or package insert, for marketed products)				
Verification of laboratory certification and laboratory normal ranges				
Study Manual, if available				
Shipping records for investigation product				
Decoding procedures for blinded trials				
Financial disclosure forms				
CVs/licenses				
Sponsor-specific documents and communications				
Reviewer initials				

Attach a separate sheet with comments if any problems found.

Study Monitor Visit Log

Protocol____________________ **Protocol date** __________ **Sponsor** ____________________

Name	Job Title	Date(s) of Visit	Signature	Study Coordinator Initials

Use additional sheets as needed. Keep with study documents file.

Study Personnel Log

Protocol____________________ **Protocol date** __________ **Sponsor** ________________________

Name	Job Title	Initials	Start Date of Study Responsibility	End Date of Study Responsibility	Signature

Use additional sheets as needed. Update when personnel changes occur.
Keep with study documents file.

Study Subject/Chart Master List

Patient name	Chart #	Protocol Number	Subject Number/Initials

Study Subject Visit Tracking Log

Protocol ______________________ **Sponsor** ______________________

Subject	Consent Date	Baseline	Week 1	Week 2	Week 4	Final Status	Comments

Subject Identification Code List

Protocol title ____________________ **Investigator** ____________________

Protocol date ____________________ **Coordinator** ____________________

Subject Name	Address	Telephone	Soc. Security Number	Chart Number	Subject Identification

Use additional sheets as needed. Update when information (address, telephone number) for a subject changes.
Keep with study documents file.

Telephone Communication Record

Protocol ______________________ **Investigator** ___________________

Person initiating the call: ____________ Date: ________________________

Organization: __________________ Time: ________________________

Call to: ________________________

Organization: __________________ Phone number: _________________

Purpose of call:

Response/Comments:

Completed telephone reports are to be filed in the study file.

Training Verification Form

Training Program: ______________________________ **Date:** _________________

I verify that I was trained on this material, that I understood the material, and that I will follow all SOPs and guidelines included in the training.

Name (printed): ____

Signature: ______________________________________ **Date:** _________________

Training Verification Master List

Training Program: ______________________________ **Date:** _________________

The following people were trained on the attached material.

Name (printed)	Signature	Date

Attach additional sheets as necessary.
Attach a copy of the training materials to the form before filing.

Study Subject Visit Tracking Log

	Acceptable Visit Date			
Baseline Visit Date	**Week 1 Visit (± 1 day)**	**Week 2 Visit (± 1 day)**	**Week 4 Visit (± 1 day)**	**Week 8 Visit (± 1 day)**
02/01/09	02/07/09–02/9/09	02/14/09–2/16/09	02/27/09–02/29/09	3/26/09–3/28/09
02/02/09	02/08/09–02/10/09	02/15/09–2/17/09	02/28/09–03/01/09	3/27/09–3/29/09
02/03/09	02/09/09–02/11/09	02/16/09–2/18/09	02/29/09–03/02/09	3/28/09–3/30/09
02/04/09	02/10/09–02/12/09	02/17/09–2/19/09	03/01/09–03/03/09	3/29/09–3/31/09
02/05/09	02/11/09–02/13/09	02/18/09–2/20/09	03/02/09–03/04/09	3/30/09–04/01/09
02/06/09	02/12/09–02/14/09	02/19/09–2/21/09	03/03/09–03/05/09	3/31/09–04/02/09
02/07/09	02/13/09–02/15/09	02/20/09–2/22/09	03/04/09–03/06/09	04/01/09–04/03/09
02/08/09	02/14/09–02/16/09	02/21/09–2/23/09	03/05/09–03/07/09	04/02/09–04/04/09
02/09/09	02/15/09–02/17/09	02/22/09–2/24/09	03/06/09–03/08/09	04/03/09–04/05/09

APPENDIX E

Code of Federal Regulations, Title 21—Food and Drugs

Chapter 1—Food and Drug Administration, Department of Health and Human Services

PART 11—ELECTRONIC RECORDS; ELECTRONIC SIGNATURES

Authority: 21 U.S.C. 321-393; 42 U.S.C. 262.
Source: 62 FR 13464, Mar. 20, 1997, unless otherwise noted.

Subpart A—General Provisions

§ 11.1 Scope.

(a) The regulations in this part set forth the criteria under which the agency considers electronic records, electronic signatures, and handwritten signatures executed to electronic records to be trustworthy, reliable, and generally equivalent to paper records and handwritten signatures executed on paper.

(b) This part applies to records in electronic form that are created, modified, maintained, archived, retrieved, or transmitted, under any records requirements set forth in agency regulations. This part also applies to electronic records submitted to the agency under requirements of the Federal Food, Drug, and Cosmetic Act and the Public Health Service Act, even if such records are not specifically identified in agency regulations. However, this part does not apply to paper records that are, or have been, transmitted by electronic means.

(c) Where electronic signatures and their associated electronic records meet the requirements of this part, the agency will consider the electronic signatures to be equivalent to full handwritten signatures, initials, and other general signings as required by agency regulations, unless specifically excepted by regulation(s) effective on or after August 20, 1997.

(d) Electronic records that meet the requirements of this part may be used in lieu of paper records, in accordance with § 11.2, unless paper records are specifically required.

(e) Computer systems (including hardware and software), controls, and attendant documentation maintained under this part shall be readily available for, and subject to, FDA inspection.

(f) This part does not apply to records required to be established or maintained by §§ 1.326 through 1.368 of this chapter. Records that satisfy the requirements of part 1, subpart J of this chapter, but that also are required under other applicable statutory provisions or regulations, remain subject to this part.

(g) This part does not apply to electronic signatures obtained under § 101.11(d) of this chapter.

(h) This part does not apply to electronic signatures obtained under § 101.8(d) of this chapter.

(i) This part does not apply to records required to be established or maintained by part 117 of this chapter. Records that satisfy the requirements of part 117 of this chapter, but that also are required under other applicable statutory provisions or regulations, remain subject to this part.

(j) This part does not apply to records required to be established or maintained by part 507 of this chapter. Records that satisfy the requirements of part 507 of this chapter, but that also are required under other applicable statutory provisions or regulations, remain subject to this part.

(k) This part does not apply to records required to be established or maintained by part 112 of this chapter. Records that satisfy the requirements of part 112 of this chapter, but that also are required under other applicable statutory provisions or regulations, remain subject to this part.

(l) This part does not apply to records required to be established or maintained by subpart L of part 1 of this chapter. Records that satisfy the requirements of subpart L of part 1 of this chapter, but that also are required under other applicable statutory provisions or regulations, remain subject to this part.

(m) This part does not apply to records required to be established or maintained by subpart M of part 1 of this chapter. Records that satisfy the requirements of subpart M of part 1 of this chapter, but that also are required under other applicable statutory provisions or regulations, remain subject to this part.

(n) This part does not apply to records required to be established or maintained by subpart O of part 1 of this chapter. Records that satisfy the requirements of subpart O of part 1 of this chapter, but that also are required under other applicable statutory provisions or regulations, remain subject to this part.

(o) This part does not apply to records required to be established or maintained by part 121 of this chapter. Records that satisfy the requirements of part 121 of this chapter, but that also are required under other applicable statutory provisions or regulations, remain subject to this part.

[62 FR 13464, Mar. 20, 1997, as amended at 69 FR 71655, Dec. 9, 2004; 79 FR 71253, 71291, Dec. 1, 2014; 80 FR 71253, June 19, 2015; 80 FR 56144, 56336, Sept. 17, 2015; 80 FR 74352, 74547, 74667, Nov. 27, 2015; 81 FR 20170, Apr. 6, 2016; 81 FR 34218, May 27, 2016]

§ 11.2 Implementation.

(a) For records required to be maintained but not submitted to the agency, persons may use electronic records in lieu of paper records or electronic signatures in lieu of traditional signatures, in whole or in part, provided that the requirements of this part are met.

(b) For records submitted to the agency, persons may use electronic records in lieu of paper records or electronic signatures in lieu of traditional signatures, in whole or in part, provided that:

(1) The requirements of this part are met; and

(2) The document or parts of a document to be submitted have been identified in public docket No. 92S-0251 as being the type of submission the agency accepts in electronic form. This docket will identify specifically what types of documents or parts of documents are acceptable for submission in electronic form without paper records and the agency receiving unit(s) (e.g., specific center, office, division, branch) to which such submissions may be made. Documents to agency receiving unit(s) not specified in the public docket will not be considered as official if they are submitted in electronic

form; paper forms of such documents will be considered as official and must accompany any electronic records. Persons are expected to consult with the intended agency receiving unit for details on how (e.g., method of transmission, media, file formats, and technical protocols) and whether to proceed with the electronic submission.

§ 11.3 Definitions.

(a) The definitions and interpretations of terms contained in section 201 of the act apply to those terms when used in this part.

(b) The following definitions of terms also apply to this part:

(1) *Act* means the Federal Food, Drug, and Cosmetic Act (secs. 201-903 (21 U.S.C. 321-393)).

(2) *Agency* means the Food and Drug Administration.

(3) *Biometrics* means a method of verifying an individual's identity based on measurement of the individual's physical feature(s) or repeatable action(s) where those features and/or actions are both unique to that individual and measurable.

(4) *Closed system* means an environment in which system access is controlled by persons who are responsible for the content of electronic records that are on the system.

(5) *Digital signature* means an electronic signature based upon cryptographic methods of originator authentication, computed by using a set of rules and a set of parameters such that the identity of the signer and the integrity of the data can be verified.

(6) *Electronic record* means any combination of text, graphics, data, audio, pictorial, or other information representation in digital form that is created, modified, maintained, archived, retrieved, or distributed by a computer system.

(7) *Electronic signature* means a computer data compilation of any symbol or series of symbols executed, adopted, or authorized by an individual to be the legally binding equivalent of the individual's handwritten signature.

(8) *Handwritten signature* means the scripted name or legal mark of an individual handwritten by that individual and executed or adopted with the present intention to authenticate a writing in a permanent form. The act of signing with a writing or marking instrument such as a pen or stylus is preserved. The scripted name or legal mark, while conventionally applied to paper, may also be applied to other devices that capture the name or mark.

(9) *Open system* means an environment in which system access is not controlled by persons who are responsible for the content of electronic records that are on the system.

Subpart B—Electronic Records

§ 11.10 Controls for closed systems.

Persons who use closed systems to create, modify, maintain, or transmit electronic records shall employ procedures and controls designed to ensure the authenticity, integrity, and, when appropriate, the confidentiality of electronic records, and to ensure that the signer cannot readily repudiate the signed record as not genuine. Such procedures and controls shall include the following:

(a) Validation of systems to ensure accuracy, reliability, consistent intended performance, and the ability to discern invalid or altered records.

(b) The ability to generate accurate and complete copies of records in both human readable and electronic form suitable for inspection, review, and copying by the agency. Persons should contact the agency if there are any questions regarding the ability of the agency to perform such review and copying of the electronic records.

(c) Protection of records to enable their accurate and ready retrieval throughout the records retention period.

(d) Limiting system access to authorized individuals.

(e) Use of secure, computer-generated, time-stamped audit trails to independently record the date and time of operator entries and actions that create, modify, or delete electronic records. Record changes shall not obscure previously recorded information. Such audit trail documentation shall be retained for a period at least as long as that required for the subject electronic records and shall be available for agency review and copying.

(f) Use of operational system checks to enforce permitted sequencing of steps and events, as appropriate.

(g) Use of authority checks to ensure that only authorized individuals can use the system, electronically sign a record, access the operation or computer system input or output device, alter a record, or perform the operation at hand.

(h) Use of device (e.g., terminal) checks to determine, as appropriate, the validity of the source of data input or operational instruction.

(i) Determination that persons who develop, maintain, or use electronic record/electronic signature systems have the education, training, and experience to perform their assigned tasks.

(j) The establishment of, and adherence to, written policies that hold individuals accountable and responsible for actions initiated under their electronic signatures, in order to deter record and signature falsification.

(k) Use of appropriate controls over systems documentation including:

(1) Adequate controls over the distribution of, access to, and use of documentation for system operation and maintenance.

(2) Revision and change control procedures to maintain an audit trail that documents time-sequenced development and modification of systems documentation.

§ 11.30 Controls for open systems.

Persons who use open systems to create, modify, maintain, or transmit electronic records shall employ procedures and controls designed to ensure the authenticity, integrity, and, as appropriate, the confidentiality of electronic records from the point of their creation to the point of their receipt. Such procedures and controls shall include those identified in § 11.10, as appropriate, and additional measures such as document encryption and use of appropriate digital signature standards to ensure, as necessary under the circumstances, record authenticity, integrity, and confidentiality.

§ 11.50 Signature manifestations.

(a) Signed electronic records shall contain information associated with the signing that clearly indicates all of the following:

(1) The printed name of the signer;

(2) The date and time when the signature was executed; and

(3) The meaning (such as review, approval, responsibility, or authorship) associated with the signature.

(b) The items identified in paragraphs (a)(1), (a)(2), and (a)(3) of this section shall be subject to the same controls as for electronic records and shall be included as part of any human readable form of the electronic record (such as electronic display or printout).

§11.70 Signature/record linking.

Electronic signatures and handwritten signatures executed to electronic records shall be linked to their respective electronic records to ensure that the signatures cannot be excised, copied, or otherwise transferred to falsify an electronic record by ordinary means.

Subpart C—Electronic Signatures

§11.100 General requirements.

(a) Each electronic signature shall be unique to one individual and shall not be reused by, or reassigned to, anyone else.

(b) Before an organization establishes, assigns, certifies, or otherwise sanctions an individual's electronic signature, or any element of such electronic signature, the organization shall verify the identity of the individual.

(c) Persons using electronic signatures shall, prior to or at the time of such use, certify to the agency that the electronic signatures in their system, used on or after August 20, 1997, are intended to be the legally binding equivalent of traditional handwritten signatures.

(1) The certification shall be submitted in paper form and signed with a traditional handwritten signature, to the Office of Regional Operations (HFC-100), 5600 Fishers Lane, Rockville, MD 20857.

(2) Persons using electronic signatures shall, upon agency request, provide additional certification or testimony that a specific electronic signature is the legally binding equivalent of the signer's handwritten signature.

§11.200 Electronic signature components and controls.

(a) Electronic signatures that are not based upon biometrics shall:

(1) Employ at least two distinct identification components such as an identification code and password.

(i) When an individual executes a series of signings during a single, continuous period of controlled system access, the first signing shall be executed using all electronic signature components; subsequent signings shall be executed using at least one electronic signature component that is only executable by, and designed to be used only by, the individual.

(ii) When an individual executes one or more signings not performed during a single, continuous period of controlled system access, each signing shall be executed using all of the electronic signature components.

(2) Be used only by their genuine owners; and

(3) Be administered and executed to ensure that attempted use of an individual's electronic signature by anyone other than its genuine owner requires collaboration of two or more individuals.

(b) Electronic signatures based upon biometrics shall be designed to ensure that they cannot be used by anyone other than their genuine owners.

§11.300 Controls for identification codes/passwords.

Persons who use electronic signatures based upon use of identification codes in combination with passwords shall employ controls to ensure their security and integrity. Such controls shall include:

(a) Maintaining the uniqueness of each combined identification code and password, such that no two individuals have the same combination of identification code and password.

(b) Ensuring that identification code and password issuances are periodically checked, recalled, or revised (e.g., to cover such events as password aging).

(c) Following loss management procedures to electronically deauthorize lost, stolen, missing, or otherwise potentially compromised tokens, cards, and other devices that bear or generate identification code or password information, and to issue temporary or permanent replacements using suitable, rigorous controls.

(d) Use of transaction safeguards to prevent unauthorized use of passwords and/or identification codes, and to detect and report in an immediate and urgent manner any attempts at their unauthorized use to the system security unit, and, as appropriate, to organizational management.

(e) Initial and periodic testing of devices, such as tokens or cards, that bear or generate identification code or password information to ensure that they function properly and have not been altered in an unauthorized manner.

• • •

PART 50—PROTECTION OF HUMAN SUBJECTS

Authority: 21 U.S.C 321, 343, 346, 346a, 348, 350a, 350b, 352, 353, 355, 360, 360c-360f, 360h-360j, 371, 379e, 381; 42 U.S.C. 216, 241, 262, 263b-263n.
Source: 45 FR 36390, May 30, 1980, unless otherwise noted.

Subpart A—General Provisions

§ 50.1 Scope.

(a) This part applies to all clinical investigations regulated by the Food and Drug Administration under sections 505(i) and 520(g) of the Federal Food, Drug, and Cosmetic Act, as well as clinical investigations that support applications for research or marketing permits for products regulated by the Food and Drug Administration, including foods, including dietary supplements, that bear a nutrient content claim or a health claim, infant formulas, food and color additives, drugs for human use, medical devices for human use, biological products for human use, and electronic products. Additional specific obligations and commitments of, and standards of conduct for, persons who sponsor or monitor clinical investigations involving particular test articles may also be found in other parts (e.g., parts 312 and 812). Compliance with these parts is intended to protect the rights and safety of subjects involved in investigations filed with the Food and Drug Administration pursuant to sections 403, 406, 409, 412, 413, 502, 503, 505, 510, 513-516, 518-520, 721, and 801 of the Federal Food, Drug, and Cosmetic Act and sections 351 and 354-360F of the Public Health Service Act.

(b) References in this part to regulatory sections of the Code of Federal Regulations are to chapter I of title 21, unless otherwise noted.

[45 FR 36390, May 30, 1980; 46 FR 8979, Jan. 27, 1981, as amended at 63 FR 26697, May 13, 1998; 64 FR 399, Jan. 5, 1999; 66 FR 20597, Apr. 24, 2001]

§ 50.3 Definitions.

As used in this part:

(a) *Act* means the Federal Food, Drug, and Cosmetic Act, as amended (secs. 201-902, 52 Stat. 1040 et seq. as amended (21 U.S.C. 321-392)).

(b) *Application for research or marketing permit* includes:

(1) A color additive petition, described in part 71.

(2) A food additive petition, described in parts 171 and 571.

(3) Data and information about a substance submitted as part of the procedures for establishing that the substance is generally recognized as safe for use that results or may reasonably be expected to result, directly or indirectly, in its becoming a component or otherwise affecting the characteristics of any food, described in §§ 170.30 and 570.30.

(4) Data and information about a food additive submitted as part of the procedures for food additives permitted to be used on an interim basis pending additional study, described in § 180.1.

(5) Data and information about a substance submitted as part of the procedures for establishing a tolerance for unavoidable contaminants in food and food-packaging materials, described in section 406 of the act.

(6) An investigational new drug application, described in part 312 of this chapter.

(7) A new drug application, described in part 314.

(8) Data and information about the bioavailability or bioequivalence of drugs for human use submitted as part of the procedures for issuing, amending, or repealing a bioequivalence requirement, described in part 320.

(9) Data and information about an over-the-counter drug for human use submitted as part of the procedures for classifying these drugs as generally recognized as safe and effective and not misbranded, described in part 330.

(10) Data and information about a prescription drug for human use submitted as part of the procedures for classifying these drugs as generally recognized as safe and effective and not misbranded, described in this chapter.

(11) [Reserved]

(12) An application for a biologics license, described in part 601 of this chapter.

(13) Data and information about a biological product submitted as part of the procedures for determining that licensed biological products are safe and effective and not misbranded, described in part 601.

(14) Data and information about an in vitro diagnostic product submitted as part of the procedures for establishing, amending, or repealing a standard for these products, described in part 809.

(15) *An Application for an Investigational Device Exemption*, described in part 812.

(16) Data and information about a medical device submitted as part of the procedures for classifying these devices, described in section 513.

(17) Data and information about a medical device submitted as part of the procedures for establishing, amending, or repealing a standard for these devices, described in section 514.

(18) An application for premarket approval of a medical device, described in section 515.

(19) A product development protocol for a medical device, described in section 515.

(20) Data and information about an electronic product submitted as part of the procedures for establishing, amending, or repealing a standard for these products, described in section 358 of the Public Health Service Act.

(21) Data and information about an electronic product submitted as part of the procedures for obtaining a variance from any electronic product performance standard, as described in § 1010.4.

(22) Data and information about an electronic product submitted as part of the procedures for granting, amending, or extending an exemption from a radiation safety performance standard, as described in § 1010.5.

(23) Data and information about a clinical study of an infant formula when submitted as part of an infant formula notification under section 412(c) of the Federal Food, Drug, and Cosmetic Act.

(24) Data and information submitted in a petition for a nutrient content claim, described in § 101.69 of this chapter, or for a health claim, described in § 101.70 of this chapter.

(25) Data and information from investigations involving children submitted in a new dietary ingredient notification, described in § 190.6 of this chapter.

(c) *Clinical investigation* means any experiment that involves a test article and one or more human subjects and that either is subject to requirements for prior submission to the Food and Drug Administration under section 505(i) or 520(g) of the act, or is not subject to requirements for prior submission to the Food and Drug Administration under these sections of the act, but the results of which are intended to be submitted later to, or held for inspection by, the Food and Drug Administration as part of an application for a research or marketing permit. The term does not include experiments that are subject to the provisions of part 58 of this chapter, regarding nonclinical laboratory studies.

(d) *Investigator* means an individual who actually conducts a clinical investigation, i.e., under whose immediate direction the test article is administered or dispensed to, or used involving, a subject, or, in the event of an investigation conducted by a team of individuals, is the responsible leader of that team.

(e) *Sponsor* means a person who initiates a clinical investigation, but who does not actually conduct the investigation, i.e., the test article is administered or dispensed to or used involving, a subject under the immediate direction of another individual. A person other than an individual (e.g., corporation or agency) that uses one or more of its own employees to conduct a clinical investigation it has initiated is considered to be a sponsor (not a sponsor-investigator), and the employees are considered to be investigators.

(f) *Sponsor-investigator* means an individual who both initiates and actually conducts, alone or with others, a clinical investigation, i.e., under whose immediate direction the test article is administered or dispensed to, or used involving, a subject. The term does not include any person other than an individual, e.g., corporation or agency.

(g) *Human subject* means an individual who is or becomes a participant in research, either as a recipient of the test article or as a control. A subject may be either a healthy human or a patient.

(h) *Institution* means any public or private entity or agency (including Federal, State, and other agencies). The word facility as used in section 520(g) of the act is deemed to be synonymous with the term *institution* for purposes of this part.

(i) *Institutional review board* (IRB) means any board, committee, or other group formally designated by an institution to review biomedical research involving humans as subjects, to approve the initiation of and conduct periodic review of such research. The term has the same meaning as the phrase *institutional review committee* as used in section 520(g) of the act.

(j) *Test article* means any drug (including a biological product for human use), medical device for human use, human food additive, color additive, electronic product, or any other article subject to regulation under the act or under sections 351 and 354-360F of the Public Health Service Act (42 U.S.C. 262 and 263b-263n).

(k) *Minimal risk* means that the probability and magnitude of harm or discomfort anticipated in the research are not greater in and of themselves than those ordinarily encountered in daily life or during the performance of routine physical or psychological examinations or tests.

(l) *Legally authorized representative* means an individual or judicial or other body authorized under applicable law to consent on behalf of a prospective subject to the subject's particpation in the procedure(s) involved in the research.

(m) *Family member* means any one of the following legally competent persons: Spouse; parents; children (including adopted children); brothers, sisters, and spouses of brothers and sisters; and any individual related by blood or affinity whose close association with the subject is the equivalent of a family relationship.

(n) *Assent* means a child's affirmative agreement to participate in a clinical investigation. Mere failure to object should not, absent affirmative agreement, be construed as assent.

(o) *Children* means persons who have not attained the legal age for consent to treatments or procedures involved in clinical investigations, under the applicable law of the jurisdiction in which the clinical investigation will be conducted.

(p) *Parent* means a child's biological or adoptive parent.

(q) *Ward* means a child who is placed in the legal custody of the State or other agency, institution, or entity, consistent with applicable Federal, State, or local law.

(r) *Permission* means the agreement of parent(s) or guardian to the participation of their child or ward in a clinical investigation.

(s) *Guardian* means an individual who is authorized under applicable State or local law to consent on behalf of a child to general medical care.

[45 FR 36390, May 30, 1980, as amended at 46 FR 8950, Jan. 27, 1981; 54 FR 9038, Mar. 3, 1989; 56 FR 28028, June 18, 1991; 61 FR 51528, Oct. 2, 1996; 62 FR 39440, July 23, 1997; 64 FR 399, Jan. 5, 1999; 64 FR 56448, Oct. 20, 1999; 66 FR 20597, Apr. 24, 2001; 78 FR 12950, Feb. 26, 2013]

Subpart B—Informed Consent of Human Subjects

Source: 46 FR 8951, Jan. 27, 1981, unless otherwise noted.

§ 50.20 General requirements for informed consent.

Except as provided in §§ 50.23 and 50.24, no investigator may involve a human being as a subject in research covered by these regulations unless the investigator has obtained the legally effective informed consent of the subject or the subject's legally authorized representative. An investigator shall seek such consent only under circumstances that provide the prospective subject or the representative sufficient opportunity to consider whether or not to participate and that minimize the possibility of coercion or undue influence. The information that is given to the subject or the representative shall be in language understandable to the subject or the representative. No informed consent, whether oral or written, may include any exculpatory language through which the subject or the representative is made to waive or appear to waive any of the subject's legal rights, or releases or appears to release the investigator, the sponsor, the institution, or its agents from liability for negligence.

[46 FR 8951, Jan. 27, 1981, as amended at 64 FR 10942, Mar. 8, 1999]

§ 50.23 Exception from general requirements.

(a) The obtaining of informed consent shall be deemed feasible unless, before use of the test article (except as provided in paragraph (b) of this section), both the investigator and a physician who is not otherwise participating in the clinical investigation certify in writing all of the following:

(1) The human subject is confronted by a life-threatening situation necessitating the use of the test article.

(2) Informed consent cannot be obtained from the subject because of an inability to communicate with, or obtain legally effective consent from, the subject.

(3) Time is not sufficient to obtain consent from the subject's legal representative.

(4) There is available no alternative method of approved or generally recognized therapy that provides an equal or greater likelihood of saving the life of the subject.

(b) If immediate use of the test article is, in the investigator's opinion, required to preserve the life of the subject, and time is not sufficient to obtain the independent determination required in paragraph (a) of this section in advance of using the test article, the determinations of the clinical investigator shall be made and, within 5 working days after the use of the article, be reviewed and evaluated in writing by a physician who is not participating in the clinical investigation.

(c) The documentation required in paragraph (a) or (b) of this section shall be submitted to the IRB within 5 working days after the use of the test article.

(d)(1) Under 10 U.S.C. 1107(f) the President may waive the prior consent requirement for the administration of an investigational new drug to a member of the armed forces in connection with the member's participation in a particular military operation. The statute specifies that only the President may waive informed consent in this connection and the President may grant such a waiver only if the President determines in writing that obtaining consent: Is not feasible; is contrary to the best interests of the military member; or is not in the interests of national security. The statute further provides that in making a determination to waive prior informed consent on the ground that it is not feasible or the ground that it is contrary to the best interests of the military members involved, the President shall apply the standards and criteria that are set forth in the relevant FDA regulations for a waiver of the prior informed consent requirements of section 505(i)(4) of the Federal Food, Drug, and Cosmetic Act (21 U.S.C. 355(i)(4)). Before such a determination may be made that obtaining informed consent from military personnel prior to the use of an investigational drug (including an antibiotic or biological product) in a specific protocol under an investigational new drug application (IND) sponsored by the Department of Defense (DOD) and limited to specific military personnel involved in a particular military operation is not feasible or is contrary to the best interests of the military members involved the Secretary of Defense must first request such a determination from the President, and certify and document to the President that the following standards and criteria contained in paragraphs (d)(1) through (d)(4) of this section have been met.

(i) The extent and strength of evidence of the safety and effectiveness of the investigational new drug in relation to the medical risk that could be encountered during the military operation supports the drug's administration under an IND.

(ii) The military operation presents a substantial risk that military personnel may be subject to a chemical, biological, nuclear, or other exposure likely to produce death or serious or life-threatening injury or illness.

(iii) There is no available satisfactory alternative therapeutic or preventive treatment in relation to the intended use of the investigational new drug.

(iv) Conditioning use of the investigational new drug on the voluntary participation of each member could significantly risk the safety and health of any individual member who would decline its use, the safety of other military personnel, and the accomplishment of the military mission.

(v) A duly constituted institutional review board (IRB) established and operated in accordance with the requirements of paragraphs (d)(2) and (d)(3) of this section, responsible for review of the study, has reviewed and approved the investigational new drug protocol and the administration of the investigational new drug without informed consent. DOD's request is to include the documentation required by § 56.115(a)(2) of this chapter.

(vi) DOD has explained:

(A) The context in which the investigational drug will be administered, e.g., the setting or whether it will be self-administered or it will be administered by a health professional;

(B) The nature of the disease or condition for which the preventive or therapeutic treatment is intended; and

(C) To the extent there are existing data or information available, information on conditions that could alter the effects of the investigational drug.

(vii) DOD's recordkeeping system is capable of tracking and will be used to track the proposed treatment from supplier to the individual recipient.

(viii) Each member involved in the military operation will be given, prior to the administration of the investigational new drug, a specific written information sheet (including information required by 10 U.S.C. 1107(d)) concerning the investigational new drug, the risks and benefits of its use, potential side effects, and other pertinent information about the appropriate use of the product.

(ix) Medical records of members involved in the military operation will accurately document the receipt by members of the notification required by paragraph (d)(1)(viii) of this section.

(x) Medical records of members involved in the military operation will accurately document the receipt by members of any investigational new drugs in accordance with FDA regulations including part 312 of this chapter.

(xi) DOD will provide adequate followup to assess whether there are beneficial or adverse health consequences that result from the use of the investigational product.

(xii) DOD is pursuing drug development, including a time line, and marketing approval with due diligence.

(xiii) FDA has concluded that the investigational new drug protocol may proceed subject to a decision by the President on the informed consent waiver request.

(xiv) DOD will provide training to the appropriate medical personnel and potential recipients on the specific investigational new drug to be administered prior to its use.

(xv) DOD has stated and justified the time period for which the waiver is needed, not to exceed one year, unless separately renewed under these standards and criteria.

(xvi) DOD shall have a continuing obligation to report to the FDA and to the President any changed circumstances relating to these standards and criteria (including the time period referred to in paragraph (d)(1)(xv) of this section) or that otherwise might affect the determination to use an investigational new drug without informed consent.

(xvii) DOD is to provide public notice as soon as practicable and consistent with classification requirements through notice in the Federal Register describing each waiver of informed consent determination, a summary of the most updated scientific information on the products used, and other pertinent information.

(xviii) Use of the investigational drug without informed consent otherwise conforms with applicable law.

(2) The duly constituted institutional review board, described in paragraph (d)(1)(v) of this section, must include at least 3 nonaffiliated members who shall not be employees or officers of the Federal Government (other than for purposes of membership on the IRB) and shall be required to obtain any necessary security clearances. This IRB shall review the proposed IND protocol at a convened meeting at which a majority of the members are present including at least one member whose primary concerns are in nonscientific areas and, if feasible, including a majority of the nonaffiliated members. The information required by § 56.115(a)(2) of this chapter is to be provided to the Secretary of Defense for further review.

(3) The duly constituted institutional review board, described in paragraph (d)(1)(v) of this section, must review and approve:

(i) The required information sheet;

(ii) The adequacy of the plan to disseminate information, including distribution of the information sheet to potential recipients, on the investigational product (e.g., in forms other than written);

(iii) The adequacy of the information and plans for its dissemination to health care providers, including potential side effects, contraindications, potential interactions, and other pertinent considerations; and

(iv) An informed consent form as required by part 50 of this chapter, in those circumstances in which DOD determines that informed consent may be obtained from some or all personnel involved.

(4) DOD is to submit to FDA summaries of institutional review board meetings at which the proposed protocol has been reviewed.

(5) Nothing in these criteria or standards is intended to preempt or limit FDA's and DOD's authority or obligations under applicable statutes and regulations.

(e)(1) Obtaining informed consent for investigational in vitro diagnostic devices used to identify chemical, biological, radiological, or nuclear agents will be deemed feasible unless, before use of the test article, both the investigator (e.g., clinical laboratory director or other responsible individual) and a physician who is not otherwise participating in the clinical investigation make the determinations and later certify in writing all of the following:

(i) The human subject is confronted by a life-threatening situation necessitating the use of the investigational in vitro diagnostic device to identify a chemical, biological, radiological, or nuclear agent that would suggest a terrorism event or other public health emergency.

(ii) Informed consent cannot be obtained from the subject because:

(A) There was no reasonable way for the person directing that the specimen be collected to know, at the time the specimen was collected, that there would be a need to use the investigational in vitro diagnostic device on that subject's specimen; and

(B) Time is not sufficient to obtain consent from the subject without risking the life of the subject.

(iii) Time is not sufficient to obtain consent from the subject's legally authorized representative.

(iv) There is no cleared or approved available alternative method of diagnosis, to identify the chemical, biological, radiological, or nuclear agent that provides an equal or greater likelihood of saving the life of the subject.

(2) If use of the investigational device is, in the opinion of the investigator (e.g., clinical laboratory director or other responsible person), required to preserve the life of the subject, and time is not sufficient to obtain the independent determination required in paragraph (e)(1) of this section in advance of using the investigational device, the determinations of the investigator shall be made and, within 5 working days after the use of the device, be reviewed and evaluated in writing by a physician who is not participating in the clinical investigation.

(3) The investigator must submit the written certification of the determinations made by the investigator and an independent physician required in paragraph (e)(1) or (e)(2) of this section to the IRB and FDA within 5 working days after the use of the device.

(4) An investigator must disclose the investigational status of the in vitro diagnostic device and what is known about the performance characteristics of the device in the report to the subject's health care provider and in any report to public health authorities. The investigator must provide the IRB with the information required in § 50.25 (except for the information described in § 50.25(a)(8)) and the procedures that will be used to provide this information to each subject or the subject's legally authorized representative at the time the test results are provided to the subject's health care provider and public health authorities.

(5) The IRB is responsible for ensuring the adequacy of the information required in section 50.25 (except for the information described in § 50.25(a)(8)) and for ensuring that procedures are in place to provide this information to each subject or the subject's legally authorized representative.

(6) No State or political subdivision of a State may establish or continue in effect any law, rule, regulation or other requirement that informed consent be obtained before an investigational in vitro diagnostic device may be used to identify chemical, biological, radiological, or nuclear agent in suspected terrorism events and other potential public health emergencies that is different from, or in addition to, the requirements of this regulation.

[46 FR 8951, Jan. 27, 1981, as amended at 55 FR 52817, Dec. 21, 1990; 64 FR 399, Jan. 5, 1999; 64 FR 54188, Oct. 5, 1999; 71 FR 32833, June 7, 2006; 76 FR 36993, June 24, 2011]

§ 50.24 Exception from informed consent requirements for emergency research.

(a) The IRB responsible for the review, approval, and continuing review of the clinical investigation described in this section may approve that investigation without requiring that informed consent of all research subjects be obtained if the IRB (with the concurrence of a licensed physician who is a member of or consultant to the IRB and who is not otherwise participating in the clinical investigation) finds and documents each of the following:

(1) The human subjects are in a life-threatening situation, available treatments are unproven or unsatisfactory, and the collection of valid scientific evidence, which may include evidence obtained through randomized placebo-controlled investigations, is necessary to determine the safety and effectiveness of particular interventions.

(2) Obtaining informed consent is not feasible because:

(i) The subjects will not be able to give their informed consent as a result of their medical condition;

(ii) The intervention under investigation must be administered before consent from the subjects' legally authorized representatives is feasible; and

(iii) There is no reasonable way to identify prospectively the individuals likely to become eligible for participation in the clinical investigation.

(3) Participation in the research holds out the prospect of direct benefit to the subjects because:

(i) Subjects are facing a life-threatening situation that necessitates intervention;

(ii) Appropriate animal and other preclinical studies have been conducted, and the information derived from those studies and related evidence support the potential for the intervention to provide a direct benefit to the individual subjects; and

(iii) Risks associated with the investigation are reasonable in relation to what is known about the medical condition of the potential class of subjects, the risks and benefits of standard therapy, if any, and what is known about the risks and benefits of the proposed intervention or activity.

(4) The clinical investigation could not practicably be carried out without the waiver.

(5) The proposed investigational plan defines the length of the potential therapeutic window based on scientific evidence, and the investigator has committed to attempting to contact a legally authorized representative for each subject within that window of time and, if feasible, to asking the legally authorized representative contacted for consent within that window rather than proceeding without consent. The investigator will summarize efforts made to contact legally authorized representatives and make this information available to the IRB at the time of continuing review.

(6) The IRB has reviewed and approved informed consent procedures and an informed consent document consistent with § 50.25. These procedures and the informed consent document are to be used with subjects or their legally authorized representatives in situations where use of such procedures and documents is feasible. The IRB has reviewed and approved procedures and information to be used when providing an opportunity for a family member to object to a subject's participation in the clinical investigation consistent with paragraph (a)(7)(v) of this section.

(7) Additional protections of the rights and welfare of the subjects will be provided, including, at least:

(i) Consultation (including, where appropriate, consultation carried out by the IRB) with representatives of the communities in which the clinical investigation will be conducted and from which the subjects will be drawn;

(ii) Public disclosure to the communities in which the clinical investigation will be conducted and from which the subjects will be drawn, prior to initiation of the clinical investigation, of plans for the investigation and its risks and expected benefits;

(iii) Public disclosure of sufficient information following completion of the clinical investigation to apprise the community and researchers of the study, including the demographic characteristics of the research population, and its results;

(iv) Establishment of an independent data monitoring committee to exercise oversight of the clinical investigation; and

(v) If obtaining informed consent is not feasible and a legally authorized representative is not reasonably available, the investigator has committed, if feasible, to attempting to contact within the therapeutic window the subject's family member who is not a legally authorized representative, and asking whether he or she objects to the subject's participation in the clinical investigation. The investigator will summarize efforts made to contact family members and make this information available to the IRB at the time of continuing review.

(b) The IRB is responsible for ensuring that procedures are in place to inform, at the earliest feasible opportunity, each subject, or if the subject remains incapacitated, a legally authorized representative of the subject, or if such a representative is not reasonably available, a family member, of the subject's inclusion in the clinical investigation, the details of the investigation and other information contained in the informed consent document. The IRB shall also ensure that there is a procedure to inform the subject, or if the subject remains incapacitated, a legally authorized representative of the subject, or if such a representative is not reasonably available, a family member, that he or she may discontinue the subject's participation at any time without penalty or loss of benefits to which the subject is otherwise entitled. If a legally authorized representative or family member is told about the clinical investigation and the subject's condition improves, the subject is also to be informed as soon as feasible. If a subject is entered into a clinical investigation with waived consent and the subject dies before a legally authorized representative or family member can be contacted, information about the clinical investigation is to be provided to the subject's legally authorized representative or family member, if feasible.

(c) The IRB determinations required by paragraph (a) of this section and the documentation required by paragraph (e) of this section are to be retained by the IRB for at least 3 years after completion of the clinical investigation, and the records shall be accessible for inspection and copying by FDA in accordance with § 56.115(b) of this chapter.

(d) Protocols involving an exception to the informed consent requirement under this section must be performed under a separate investigational new drug application (IND) or investigational device exemption (IDE) that clearly identifies such protocols as protocols that may include subjects who are unable to consent. The submission of those protocols in a separate IND/IDE is required even if an IND for the same drug product or an IDE for the same device already exists. Applications for investigations under this section may not be submitted as amendments under §§ 312.30 or 812.35 of this chapter.

(e) If an IRB determines that it cannot approve a clinical investigation because the investigation does not meet the criteria in the exception provided under paragraph (a) of this section or because of other relevant ethical concerns, the IRB must document its findings and provide these findings promptly in writing to the clinical investigator and to the sponsor of the clinical investigation. The sponsor of the clinical investigation must promptly disclose this information to FDA and to the sponsor's clinical investigators who are participating or are asked to participate in this or a substantially equivalent clinical investigation of the sponsor, and to other IRB's that have been, or are, asked to review this or a substantially equivalent investigation by that sponsor.

[61 FR 51528, Oct. 2, 1996]

§ 50.25 Elements of informed consent.

(a) Basic elements of informed consent. In seeking informed consent, the following information shall be provided to each subject:

(1) A statement that the study involves research, an explanation of the purposes of the research and the expected duration of the subject's participation, a description of the procedures to be followed, and identification of any procedures which are experimental.

(2) A description of any reasonably foreseeable risks or discomforts to the subject.

(3) A description of any benefits to the subject or to others which may reasonably be expected from the research.

(4) A disclosure of appropriate alternative procedures or courses of treatment, if any, that might be advantageous to the subject.

(5) A statement describing the extent, if any, to which confidentiality of records identifying the subject will be maintained and that notes the possibility that the Food and Drug Administration may inspect the records.

(6) For research involving more than minimal risk, an explanation as to whether any compensation and an explanation as to whether any medical treatments are available if injury occurs and, if so, what they consist of, or where further information may be obtained.

(7) An explanation of whom to contact for answers to pertinent questions about the research and research subjects' rights, and whom to contact in the event of a research-related injury to the subject.

(8) A statement that participation is voluntary, that refusal to participate will involve no penalty or loss of benefits to which the subject is otherwise entitled, and that the subject may discontinue participation at any time without penalty or loss of benefits to which the subject is otherwise entitled.

(b) *Additional elements of informed consent.* When appropriate, one or more of the following elements of information shall also be provided to each subject:

(1) A statement that the particular treatment or procedure may involve risks to the subject (or to the embryo or fetus, if the subject is or may become pregnant) which are currently unforeseeable.

(2) Anticipated circumstances under which the subject's participation may be terminated by the investigator without regard to the subject's consent.

(3) Any additional costs to the subject that may result from participation in the research.

(4) The consequences of a subject's decision to withdraw from the research and procedures for orderly termination of participation by the subject.

(5) A statement that significant new findings developed during the course of the research which may relate to the subject's willingness to continue participation will be provided to the subject.

(6) The approximate number of subjects involved in the study.

(c) When seeking informed consent for applicable clinical trials, as defined in 42 U.S.C. 282(j)(1)(A), the following statement shall be provided to each clinical trial subject in informed consent documents and processes. This will notify the clinical trial subject that clinical trial information has been or will be submitted for inclusion in the clinical trial registry databank under paragraph (j) of section 402 of the Public Health Service Act. The statement is: "A description of this clinical trial will be available on *http://www.ClinicalTrials.gov*, as required by U.S. Law. This

Web site will not include information that can identify you. At most, the Web site will include a summary of the results. You can search this Web site at any time."

(d) The informed consent requirements in these regulations are not intended to preempt any applicable Federal, State, or local laws which require additional information to be disclosed for informed consent to be legally effective.

(e) Nothing in these regulations is intended to limit the authority of a physician to provide emergency medical care to the extent the physician is permitted to do so under applicable Federal, State, or local law.

[46 FR 8951, Jan. 27, 1981, as amended at 76 FR 270, Jan. 4, 2011]

§ 50.27 Documentation of informed consent.

(a) Except as provided in § 56.109(c), informed consent shall be documented by the use of a written consent form approved by the IRB and signed and dated by the subject or the subject's legally authorized representative at the time of consent. A copy shall be given to the person signing the form.

(b) Except as provided in § 56.109(c), the consent form may be either of the following:

(1) A written consent document that embodies the elements of informed consent required by § 50.25. This form may be read to the subject or the subject's legally authorized representative, but, in any event, the investigator shall give either the subject or the representative adequate opportunity to read it before it is signed.

(2) A *short form* written consent document stating that the elements of informed consent required by § 50.25 have been presented orally to the subject or the subject's legally authorized representative. When this method is used, there shall be a witness to the oral presentation. Also, the IRB shall approve a written summary of what is to be said to the subject or the representative. Only the short form itself is to be signed by the subject or the representative. However, the witness shall sign both the short form and a copy of the summary, and the person actually obtaining the consent shall sign a copy of the summary. A copy of the summary shall be given to the subject or the representative in addition to a copy of the short form.

[46 FR 8951, Jan. 27, 1981, as amended at 61 FR 57280, Nov. 5, 1996]

Subpart C [Reserved]

Subpart D—Additional Safeguards for Children in Clinical Investigations

Source: 66 FR 20598, Apr. 24, 2001, unless otherwise noted.

§ 50.50 IRB duties.

In addition to other responsibilities assigned to IRBs under this part and part 56 of this chapter, each IRB must review clinical investigations involving children as subjects covered by this subpart D and approve only those clinical investigations that satisfy the criteria described in § 50.51, § 50.52, or § 50.53 and the conditions of all other applicable sections of this subpart D.

§ 50.51 Clinical investigations not involving greater than minimal risk.

Any clinical investigation within the scope described in §§ 50.1 and 56.101 of this chapter in which no greater than minimal risk to children is presented may involve children as subjects only if the IRB finds that:

(a) No greater than minimal risk to children is presented; and

(b) Adequate provisions are made for soliciting the assent of the children and the permission of their parents or guardians as set forth in § 50.55.

[78 FR 12951, Feb. 26, 2013]

§ 50.52 Clinical investigations involving greater than minimal risk but presenting the prospect of direct benefit to individual subjects.

Any clinical investigation within the scope described in §§ 50.1 and 56.101 of this chapter in which more than minimal risk to children is presented by an intervention or procedure that holds out the prospect of direct benefit for the individual subject, or by a monitoring procedure that is likely to contribute to the subject's well-being, may involve children as subjects only if the IRB finds that:

(a) The risk is justified by the anticipated benefit to the subjects;

(b) The relation of the anticipated benefit to the risk is at least as favorable to the subjects as that presented by available alternative approaches; and

(c) Adequate provisions are made for soliciting the assent of the children and permission of their parents or guardians as set forth in § 50.55.

[66 FR 20598, Apr. 24, 2001, as amended at 78 FR 12951, Feb. 26, 2013]

§ 50.53 Clinical investigations involving greater than minimal risk and no prospect of direct benefit to individual subjects, but likely to yield generalizable knowledge about the subjects' disorder or condition.

Any clinical investigation within the scope described in §§ 50.1 and 56.101 of this chapter in which more than minimal risk to children is presented by an intervention or procedure that does not hold out the prospect of direct benefit for the individual subject, or by a monitoring procedure that is not likely to contribute to the well-being of the subject, may involve children as subjects only if the IRB finds that:

(a) The risk represents a minor increase over minimal risk;

(b) The intervention or procedure presents experiences to subjects that are reasonably commensurate with those inherent in their actual or expected medical, dental, psychological, social, or educational situations;

(c) The intervention or procedure is likely to yield generalizable knowledge about the subjects' disorder or condition that is of vital importance for the understanding or amelioration of the subjects' disorder or condition; and

(d) Adequate provisions are made for soliciting the assent of the children and permission of their parents or guardians as set forth in § 50.55.

[66 FR 20598, Apr. 24, 2001, as amended at 78 FR 12951, Feb. 26, 2013]

§ 50.54 Clinical investigations not otherwise approvable that present an opportunity to understand, prevent, or alleviate a serious problem affecting the health or welfare of children.

If an IRB does not believe that a clinical investigation within the scope described in §§ 50.1 and 56.101 of this chapter and involving children as subjects meets the requirements of § 50.51, § 50.52, or § 50.53, the clinical investigation may proceed only if:

(a) The IRB finds that the clinical investigation presents a reasonable opportunity to further the understanding, prevention, or alleviation of a serious problem affecting the health or welfare of children; and

(b) The Commissioner of Food and Drugs, after consultation with a panel of experts in pertinent disciplines (for example: science, medicine, education, ethics, law) and following opportunity for public review and comment, determines either:

(1) That the clinical investigation in fact satisfies the conditions of § 50.51, § 50.52, or § 50.53, as applicable, or

(2) That the following conditions are met:

(i) The clinical investigation presents a reasonable opportunity to further the understanding, prevention, or alleviation of a serious problem affecting the health or welfare of children;

(ii) The clinical investigation will be conducted in accordance with sound ethical principles; and

(iii) Adequate provisions are made for soliciting the assent of children and the permission of their parents or guardians as set forth in § 50.55.

[66 FR 20598, Apr. 24, 2001, as amended at 78 FR 12951, Feb. 26, 2013]

§ 50.55 Requirements for permission by parents or guardians and for assent by children.

(a) In addition to the determinations required under other applicable sections of this subpart D, the IRB must determine that adequate provisions are made for soliciting the assent of the children when in the judgment of the IRB the children are capable of providing assent.

(b) In determining whether children are capable of providing assent, the IRB must take into account the ages, maturity, and psychological state of the children involved. This judgment may be made for all children to be involved in clinical investigations under a particular protocol, or for each child, as the IRB deems appropriate.

(c) The assent of the children is not a necessary condition for proceeding with the clinical investigation if the IRB determines:

(1) That the capability of some or all of the children is so limited that they cannot reasonably be consulted, or

(2) That the intervention or procedure involved in the clinical investigation holds out a prospect of direct benefit that is important to the health or well-being of the children and is available only in the context of the clinical investigation.

(d) Even where the IRB determines that the subjects are capable of assenting, the IRB may still waive the assent requirement if it finds and documents that:

(1) The clinical investigation involves no more than minimal risk to the subjects;

(2) The waiver will not adversely affect the rights and welfare of the subjects;

(3) The clinical investigation could not practicably be carried out without the waiver; and

(4) Whenever appropriate, the subjects will be provided with additional pertinent information after participation.

(e) In addition to the determinations required under other applicable sections of this subpart D, the IRB must determine, in accordance with and to the extent that consent is required under part 50, that the permission of each child's parents or guardian is granted.

(1) Where parental permission is to be obtained, the IRB may find that the permission of one parent is sufficient for clinical investigations to be conducted under § 50.51 or § 50.52.

(2) Where clinical investigations are covered by § 50.53 or § 50.54 and permission is to be obtained from parents, both parents must give their permission unless one parent is deceased, unknown, incompetent, or not reasonably available, or when only one parent has legal responsibility for the care and custody of the child.

(f) Permission by parents or guardians must be documented in accordance with and to the extent required by § 50.27.

(g) When the IRB determines that assent is required, it must also determine whether and how assent must be documented.

[66 FR 20598, Apr. 24, 2001, as amended at 78 FR 12951, Feb. 26, 2013]

§ 50.56 Wards.

(a) Children who are wards of the State or any other agency, institution, or entity can be included in clinical investigations approved under § 50.53 or § 50.54 only if such clinical investigations are:

(1) Related to their status as wards; or

(2) Conducted in schools, camps, hospitals, institutions, or similar settings in which the majority of children involved as subjects are not wards.

(b) If the clinical investigation is approved under paragraph (a) of this section, the IRB must require appointment of an advocate for each child who is a ward.

(1) The advocate will serve in addition to any other individual acting on behalf of the child as guardian or in loco parentis.

(2) One individual may serve as advocate for more than one child.

(3) The advocate must be an individual who has the background and experience to act in, and agrees to act in, the best interest of the child for the duration of the child's participation in the clinical investigation.

(4) The advocate must not be associated in any way (except in the role as advocate or member of the IRB) with the clinical investigation, the investigator(s), or the guardian organization.

• • •

PART 54—FINANCIAL DISCLOSURE BY CLINICAL INVESTIGATORS

Authority: 21 U.S.C. 321, 331, 351, 352, 353, 355, 360, 360c-360j, 371, 372, 373, 374, 375, 376, 379; 42 U.S.C. 262.
Source: 63 FR 5250, Feb. 2, 1998, unless otherwise noted.

§ 54.1 Purpose.

(a) The Food and Drug Administration (FDA) evaluates clinical studies submitted in marketing applications, required by law, for new human drugs and biological products and marketing applications and reclassification petitions for medical devices.

(b) The agency reviews data generated in these clinical studies to determine whether the applications are approvable under the statutory requirements. FDA may consider clinical studies inadequate and the data inadequate if, among other things, appropriate steps have not been taken in the design, conduct, reporting, and analysis of the studies to minimize bias. One potential source of bias in clinical studies is a financial interest of the clinical investigator in the outcome of the study because of the way payment is arranged (e.g., a royalty) or because the investigator has a proprietary interest in the product (e.g., a patent) or because the investigator has an equity interest in the sponsor of the covered study. This section and conforming regulations require an applicant whose submission relies in part on clinical data to disclose certain financial arrangements between sponsor(s) of the covered studies and the clinical investigators and certain interests of the clinical investigators in the product under study or in the sponsor of the covered studies. FDA will use this information, in conjunction with information about the design and purpose of the study, as well as information obtained through on-site inspections, in the agency's assessment of the reliability of the data.

§ 54.2 Definitions.

For the purposes of this part:

(a) *Compensation affected by the outcome of clinical studies* means compensation that could be higher for a favorable outcome than for an unfavorable outcome, such as compensation that is explicitly greater for a favorable result or compensation to the investigator in the form of an equity interest in the sponsor of a covered study or in the form of compensation tied to sales of the product, such as a royalty interest.

(b) *Significant equity interest in the sponsor of a covered study* means any ownership interest, stock options, or other financial interest whose value cannot be readily determined through reference to public prices (generally, interests in a nonpublicly traded corporation), or any equity interest in a publicly traded corporation that exceeds $50,000 during the time the clinical investigator is carrying out the study and for 1 year following completion of the study.

(c) *Proprietary interest in the tested product* means property or other financial interest in the product including, but not limited to, a patent, trademark, copyright or licensing agreement.

(d) *Clinical investigator* means only a listed or identified investigator or subinvestigator who is directly involved in the treatment or evaluation of research subjects. The term also includes the spouse and each dependent child of the investigator.

(e) *Covered clinical study* means any study of a drug or device in humans submitted in a marketing application or reclassification petition subject to this part that the applicant or FDA relies on to establish that the product is effective (including studies that show equivalence to an effective product) or any study in which a single investigator makes a significant contribution to the demonstration of safety. This would, in general, not include phase I tolerance studies or pharmacokinetic studies, most clinical pharmacology studies (unless they are critical to an efficacy determination), large open safety studies conducted at multiple sites, treatment protocols, and parallel track protocols. An applicant may consult with FDA as to which clinical studies constitute "covered clinical studies" for purposes of complying with financial disclosure requirements.

(f) *Significant payments* of other sorts means payments made by the sponsor of a covered study to the investigator or the institution to support activities of the investigator that have a monetary value of more than $25,000, exclusive of the costs of conducting the clinical study or other clinical studies, (e.g., a grant to fund ongoing research, compensation in the form of equipment or retainers for ongoing consultation or honoraria) during the time the clinical investigator is carrying out the study and for 1 year following the completion of the study.

(g) *Applicant* means the party who submits a marketing application to FDA for approval of a drug, device, or biologic product. The applicant is responsible for submitting the appropriate certification and disclosure statements required in this part.

(h) *Sponsor of the covered clinical study* means the party supporting a particular study at the time it was carried out.

[63 FR 5250, Feb. 2, 1998, as amended at 63 FR 72181, Dec. 31, 1998]

§ 54.3 Scope.

The requirements in this part apply to any applicant who submits a marketing application for a human drug, biological product, or device and who submits covered clinical studies. The applicant is responsible for making the appropriate certification or disclosure statement where the applicant either contracted with one or more clinical investigators to conduct the studies or submitted studies conducted by others not under contract to the applicant.

§ 54.4 Certification and disclosure requirements.

For purposes of this part, an applicant must submit a list of all clinical investigators who conducted covered clinical studies to determine whether the applicant's product meets FDA's marketing requirements, identifying those clinical investigators who are full-time or part-time employees of the sponsor of each covered study. The applicant must also completely and accurately disclose or certify information concerning the financial interests of a clinical investigator who is not a full-time or part-time employee of the sponsor for each covered clinical study. Clinical investigators subject to investigational new drug or investigational device exemption regulations must provide the sponsor of the study with sufficient accurate information needed to allow subsequent disclosure or certification. The applicant is required to submit for each clinical investigator who participates in a covered study, either a certification that none of the financial arrangements described in § 54.2 exist, or disclose the nature of those arrangements to the agency. Where the applicant acts with due diligence to obtain the information required in this section but is unable to do so, the applicant shall certify that despite the applicant's due diligence in attempting to obtain the information, the applicant was unable to obtain the information and shall include the reason.

(a) The applicant (of an application submitted under sections 505, 506, 510(k), 513, or 515 of the Federal Food, Drug, and Cosmetic Act, or section 351 of the Public Health Service Act) that relies in whole or in part on clinical studies shall submit, for each clinical investigator who participated in a covered clinical study, either a certification described in paragraph (a)(1) of this section or a disclosure statement described in paragraph (a)(3) of this section.

(1) Certification: The applicant covered by this section shall submit for all clinical investigators (as defined in § 54.2(d)), to whom the certification applies, a completed Form FDA 3454 attesting to the absence of financial interests and arrangements described in paragraph (a)(3) of this section. The form shall be dated and signed by the chief financial officer or other responsible corporate official or representative.

(2) If the certification covers less than all covered clinical data in the application, the applicant shall include in the certification a list of the studies covered by this certification.

(3) Disclosure Statement: For any clinical investigator defined in § 54.2(d) for whom the applicant does not submit the certification described in paragraph (a)(1) of this section, the applicant shall submit a completed Form FDA 3455 disclosing completely and accurately the following:

(i) Any financial arrangement entered into between the sponsor of the covered study and the clinical investigator involved in the conduct of a covered clinical trial, whereby the value of the compensation to the clinical investigator for conducting the study could be influenced by the outcome of the study;

(ii) Any significant payments of other sorts from the sponsor of the covered study, such as a grant to fund ongoing research, compensation in the form of equipment, retainer for ongoing consultation, or honoraria;

(iii) Any proprietary interest in the tested product held by any clinical investigator involved in a study;

(iv) Any significant equity interest in the sponsor of the covered study held by any clinical investigator involved in any clinical study; and

(v) Any steps taken to minimize the potential for bias resulting from any of the disclosed arrangements, interests, or payments.

(b) The clinical investigator shall provide to the sponsor of the covered study sufficient accurate financial information to allow the sponsor to submit complete and accurate certification or disclosure statements as required in paragraph (a) of this section. The investigator shall promptly update this information if any relevant changes occur in the course of the investigation or for 1 year following completion of the study.

(c) Refusal to file application. FDA may refuse to file any marketing application described in paragraph (a) of this section that does not contain the information required by this section or a certification by the applicant that the applicant has acted with due diligence to obtain the information but was unable to do so and stating the reason.

[63 FR 5250, Feb. 2, 1998; 63 FR 35134, June 29, 1998, as amended at 64 FR 399, Jan. 5, 1999]

§ 54.5 Agency evaluation of financial interests.

(a) *Evaluation of disclosure statement.* FDA will evaluate the information disclosed under § 54.4(a)(2) about each covered clinical study in an application to determine the impact of any disclosed financial interests on the reliability of the study. FDA may consider both the size and nature of a disclosed financial interest (including the potential increase in the value of the interest if the product is approved) and steps that have been taken to minimize the potential for bias.

(b) *Effect of study design.* In assessing the potential of an investigator's financial interests to bias a study, FDA will take into account the design and purpose of the study. Study designs that utilize such approaches as multiple investigators (most of whom do not have a disclosable interest), blinding, objective endpoints, or measurement of endpoints by someone other than the investigator may adequately protect against any bias created by a disclosable financial interest.

(c) Agency actions to ensure reliability of data. If FDA determines that the financial interests of any clinical investigator raise a serious question about the integrity of the data, FDA will take any action it deems necessary to ensure the reliability of the data including:

(1) Initiating agency audits of the data derived from the clinical investigator in question;

(2) Requesting that the applicant submit further analyses of data, e.g., to evaluate the effect of the clinical investigator's data on overall study outcome;

(3) Requesting that the applicant conduct additional independent studies to confirm the results of the questioned study; and

(4) Refusing to treat the covered clinical study as providing data that can be the basis for an agency action.

§ 54.6 Recordkeeping and record retention.

(a) *Financial records of clinical investigators to be retained.* An applicant who has submitted a marketing application containing covered clinical studies shall keep on file certain information pertaining to the financial interests of clinical investigators who conducted studies on which the application relies and who are not full or part-time employees of the applicant, as follows:

(1) Complete records showing any financial interest or arrangement as described in § 54.4(a)(3)(i) paid to such clinical investigators by the sponsor of the covered study.

(2) Complete records showing significant payments of other sorts, as described in § 54.4(a)(3)(ii), made by the sponsor of the covered clinical study to the clinical investigator.

(3) Complete records showing any financial interests held by clinical investigators as set forth in § 54.4(a)(3)(iii) and (a)(3)(iv).

(b) Requirements for maintenance of clinical investigators' financial records. (1) For any application submitted for a covered product, an applicant shall retain records as described in paragraph (a) of this section for 2 years after the date of approval of the application.

(2) The person maintaining these records shall, upon request from any properly authorized officer or employee of FDA, at reasonable times, permit such officer or employee to have access to and copy and verify these records.

• • •

PART 56—INSTITUTIONAL REVIEW BOARDS

Authority: 21 U.S.C. 321, 343, 346, 346a, 348, 350a, 350b, 351, 352, 353, 355, 360, 360c-360f, 360h, 360i, 360j, 360hh-360ss, 371, 379e, 381; 42 U.S.C. 216, 241, 262.

Source: 46 FR 8975, Jan. 27, 1981, unless otherwise noted.

Subpart A—General Provisions

§ 56.101 Scope.

(a) This part contains the general standards for the composition, operation, and responsibility of an Institutional Review Board (IRB) that reviews clinical investigations regulated by the Food and Drug Administration under sections 505(i) and 520(g) of the act, as well as clinical investigations that support applications for research or marketing permits for products regulated by the Food and Drug Administration, including foods, including dietary supplements, that bear a nutrient content claim or a health claim, infant formulas, food and color additives, drugs for human use, medical devices for human use, biological products for human use, and electronic products. Compliance with this part is intended to protect the rights and welfare of human subjects involved in such investigations.

(b) References in this part to regulatory sections of the Code of Federal Regulations are to chapter I of title 21, unless otherwise noted.

[46 FR 8975, Jan. 27, 1981, as amended at 64 FR 399, Jan. 5, 1999; 66 FR 20599, Apr. 24, 2001]

§ 56.102 Definitions.

As used in this part:

(a) Act means the Federal Food, Drug, and Cosmetic Act, as amended (secs. 201-902, 52 Stat. 1040 et seq., as amended (21 U.S.C. 321-392)).

(b) *Application for research or marketing permit* includes:

(1) A color additive petition, described in part 71.

(2) Data and information regarding a substance submitted as part of the procedures for establishing that a substance is generally recognized as safe for a use which results or may reasonably be expected to result, directly or indirectly, in its becoming a component or otherwise affecting the characteristics of any food, described in § 170.35.

(3) A food additive petition, described in part 171.

(4) Data and information regarding a food additive submitted as part of the procedures regarding food additives permitted to be used on an interim basis pending additional study, described in § 180.1.

(5) Data and information regarding a substance submitted as part of the procedures for establishing a tolerance for unavoidable contaminants in food and food-packaging materials, described in section 406 of the act.

(6) An investigational new drug application, described in part 312 of this chapter.

(7) A new drug application, described in part 314.

(8) Data and information regarding the bioavailability or bioequivalence of drugs for human use submitted as part of the procedures for issuing, amending, or repealing a bioequivalence requirement, described in part 320.

(9) Data and information regarding an over-the-counter drug for human use submitted as part of the procedures for classifying such drugs as generally recognized as safe and effective and not misbranded, described in part 330.

(10) An application for a biologics license, described in part 601 of this chapter.

(11) Data and information regarding a biological product submitted as part of the procedures for determining that licensed biological products are safe and effective and not misbranded, as described in part 601 of this chapter.

(12) An Application for an Investigational Device Exemption, described in part 812.

(13) Data and information regarding a medical device for human use submitted as part of the procedures for classifying such devices, described in part 860.

(14) Data and information regarding a medical device for human use submitted as part of the procedures for establishing, amending, or repealing a standard for such device, described in part 861.

(15) An application for premarket approval of a medical device for human use, described in section 515 of the act.

(16) A product development protocol for a medical device for human use, described in section 515 of the act.

(17) Data and information regarding an electronic product submitted as part of the procedures for establishing, amending, or repealing a standard for such products, described in section 358 of the Public Health Service Act.

(18) Data and information regarding an electronic product submitted as part of the procedures for obtaining a variance from any electronic product performance standard, as described in § 1010.4.

(19) Data and information regarding an electronic product submitted as part of the procedures for granting, amending, or extending an exemption from a radiation safety performance standard, as described in § 1010.5.

(20) Data and information regarding an electronic product submitted as part of the procedures for obtaining an exemption from notification of a radiation safety defect or failure of compliance with a radiation safety performance standard, described in subpart D of part 1003.

(21) Data and information about a clinical study of an infant formula when submitted as part of an infant formula notification under section 412(c) of the Federal Food, Drug, and Cosmetic Act.

(22) Data and information submitted in a petition for a nutrient content claim, described in § 101.69 of this chapter, and for a health claim, described in § 101.70 of this chapter.

(23) Data and information from investigations involving children submitted in a new dietary ingredient notification, described in § 190.6 of this chapter.

(c) *Clinical investigation* means any experiment that involves a test article and one or more human subjects, and that either must meet the requirements for prior submission to the Food and Drug Administration under section 505(i) or 520(g) of the act, or need not meet the requirements for prior submission to the Food and Drug Administration under these sections of the act, but the results of which are intended to be later submitted to, or held for inspection by, the Food and Drug Administration as part of an application for a research or marketing permit. The term does not include experiments that must meet the provisions of part 58, regarding nonclinical laboratory studies. The terms *research, clinical research, clinical study, study,* and *clinical investigation* are deemed to be synonymous for purposes of this part.

(d) *Emergency use* means the use of a test article on a human subject in a life-threatening situation in which no standard acceptable treatment is available, and in which there is not sufficient time to obtain IRB approval.

(e) *Human subject* means an individual who is or becomes a participant in research, either as a recipient of the test article or as a control. A subject may be either a healthy individual or a patient.

(f) *Institution* means any public or private entity or agency (including Federal, State, and other agencies). The term facility as used in section 520(g) of the act is deemed to be synonymous with the term *institution* for purposes of this part.

(g) *Institutional Review Board (IRB)* means any board, committee, or other group formally designated by an institution to review, to approve the initiation of, and to conduct periodic review of, biomedical research involving human subjects. The primary purpose of such review is to assure the protection of the rights and welfare of the human subjects. The term has the same meaning as the phrase institutional review committee as used in section 520(g) of the act.

(h) *Investigator* means an individual who actually conducts a clinical investigation (i.e., under whose immediate direction the test article is administered or dispensed to, or used involving, a subject) or, in the event of an investigation conducted by a team of individuals, is the responsible leader of that team.

(i) *Minimal risk* means that the probability and magnitude of harm or discomfort anticipated in the research are not greater in and of themselves than those ordinarily encountered in daily life or during the performance of routine physical or psychological examinations or tests.

(j) *Sponsor* means a person or other entity that initiates a clinical investigation, but that does not actually conduct the investigation, i.e., the test article is administered or dispensed to, or used involving, a subject under the immediate direction of another individual. A person other than an individual (e.g., a corporation or agency) that uses one or more of its own employees to conduct an investigation that it has initiated is considered to be a sponsor (not a sponsor-investigator), and the employees are considered to be investigators.

(k) *Sponsor-investigator* means an individual who both initiates and actually conducts, alone or with others, a clinical investigation, i.e., under whose immediate direction the test article is administered or dispensed to, or used involving, a subject. The term does not include any person other than an individual, e.g., it does not include a corporation or agency. The obligations of a sponsor-investigator under this part include both those of a sponsor and those of an investigator.

(l) *Test article* means any drug for human use, biological product for human use, medical device for human use, human food additive, color additive, electronic product, or any other article subject to regulation under the act or under sections 351 or 354-360F of the Public Health Service Act.

(m) *IRB approval* means the determination of the IRB that the clinical investigation has been reviewed and may be conducted at an institution within the constraints set forth by the IRB and by other institutional and Federal requirements.

[46 FR 8975, Jan. 27, 1981, as amended at 54 FR 9038, Mar. 3, 1989; 56 FR 28028, June 18, 1991; 64 FR 399, Jan. 5, 1999; 64 FR 56448, Oct. 20, 1999; 65 FR 52302, Aug. 29, 2000; 66 FR 20599, Apr. 24, 2001; 74 FR 2368, Jan. 15, 2009]

§ 56.103 Circumstances in which IRB review is required.

(a) Except as provided in §§ 56.104 and 56.105, any clinical investigation which must meet the requirements for prior submission (as required in parts 312, 812, and 813) to the Food and Drug Administration shall not be initiated unless that investigation has been reviewed and approved by, and remains subject to continuing review by, an IRB meeting the requirements of this part.

(b) Except as provided in §§ 56.104 and 56.105, the Food and Drug Administration may decide not to consider in support of an application for a research or marketing permit any data or information that has been derived from a clinical investigation that has not been approved by, and that was not subject to initial and continuing review by, an IRB meeting the requirements of this part. The determination that a clinical investigation may not be considered in support of an application for a research or marketing permit does not, however, relieve the applicant for such a permit of any obligation under any other applicable regulations to submit the results of the investigation to the Food and Drug Administration.

(c) Compliance with these regulations will in no way render inapplicable pertinent Federal, State, or local laws or regulations.

[46 FR 8975, Jan. 27, 1981; 46 FR 14340, Feb. 27, 1981]

§ 56.104 Exemptions from IRB requirement.

The following categories of clinical investigations are exempt from the requirements of this part for IRB review:

(a) Any investigation which commenced before July 27, 1981 and was subject to requirements for IRB review under FDA regulations before that date, provided that the investigation remains subject to review of an IRB which meets the FDA requirements in effect before July 27, 1981.

(b) Any investigation commenced before July 27, 1981 and was not otherwise subject to requirements for IRB review under Food and Drug Administration regulations before that date.

(c) Emergency use of a test article, provided that such emergency use is reported to the IRB within 5 working days. Any subsequent use of the test article at the institution is subject to IRB review.

(d) Taste and food quality evaluations and consumer acceptance studies, if wholesome foods without additives are consumed or if a food is consumed that contains a food ingredient at or below the level and for a use found to be safe, or agricultural, chemical, or environmental contaminant at or below the level found to be safe, by the Food and Drug Administration or approved by the Environmental Protection Agency or the Food Safety and Inspection Service of the U.S. Department of Agriculture.

[46 FR 8975, Jan. 27, 1981, as amended at 56 FR 28028, June 18, 1991]

§ 56.105 Waiver of IRB requirement.

On the application of a sponsor or sponsor-investigator, the Food and Drug Administration may waive any of the requirements contained in these regulations, including the requirements for IRB review, for specific research activities or for classes of research activities, otherwise covered by these regulations.

Subpart B—Organization and Personnel

§ 56.106 Registration.

(a) *Who must register?* Each IRB in the United States that reviews clinical investigations regulated by FDA under sections 505(i) or 520(g) of the act and each IRB in the United States that reviews clinical investigations that are intended to support applications for research or marketing permits for FDA-regulated products must register at a site maintained by the Department of Health and Human Services (HHS). (A research permit under section 505(i) of the act is usually known as an investigational new drug application (IND), while a research permit under section 520(g) of the act is usually known as an investigational device exemption (IDE).) An individual authorized to act on the IRB's behalf must submit the registration information. All other IRBs may register voluntarily.

(b) *What information must an IRB register?* Each IRB must provide the following information:

(1) The name, mailing address, and street address (if different from the mailing address) of the institution operating the IRB and the name, mailing address, phone number, facsimile number, and electronic mail address of the senior officer of that institution who is responsible for overseeing activities performed by the IRB;

(2) The IRB's name, mailing address, street address (if different from the mailing address), phone number, facsimile number, and electronic mail address; each IRB chairperson's name, phone number, and electronic mail address; and the name, mailing address, phone number, facsimile number, and electronic mail address of the contact person providing the registration information.

(3) The approximate number of active protocols involving FDA-regulated products reviewed. For purposes of this rule, an "active protocol" is any protocol for which an IRB conducted an initial review or a continuing review at a convened meeting or under an expedited review procedure during the preceding 12 months; and

(4) A description of the types of FDA-regulated products (such as biological products, color additives, food additives, human drugs, or medical devices) involved in the protocols that the IRB reviews.

(c) *When must an IRB register?* Each IRB must submit an initial registration. The initial registration must occur before the IRB begins to review a clinical investigation described in paragraph (a) of this section. Each IRB must renew its registration every 3 years. IRB registration becomes effective after review and acceptance by HHS.

(d) *Where can an IRB register?* Each IRB may register electronically through http://ohrp.cit.nih.gov/efile. If an IRB lacks the ability to register electronically, it must send its registration information, in writing, to the Office of Good Clinical Practice, Office of Special Medical Programs, Food and Drug Administration, 10903 New Hampshire Ave., Bldg. 32, Rm. 5129, Silver Spring, MD 20993.

(e) *How does an IRB revise its registration information?* If an IRB's contact or chair person information changes, the IRB must revise its registration information by submitting any changes in that information within 90 days of the change. An IRB's decision to review new types of FDA-regulated products (such as a decision to review studies pertaining to food additives whereas the IRB previously reviewed studies pertaining to drug products), or to discontinue reviewing clinical investigations regulated by FDA is a change that must be reported within 30 days of the change. An IRB's decision to disband is a change that must be reported within 30 days of permanent cessation of the IRB's review of research. All other information changes may be reported when the IRB renews its registration. The revised information must be sent to FDA either electronically or in writing in accordance with paragraph (d) of this section.

[74 FR 2368, Jan. 15, 2009, as amended at 78 FR 16401, Mar. 15, 2013]

§ 56.107 IRB membership.

(a) Each IRB shall have at least five members, with varying backgrounds to promote complete and adequate review of research activities commonly conducted by the institution. The IRB shall be sufficiently qualified through the experience and expertise of its members, and the diversity of the members, including consideration of race, gender, cultural backgrounds, and sensitivity to such issues as community attitudes, to promote respect for its advice and counsel in safeguarding the rights and welfare of human subjects. In addition to possessing the professional competence necessary to review the specific research activities, the IRB shall be able to ascertain the acceptability of proposed research in terms of institutional commitments and regulations, applicable law, and standards of professional conduct and practice. * * * The IRB shall therefore include persons knowledgeable in these areas. If an IRB regularly reviews research that involves a vulnerable category of subjects, such as children, prisoners, pregnant women, or handicapped or mentally disabled persons, consideration shall be given to the inclusion of one or more individuals who are knowledgeable about and experienced in working with those subjects.

(b) Every nondiscriminatory effort will be made to ensure that no IRB consists entirely of men or entirely of women, including the instituton's consideration of qualified persons of both sexes, so long as no selection is made to the IRB on the basis of gender. No IRB may consist entirely of members of one profession.

(c) Each IRB shall include at least one member whose primary concerns are in the scientific area and at least one member whose primary concerns are in nonscientific areas.

(d) Each IRB shall include at least one member who is not otherwise affiliated with the institution and who is not part of the immediate family of a person who is affiliated with the institution.

(e) No IRB may have a member participate in the IRB's initial or continuing review of any project in which the member has a conflicting interest, except to provide information requested by the IRB.

(f) An IRB may, in its discretion, invite individuals with competence in special areas to assist in the review of complex issues which require expertise beyond or in addition to that available on the IRB. These individuals may not vote with the IRB.

[46 FR 8975, Jan. 27, 1981, as amended at 56 FR 28028, June 18, 1991; 56 FR 29756, June 28, 1991; 78 FR 16401, Mar. 15, 2013]

Subpart C—IRB Functions and Operations

§ 56.108 IRB functions and operations.

In order to fulfill the requirements of these regulations, each IRB shall:

(a) Follow written procedures: (1) For conducting its initial and continuing review of research and for reporting its findings and actions to the investigator and the institution; (2) for determining which projects require review more often than annually and which projects need verification from sources other than the investigator that no material changes have occurred since previous IRB review; (3) for ensuring prompt reporting to the IRB of changes in research activity; and (4) for ensuring that changes in approved research, during the period for which IRB approval has already been given, may not be initiated without IRB review and approval except where necessary to eliminate apparent immediate hazards to the human subjects.

(b) Follow written procedures for ensuring prompt reporting to the IRB, appropriate institutional officials, and the Food and Drug Administration of: (1) Any unanticipated problems involving risks to human subjects or others; (2) any instance of serious or continuing noncompliance with these regulations or the requirements or determinations of the IRB; or (3) any suspension or termination of IRB approval.

(c) Except when an expedited review procedure is used (see § 56.110), review proposed research at convened meetings at which a majority of the members of the IRB are present, including at least one member whose primary concerns are in nonscientific areas. In order for the research to be approved, it shall receive the approval of a majority of those members present at the meeting.

[46 FR 8975, Jan. 27, 1981, as amended at 56 FR 28028, June 18, 1991; 67 FR 9585, Mar. 4, 2002]

§ 56.109 IRB review of research.

(a) An IRB shall review and have authority to approve, require modifications in (to secure approval), or disapprove all research activities covered by these regulations.

(b) An IRB shall require that information given to subjects as part of informed consent is in accordance with § 50.25. The IRB may require that information, in addition to that specifically mentioned in § 50.25, be given to the subjects when in the IRB's judgment the information would meaningfully add to the protection of the rights and welfare of subjects.

(c) An IRB shall require documentation of informed consent in accordance with § 50.27 of this chapter, except as follows:

(1) The IRB may, for some or all subjects, waive the requirement that the subject, or the subject's legally authorized representative, sign a written consent form if it finds that the research presents no

more than minimal risk of harm to subjects and involves no procedures for which written consent is normally required outside the research context; or

(2) The IRB may, for some or all subjects, find that the requirements in § 50.24 of this chapter for an exception from informed consent for emergency research are met.

(d) In cases where the documentation requirement is waived under paragraph (c)(1) of this section, the IRB may require the investigator to provide subjects with a written statement regarding the research.

(e) An IRB shall notify investigators and the institution in writing of its decision to approve or disapprove the proposed research activity, or of modifications required to secure IRB approval of the research activity. If the IRB decides to disapprove a research activity, it shall include in its written notification a statement of the reasons for its decision and give the investigator an opportunity to respond in person or in writing. For investigations involving an exception to informed consent under § 50.24 of this chapter, an IRB shall promptly notify in writing the investigator and the sponsor of the research when an IRB determines that it cannot approve the research because it does not meet the criteria in the exception provided under § 50.24(a) of this chapter or because of other relevant ethical concerns. The written notification shall include a statement of the reasons for the IRB's determination.

(f) An IRB shall conduct continuing review of research covered by these regulations at intervals appropriate to the degree of risk, but not less than once per year, and shall have authority to observe or have a third party observe the consent process and the research.

(g) An IRB shall provide in writing to the sponsor of research involving an exception to informed consent under § 50.24 of this chapter a copy of information that has been publicly disclosed under § 50.24(a)(7)(ii) and (a)(7)(iii) of this chapter. The IRB shall provide this information to the sponsor promptly so that the sponsor is aware that such disclosure has occurred. Upon receipt, the sponsor shall provide copies of the information disclosed to FDA.

(h) When some or all of the subjects in a study are children, an IRB must determine that the research study is in compliance with part 50, subpart D of this chapter, at the time of its initial review of the research. When some or all of the subjects in a study that was ongoing on April 30, 2001, are children, an IRB must conduct a review of the research to determine compliance with part 50, subpart D of this chapter, either at the time of continuing review or, at the discretion of the IRB, at an earlier date.

[46 FR 8975, Jan. 27, 1981, as amended at 61 FR 51529, Oct. 2, 1996; 66 FR 20599, Apr. 24, 2001; 78 FR 12951, Feb. 26, 2013]

§ 56.110 Expedited review procedures for certain kinds of research involving no more than minimal risk, and for minor changes in approved research.

(a) The Food and Drug Administration has established, and published in the Federal Register, a list of categories of research that may be reviewed by the IRB through an expedited review procedure. The list will be amended, as appropriate, through periodic republication in the Federal Register.

(b) An IRB may use the expedited review procedure to review either or both of the following: (1) Some or all of the research appearing on the list and found by the reviewer(s) to involve no more than minimal risk, (2) minor changes in previously approved research during the period (of 1 year or less) for which approval is authorized. Under an expedited review procedure, the review may be carried out by the IRB chairperson or by one or more experienced reviewers designated by the IRB chairperson from among the members of the IRB. In reviewing the research, the reviewers may exercise all of the authorities of the IRB except that the reviewers may not disapprove the research. A research activity may be disapproved only after review in accordance with the nonexpedited review procedure set forth in § 56.108(c).

(c) Each IRB which uses an expedited review procedure shall adopt a method for keeping all members advised of research proposals which have been approved under the procedure.

(d) The Food and Drug Administration may restrict, suspend, or terminate an institution's or IRB's use of the expedited review procedure when necessary to protect the rights or welfare of subjects.

[46 FR 8975, Jan. 27, 1981, as amended at 56 FR 28029, June 18, 1991]

§ 56.111 Criteria for IRB approval of research.

(a) In order to approve research covered by these regulations the IRB shall determine that all of the following requirements are satisfied:

(1) Risks to subjects are minimized: (i) By using procedures which are consistent with sound research design and which do not unnecessarily expose subjects to risk, and (ii) whenever appropriate, by using procedures already being performed on the subjects for diagnostic or treatment purposes.

(2) Risks to subjects are reasonable in relation to anticipated benefits, if any, to subjects, and the importance of the knowledge that may be expected to result. In evaluating risks and benefits, the IRB should consider only those risks and benefits that may result from the research (as distinguished from risks and benefits of therapies that subjects would receive even if not participating in the research). The IRB should not consider possible long-range effects of applying knowledge gained in the research (for example, the possible effects of the research on public policy) as among those research risks that fall within the purview of its responsibility.

(3) Selection of subjects is equitable. In making this assessment the IRB should take into account the purposes of the research and the setting in which the research will be conducted and should be particularly cognizant of the special problems of research involving vulnerable populations, such as children, prisoners, pregnant women, handicapped, or mentally disabled persons, or economically or educationally disadvantaged persons.

(4) Informed consent will be sought from each prospective subject or the subject's legally authorized representative, in accordance with and to the extent required by part 50.

(5) Informed consent will be appropriately documented, in accordance with and to the extent required by § 50.27.

(6) Where appropriate, the research plan makes adequate provision for monitoring the data collected to ensure the safety of subjects.

(7) Where appropriate, there are adequate provisions to protect the privacy of subjects and to maintain the confidentiality of data.

(b) When some or all of the subjects, such as children, prisoners, pregnant women, handicapped, or mentally disabled persons, or economically or educationally disadvantaged persons, are likely to be vulnerable to coercion or undue influence additional safeguards have been included in the study to protect the rights and welfare of these subjects.

(c) In order to approve research in which some or all of the subjects are children, an IRB must determine that all research is in compliance with part 50, subpart D of this chapter.

[46 FR 8975, Jan. 27, 1981, as amended at 56 FR 28029, June 18, 1991; 66 FR 20599, Apr. 24, 2001]

§ 56.112 Review by institution.

Research covered by these regulations that has been approved by an IRB may be subject to further appropriate review and approval or disapproval by officials of the institution. However, those officials may not approve the research if it has not been approved by an IRB.

§ 56.113 Suspension or termination of IRB approval of research.

An IRB shall have authority to suspend or terminate approval of research that is not being conducted in accordance with the IRB's requirements or that has been associated with unexpected serious harm to subjects. Any suspension or termination of approval shall include a statement of the reasons for the IRB's action and shall be reported promptly to the investigator, appropriate institutional officials, and the Food and Drug Administration.

§ 56.114 Cooperative research.

In complying with these regulations, institutions involved in multi-institutional studies may use joint review, reliance upon the review of another qualified IRB, or similar arrangements aimed at avoidance of duplication of effort.

Subpart D—Records and Reports

§ 56.115 IRB records.

(a) An institution, or where appropriate an IRB, shall prepare and maintain adequate documentation of IRB activities, including the following:

(1) Copies of all research proposals reviewed, scientific evaluations, if any, that accompany the proposals, approved sample consent documents, progress reports submitted by investigators, and reports of injuries to subjects.

(2) Minutes of IRB meetings which shall be in sufficient detail to show attendance at the meetings; actions taken by the IRB; the vote on these actions including the number of members voting for, against, and abstaining; the basis for requiring changes in or disapproving research; and a written summary of the discussion of controverted issues and their resolution.

(3) Records of continuing review activities.

(4) Copies of all correspondence between the IRB and the investigators.

(5) A list of IRB members identified by name; earned degrees; representative capacity; indications of experience such as board certifications, licenses, etc., sufficient to describe each member's chief anticipated contributions to IRB deliberations; and any employment or other relationship between each member and the institution; for example: full-time employee, part-time employee, a member of governing panel or board, stockholder, paid or unpaid consultant.

(6) Written procedures for the IRB as required by § 56.108 (a) and (b).

(7) Statements of significant new findings provided to subjects, as required by § 50.25.

(b) The records required by this regulation shall be retained for at least 3 years after completion of the research, and the records shall be accessible for inspection and copying by authorized representatives of the Food and Drug Administration at reasonable times and in a reasonable manner.

(c) The Food and Drug Administration may refuse to consider a clinical investigation in support of an application for a research or marketing permit if the institution or the IRB that reviewed the investigation refuses to allow an inspection under this section.

[46 FR 8975, Jan. 27, 1981, as amended at 56 FR 28029, June 18, 1991; 67 FR 9585, Mar. 4, 2002]

Subpart E—Administrative Actions for Noncompliance

§ 56.120 Lesser administrative actions.

(a) If apparent noncompliance with these regulations in the operation of an IRB is observed by an FDA investigator during an inspection, the inspector will present an oral or written summary of observations to an appropriate representative of the IRB. The Food and Drug Administration may subsequently send a letter describing the noncompliance to the IRB and to the parent institution. The agency will require that the IRB or the parent institution respond to this letter within a time period specified by FDA and describe the corrective actions that will be taken by the IRB, the institution, or both to achieve compliance with these regulations.

(b) On the basis of the IRB's or the institution's response, FDA may schedule a reinspection to confirm the adequacy of corrective actions. In addition, until the IRB or the parent institution takes appropriate corrective action, the Agency may require the IRB to:

(1) Withhold approval of new studies subject to the requirements of this part that are conducted at the institution or reviewed by the IRB;

(2) Direct that no new subjects be added to ongoing studies subject to this part; or

(3) Terminate ongoing studies subject to this part when doing so would not endanger the subjects.

(c) When the apparent noncompliance creates a significant threat to the rights and welfare of human subjects, FDA may notify relevant State and Federal regulatory agencies and other parties with a direct interest in the Agency's action of the deficiencies in the operation of the IRB.

(d) The parent institution is presumed to be responsible for the operation of an IRB, and the Food and Drug Administration will ordinarily direct any administrative action under this subpart against the institution. However, depending on the evidence of responsibility for deficiencies, determined during the investigation, the Food and Drug Administration may restrict its administrative actions to the IRB or to a component of the parent institution determined to be responsible for formal designation of the IRB.

[46 FR 8975, Jan. 27, 1981, as amended at 81 FR 19035, Apr. 4, 2016]

§ 56.121 Disqualification of an IRB or an institution.

(a) Whenever the IRB or the institution has failed to take adequate steps to correct the noncompliance stated in the letter sent by the agency under § 56.120(a), and the Commissioner of Food and Drugs determines that this noncompliance may justify the disqualification of the IRB or of the parent institution, the Commissioner will institute proceedings in accordance with the requirements for a regulatory hearing set forth in part 16.

(b) The Commissioner may disqualify an IRB or the parent institution if the Commissioner determines that:

(1) The IRB has refused or repeatedly failed to comply with any of the regulations set forth in this part, and

(2) The noncompliance adversely affects the rights or welfare of the human subjects in a clinical investigation.

(c) If the Commissioner determines that disqualification is appropriate, the Commissioner will issue an order that explains the basis for the determination and that prescribes any actions to be taken with regard to ongoing clinical research conducted under the review of the IRB. The Food and Drug Administration will send notice of the disqualification to the IRB and the parent institution. Other parties with a direct interest, such as sponsors and clinical investigators, may also be sent a notice of the disqualification. In addition, the agency may elect to publish a notice of its action in the Federal Register.

(d) The Food and Drug Administration will not approve an application for a research permit for a clinical investigation that is to be under the review of a disqualified IRB or that is to be conducted at a disqualified institution, and it may refuse to consider in support of a marketing permit the data from a clinical investigation that was reviewed by a disqualified IRB as conducted at a disqualified institution, unless the IRB or the parent institution is reinstated as provided in § 56.123.

§ 56.122 Public disclosure of information regarding revocation.

A determination that the Food and Drug Administration has disqualified an institution and the administrative record regarding that determination are disclosable to the public under part 20.

§ 56.123 Reinstatement of an IRB or an institution.

An IRB or an institution may be reinstated if the Commissioner determines, upon an evaluation of a written submission from the IRB or institution that explains the corrective action that the institution or IRB plans to take, that the IRB or institution has provided adequate assurance that it will operate in compliance with the standards set forth in this part. Notification of reinstatement shall be provided to all persons notified under § 56.121(c).

§ 56.124 Actions alternative or additional to disqualification.

Disqualification of an IRB or of an institution is independent of, and neither in lieu of nor a precondition to, other proceedings or actions authorized by the act. The Food and Drug Administration may, at any time, through the Department of Justice institute any appropriate judicial proceedings (civil or criminal) and any other appropriate regulatory action, in addition to or in lieu of, and before, at the time of, or after, disqualification. The agency may also refer pertinent matters to another Federal, State, or local government agency for any action that that agency determines to be appropriate.

• • •

SUBCHAPTER D—DRUGS FOR HUMAN USE

PART 312—INVESTIGATIONAL NEW DRUG APPLICATION

Authority: 21 U.S.C. 321, 331, 351, 352, 353, 355, 360bbb, 371; 42 U.S.C. 262.
Source: 52 FR 8831, Mar. 19, 1987, unless otherwise noted.
Editorial note: Nomenclature changes to part 312 appear at 69 FR 13717, Mar. 24, 2004.

Subpart A—General Provisions

§ 312.1 Scope.

(a) This part contains procedures and requirements governing the use of investigational new drugs, including procedures and requirements for the submission to, and review by, the Food and Drug Administration of investigational new drug applications (IND's). An investigational new drug for which an IND is in effect in accordance with this part is exempt from the premarketing approval requirements that are otherwise applicable and may be shipped lawfully for the purpose of conducting clinical investigations of that drug.

(b) References in this part to regulations in the Code of Federal Regulations are to chapter I of title 21, unless otherwise noted.

§ 312.2 Applicability.

(a) *Applicability*. Except as provided in this section, this part applies to all clinical investigations of products that are subject to section 505 of the Federal Food, Drug, and Cosmetic Act or to the licensing provisions of the Public Health Service Act (58 Stat. 632, as amended (42 U.S.C. 201 et seq.)).

(b) *Exemptions*. (1) The clinical investigation of a drug product that is lawfully marketed in the United States is exempt from the requirements of this part if all the following apply:

(i) The investigation is not intended to be reported to FDA as a well-controlled study in support of a new indication for use nor intended to be used to support any other significant change in the labeling for the drug;

(ii) If the drug that is undergoing investigation is lawfully marketed as a prescription drug product, the investigation is not intended to support a significant change in the advertising for the product;

(iii) The investigation does not involve a route of administration or dosage level or use in a patient population or other factor that significantly increases the risks (or decreases the acceptability of the risks) associated with the use of the drug product;

(iv) The investigation is conducted in compliance with the requirements for institutional review set forth in part 56 and with the requirements for informed consent set forth in part 50; and

(v) The investigation is conducted in compliance with the requirements of § 312.7.

(2)(i) A clinical investigation involving an in vitro diagnostic biological product listed in paragraph (b)(2)(ii) of this section is exempt from the requirements of this part if (a) it is intended to be used in a diagnostic procedure that confirms the diagnosis made by another, medically established, diagnostic product or procedure and (b) it is shipped in compliance with § 312.160.

(ii) In accordance with paragraph (b)(2)(i) of this section, the following products are exempt from the requirements of this part: (a) blood grouping serum; (b) reagent red blood cells; and (c) anti-human globulin.

(3) A drug intended solely for tests in vitro or in laboratory research animals is exempt from the requirements of this part if shipped in accordance with § 312.160.

(4) FDA will not accept an application for an investigation that is exempt under the provisions of paragraph (b)(1) of this section.

(5) A clinical investigation involving use of a placebo is exempt from the requirements of this part if the investigation does not otherwise require submission of an IND.

(6) A clinical investigation involving an exception from informed consent under § 50.24 of this chapter is not exempt from the requirements of this part.

(c) *Bioavailability studies.* The applicability of this part to in vivo bioavailability studies in humans is subject to the provisions of § 320.31.

(d) *Unlabeled indication.* This part does not apply to the use in the practice of medicine for an unlabeled indication of a new drug product approved under part 314 or of a licensed biological product.

(e) *Guidance.* FDA may, on its own initiative, issue guidance on the applicability of this part to particular investigational uses of drugs. On request, FDA will advise on the applicability of this part to a planned clinical investigation.

[52 FR 8831, Mar. 19, 1987, as amended at 61 FR 51529, Oct. 2, 1996; 64 FR 401, Jan. 5, 1999]

§ 312.3 Definitions and interpretations.

(a) The definitions and interpretations of terms contained in section 201 of the Act apply to those terms when used in this part:

(b) The following definitions of terms also apply to this part:

Act means the Federal Food, Drug, and Cosmetic Act (secs. 201-902, 52 Stat. 1040 et seq., as amended (21 U.S.C. 301-392)).

Clinical investigation means any experiment in which a drug is administered or dispensed to, or used involving, one or more human subjects. For the purposes of this part, an experiment is any use of a drug except for the use of a marketed drug in the course of medical practice.

Contract research organization means a person that assumes, as an independent contractor with the sponsor, one or more of the obligations of a sponsor, e.g., design of a protocol, selection or monitoring of investigations, evaluation of reports, and preparation of materials to be submitted to the Food and Drug Administration.

FDA means the Food and Drug Administration.

IND means an investigational new drug application. For purposes of this part, "IND" is synonymous with "Notice of Claimed Investigational Exemption for a New Drug."

Independent ethics committee (IEC) means a review panel that is responsible for ensuring the protection of the rights, safety, and well-being of human subjects involved in a clinical investigation and is adequately constituted to provide assurance of that protection. An institutional review board (IRB), as defined in § 56.102(g) of this chapter and subject to the requirements of part 56 of this chapter, is one type of IEC.

Investigational new drug means a new drug or biological drug that is used in a clinical investigation. The term also includes a biological product that is used in vitro for diagnostic purposes. The terms "investigational drug" and "investigational new drug" are deemed to be synonymous for purposes of this part.

Investigator means an individual who actually conducts a clinical investigation (i.e., under whose immediate direction the drug is administered or dispensed to a subject). In the event an investigation is conducted by a team of individuals, the investigator is the responsible leader of the team. "Subinvestigator" includes any other individual member of that team.

Marketing application means an application for a new drug submitted under section 505(b) of the act or a biologics license application for a biological product submitted under the Public Health Service Act.

Sponsor means a person who takes responsibility for and initiates a clinical investigation. The sponsor may be an individual or pharmaceutical company, governmental agency, academic institution, private organization, or other organization. The sponsor does not actually conduct the investigation unless the sponsor is a sponsor-investigator. A person other than an individual that uses one or more of its own employees to conduct an investigation that it has initiated is a sponsor, not a sponsor-investigator, and the employees are investigators.

Sponsor-Investigator means an individual who both initiates and conducts an investigation, and under whose immediate direction the investigational drug is administered or dispensed. The term does not include any person other than an individual. The requirements applicable to a sponsor-investigator under this part include both those applicable to an investigator and a sponsor.

Subject means a human who participates in an investigation, either as a recipient of the investigational new drug or as a control. A subject may be a healthy human or a patient with a disease.

[52 FR 8831, Mar. 19, 1987, as amended at 64 FR 401, Jan. 5, 1999; 64 FR 56449, Oct. 20, 1999; 73 FR 22815, Apr. 28, 2008]

§ 312.6 Labeling of an investigational new drug.

(a) The immediate package of an investigational new drug intended for human use shall bear a label with the statement "Caution: New Drug—Limited by Federal (or United States) law to investigational use."

(b) The label or labeling of an investigational new drug shall not bear any statement that is false or misleading in any particular and shall not represent that the investigational new drug is safe or effective for the purposes for which it is being investigated.

(c) The appropriate FDA Center Director, according to the procedures set forth in §§ 201.26 or 610.68 of this chapter, may grant an exception or alternative to the provision in paragraph (a) of this section, to the extent that this provision is not explicitly required by statute, for specified lots, batches, or other units of a human drug product that is or will be included in the Strategic National Stockpile.

[52 FR 8831, Mar. 19, 1987, as amended at 72 FR 73599, Dec. 28, 2007]

§ 312.7 Promotion of investigational drugs.

(a) *Promotion of an investigational new drug.* A sponsor or investigator, or any person acting on behalf of a sponsor or investigator, shall not represent in a promotional context that an investigational new drug is safe or effective for the purposes for which it is under investigation or otherwise promote the drug. This provision is not intended to restrict the full exchange of scientific information concerning the drug, including dissemination of scientific findings in scientific or lay media. Rather, its intent is to restrict promotional claims of safety or effectiveness of the drug for a use for which it is under investigation and to preclude commercialization of the drug before it is approved for commercial distribution.

(b) *Commercial distribution of an investigational new drug.* A sponsor or investigator shall not commercially distribute or test market an investigational new drug.

(c) *Prolonging an investigation.* A sponsor shall not unduly prolong an investigation after finding that the results of the investigation appear to establish sufficient data to support a marketing application.

[52 FR 8831, Mar. 19, 1987, as amended at 52 FR 19476, May 22, 1987; 67 FR 9585, Mar. 4, 2002; 74 FR 40899, Aug. 13, 2009]

§ 312.8 Charging for investigational drugs under an IND.

(a) *General criteria for charging.* (1) A sponsor must meet the applicable requirements in paragraph (b) of this section for charging in a clinical trial or paragraph (c) of this section for charging for expanded access to an investigational drug for treatment use under subpart I of this part, except that sponsors need not fulfill the requirements in this section to charge for an approved drug obtained from another entity not affiliated with the sponsor for use as part of the clinical trial evaluation (e.g., in a clinical trial of a new use of the approved drug, for use of the approved drug as an active control).

(2) A sponsor must justify the amount to be charged in accordance with paragraph (d) of this section.

(3) A sponsor must obtain prior written authorization from FDA to charge for an investigational drug.

(4) FDA will withdraw authorization to charge if it determines that charging is interfering with the development of a drug for marketing approval or that the criteria for the authorization are no longer being met.

(b) *Charging in a clinical trial*—(1) *Charging for a sponsor's drug.* A sponsor who wishes to charge for its investigational drug, including investigational use of its approved drug, must:

(i) Provide evidence that the drug has a potential clinical benefit that, if demonstrated in the clinical investigations, would provide a significant advantage over available products in the diagnosis, treatment, mitigation, or prevention of a disease or condition;

(ii) Demonstrate that the data to be obtained from the clinical trial would be essential to establishing that the drug is effective or safe for the purpose of obtaining initial approval of a drug, or would support a significant change in the labeling of an approved drug (e.g., new indication, inclusion of comparative safety information); and

(iii) Demonstrate that the clinical trial could not be conducted without charging because the cost of the drug is extraordinary to the sponsor. The cost may be extraordinary due to manufacturing complexity, scarcity of a natural resource, the large quantity of drug needed (e.g., due to the size or duration of the trial), or some combination of these or other extraordinary circumstances (e.g., resources available to a sponsor).

(2) *Duration of charging in a clinical trial.* Unless FDA specifies a shorter period, charging may continue for the length of the clinical trial.

(c) *Charging for expanded access to investigational drug for treatment use.* (1) A sponsor who wishes to charge for expanded access to an investigational drug for treatment use under subpart I of this part must provide reasonable assurance that charging will not interfere with developing the drug for marketing approval.

(2) For expanded access under § 312.320 (treatment IND or treatment protocol), such assurance must include:

(i) Evidence of sufficient enrollment in any ongoing clinical trial(s) needed for marketing approval to reasonably assure FDA that the trial(s) will be successfully completed as planned;

(ii) Evidence of adequate progress in the development of the drug for marketing approval; and

(iii) Information submitted under the general investigational plan (§ 312.23(a)(3)(iv)) specifying the drug development milestones the sponsor plans to meet in the next year.

(3) The authorization to charge is limited to the number of patients authorized to receive the drug under the treatment use, if there is a limitation.

(4) Unless FDA specifies a shorter period, charging for expanded access to an investigational drug for treatment use under subpart I of this part may continue for 1 year from the time of FDA authorization. A sponsor may request that FDA reauthorize charging for additional periods.

(d) *Costs recoverable when charging for an investigational drug.* (1) A sponsor may recover only the direct costs of making its investigational drug available.

(i) Direct costs are costs incurred by a sponsor that can be specifically and exclusively attributed to providing the drug for the investigational use for which FDA has authorized cost recovery. Direct costs include costs per unit to manufacture the drug (e.g., raw materials, labor, and nonreusable supplies and equipment used to manufacture the quantity of drug needed for the use for which charging is authorized) or costs to acquire the drug from another manufacturing source, and direct costs to ship and handle (e.g., store) the drug.

(ii) Indirect costs include costs incurred primarily to produce the drug for commercial sale (e.g., costs for facilities and equipment used to manufacture the supply of investigational drug, but that are primarily intended to produce large quantities of drug for eventual commercial sale) and research and development, administrative, labor, or other costs that would be incurred even if the clinical trial or treatment use for which charging is authorized did not occur.

(2) For expanded access to an investigational drug for treatment use under §§ 312.315 (intermediate-size patient populations) and 312.320 (treatment IND or treatment protocol), in addition to the direct costs described in paragraph (d)(1)(i) of this section, a sponsor may recover the costs of monitoring the expanded access IND or protocol, complying with IND reporting requirements, and other administrative costs directly associated with the expanded access IND.

(3) To support its calculation for cost recovery, a sponsor must provide supporting documentation to show that the calculation is consistent with the requirements of paragraphs (d)(1) and, if applicable, (d)(2) of this section. The documentation must be accompanied by a statement that an independent certified public accountant has reviewed and approved the calculations.

[74 FR 40899, Aug. 13, 2009]

§312.10 Waivers.

(a) A sponsor may request FDA to waive applicable requirement under this part. A waiver request may be submitted either in an IND or in an information amendment to an IND. In an emergency, a request may be made by telephone or other rapid communication means. A waiver request is required to contain at least one of the following:

(1) An explanation why the sponsor's compliance with the requirement is unnecessary or cannot be achieved;

(2) A description of an alternative submission or course of action that satisfies the purpose of the requirement; or

(3) Other information justifying a waiver.

(b) FDA may grant a waiver if it finds that the sponsor's noncompliance would not pose a significant and unreasonable risk to human subjects of the investigation and that one of the following is met:

(1) The sponsor's compliance with the requirement is unnecessary for the agency to evaluate the application, or compliance cannot be achieved;

(2) The sponsor's proposed alternative satisfies the requirement; or

(3) The applicant's submission otherwise justifies a waiver.

[52 FR 8831, Mar. 19, 1987, as amended at 52 FR 23031, June 17, 1987; 67 FR 9585, Mar. 4, 2002]

Subpart B—Investigational New Drug Application (IND)

§312.20 Requirement for an IND.

(a) A sponsor shall submit an IND to FDA if the sponsor intends to conduct a clinical investigation with an investigational new drug that is subject to §312.2(a).

(b) A sponsor shall not begin a clinical investigation subject to §312.2(a) until the investigation is subject to an IND which is in effect in accordance with §312.40.

(c) A sponsor shall submit a separate IND for any clinical investigation involving an exception from informed consent under §50.24 of this chapter. Such a clinical investigation is not permitted to proceed without the prior written authorization from FDA. FDA shall provide a written determination 30 days after FDA receives the IND or earlier.

[52 FR 8831, Mar. 19, 1987, as amended at 61 FR 51529, Oct. 2, 1996; 62 FR 32479, June 16, 1997]

§312.21 Phases of an investigation.

An IND may be submitted for one or more phases of an investigation. The clinical investigation of a previously untested drug is generally divided into three phases. Although in general the phases are conducted sequentially, they may overlap. These three phases of an investigation are a follows:

(a) *Phase 1.* (1) Phase 1 includes the initial introduction of an investigational new drug into humans. Phase 1 studies are typically closely monitored and may be conducted in patients or normal volunteer subjects. These studies are designed to determine the metabolism and pharmacologic actions of the drug in humans, the side effects associated with increasing doses, and, if possible, to gain early evidence on effectiveness. During Phase 1, sufficient information about the drug's pharmacokinetics and pharmacological effects should be obtained to permit the design of well-controlled, scientifically valid, Phase 2 studies. The total number of subjects and patients included in Phase 1 studies varies with the drug, but is generally in the range of 20 to 80.

(2) Phase 1 studies also include studies of drug metabolism, structure-activity relationships, and mechanism of action in humans, as well as studies in which investigational drugs are used as research tools to explore biological phenomena or disease processes.

(b) *Phase 2.* Phase 2 includes the controlled clinical studies conducted to evaluate the effectiveness of the drug for a particular indication or indications in patients with the disease or condition under study and to determine the common short-term side effects and risks associated with the drug. Phase 2 studies are typically well controlled, closely monitored, and conducted in a relatively small number of patients, usually involving no more than several hundred subjects.

(c) *Phase 3.* Phase 3 studies are expanded controlled and uncontrolled trials. They are performed after preliminary evidence suggesting effectiveness of the drug has been obtained, and are intended to gather the additional information about effectiveness and safety that is needed to evaluate the overall benefit-risk relationship of the drug and to provide an adequate basis for physician labeling. Phase 3 studies usually include from several hundred to several thousand subjects.

§ 312.22 General principles of the IND submission.

(a) FDA's primary objectives in reviewing an IND are, in all phases of the investigation, to assure the safety and rights of subjects, and, in Phase 2 and 3, to help assure that the quality of the scientific evaluation of drugs is adequate to permit an evaluation of the drug's effectiveness and safety. Therefore, although FDA's review of Phase 1 submissions will focus on assessing the safety of Phase 1 investigations, FDA's review of Phases 2 and 3 submissions will also include an assessment of the scientific quality of the clinical investigations and the likelihood that the investigations will yield data capable of meeting statutory standards for marketing approval.

(b) The amount of information on a particular drug that must be submitted in an IND to assure the accomplishment of the objectives described in paragraph (a) of this section depends upon such factors as the novelty of the drug, the extent to which it has been studied previously, the known or suspected risks, and the developmental phase of the drug.

(c) The central focus of the initial IND submission should be on the general investigational plan and the protocols for specific human studies. Subsequent amendments to the IND that contain new or revised protocols should build logically on previous submissions and should be supported by additional information, including the results of animal toxicology studies or other human studies as appropriate. Annual reports to the IND should serve as the focus for reporting the status of studies being conducted under the IND and should update the general investigational plan for the coming year.

(d) The IND format set forth in § 312.23 should be followed routinely by sponsors in the interest of fostering an efficient review of applications. Sponsors are expected to exercise considerable discretion, however, regarding the content of information submitted in each section, depending upon the kind of drug being studied and the nature of the available information. Section 312.23 outlines the information needed for a commercially sponsored IND for a new molecular entity. A sponsor-investigator who uses, as a research tool, an investigational new drug that is already subject to a manufacturer's IND or marketing application should follow the same general format, but ordinarily may, if authorized by the manufacturer, refer to the manufacturer's IND or marketing application in providing the technical information supporting the proposed clinical investigation. A sponsor-investigator who uses an investigational drug not subject to a manufacturer's IND or marketing application is ordinarily required to submit all technical information supporting the IND, unless such information may be referenced from the scientific literature.

§ 312.23 IND content and format.

(a) A sponsor who intends to conduct a clinical investigation subject to this part shall submit an "Investigational New Drug Application" (IND) including, in the following order:

(1) *Cover sheet (Form FDA-1571).* A cover sheet for the application containing the following:

(i) The name, address, and telephone number of the sponsor, the date of the application, and the name of the investigational new drug.

(ii) Identification of the phase or phases of the clinical investigation to be conducted.

(iii) A commitment not to begin clinical investigations until an IND covering the investigations is in effect.

(iv) A commitment that an Institutional Review Board (IRB) that complies with the requirements set forth in part 56 will be responsible for the initial and continuing review and approval of each of the studies in the proposed clinical investigation and that the investigator will report to the IRB proposed changes in the research activity in accordance with the requirements of part 56.

(v) A commitment to conduct the investigation in accordance with all other applicable regulatory requirements.

(vi) The name and title of the person responsible for monitoring the conduct and progress of the clinical investigations.

(vii) The name(s) and title(s) of the person(s) responsible under § 312.32 for review and evaluation of information relevant to the safety of the drug.

(viii) If a sponsor has transferred any obligations for the conduct of any clinical study to a contract research organization, a statement containing the name and address of the contract research organization, identification of the clinical study, and a listing of the obligations transferred. If all obligations governing the conduct of the study have been transferred, a general statement of this transfer—in lieu of a listing of the specific obligations transferred—may be submitted.

(ix) The signature of the sponsor or the sponsor's authorized representative. If the person signing the application does not reside or have a place of business within the United States, the IND is required to contain the name and address of, and be countersigned by, an attorney, agent, or other authorized official who resides or maintains a place of business within the United States.

(2) *A table of contents.*

(3) *Introductory statement and general investigational plan.* (i) A brief introductory statement giving the name of the drug and all active ingredients, the drug's pharmacological class, the structural formula of the drug (if known), the formulation of the dosage form(s) to be used, the route of administration, and the broad objectives and planned duration of the proposed clinical investigation(s).

(ii) A brief summary of previous human experience with the drug, with reference to other IND's if pertinent, and to investigational or marketing experience in other countries that may be relevant to the safety of the proposed clinical investigation(s).

(iii) If the drug has been withdrawn from investigation or marketing in any country for any reason related to safety or effectiveness, identification of the country(ies) where the drug was withdrawn and the reasons for the withdrawal.

(iv) A brief description of the overall plan for investigating the drug product for the following year. The plan should include the following: (a) The rationale for the drug or the research study; (b) the indication(s) to be studied; (c) the general approach to be followed in evaluating the drug; (d) the kinds of clinical trials to be conducted in the first year following the submission (if plans are not developed for the entire year, the sponsor should so indicate); (e) the estimated number of patients to be given the drug in those studies; and (f) any risks of particular severity or seriousness anticipated on the basis of the toxicological data in animals or prior studies in humans with the drug or related drugs.

(4) [Reserved]

(5) *Investigator's brochure.* If required under § 312.55, a copy of the investigator's brochure, containing the following information:

(i) A brief description of the drug substance and the formulation, including the structural formula, if known.

(ii) A summary of the pharmacological and toxicological effects of the drug in animals and, to the extent known, in humans.

(iii) A summary of the pharmacokinetics and biological disposition of the drug in animals and, if known, in humans.

(iv) A summary of information relating to safety and effectiveness in humans obtained from prior clinical studies. (Reprints of published articles on such studies may be appended when useful.)

(v) A description of possible risks and side effects to be anticipated on the basis of prior experience with the drug under investigation or with related drugs, and of precautions or special monitoring to be done as part of the investigational use of the drug.

(6) *Protocols.* (i) A protocol for each planned study. (Protocols for studies not submitted initially in the IND should be submitted in accordance with § 312.30(a).) In general, protocols for Phase 1 studies may be less detailed and more flexible than protocols for Phase 2 and 3 studies. Phase 1 protocols should be directed primarily at providing an outline of the investigation—an estimate of the number of patients to be involved, a description of safety exclusions, and a description of the dosing plan including duration, dose, or method to be used in determining dose—and should specify in detail only those elements of the study that are critical to safety, such as necessary monitoring of vital signs and blood chemistries. Modifications of the experimental design of Phase 1 studies that do not affect critical safety assessments are required to be reported to FDA only in the annual report.

(ii) In Phases 2 and 3, detailed protocols describing all aspects of the study should be submitted. A protocol for a Phase 2 or 3 investigation should be designed in such a way that, if the sponsor anticipates that some deviation from the study design may become necessary as the investigation progresses, alternatives or contingencies to provide for such deviation are built into the protocols at the outset. For example, a protocol for a controlled short-term study might include a plan for an early crossover of nonresponders to an alternative therapy.

(iii) A protocol is required to contain the following, with the specific elements and detail of the protocol reflecting the above distinctions depending on the phase of study:

(a) A statement of the objectives and purpose of the study.

(b) The name and address and a statement of the qualifications (curriculum vitae or other statement of qualifications) of each investigator, and the name of each subinvestigator (e.g., research fellow, resident) working under the supervision of the investigator; the name and address of the research facilities to be used; and the name and address of each reviewing Institutional Review Board.

(c) The criteria for patient selection and for exclusion of patients and an estimate of the number of patients to be studied.

(d) A description of the design of the study, including the kind of control group to be used, if any, and a description of methods to be used to minimize bias on the part of subjects, investigators, and analysts.

(e) The method for determining the dose(s) to be administered, the planned maximum dosage, and the duration of individual patient exposure to the drug.

(f) A description of the observations and measurements to be made to fulfill the objectives of the study.

(g) A description of clinical procedures, laboratory tests, or other measures to be taken to monitor the effects of the drug in human subjects and to minimize risk.

(7) *Chemistry, manufacturing, and control information.* (i) As appropriate for the particular investigations covered by the IND, a section describing the composition, manufacture, and control of the drug substance and the drug product. Although in each phase of the investigation sufficient information is required to be submitted to assure the proper identification, quality, purity, and strength

of the investigational drug, the amount of information needed to make that assurance will vary with the phase of the investigation, the proposed duration of the investigation, the dosage form, and the amount of information otherwise available. FDA recognizes that modifications to the method of preparation of the new drug substance and dosage form and changes in the dosage form itself are likely as the investigation progresses. Therefore, the emphasis in an initial Phase 1 submission should generally be placed on the identification and control of the raw materials and the new drug substance. Final specifications for the drug substance and drug product are not expected until the end of the investigational process.

(ii) It should be emphasized that the amount of information to be submitted depends upon the scope of the proposed clinical investigation. For example, although stability data are required in all phases of the IND to demonstrate that the new drug substance and drug product are within acceptable chemical and physical limits for the planned duration of the proposed clinical investigation, if very short-term tests are proposed, the supporting stability data can be correspondingly limited.

(iii) As drug development proceeds and as the scale or production is changed from the pilot-scale production appropriate for the limited initial clinical investigations to the larger-scale production needed for expanded clinical trials, the sponsor should submit information amendments to supplement the initial information submitted on the chemistry, manufacturing, and control processes with information appropriate to the expanded scope of the investigation.

(iv) Reflecting the distinctions described in this paragraph (a)(7), and based on the phase(s) to be studied, the submission is required to contain the following:

(a) *Drug substance.* A description of the drug substance, including its physical, chemical, or biological characteristics; the name and address of its manufacturer; the general method of preparation of the drug substance; the acceptable limits and analytical methods used to assure the identity, strength, quality, and purity of the drug substance; and information sufficient to support stability of the drug substance during the toxicological studies and the planned clinical studies. Reference to the current edition of the United States Pharmacopeia—National Formulary may satisfy relevant requirements in this paragraph.

(b) *Drug product.* A list of all components, which may include reasonable alternatives for inactive compounds, used in the manufacture of the investigational drug product, including both those components intended to appear in the drug product and those which may not appear but which are used in the manufacturing process, and, where applicable, the quantitative composition of the investigational drug product, including any reasonable variations that may be expected during the investigational stage; the name and address of the drug product manufacturer; a brief general description of the manufacturing and packaging procedure as appropriate for the product; the acceptable limits and analytical methods used to assure the identity, strength, quality, and purity of the drug product; and information sufficient to assure the product's stability during the planned clinical studies. Reference to the current edition of the United States Pharmacopeia—National Formulary may satisfy certain requirements in this paragraph.

(c) A brief general description of the composition, manufacture, and control of any placebo used in a controlled clinical trial.

(d) *Labeling*. A copy of all labels and labeling to be provided to each investigator.

(e) *Environmental analysis requirements.* A claim for categorical exclusion under § 25.30 or 25.31 or an environmental assessment under § 25.40.

(8) *Pharmacology and toxicology information.* Adequate information about pharmacological and toxicological studies of the drug involving laboratory animals or in vitro, on the basis of which the sponsor has concluded that it is reasonably safe to conduct the proposed clinical investigations. The kind, duration, and scope of animal and other tests required varies with the duration and nature of the proposed clinical investigations. Guidance documents are available from FDA that describe

ways in which these requirements may be met. Such information is required to include the identification and qualifications of the individuals who evaluated the results of such studies and concluded that it is reasonably safe to begin the proposed investigations and a statement of where the investigations were conducted and where the records are available for inspection. As drug development proceeds, the sponsor is required to submit informational amendments, as appropriate, with additional information pertinent to safety.

(i) *Pharmacology and drug disposition.* A section describing the pharmacological effects and mechanism(s) of action of the drug in animals, and information on the absorption, distribution, metabolism, and excretion of the drug, if known.

(ii) *Toxicology.* (a) An integrated summary of the toxicological effects of the drug in animals and in vitro. Depending on the nature of the drug and the phase of the investigation, the description is to include the results of acute, subacute, and chronic toxicity tests; tests of the drug's effects on reproduction and the developing fetus; any special toxicity test related to the drug's particular mode of administration or conditions of use (e.g., inhalation, dermal, or ocular toxicology); and any in vitro studies intended to evaluate drug toxicity.

(b) For each toxicology study that is intended primarily to support the safety of the proposed clinical investigation, a full tabulation of data suitable for detailed review.

(iii) For each nonclinical laboratory study subject to the good laboratory practice regulations under part 58, a statement that the study was conducted in compliance with the good laboratory practice regulations in part 58, or, if the study was not conducted in compliance with those regulations, a brief statement of the reason for the noncompliance.

(9) *Previous human experience with the investigational drug.* A summary of previous human experience known to the applicant, if any, with the investigational drug. The information is required to include the following:

(i) If the investigational drug has been investigated or marketed previously, either in the United States or other countries, detailed information about such experience that is relevant to the safety of the proposed investigation or to the investigation's rationale. If the drug has been the subject of controlled trials, detailed information on such trials that is relevant to an assessment of the drug's effectiveness for the proposed investigational use(s) should also be provided. Any published material that is relevant to the safety of the proposed investigation or to an assessment of the drug's effectiveness for its proposed investigational use should be provided in full. Published material that is less directly relevant may be supplied by a bibliography.

(ii) If the drug is a combination of drugs previously investigated or marketed, the information required under paragraph (a)(9)(i) of this section should be provided for each active drug component. However, if any component in such combination is subject to an approved marketing application or is otherwise lawfully marketed in the United States, the sponsor is not required to submit published material concerning that active drug component unless such material relates directly to the proposed investigational use (including publications relevant to component-component interaction).

(iii) If the drug has been marketed outside the United States, a list of the countries in which the drug has been marketed and a list of the countries in which the drug has been withdrawn from marketing for reasons potentially related to safety or effectiveness.

(10) *Additional information.* In certain applications, as described below, information on special topics may be needed. Such information shall be submitted in this section as follows:

(i) *Drug dependence and abuse potential.* If the drug is a psychotropic substance or otherwise has abuse potential, a section describing relevant clinical studies and experience and studies in test animals.

(ii) *Radioactive drugs.* If the drug is a radioactive drug, sufficient data from animal or human studies to allow a reasonable calculation of radiation-absorbed dose to the whole body and critical organs upon administration to a human subject. Phase 1 studies of radioactive drugs must include studies which will obtain sufficient data for dosimetry calculations.

(iii) *Pediatric studies.* Plans for assessing pediatric safety and effectiveness.

(iv) *Other information.* A brief statement of any other information that would aid evaluation of the proposed clinical investigations with respect to their safety or their design and potential as controlled clinical trials to support marketing of the drug.

(11) Relevant information. If requested by FDA, any other relevant information needed for review of the application.

(b) *Information previously submitted.* The sponsor ordinarily is not required to resubmit information previously submitted, but may incorporate the information by reference. A reference to information submitted previously must identify the file by name, reference number, volume, and page number where the information can be found. A reference to information submitted to the agency by a person other than the sponsor is required to contain a written statement that authorizes the reference and that is signed by the person who submitted the information.

(c) *Material in a foreign language.* The sponsor shall submit an accurate and complete English translation of each part of the IND that is not in English. The sponsor shall also submit a copy of each original literature publication for which an English translation is submitted.

(d) *Number of copies.* The sponsor shall submit an original and two copies of all submissions to the IND file, including the original submission and all amendments and reports.

(e) *Numbering of IND submissions.* Each submission relating to an IND is required to be numbered serially using a single, three-digit serial number. The initial IND is required to be numbered 000; each subsequent submission (e.g., amendment, report, or correspondence) is required to be numbered chronologically in sequence.

(f) *Identification of exception from informed consent.* If the investigation involves an exception from informed consent under § 50.24 of this chapter, the sponsor shall prominently identify on the cover sheet that the investigation is subject to the requirements in § 50.24 of this chapter.

[52 FR 8831, Mar. 19, 1987, as amended at 52 FR 23031, June 17, 1987; 53 FR 1918, Jan. 25, 1988; 61 FR
[52 FR 8831, Mar. 19, 1987, as amended at 52 FR 23031, June 17, 1987; 53 FR 1918, Jan. 25, 1988; 61 FR
51529, Oct. 2, 1996; 62 FR 40599, July 29, 1997; 63 FR 66669, Dec. 2, 1998; 65 FR 56479, Sept. 19, 2000; 67 FR 9585, Mar. 4, 2002]

§ 312.30 Protocol amendments.

Once an IND is in effect, a sponsor shall amend it as needed to ensure that the clinical investigations are conducted according to protocols included in the application. This section sets forth the provisions under which new protocols may be submitted and changes in previously submitted protocols may be made. Whenever a sponsor intends to conduct a clinical investigation with an exception from informed consent for emergency research as set forth in § 50.24 of this chapter, the sponsor shall submit a separate IND for such investigation.

(a) *New protocol.* Whenever a sponsor intends to conduct a study that is not covered by a protocol already contained in the IND, the sponsor shall submit to FDA a protocol amendment containing the protocol for the study. Such study may begin provided two conditions are met: (1) The sponsor has submitted the protocol to FDA for its review; and (2) the protocol has been approved by the Institutional Review Board (IRB) with responsibility for review and approval of the study in accordance with the requirements of part 56. The sponsor may comply with these two conditions in either order.

(b) *Changes in a protocol.* (1) A sponsor shall submit a protocol amendment describing any change in a Phase 1 protocol that significantly affects the safety of subjects or any change in a Phase 2 or 3 protocol that significantly affects the safety of subjects, the scope of the investigation, or the scientific quality of the study. Examples of changes requiring an amendment under this paragraph include:

(i) Any increase in drug dosage or duration of exposure of individual subjects to the drug beyond that in the current protocol, or any significant increase in the number of subjects under study.

(ii) Any significant change in the design of a protocol (such as the addition or dropping of a control group).

(iii) The addition of a new test or procedure that is intended to improve monitoring for, or reduce the risk of, a side effect or adverse event; or the dropping of a test intended to monitor safety.

(2)(i) A protocol change under paragraph (b)(1) of this section may be made provided two conditions are met:

(a) The sponsor has submitted the change to FDA for its review; and

(b) The change has been approved by the IRB with responsibility for review and approval of the study. The sponsor may comply with these two conditions in either order.

(ii) Notwithstanding paragraph (b)(2)(i) of this section, a protocol change intended to eliminate an apparent immediate hazard to subjects may be implemented immediately provided FDA is subsequently notified by protocol amendment and the reviewing IRB is notified in accordance with § 56.104(c).

(c) *New investigator.* A sponsor shall submit a protocol amendment when a new investigator is added to carry out a previously submitted protocol, except that a protocol amendment is not required when a licensed practitioner is added in the case of a treatment protocol under § 312.315 or § 312.320. Once the investigator is added to the study, the investigational drug may be shipped to the investigator and the investigator may begin participating in the study. The sponsor shall notify FDA of the new investigator within 30 days of the investigator being added.

(d) *Content and format.* A protocol amendment is required to be prominently identified as such (i.e., "Protocol Amendment: New Protocol", "Protocol Amendment: Change in Protocol", or "Protocol Amendment: New Investigator"), and to contain the following:

(1)(i) In the case of a new protocol, a copy of the new protocol and a brief description of the most clinically significant differences between it and previous protocols.

(ii) In the case of a change in protocol, a brief description of the change and reference (date and number) to the submission that contained the protocol.

(iii) In the case of a new investigator, the investigator's name, the qualifications to conduct the investigation, reference to the previously submitted protocol, and all additional information about the investigator's study as is required under § 312.23(a)(6)(iii)(b).

(2) Reference, if necessary, to specific technical information in the IND or in a concurrently submitted information amendment to the IND that the sponsor relies on to support any clinically significant change in the new or amended protocol. If the reference is made to supporting information already in the IND, the sponsor shall identify by name, reference number, volume, and page number the location of the information.

(3) If the sponsor desires FDA to comment on the submission, a request for such comment and the specific questions FDA's response should address.

(e) *When submitted.* A sponsor shall submit a protocol amendment for a new protocol or a change in protocol before its implementation. Protocol amendments to add a new investigator or to provide additional information about investigators may be grouped and submitted at 30-day intervals.

When several submissions of new protocols or protocol changes are anticipated during a short period, the sponsor is encouraged, to the extent feasible, to include these all in a single submission.

[52 FR 8831, Mar. 19, 1987, as amended at 52 FR 23031, June 17, 1987; 53 FR 1918, Jan. 25, 1988; 61 FR 51530, Oct. 2, 1996; 67 FR 9585, Mar. 4, 2002; 74 FR 40942, Aug. 13, 2009]

§ 312.31 Information amendments.

(a) *Requirement for information amendment.* A sponsor shall report in an information amendment essential information on the IND that is not within the scope of a protocol amendment, IND safety reports, or annual report. Examples of information requiring an information amendment include:

(1) New toxicology, chemistry, or other technical information; or

(2) A report regarding the discontinuance of a clinical investigation.

(b) *Content and format of an information amendment.* An information amendment is required to bear prominent identification of its contents (e.g., "Information Amendment: Chemistry, Manufacturing, and Control", "Information Amendment: Pharmacology-Toxicology", "Information Amendment: Clinical"), and to contain the following:

(1) A statement of the nature and purpose of the amendment.

(2) An organized submission of the data in a format appropriate for scientific review.

(3) If the sponsor desires FDA to comment on an information amendment, a request for such comment.

(c) *When submitted.* Information amendments to the IND should be submitted as necessary but, to the extent feasible, not more than every 30 days.

[52 FR 8831, Mar. 19, 1987, as amended at 52 FR 23031, June 17, 1987; 53 FR 1918, Jan. 25, 1988; 67 FR 9585, Mar. 4, 2002]

§ 312.32 IND safety reporting.

(a) *Definitions.* The following definitions of terms apply to this section:

Adverse event means any untoward medical occurrence associated with the use of a drug in humans, whether or not considered drug related.

Life-threatening adverse event or life-threatening suspected adverse reaction. An adverse event or suspected adverse reaction is considered "life-threatening" if, in the view of either the investigator or sponsor, its occurrence places the patient or subject at immediate risk of death. It does not include an adverse event or suspected adverse reaction that, had it occurred in a more severe form, might have caused death.

Serious adverse event or *serious suspected adverse reaction*. An adverse event or suspected adverse reaction is considered "serious" if, in the view of either the investigator or sponsor, it results in any of the following outcomes: Death, a life-threatening adverse event, inpatient hospitalization or prolongation of existing hospitalization, a persistent or significant incapacity or substantial disruption of the ability to conduct normal life functions, or a congenital anomaly/birth defect. Important medical events that may not result in death, be life-threatening, or require hospitalization may be considered serious when, based upon appropriate medical judgment, they may jeopardize the patient or subject and may require medical or surgical intervention to prevent one of the outcomes listed in this definition. Examples of such medical events include allergic bronchospasm requiring intensive treatment in an emergency room or at home, blood dyscrasias or convulsions that do not result in inpatient hospitalization, or the development of drug dependency or drug abuse.

Suspected adverse reaction means any adverse event for which there is a reasonable possibility that the drug caused the adverse event. For the purposes of IND safety reporting, "reasonable possibility" means there is evidence to suggest a causal relationship between the drug and the adverse event. Suspected adverse reaction implies a lesser degree of certainty about causality than adverse reaction, which means any adverse event caused by a drug.

Unexpected adverse event or unexpected suspected adverse reaction. An adverse event or suspected adverse reaction is considered "unexpected" if it is not listed in the investigator brochure or is not listed at the specificity or severity that has been observed; or, if an investigator brochure is not required or available, is not consistent with the risk information described in the general investigational plan or elsewhere in the current application, as amended. For example, under this definition, hepatic necrosis would be unexpected (by virtue of greater severity) if the investigator brochure referred only to elevated hepatic enzymes or hepatitis. Similarly, cerebral thromboembolism and cerebral vasculitis would be unexpected (by virtue of greater specificity) if the investigator brochure listed only cerebral vascular accidents. "Unexpected," as used in this definition, also refers to adverse events or suspected adverse reactions that are mentioned in the investigator brochure as occurring with a class of drugs or as anticipated from the pharmacological properties of the drug, but are not specifically mentioned as occurring with the particular drug under investigation.

(b) Review of safety information. The sponsor must promptly review all information relevant to the safety of the drug obtained or otherwise received by the sponsor from foreign or domestic sources, including information derived from any clinical or epidemiological investigations, animal or in vitro studies, reports in the scientific literature, and unpublished scientific papers, as well as reports from foreign regulatory authorities and reports of foreign commercial marketing experience for drugs that are not marketed in the United States.

(c)(1) IND safety reports. The sponsor must notify FDA and all participating investigators (i.e., all investigators to whom the sponsor is providing drug under its INDs or under any investigator's IND) in an IND safety report of potential serious risks, from clinical trials or any other source, as soon as possible, but in no case later than 15 calendar days after the sponsor determines that the information qualifies for reporting under paragraph (c)(1)(i), (c)(1)(ii), (c)(1)(iii), or (c)(1)(iv) of this section. In each IND safety report, the sponsor must identify all IND safety reports previously submitted to FDA concerning a similar suspected adverse reaction, and must analyze the significance of the suspected adverse reaction in light of previous, similar reports or any other relevant information.

(i) Serious and unexpected suspected adverse reaction. The sponsor must report any suspected adverse reaction that is both serious and unexpected. The sponsor must report an adverse event as a suspected adverse reaction only if there is evidence to suggest a causal relationship between the drug and the adverse event, such as:

(A) A single occurrence of an event that is uncommon and known to be strongly associated with drug exposure (e.g., angioedema, hepatic injury, Stevens-Johnson Syndrome);

(B) One or more occurrences of an event that is not commonly associated with drug exposure, but is otherwise uncommon in the population exposed to the drug (e.g., tendon rupture);

(C) An aggregate analysis of specific events observed in a clinical trial (such as known consequences of the underlying disease or condition under investigation or other events that commonly occur in the study population independent of drug therapy) that indicates those events occur more frequently in the drug treatment group than in a concurrent or historical control group.

(ii) Findings from other studies. The sponsor must report any findings from epidemiological studies, pooled analysis of multiple studies, or clinical studies (other than those reported under paragraph (c)(1)(i) of this section), whether or not conducted under an IND, and whether or not conducted by the sponsor, that suggest a significant risk in humans exposed to the drug. Ordinarily, such a finding would result in a safety-related change in the protocol, informed consent, investigator brochure (excluding routine updates of these documents), or other aspects of the overall conduct of the clinical investigation.

(iii) Findings from animal or in vitro testing. The sponsor must report any findings from animal or in vitro testing, whether or not conducted by the sponsor, that suggest a significant risk in humans exposed to the drug, such as reports of mutagenicity, teratogenicity, or carcinogenicity, or reports of significant organ toxicity at or near the expected human exposure. Ordinarily, any such findings would result in a safety-related change in the protocol, informed consent, investigator brochure (excluding routine updates of these documents), or other aspects of the overall conduct of the clinical investigation.

(iv) Increased rate of occurrence of serious suspected adverse reactions. The sponsor must report any clinically important increase in the rate of a serious suspected adverse reaction over that listed in the protocol or investigator brochure.

(v) Submission of IND safety reports. The sponsor must submit each IND safety report in a narrative format or on FDA Form 3500A or in an electronic format that FDA can process, review, and archive. FDA will periodically issue guidance on how to provide the electronic submission (e.g., method of transmission, media, file formats, preparation and organization of files). The sponsor may submit foreign suspected adverse reactions on a Council for International Organizations of Medical Sciences (CIOMS) I Form instead of a FDA Form 3500A. Reports of overall findings or pooled analyses from published and unpublished in vitro, animal, epidemiological, or clinical studies must be submitted in a narrative format. Each notification to FDA must bear prominent identification of its contents, i.e., "IND Safety Report," and must be transmitted to the review division in the Center for Drug Evaluation and Research or in the Center for Biologics Evaluation and Research that has responsibility for review of the IND. Upon request from FDA, the sponsor must submit to FDA any additional data or information that the agency deems necessary, as soon as possible, but in no case later than 15 calendar days after receiving the request.

(2) Unexpected fatal or life-threatening suspected adverse reaction reports. The sponsor must also notify FDA of any unexpected fatal or life-threatening suspected adverse reaction as soon as possible but in no case later than 7 calendar days after the sponsor's initial receipt of the information.

(3) Reporting format or frequency. FDA may require a sponsor to submit IND safety reports in a format or at a frequency different than that required under this paragraph. The sponsor may also propose and adopt a different reporting format or frequency if the change is agreed to in advance by the director of the FDA review division that has responsibility for review of the IND.

(4) Investigations of marketed drugs. A sponsor of a clinical study of a drug marketed or approved in the United States that is conducted under an IND is required to submit IND safety reports for suspected adverse reactions that are observed in the clinical study, at domestic or foreign study sites. The sponsor must also submit safety information from the clinical study as prescribed by the postmarketing safety reporting requirements (e.g., §§ 310.305, 314.80, and 600.80 of this chapter).

(5) Reporting study endpoints. Study endpoints (e.g., mortality or major morbidity) must be reported to FDA by the sponsor as described in the protocol and ordinarily would not be reported under paragraph (c) of this section. However, if a serious and unexpected adverse event occurs for which there is evidence suggesting a causal relationship between the drug and the event (e.g., death from anaphylaxis), the event must be reported under § 312.32(c)(1)(i) as a serious and unexpected suspected adverse reaction even if it is a component of the study endpoint (e.g., all-cause mortality).

(d) Followup. (1) The sponsor must promptly investigate all safety information it receives.

(2) Relevant followup information to an IND safety report must be submitted as soon as the information is available and must be identified as such, i.e., "Followup IND Safety Report."

(3) If the results of a sponsor's investigation show that an adverse event not initially determined to be reportable under paragraph (c) of this section is so reportable, the sponsor must report such suspected adverse reaction in an IND safety report as soon as possible, but in no case later than 15 calendar days after the determination is made.

(e) *Disclaimer.* A safety report or other information submitted by a sponsor under this part (and any release by FDA of that report or information) does not necessarily reflect a conclusion by the sponsor or FDA that the report or information constitutes an admission that the drug caused or contributed to an adverse event. A sponsor need not admit, and may deny, that the report or information submitted by the sponsor constitutes an admission that the drug caused or contributed to an adverse event.

[75 FR 59961, Sept. 29, 2010]

§312.33 Annual reports.

A sponsor shall within 60 days of the anniversary date that the IND went into effect, submit a brief report of the progress of the investigation that includes:

(a) *Individual study information.* A brief summary of the status of each study in progress and each study completed during the previous year. The summary is required to include the following information for each study:

(1) The title of the study (with any appropriate study identifiers such as protocol number), its purpose, a brief statement identifying the patient population, and a statement as to whether the study is completed.

(2) The total number of subjects initially planned for inclusion in the study; the number entered into the study to date, tabulated by age group, gender, and race; the number whose participation in the study was completed as planned; and the number who dropped out of the study for any reason.

(3) If the study has been completed, or if interim results are known, a brief description of any available study results.

(b) *Summary information.* Information obtained during the previous year's clinical and nonclinical investigations, including:

(1) A narrative or tabular summary showing the most frequent and most serious adverse experiences by body system.

(2) A summary of all IND safety reports submitted during the past year.

(3) A list of subjects who died during participation in the investigation, with the cause of death for each subject.

(4) A list of subjects who dropped out during the course of the investigation in association with any adverse experience, whether or not thought to be drug related.

(5) A brief description of what, if anything, was obtained that is pertinent to an understanding of the drug's actions, including, for example, information about dose response, information from controlled trials, and information about bioavailability.

(6) A list of the preclinical studies (including animal studies) completed or in progress during the past year and a summary of the major preclinical findings.

(7) A summary of any significant manufacturing or microbiological changes made during the past year.

(c) A description of the general investigational plan for the coming year to replace that submitted 1 year earlier. The general investigational plan shall contain the information required under §312.23(a)(3)(iv).

(d) If the investigator brochure has been revised, a description of the revision and a copy of the new brochure.

(e) A description of any significant Phase 1 protocol modifications made during the previous year and not previously reported to the IND in a protocol amendment.

(f) A brief summary of significant foreign marketing developments with the drug during the past year, such as approval of marketing in any country or withdrawal or suspension from marketing in any country.

(g) If desired by the sponsor, a log of any outstanding business with respect to the IND for which the sponsor requests or expects a reply, comment, or meeting.

[52 FR 8831, Mar. 19, 1987, as amended at 52 FR 23031, June 17, 1987; 63 FR 6862, Feb. 11, 1998; 67 FR 9585, Mar. 4, 2002]

§ 312.38 Withdrawal of an IND.

(a) At any time a sponsor may withdraw an effective IND without prejudice.

(b) If an IND is withdrawn, FDA shall be so notified, all clinical investigations conducted under the IND shall be ended, all current investigators notified, and all stocks of the drug returned to the sponsor or otherwise disposed of at the request of the sponsor in accordance with § 312.59.

(c) If an IND is withdrawn because of a safety reason, the sponsor shall promptly so inform FDA, all participating investigators, and all reviewing Institutional Review Boards, together with the reasons for such withdrawal.

[52 FR 8831, Mar. 19, 1987, as amended at 52 FR 23031, June 17, 1987; 67 FR 9586, Mar. 4, 2002]

Subpart C—Administrative Actions

§ 312.40 General requirements for use of an investigational new drug in a clinical investigation.

(a) An investigational new drug may be used in a clinical investigation if the following conditions are met:

(1) The sponsor of the investigation submits an IND for the drug to FDA; the IND is in effect under paragraph (b) of this section; and the sponsor complies with all applicable requirements in this part and parts 50 and 56 with respect to the conduct of the clinical investigations; and

(2) Each participating investigator conducts his or her investigation in compliance with the requirements of this part and parts 50 and 56.

(b) An IND goes into effect:

(1) Thirty days after FDA receives the IND, unless FDA notifies the sponsor that the investigations described in the IND are subject to a clinical hold under § 312.42; or

(2) On earlier notification by FDA that the clinical investigations in the IND may begin. FDA will notify the sponsor in writing of the date it receives the IND.

(c) A sponsor may ship an investigational new drug to investigators named in the IND:

(1) Thirty days after FDA receives the IND; or

(2) On earlier FDA authorization to ship the drug.

(d) An investigator may not administer an investigational new drug to human subjects until the IND goes into effect under paragraph (b) of this section.

§ 312.41 Comment and advice on an IND.

(a) FDA may at any time during the course of the investigation communicate with the sponsor orally or in writing about deficiencies in the IND or about FDA's need for more data or information.

(b) On the sponsor's request, FDA will provide advice on specific matters relating to an IND. Examples of such advice may include advice on the adequacy of technical data to support an investigational plan, on the design of a clinical trial, and on whether proposed investigations are likely to produce the data and information that is needed to meet requirements for a marketing application.

(c) Unless the communication is accompanied by a clinical hold order under § 312.42, FDA communications with a sponsor under this section are solely advisory and do not require any modification in the planned or ongoing clinical investigations or response to the agency.

[52 FR 8831, Mar. 19, 1987, as amended at 52 FR 23031, June 17, 1987; 67 FR 9586, Mar. 4, 2002]

§ 312.42 Clinical holds and requests for modification.

(a) *General.* A clinical hold is an order issued by FDA to the sponsor to delay a proposed clinical investigation or to suspend an ongoing investigation. The clinical hold order may apply to one or more of the investigations covered by an IND. When a proposed study is placed on clinical hold, subjects may not be given the investigational drug. When an ongoing study is placed on clinical hold, no new subjects may be recruited to the study and placed on the investigational drug; patients already in the study should be taken off therapy involving the investigational drug unless specifically permitted by FDA in the interest of patient safety.

(b) *Grounds for imposition of clinical hold*—(1) *Clinical hold of a Phase 1 study under an IND.* FDA may place a proposed or ongoing Phase 1 investigation on clinical hold if it finds that:

(i) Human subjects are or would be exposed to an unreasonable and significant risk of illness or injury;

(ii) The clinical investigators named in the IND are not qualified by reason of their scientific training and experience to conduct the investigation described in the IND;

(iii) The investigator brochure is misleading, erroneous, or materially incomplete; or

(iv) The IND does not contain sufficient information required under § 312.23 to assess the risks to subjects of the proposed studies.

(v) The IND is for the study of an investigational drug intended to treat a life-threatening disease or condition that affects both genders, and men or women with reproductive potential who have the disease or condition being studied are excluded from eligibility because of a risk or potential risk from use of the investigational drug of reproductive toxicity (*i.e.*, affecting reproductive organs) or developmental toxicity (*i.e.*, affecting potential offspring). The phrase "women with reproductive potential" does not include pregnant women. For purposes of this paragraph, "life-threatening illnesses or diseases" are defined as "diseases or conditions where the likelihood of death is high unless the course of the disease is interrupted." The clinical hold would not apply under this paragraph to clinical studies conducted:

(A) Under special circumstances, such as studies pertinent only to one gender (e.g., studies evaluating the excretion of a drug in semen or the effects on menstrual function);

(B) Only in men or women, as long as a study that does not exclude members of the other gender with reproductive potential is being conducted concurrently, has been conducted, or will take place within a reasonable time agreed upon by the agency; or

(C) Only in subjects who do not suffer from the disease or condition for which the drug is being studied.

(2) *Clinical hold of a Phase 2 or 3 study under an IND.* FDA may place a proposed or ongoing Phase 2 or 3 investigation on clinical hold if it finds that:

(i) Any of the conditions in paragraphs (b)(1)(i) through (b)(1)(v) of this section apply; or

(ii) The plan or protocol for the investigation is clearly deficient in design to meet its stated objectives.

(3) *Clinical hold of an expanded access IND or expanded access protocol.* FDA may place an expanded access IND or expanded access protocol on clinical hold under the following conditions:

(i) *Final use.* FDA may place a proposed expanded access IND or treatment use protocol on clinical hold if it is determined that:

(A) The pertinent criteria in subpart I of this part for permitting the expanded access use to begin are not satisfied; or

(B) The expanded access IND or expanded access protocol does not comply with the requirements for expanded access submissions in subpart I of this part.

(ii) *Ongoing use.* FDA may place an ongoing expanded access IND or expanded access protocol on clinical hold if it is determined that the pertinent criteria in subpart I of this part for permitting the expanded access are no longer satisfied.

(4) *Clinical hold of any study that is not designed to be adequate and well-controlled.* FDA may place a proposed or ongoing investigation that is not designed to be adequate and well-controlled on clinical hold if it finds that:

(i) Any of the conditions in paragraph (b)(1) or (b)(2) of this section apply; or

(ii) There is reasonable evidence the investigation that is not designed to be adequate and well-controlled is impeding enrollment in, or otherwise interfering with the conduct or completion of, a study that is designed to be an adequate and well-controlled investigation of the same or another investigational drug; or

(iii) Insufficient quantities of the investigational drug exist to adequately conduct both the investigation that is not designed to be adequate and well-controlled and the investigations that are designed to be adequate and well-controlled; or

(iv) The drug has been studied in one or more adequate and well-controlled investigations that strongly suggest lack of effectiveness; or

(v) Another drug under investigation or approved for the same indication and available to the same patient population has demonstrated a better potential benefit/risk balance; or

(vi) The drug has received marketing approval for the same indication in the same patient population; or

(vii) The sponsor of the study that is designed to be an adequate and well-controlled investigation is not actively pursuing marketing approval of the investigational drug with due diligence; or

(viii) The Commissioner determines that it would not be in the public interest for the study to be conducted or continued. FDA ordinarily intends that clinical holds under paragraphs (b)(4)(ii), (b)(4)(iii) and (b)(4)(v) of this section would only apply to additional enrollment in nonconcurrently controlled trials rather than eliminating continued access to individuals already receiving the investigational drug.

(5) *Clinical hold of any investigation involving an exception from informed consent under § 50.24 of this chapter.* FDA may place a proposed or ongoing investigation involving an exception from informed consent under § 50.24 of this chapter on clinical hold if it is determined that:

(i) Any of the conditions in paragraphs (b)(1) or (b)(2) of this section apply; or

(ii) The pertinent criteria in § 50.24 of this chapter for such an investigation to begin or continue are not submitted or not satisfied.

(6) Clinical hold of any investigation involving an exception from informed consent under § 50.23(d) of this chapter. FDA may place a proposed or ongoing investigation involving an exception from informed consent under § 50.23(d) of this chapter on clinical hold if it is determined that:

(i) Any of the conditions in paragraphs (b)(1) or (b)(2) of this section apply; or

(ii) A determination by the President to waive the prior consent requirement for the administration of an investigational new drug has not been made.

(c) Discussion of deficiency. Whenever FDA concludes that a deficiency exists in a clinical investigation that may be grounds for the imposition of clinical hold FDA will, unless patients are exposed to immediate and serious risk, attempt to discuss and satisfactorily resolve the matter with the sponsor before issuing the clinical hold order.

(d) *Imposition of clinical hold.* The clinical hold order may be made by telephone or other means of rapid communication or in writing. The clinical hold order will identify the studies under the IND to which the hold applies, and will briefly explain the basis for the action. The clinical hold order will be made by or on behalf of the Division Director with responsibility for review of the IND. As soon as possible, and no more than 30 days after imposition of the clinical hold, the Division Director will provide the sponsor a written explanation of the basis for the hold.

(e) *Resumption of clinical investigations.* An investigation may only resume after FDA (usually the Division Director, or the Director's designee, with responsibility for review of the IND) has notified the sponsor that the investigation may proceed. Resumption of the affected investigation(s) will be authorized when the sponsor corrects the deficiency(ies) previously cited or otherwise satisfies the agency that the investigation(s) can proceed. FDA may notify a sponsor of its determination regarding the clinical hold by telephone or other means of rapid communication. If a sponsor of an IND that has been placed on clinical hold requests in writing that the clinical hold be removed and submits a complete response to the issue(s) identified in the clinical hold order, FDA shall respond in writing to the sponsor within 30-calendar days of receipt of the request and the complete response. FDA's response will either remove or maintain the clinical hold, and will state the reasons for such determination. Notwithstanding the 30-calendar day response time, a sponsor may not proceed with a clinical trial on which a clinical hold has been imposed until the sponsor has been notified by FDA that the hold has been lifted.

(f) *Appeal.* If the sponsor disagrees with the reasons cited for the clinical hold, the sponsor may request reconsideration of the decision in accordance with § 312.48.

(g) *Conversion of IND on clinical hold to inactive status.* If all investigations covered by an IND remain on clinical hold for 1 year or more, the IND may be placed on inactive status by FDA under § 312.45.

[52 FR 8831, Mar. 19, 1987, as amended at 52 FR 19477, May 22, 1987; 57 FR 13249, Apr. 15, 1992; 61 FR 51530, Oct. 2, 1996; 63 FR 68678, Dec. 14, 1998; 64 FR 54189, Oct. 5, 1999; 65 FR 34971, June 1, 2000; 74 FR 40942, Aug. 13, 2009]

§ 312.44 Termination.

(a) *General.* This section describes the procedures under which FDA may terminate an IND. If an IND is terminated, the sponsor shall end all clinical investigations conducted under the IND and recall or otherwise provide for the disposition of all unused supplies of the drug. A termination action may be based on deficiencies in the IND or in the conduct of an investigation under an IND. Except as provided in paragraph (d) of this section, a termination shall be preceded by a proposal to terminate by FDA and an opportunity for the sponsor to respond. FDA will, in general, only initiate an action under this section after first attempting to resolve differences informally or, when appropriate, through the clinical hold procedures described in § 312.42.

(b) *Grounds for termination*—(1) *Phase 1.* FDA may propose to terminate an IND during Phase 1 if it finds that:

(i) Human subjects would be exposed to an unreasonable and significant risk of illness or injury.

(ii) The IND does not contain sufficient information required under § 312.23 to assess the safety to subjects of the clinical investigations.

(iii) The methods, facilities, and controls used for the manufacturing, processing, and packing of the investigational drug are inadequate to establish and maintain appropriate standards of identity, strength, quality, and purity as needed for subject safety.

(iv) The clinical investigations are being conducted in a manner substantially different than that described in the protocols submitted in the IND.

(v) The drug is being promoted or distributed for commercial purposes not justified by the requirements of the investigation or permitted by § 312.7.

(vi) The IND, or any amendment or report to the IND, contains an untrue statement of a material fact or omits material information required by this part.

(vii) The sponsor fails promptly to investigate and inform the Food and Drug Administration and all investigators of serious and unexpected adverse experiences in accordance with § 312.32 or fails to make any other report required under this part.

(viii) The sponsor fails to submit an accurate annual report of the investigations in accordance with § 312.33.

(ix) The sponsor fails to comply with any other applicable requirement of this part, part 50, or part 56.

(x) The IND has remained on inactive status for 5 years or more.

(xi) The sponsor fails to delay a proposed investigation under the IND or to suspend an ongoing investigation that has been placed on clinical hold under § 312.42(b)(4).

(2) *Phase 2 or 3.* FDA may propose to terminate an IND during Phase 2 or Phase 3 if FDA finds that:

(i) Any of the conditions in paragraphs (b)(1)(i) through (b)(1)(xi) of this section apply; or

(ii) The investigational plan or protocol(s) is not reasonable as a bona fide scientific plan to determine whether or not the drug is safe and effective for use; or

(iii) There is convincing evidence that the drug is not effective for the purpose for which it is being investigated.

(3) FDA may propose to terminate a treatment IND if it finds that:

(i) Any of the conditions in paragraphs (b)(1)(i) through (x) of this section apply; or

(ii) Any of the conditions in § 312.42(b)(3) apply.

(c) *Opportunity for sponsor response.* (1) If FDA proposes to terminate an IND, FDA will notify the sponsor in writing, and invite correction or explanation within a period of 30 days.

(2) On such notification, the sponsor may provide a written explanation or correction or may request a conference with FDA to provide the requested explanation or correction. If the sponsor does not respond to the notification within the allocated time, the IND shall be terminated.

(3) If the sponsor responds but FDA does not accept the explanation or correction submitted, FDA shall inform the sponsor in writing of the reason for the nonacceptance and provide the sponsor with an opportunity for a regulatory hearing before FDA under part 16 on the question of whether the IND should be terminated. The sponsor's request for a regulatory hearing must be made within 10 days of the sponsor's receipt of FDA's notification of nonacceptance.

(d) *Immediate termination of IND.* Notwithstanding paragraphs (a) through (c) of this section, if at any time FDA concludes that continuation of the investigation presents an immediate and substantial danger to the health of individuals, the agency shall immediately, by written notice to the sponsor from the Director of the Center for Drug Evaluation and Research or the Director of the Center for Biologics Evaluation and Research, terminate the IND. An IND so terminated is subject to reinstatement by the Director on the basis of additional submissions that eliminate such danger. If an IND is terminated under this paragraph, the agency will afford the sponsor an opportunity for a regulatory hearing under part 16 on the question of whether the IND should be reinstated.

[52 FR 8831, Mar. 19, 1987, as amended at 52 FR 23031, June 17, 1987; 55 FR 11579, Mar. 29, 1990; 57 FR 13249, Apr. 15, 1992; 67 FR 9586, Mar. 4, 2002]

§312.45 Inactive status.

(a) If no subjects are entered into clinical studies for a period of 2 years or more under an IND, or if all investigations under an IND remain on clinical hold for 1 year or more, the IND may be placed by FDA on inactive status. This action may be taken by FDA either on request of the sponsor or on FDA's own initiative. If FDA seeks to act on its own initiative under this section, it shall first notify the sponsor in writing of the proposed inactive status. Upon receipt of such notification, the sponsor shall have 30 days to respond as to why the IND should continue to remain active.

(b) If an IND is placed on inactive status, all investigators shall be so notified and all stocks of the drug shall be returned or otherwise disposed of in accordance with §312.59.

(c) A sponsor is not required to submit annual reports to an IND on inactive status. An inactive IND is, however, still in effect for purposes of the public disclosure of data and information under §312.130.

(d) A sponsor who intends to resume clinical investigation under an IND placed on inactive status shall submit a protocol amendment under §312.30 containing the proposed general investigational plan for the coming year and appropriate protocols. If the protocol amendment relies on information previously submitted, the plan shall reference such information. Additional information supporting the proposed investigation, if any, shall be submitted in an information amendment. Notwithstanding the provisions of §312.30, clinical investigations under an IND on inactive status may only resume (1) 30 days after FDA receives the protocol amendment, unless FDA notifies the sponsor that the investigations described in the amendment are subject to a clinical hold under §312.42, or (2) on earlier notification by FDA that the clinical investigations described in the protocol amendment may begin.

(e) An IND that remains on inactive status for 5 years or more may be terminated under §312.44.

[52 FR 8831, Mar. 19, 1987, as amended at 52 FR 23031, June 17, 1987; 67 FR 9586, Mar. 4, 2002]

§312.47 Meetings.

(a) *General.* Meetings between a sponsor and the agency are frequently useful in resolving questions and issues raised during the course of a clinical investigation. FDA encourages such meetings to the extent that they aid in the evaluation of the drug and in the solution of scientific problems concerning the drug, to the extent that FDA's resources permit. The general principle underlying the conduct of such meetings is that there should be free, full, and open communication about any scientific or medical question that may arise during the clinical investigation. These meetings shall be conducted and documented in accordance with part 10.

(b) *"End-of-Phase 2" meetings and meetings held before submission of a marketing application.* At specific times during the drug investigation process, meetings between FDA and a sponsor can be especially helpful in minimizing wasteful expenditures of time and money and thus in speeding the drug development and evaluation process. In particular, FDA has found that meetings at the end of Phase 2 of an investigation (end-of-Phase 2 meetings) are of considerable assistance in planning later studies and that meetings held near completion of Phase 3 and before submission of a marketing application ("pre-NDA" meetings) are helpful in developing methods of presentation and submission of data in the marketing application that facilitate review and allow timely FDA response.

(1) *End-of-Phase 2 meetings*—(i) *Purpose.* The purpose of an end-of-phase 2 meeting is to determine the safety of proceeding to Phase 3, to evaluate the Phase 3 plan and protocols and the adequacy of current studies and plans to assess pediatric safety and effectiveness, and to identify any additional information necessary to support a marketing application for the uses under investigation.

(ii) *Eligibility for meeting.* While the end-of-Phase 2 meeting is designed primarily for IND's involving new molecular entities or major new uses of marketed drugs, a sponsor of any IND may request and obtain an end-of-Phase 2 meeting.

(iii) *Timing.* To be most useful to the sponsor, end-of-Phase 2 meetings should be held before major commitments of effort and resources to specific Phase 3 tests are made. The scheduling of an end-of-Phase 2 meeting is not, however, intended to delay the transition of an investigation from Phase 2 to Phase 3.

(iv) *Advance information.* At least 1 month in advance of an end-of-Phase 2 meeting, the sponsor should submit background information on the sponsor's plan for Phase 3, including summaries of the Phase 1 and 2 investigations, the specific protocols for Phase 3 clinical studies, plans for any additional nonclinical studies, plans for pediatric studies, including a time line for protocol finalization, enrollment, completion, and data analysis, or information to support any planned request for waiver or deferral of pediatric studies, and, if available, tentative labeling for the drug. The recommended contents of such a submission are described more fully in FDA Staff Manual Guide 4850.7 that is publicly available under FDA's public information regulations in part 20.

(v) *Conduct of meeting.* Arrangements for an end-of-Phase 2 meeting are to be made with the division in FDA's Center for Drug Evaluation and Research or the Center for Biologics Evaluation and Research which is responsible for review of the IND. The meeting will be scheduled by FDA at a time convenient to both FDA and the sponsor. Both the sponsor and FDA may bring consultants to the meeting. The meeting should be directed primarily at establishing agreement between FDA and the sponsor of the overall plan for Phase 3 and the objectives and design of particular studies. The adequacy of the technical information to support Phase 3 studies and/or a marketing application may also be discussed. FDA will also provide its best judgment, at that time, of the pediatric studies that will be required for the drug product and whether their submission will be deferred until after approval. Agreements reached at the meeting on these matters will be recorded in minutes of the conference that will be taken by FDA in accordance with § 10.65 and provided to the sponsor. The minutes along with any other written material provided to the sponsor will serve as a permanent record of any agreements reached. Barring a significant scientific development that requires otherwise, studies conducted in accordance with the agreement shall be presumed to be sufficient in objective and design for the purpose of obtaining marketing approval for the drug.

(2) *"Pre-NDA" and "pre-BLA" meetings.* FDA has found that delays associated with the initial review of a marketing application may be reduced by exchanges of information about a proposed marketing application. The primary purpose of this kind of exchange is to uncover any major unresolved problems, to identify those studies that the sponsor is relying on as adequate and well-controlled to establish the drug's effectiveness, to identify the status of ongoing or needed studies adequate to assess pediatric safety and effectiveness, to acquaint FDA reviewers with the general information to be submitted in the marketing application (including technical information), to discuss appropriate methods for statistical analysis of the data, and to discuss the best approach to the presentation and formatting of data in the marketing application. Arrangements for such a meeting are to be initiated by the sponsor with the division responsible for review of the IND. To permit FDA to provide the sponsor with the most useful advice on preparing a marketing application, the sponsor should submit to FDA's reviewing division at least 1 month in advance of the meeting the following information:

(i) A brief summary of the clinical studies to be submitted in the application.

(ii) A proposed format for organizing the submission, including methods for presenting the data.

(iii) Information on the status of needed or ongoing pediatric studies.

(iv) Any other information for discussion at the meeting.

[52 FR 8831, Mar. 19, 1987, as amended at 52 FR 23031, June 17, 1987; 55 FR 11580, Mar. 29, 1990; 63 FR 66669, Dec. 2, 1998; 67 FR 9586, Mar. 4, 2002]

§ 312.48 Dispute resolution.

(a) *General.* The Food and Drug Administration is committed to resolving differences between sponsors and FDA reviewing divisions with respect to requirements for IND's as quickly and amicably as possible through the cooperative exchange of information and views.

(b) *Administrative and procedural issues.* When administrative or procedural disputes arise, the sponsor should first attempt to resolve the matter with the division in FDA's Center for Drug Evaluation and Research or Center for Biologics Evaluation and Research which is responsible for review of the IND, beginning with the consumer safety officer assigned to the application. If the dispute is not resolved, the sponsor may raise the matter with the person designated as ombudsman, whose function shall be to investigate what has happened and to facilitate a timely and equitable resolution. Appropriate issues to raise with the ombudsman include resolving difficulties in scheduling meetings and obtaining timely replies to inquiries. Further details on this procedure are contained in FDA Staff Manual Guide 4820.7 that is publicly available under FDA's public information regulations in part 20.

(c) *Scientific and medical disputes.* (1) When scientific or medical disputes arise during the drug investigation process, sponsors should discuss the matter directly with the responsible reviewing officials. If necessary, sponsors may request a meeting with the appropriate reviewing officials and management representatives in order to seek a resolution. Requests for such meetings shall be directed to the director of the division in FDA's Center for Drug Evaluation and Research or Center for Biologics Evaluation and Research which is responsible for review of the IND. FDA will make every attempt to grant requests for meetings that involve important issues and that can be scheduled at mutually convenient times.

(2) The "end-of-Phase 2" and "pre-NDA" meetings described in § 312.47(b) will also provide a timely forum for discussing and resolving scientific and medical issues on which the sponsor disagrees with the agency.

(3) In requesting a meeting designed to resolve a scientific or medical dispute, applicants may suggest that FDA seek the advice of outside experts, in which case FDA may, in its discretion, invite to the meeting one or more of its advisory committee members or other consultants, as designated by the agency. Applicants may rely on, and may bring to any meeting, their own consultants. For major scientific and medical policy issues not resolved by informal meetings, FDA may refer the matter to one of its standing advisory committees for its consideration and recommendations.

[52 FR 8831, Mar. 19, 1987, as amended at 55 FR 11580, Mar. 29, 1990]

Subpart D—Responsibilities of Sponsors and Investigators

§ 312.50 General responsibilities of sponsors.

Sponsors are responsible for selecting qualified investigators, providing them with the information they need to conduct an investigation properly, ensuring proper monitoring of the investigation(s), ensuring that the investigation(s) is conducted in accordance with the general investigational plan and protocols contained in the IND, maintaining an effective IND with respect to the investigations, and ensuring that FDA and all participating investigators are promptly informed of significant new adverse effects or risks with respect to the drug. Additional specific responsibilities of sponsors are described elsewhere in this part.

§ 312.52 Transfer of obligations to a contract research organization.

(a) A sponsor may transfer responsibility for any or all of the obligations set forth in this part to a contract research organization. Any such transfer shall be described in writing. If not all obligations are transferred, the writing is required to describe each of the obligations being assumed by the contract research organization. If all obligations are transferred, a general statement that all obligations have been transferred is acceptable. Any obligation not covered by the written description shall be deemed not to have been transferred.

(b) A contract research organization that assumes any obligation of a sponsor shall comply with the specific regulations in this chapter applicable to this obligation and shall be subject to the same regulatory action as a sponsor for failure to comply with any obligation assumed under these regulations. Thus, all references to "sponsor" in this part apply to a contract research organization to the extent that it assumes one or more obligations of the sponsor.

§ 312.53 Selecting investigators and monitors.

(a) *Selecting investigators.* A sponsor shall select only investigators qualified by training and experience as appropriate experts to investigate the drug.

(b) *Control of drug.* A sponsor shall ship investigational new drugs only to investigators participating in the investigation.

(c) *Obtaining information from the investigator.* Before permitting an investigator to begin participation in an investigation, the sponsor shall obtain the following:

(1) A signed investigator statement (Form FDA-1572) containing:

(i) The name and address of the investigator;

(ii) The name and code number, if any, of the protocol(s) in the IND identifying the study(ies) to be conducted by the investigator;

(iii) The name and address of any medical school, hospital, or other research facility where the clinical investigation(s) will be conducted;

(iv) The name and address of any clinical laboratory facilities to be used in the study;

(v) The name and address of the IRB that is responsible for review and approval of the study(ies);

(vi) A commitment by the investigator that he or she:

(a) Will conduct the study(ies) in accordance with the relevant, current protocol(s) and will only make changes in a protocol after notifying the sponsor, except when necessary to protect the safety, the rights, or welfare of subjects;

(b) Will comply with all requirements regarding the obligations of clinical investigators and all other pertinent requirements in this part;

(c) Will personally conduct or supervise the described investigation(s);

(d) Will inform any potential subjects that the drugs are being used for investigational purposes and will ensure that the requirements relating to obtaining informed consent (21 CFR part 50) and institutional review board review and approval (21 CFR part 56) are met;

(e) Will report to the sponsor adverse experiences that occur in the course of the investigation(s) in accordance with § 312.64;

(f) Has read and understands the information in the investigator's brochure, including the potential risks and side effects of the drug; and

(g) Will ensure that all associates, colleagues, and employees assisting in the conduct of the study(ies) are informed about their obligations in meeting the above commitments.

(vii) A commitment by the investigator that, for an investigation subject to an institutional review requirement under part 56, an IRB that complies with the requirements of that part will be responsible for the initial and continuing review and approval of the clinical investigation and that the investigator will promptly report to the IRB all changes in the research activity and all unanticipated problems involving risks to human subjects or others, and will not make any changes in the research without IRB approval, except where necessary to eliminate apparent immediate hazards to the human subjects.

(viii) A list of the names of the subinvestigators (e.g., research fellows, residents) who will be assisting the investigator in the conduct of the investigation(s).

(2) *Curriculum vitae.* A curriculum vitae or other statement of qualifications of the investigator showing the education, training, and experience that qualifies the investigator as an expert in the clinical investigation of the drug for the use under investigation.

(3) *Clinical protocol.* (i) For Phase 1 investigations, a general outline of the planned investigation including the estimated duration of the study and the maximum number of subjects that will be involved.

(ii) For Phase 2 or 3 investigations, an outline of the study protocol including an approximation of the number of subjects to be treated with the drug and the number to be employed as controls, if any; the clinical uses to be investigated; characteristics of subjects by age, sex, and condition; the kind of clinical observations and laboratory tests to be conducted; the estimated duration of the study; and copies or a description of case report forms to be used.

(4) *Financial disclosure information.* Sufficient accurate financial information to allow the sponsor to submit complete and accurate certification or disclosure statements required under part 54 of this chapter. The sponsor shall obtain a commitment from the clinical investigator to promptly update this information if any relevant changes occur during the course of the investigation and for 1 year following the completion of the study.

(d) *Selecting monitors.* A sponsor shall select a monitor qualified by training and experience to monitor the progress of the investigation.

[52 FR 8831, Mar. 19, 1987, as amended at 52 FR 23031, June 17, 1987; 61 FR 57280, Nov. 5, 1996; 63 FR 5252, Feb. 2, 1998; 67 FR 9586, Mar. 4, 2002]

§ 312.54 Emergency research under § 50.24 of this chapter.

(a) The sponsor shall monitor the progress of all investigations involving an exception from informed consent under § 50.24 of this chapter. When the sponsor receives from the IRB information concerning the public disclosures required by § 50.24(a)(7)(ii) and (a)(7)(iii) of this chapter, the sponsor promptly shall submit to the IND file and to Docket Number 95S-0158 in the Division of Dockets Management (HFA-305), Food and Drug Administration, 5630 Fishers Lane, rm. 1061, Rockville, MD 20852, copies of the information that was disclosed, identified by the IND number.

(b) The sponsor also shall monitor such investigations to identify when an IRB determines that it cannot approve the research because it does not meet the criteria in the exception in § 50.24(a) of this chapter or because of other relevant ethical concerns. The sponsor promptly shall provide this information in writing to FDA, investigators who are asked to participate in this or a substantially equivalent clinical investigation, and other IRB's that are asked to review this or a substantially equivalent investigation.

[61 FR 51530, Oct. 2, 1996, as amended at 68 FR 24879, May 9, 2003]

§ 312.55 Informing investigators.

(a) Before the investigation begins, a sponsor (other than a sponsor-investigator) shall give each participating clinical investigator an investigator brochure containing the information described in § 312.23(a)(5).

(b) The sponsor shall, as the overall investigation proceeds, keep each participating investigator informed of new observations discovered by or reported to the sponsor on the drug, particularly with respect to adverse effects and safe use. Such information may be distributed to investigators by means of periodically revised investigator brochures, reprints or published studies, reports or letters to clinical investigators, or other appropriate means. Important safety information is required to be relayed to investigators in accordance with § 312.32.

[52 FR 8831, Mar. 19, 1987, as amended at 52 FR 23031, June 17, 1987; 67 FR 9586, Mar. 4, 2002]

§ 312.56 Review of ongoing investigations.

(a) The sponsor shall monitor the progress of all clinical investigations being conducted under its IND.

(b) A sponsor who discovers that an investigator is not complying with the signed agreement (Form FDA-1572), the general investigational plan, or the requirements of this part or other applicable parts shall promptly either secure compliance or discontinue shipments of the investigational new drug to the investigator and end the investigator's participation in the investigation. If the investigator's participation in the investigation is ended, the sponsor shall require that the investigator dispose of or return the investigational drug in accordance with the requirements of § 312.59 and shall notify FDA.

(c) The sponsor shall review and evaluate the evidence relating to the safety and effectiveness of the drug as it is obtained from the investigator. The sponsors shall make such reports to FDA regarding information relevant to the safety of the drug as are required under § 312.32. The sponsor shall make annual reports on the progress of the investigation in accordance with § 312.33.

(d) A sponsor who determines that its investigational drug presents an unreasonable and significant risk to subjects shall discontinue those investigations that present the risk, notify FDA, all institutional review boards, and all investigators who have at any time participated in the investigation of the discontinuance, assure the disposition of all stocks of the drug outstanding as required by § 312.59, and furnish FDA with a full report of the sponsor's actions. The sponsor shall discontinue the investigation as soon as possible, and in no event later than 5 working days after making the determination that the investigation should be discontinued. Upon request, FDA will confer with a sponsor on the need to discontinue an investigation.

[52 FR 8831, Mar. 19, 1987, as amended at 52 FR 23031, June 17, 1987; 67 FR 9586, Mar. 4, 2002]

§ 312.57 Recordkeeping and record retention.

(a) A sponsor shall maintain adequate records showing the receipt, shipment, or other disposition of the investigational drug. These records are required to include, as appropriate, the name of the investigator to whom the drug is shipped, and the date, quantity, and batch or code mark of each such shipment.

(b) A sponsor shall maintain complete and accurate records showing any financial interest in § 54.4(a)(3)(i), (a)(3)(ii), (a)(3)(iii), and (a)(3)(iv) of this chapter paid to clinical investigators by the sponsor of the covered study. A sponsor shall also maintain complete and accurate records concerning all other financial interests of investigators subject to part 54 of this chapter.

(c) A sponsor shall retain the records and reports required by this part for 2 years after a marketing application is approved for the drug; or, if an application is not approved for the drug, until 2 years after shipment and delivery of the drug for investigational use is discontinued and FDA has been so notified.

(d) A sponsor shall retain reserve samples of any test article and reference standard identified in, and used in any of the bioequivalence or bioavailability studies described in, § 320.38 or § 320.63 of this chapter, and release the reserve samples to FDA upon request, in accordance with, and for the period specified in § 320.38.

[52 FR 8831, Mar. 19, 1987, as amended at 52 FR 23031, June 17, 1987; 58 FR 25926, Apr. 28, 1993; 63 FR 5252, Feb. 2, 1998; 67 FR 9586, Mar. 4, 2002]

§ 312.58 Inspection of sponsor's records and reports.

(a) *FDA inspection*. A sponsor shall upon request from any properly authorized officer or employee of the Food and Drug Administration, at reasonable times, permit such officer or employee to have access to and copy and verify any records and reports relating to a clinical investigation conducted under this part. Upon written request by FDA, the sponsor shall submit the records or reports (or copies of them) to FDA. The sponsor shall discontinue shipments of the drug to any investigator who has failed to maintain or make available records or reports of the investigation as required by this part.

(b) *Controlled substances*. If an investigational new drug is a substance listed in any schedule of the Controlled Substances Act (21 U.S.C. 801; 21 CFR part 1308), records concerning shipment, delivery, receipt, and disposition of the drug, which are required to be kept under this part or other applicable parts of this chapter shall, upon the request of a properly authorized employee of the Drug Enforcement Administration of the U.S. Department of Justice, be made available by the investigator or sponsor to whom the request is made, for inspection and copying. In addition, the sponsor shall assure that adequate precautions are taken, including storage of the investigational drug in a securely locked, substantially constructed cabinet, or other securely locked, substantially constructed enclosure, access to which is limited, to prevent theft or diversion of the substance into illegal channels of distribution.

§ 312.59 Disposition of unused supply of investigational drug.

The sponsor shall assure the return of all unused supplies of the investigational drug from each individual investigator whose participation in the investigation is discontinued or terminated. The sponsor may authorize alternative disposition of unused supplies of the investigational drug provided this alternative disposition does not expose humans to risks from the drug. The sponsor shall maintain written records of any disposition of the drug in accordance with § 312.57.

[52 FR 8831, Mar. 19, 1987, as amended at 52 FR 23031, June 17, 1987; 67 FR 9586, Mar. 4, 2002]

§ 312.60 General responsibilities of investigators.

An investigator is responsible for ensuring that an investigation is conducted according to the signed investigator statement, the investigational plan, and applicable regulations; for protecting the rights, safety, and welfare of subjects under the investigator's care; and for the control of drugs under investigation. An investigator shall, in accordance with the provisions of part 50 of this chapter, obtain the informed consent of each human subject to whom the drug is administered, except as provided in §§ 50.23 or 50.24 of this chapter. Additional specific responsibilities of clinical investigators are set forth in this part and in parts 50 and 56 of this chapter.

[52 FR 8831, Mar. 19, 1987, as amended at 61 FR 51530, Oct. 2, 1996]

§ 312.61 Control of the investigational drug.

An investigator shall administer the drug only to subjects under the investigator's personal supervision or under the supervision of a subinvestigator responsible to the investigator. The investigator shall not supply the investigational drug to any person not authorized under this part to receive it.

§ 312.62 Investigator recordkeeping and record retention.

(a) *Disposition of drug*. An investigator is required to maintain adequate records of the disposition of the drug, including dates, quantity, and use by subjects. If the investigation is terminated, suspended, discontinued, or completed, the investigator shall return the unused supplies of the drug to the sponsor, or otherwise provide for disposition of the unused supplies of the drug under § 312.59.

(b) *Case histories*. An investigator is required to prepare and maintain adequate and accurate case histories that record all observations and other data pertinent to the investigation on each individual administered the investigational drug or employed as a control in the investigation. Case histories include the case report forms and supporting data including, for example, signed and dated consent forms and medical records including, for example, progress notes of the physician, the individual's hospital chart(s), and the nurses' notes. The case history for each individual shall document that informed consent was obtained prior to participation in the study.

(c) *Record retention.* An investigator shall retain records required to be maintained under this part for a period of 2 years following the date a marketing application is approved for the drug for the indication for which it is being investigated; or, if no application is to be filed or if the application is not approved for such indication, until 2 years after the investigation is discontinued and FDA is notified.

[52 FR 8831, Mar. 19, 1987, as amended at 52 FR 23031, June 17, 1987; 61 FR 57280, Nov. 5, 1996; 67 FR 9586, Mar. 4, 2002]

§ 312.64 Investigator reports.

(a) *Progress reports.* The investigator shall furnish all reports to the sponsor of the drug who is responsible for collecting and evaluating the results obtained. The sponsor is required under § 312.33 to submit annual reports to FDA on the progress of the clinical investigations.

(b) *Safety reports.* An investigator must immediately report to the sponsor any serious adverse event, whether or not considered drug related, including those listed in the protocol or investigator brochure and must include an assessment of whether there is a reasonable possibility that the drug caused the event. Study endpoints that are serious adverse events (e.g., all-cause mortality) must be reported in accordance with the protocol unless there is evidence suggesting a causal relationship between the drug and the event (e.g., death from anaphylaxis). In that case, the investigator must immediately report the event to the sponsor. The investigator must record nonserious adverse events and report them to the sponsor according to the timetable for reporting specified in the protocol.

(c) *Final report.* An investigator shall provide the sponsor with an adequate report shortly after completion of the investigator's participation in the investigation.

(d) *Financial disclosure reports.* The clinical investigator shall provide the sponsor with sufficient accurate financial information to allow an applicant to submit complete and accurate certification or disclosure statements as required under part 54 of this chapter. The clinical investigator shall promptly update this information if any relevant changes occur during the course of the investigation and for 1 year following the completion of the study.

[52 FR 8831, Mar. 19, 1987, as amended at 52 FR 23031, June 17, 1987; 63 FR 5252, Feb. 2, 1998; 67 FR 9586, Mar. 4, 2002; 75 FR 59963, Sept. 29, 2010]

§ 312.66 Assurance of IRB review.

An investigator shall assure that an IRB that complies with the requirements set forth in part 56 will be responsible for the initial and continuing review and approval of the proposed clinical study. The investigator shall also assure that he or she will promptly report to the IRB all changes in the research activity and all unanticipated problems involving risk to human subjects or others, and that he or she will not make any changes in the research without IRB approval, except where necessary to eliminate apparent immediate hazards to human subjects.

[52 FR 8831, Mar. 19, 1987, as amended at 52 FR 23031, June 17, 1987; 67 FR 9586, Mar. 4, 2002]

§ 312.68 Inspection of investigator's records and reports.

An investigator shall upon request from any properly authorized officer or employee of FDA, at reasonable times, permit such officer or employee to have access to, and copy and verify any records or reports made by the investigator pursuant to § 312.62. The investigator is not required to divulge subject names unless the records of particular individuals require a more detailed study of the cases, or unless there is reason to believe that the records do not represent actual case studies, or do not represent actual results obtained.

§312.69 Handling of controlled substances.

If the investigational drug is subject to the Controlled Substances Act, the investigator shall take adequate precautions, including storage of the investigational drug in a securely locked, substantially constructed cabinet, or other securely locked, substantially constructed enclosure, access to which is limited, to prevent theft or diversion of the substance into illegal channels of distribution.

§312.70 Disqualification of a clinical investigator.

(a) If FDA has information indicating that an investigator (including a sponsor-investigator) has repeatedly or deliberately failed to comply with the requirements of this part, part 50 or part 56 of this chapter, or has repeatedly or deliberately submitted to FDA or to the sponsor false information in any required report, the Center for Drug Evaluation and Research or the Center for Biologics Evaluation and Research will furnish the investigator written notice of the matter complained of and offer the investigator an opportunity to explain the matter in writing, or, at the option of the investigator, in an informal conference. If an explanation is offered and accepted by the applicable Center, the Center will discontinue the disqualification proceeding. If an explanation is offered but not accepted by the applicable Center, the investigator will be given an opportunity for a regulatory hearing under part 16 of this chapter on the question of whether the investigator is eligible to receive test articles under this part and eligible to conduct any clinical investigation that supports an application for a research or marketing permit for products regulated by FDA.

(b) After evaluating all available information, including any explanation presented by the investigator, if the Commissioner determines that the investigator has repeatedly or deliberately failed to comply with the requirements of this part, part 50 or part 56 of this chapter, or has repeatedly or deliberately submitted to FDA or to the sponsor false information in any required report, the Commissioner will notify the investigator, the sponsor of any investigation in which the investigator has been named as a participant, and the reviewing institutional review boards (IRBs) that the investigator is not eligible to receive test articles under this part. The notification to the investigator, sponsor, and IRBs will provide a statement of the basis for such determination. The notification also will explain that an investigator determined to be ineligible to receive test articles under this part will be ineligible to conduct any clinical investigation that supports an application for a research or marketing permit for products regulated by FDA, including drugs, biologics, devices, new animal drugs, foods, including dietary supplements, that bear a nutrient content claim or a health claim, infant formulas, food and color additives, and tobacco products.

(c) Each application or submission to FDA under the provisions of this chapter containing data reported by an investigator who has been determined to be ineligible to receive FDA-regulated test articles is subject to examination to determine whether the investigator has submitted unreliable data that are essential to the continuation of an investigation or essential to the approval of a marketing application, or essential to the continued marketing of an FDA-regulated product.

(d) If the Commissioner determines, after the unreliable data submitted by the investigator are eliminated from consideration, that the data remaining are inadequate to support a conclusion that it is reasonably safe to continue the investigation, the Commissioner will notify the sponsor, who shall have an opportunity for a regulatory hearing under part 16 of this chapter. If a danger to the public health exists, however, the Commissioner shall terminate the IND immediately and notify the sponsor and the reviewing IRBs of the termination. In such case, the sponsor shall have an opportunity for a regulatory hearing before FDA under part 16 on the question of whether the IND should be reinstated. The determination that an investigation may not be considered in support of a research or marketing application or a notification or petition submission does not, however, relieve the sponsor of any obligation under any other applicable regulation to submit to FDA the results of the investigation.

(e) If the Commissioner determines, after the unreliable data submitted by the investigator are eliminated from consideration, that the continued approval of the product for which the data were submitted cannot be justified, the Commissioner will proceed to withdraw approval of the product in accordance with the applicable provisions of the relevant statutes.

(f) An investigator who has been determined to be ineligible under paragraph (b) of this section may be reinstated as eligible when the Commissioner determines that the investigator has presented adequate assurances that the investigator will employ all test articles, and will conduct any clinical investigation that supports an application for a research or marketing permit for products regulated by FDA, solely in compliance with the applicable provisions of this chapter.

[77 FR 25359, Apr. 30, 2012]

Subpart E—Drugs Intended to Treat Life-threatening and Severely-debilitating Illnesses

Authority: 21 U.S.C. 351, 352, 353, 355, 371; 42 U.S.C. 262.

Source: 53 FR 41523, Oct. 21, 1988, unless otherwise noted.

§ 312.80 Purpose.

The purpose of this section is to establish procedures designed to expedite the development, evaluation, and marketing of new therapies intended to treat persons with life-threatening and severely-debilitating illnesses, especially where no satisfactory alternative therapy exists. As stated § 314.105(c) of this chapter, while the statutory standards of safety and effectiveness apply to all drugs, the many kinds of drugs that are subject to them, and the wide range of uses for those drugs, demand flexibility in applying the standards. The Food and Drug Administration (FDA) has determined that it is appropriate to exercise the broadest flexibility in applying the statutory standards, while preserving appropriate guarantees for safety and effectiveness. These procedures reflect the recognition that physicians and patients are generally willing to accept greater risks or side effects from products that treat life-threatening and severely-debilitating illnesses, than they would accept from products that treat less serious illnesses. These procedures also reflect the recognition that the benefits of the drug need to be evaluated in light of the severity of the disease being treated. The procedure outlined in this section should be interpreted consistent with that purpose.

§ 312.81 Scope.

This section applies to new drug and biological products that are being studied for their safety and effectiveness in treating life-threatening or severely-debilitating diseases.

(a) For purposes of this section, the term "life-threatening" means:

(1) Diseases or conditions where the likelihood of death is high unless the course of the disease is interrupted; and

(2) Diseases or conditions with potentially fatal outcomes, where the end point of clinical trial analysis is survival.

(b) For purposes of this section, the term "severely debilitating" means diseases or conditions that cause major irreversible morbidity.

(c) Sponsors are encouraged to consult with FDA on the applicability of these procedures to specific products.

[53 FR 41523, Oct. 21, 1988, as amended at 64 FR 401, Jan. 5, 1999]

§312.82 Early consultation.

For products intended to treat life-threatening or severely-debilitating illnesses, sponsors may request to meet with FDA-reviewing officials early in the drug development process to review and reach agreement on the design of necessary preclinical and clinical studies. Where appropriate, FDA will invite to such meetings one or more outside expert scientific consultants or advisory committee members. To the extent FDA resources permit, agency reviewing officials will honor requests for such meetings

(a) *Pre-investigational new drug (IND) meetings.* Prior to the submission of the initial IND, the sponsor may request a meeting with FDA-reviewing officials. The primary purpose of this meeting is to review and reach agreement on the design of animal studies needed to initiate human testing. The meeting may also provide an opportunity for discussing the scope and design of phase 1 testing, plans for studying the drug product in pediatric populations, and the best approach for presentation and formatting of data in the IND.

(b) *End-of-phase 1 meetings.* When data from phase 1 clinical testing are available, the sponsor may again request a meeting with FDA-reviewing officials. The primary purpose of this meeting is to review and reach agreement on the design of phase 2 controlled clinical trials, with the goal that such testing will be adequate to provide sufficient data on the drug's safety and effectiveness to support a decision on its approvability for marketing, and to discuss the need for, as well as the design and timing of, studies of the drug in pediatric patients. For drugs for life-threatening diseases, FDA will provide its best judgment, at that time, whether pediatric studies will be required and whether their submission will be deferred until after approval. The procedures outlined in §312.47(b)(1) with respect to end-of-phase 2 conferences, including documentation of agreements reached, would also be used for end-of-phase 1 meetings.

[53 FR 41523, Oct. 21, 1988, as amended at 63 FR 66669, Dec. 2, 1998]

§312.83 Treatment protocols.

If the preliminary analysis of phase 2 test results appears promising, FDA may ask the sponsor to submit a treatment protocol to be reviewed under the procedures and criteria listed in §§312.305 and 312.320. Such a treatment protocol, if requested and granted, would normally remain in effect while the complete data necessary for a marketing application are being assembled by the sponsor and reviewed by FDA (unless grounds exist for clinical hold of ongoing protocols, as provided in §312.42(b)(3)(ii)).

[53 FR 41523, Oct. 21, 1988, as amended at 76 FR 13880, Mar. 15, 2011]

§312.84 Risk-benefit analysis in review of marketing applications for drugs to treat life-threatening and severely-debilitating illnesses.

(a) FDA's application of the statutory standards for marketing approval shall recognize the need for a medical risk-benefit judgment in making the final decision on approvability. As part of this evaluation, consistent with the statement of purpose in §312.80, FDA will consider whether the benefits of the drug outweigh the known and potential risks of the drug and the need to answer remaining questions about risks and benefits of the drug, taking into consideration the severity of the disease and the absence of satisfactory alternative therapy.

(b) In making decisions on whether to grant marketing approval for products that have been the subject of an end-of-phase 1 meeting under §312.82, FDA will usually seek the advice of outside expert scientific consultants or advisory committees. Upon the filing of such a marketing application under §314.101 or part 601 of this chapter, FDA will notify the members of the relevant standing advisory committee of the application's filing and its availability for review.

(c) If FDA concludes that the data presented are not sufficient for marketing approval, FDA will issue a complete response letter under §314.110 of this chapter or the biological product licensing procedures. Such letter, in describing the deficiencies in the application, will address why the results of the research design agreed to under § 312.82, or in subsequent meetings, have not provided sufficient evidence for marketing approval. Such letter will also describe any recommendations made by the advisory committee regarding the application.

(d) Marketing applications submitted under the procedures contained in this section will be subject to the requirements and procedures contained in part 314 or part 600 of this chapter, as well as those in this subpart.

[53 FR 41523, Oct. 21, 1988, as amended at 73 FR 39607, July 10, 2008]

§ 312.85 Phase 4 studies.

Concurrent with marketing approval, FDA may seek agreement from the sponsor to conduct certain postmarketing (phase 4) studies to delineate additional information about the drug's risks, benefits, and optimal use. These studies could include, but would not be limited to, studying different doses or schedules of administration than were used in phase 2 studies, use of the drug in other patient populations or other stages of the disease, or use of the drug over a longer period of time.

§ 312.86 Focused FDA regulatory research.

At the discretion of the agency, FDA may undertake focused regulatory research on critical rate-limiting aspects of the preclinical, chemical/manufacturing, and clinical phases of drug development and evaluation. When initiated, FDA will undertake such research efforts as a means for meeting a public health need in facilitating the development of therapies to treat life-threatening or severely debilitating illnesses.

§ 312.87 Active monitoring of conduct and evaluation of clinical trials.

For drugs covered under this section, the Commissioner and other agency officials will monitor the progress of the conduct and evaluation of clinical trials and be involved in facilitating their appropriate progress.

§ 312.88 Safeguards for patient safety.

All of the safeguards incorporated within parts 50, 56, 312, 314, and 600 of this chapter designed to ensure the safety of clinical testing and the safety of products following marketing approval apply to drugs covered by this section. This includes the requirements for informed consent (part 50 of this chapter) and institutional review boards (part 56 of this chapter). These safeguards further include the review of animal studies prior to initial human testing (§ 312.23), and the monitoring of adverse drug experiences through the requirements of IND safety reports (§ 312.32), safety update reports during agency review of a marketing application (§ 314.50 of this chapter), and postmarketing adverse reaction reporting (§ 314.80 of this chapter).

Subpart F—Miscellaneous

§ 312.110 Import and export requirements.

(a) *Imports.* An investigational new drug offered for import into the United States complies with the requirements of this part if it is subject to an IND that is in effect for it under § 312.40 and: (1) The consignee in the United States is the sponsor of the IND; (2) the consignee is a qualified investigator named in the IND; or (3) the consignee is the domestic agent of a foreign sponsor, is responsible for the control and distribution of the investigational drug, and the IND identifies the consignee and describes what, if any, actions the consignee will take with respect to the investigational drug.

(b) *Exports.* An investigational new drug may be exported from the United States for use in a clinical investigation under any of the following conditions:

(1) An IND is in effect for the drug under § 312.40, the drug complies with the laws of the country to which it is being exported, and each person who receives the drug is an investigator in a study submitted to and allowed to proceed under the IND; or

(2) The drug has valid marketing authorization in Australia, Canada, Israel, Japan, New Zealand, Switzerland, South Africa, or in any country in the European Union or the European Economic Area, and complies with the laws of the country to which it is being exported, section 802(b)(1)(A), (f), and (g) of the act, and § 1.101 of this chapter; or

(3) The drug is being exported to Australia, Canada, Israel, Japan, New Zealand, Switzerland, South Africa, or to any country in the European Union or the European Economic Area, and complies with the laws of the country to which it is being exported, the applicable provisions of section 802(c), (f), and (g) of the act, and § 1.101 of this chapter. Drugs exported under this paragraph that are not the subject of an IND are exempt from the label requirement in § 312.6(a); or

(4) Except as provided in paragraph (b)(5) of this section, the person exporting the drug sends a written certification to the Office of International Programs (HFG-1), Food and Drug Administration, 5600 Fishers Lane, Rockville, MD 20857, at the time the drug is first exported and maintains records documenting compliance with this paragraph. The certification shall describe the drug that is to be exported (i.e., trade name (if any), generic name, and dosage form), identify the country or countries to which the drug is to be exported, and affirm that:

(i) The drug is intended for export;

(ii) The drug is intended for investigational use in a foreign country;

(iii) The drug meets the foreign purchaser's or consignee's specifications;

(iv) The drug is not in conflict with the importing country's laws;

(v) The outer shipping package is labeled to show that the package is intended for export from the United States;

(vi) The drug is not sold or offered for sale in the United States;

(vii) The clinical investigation will be conducted in accordance with § 312.120;

(viii) The drug is manufactured, processed, packaged, and held in substantial conformity with current good manufacturing practices;

(ix) The drug is not adulterated within the meaning of section 501(a)(1), (a)(2)(A), (a)(3), (c), or (d) of the act;

(x) The drug does not present an imminent hazard to public health, either in the United States, if the drug were to be reimported, or in the foreign country; and

(xi) The drug is labeled in accordance with the foreign country's laws.

(5) In the event of a national emergency in a foreign country, where the national emergency necessitates exportation of an investigational new drug, the requirements in paragraph (b)(4) of this section apply as follows:

(i) *Situations where the investigational new drug is to be stockpiled in anticipation of a national emergency.* There may be instances where exportation of an investigational new drug is needed so that the drug may be stockpiled and made available for use by the importing country if and when a national emergency arises. In such cases:

(A) A person may export an investigational new drug under paragraph (b)(4) of this section without making an affirmation with respect to any one or more of paragraphs (b)(4)(i), (b)(4)(iv), (b)(4)(vi), (b)(4)(vii), (b)(4)(viii), and/or (b)(4)(ix) of this section, provided that he or she:

(1) Provides a written statement explaining why compliance with each such paragraph is not feasible or is contrary to the best interests of the individuals who may receive the investigational new drug;

(2) Provides a written statement from an authorized official of the importing country's government. The statement must attest that the official agrees with the exporter's statement made under paragraph (b)(5)(i)(A)(1) of this section; explain that the drug is to be stockpiled solely for use of the importing country in a national emergency; and describe the potential national emergency that warrants exportation of the investigational new drug under this provision; and

(3) Provides a written statement showing that the Secretary of Health and Human Services (the Secretary), or his or her designee, agrees with the findings of the authorized official of the importing country's government. Persons who wish to obtain a written statement from the Secretary should direct their requests to Secretary's Operations Center, Office of Emergency Operations and Security Programs, Office of Public Health Emergency Preparedness, Office of the Secretary, Department of Health and Human Services, 200 Independence Ave. SW., Washington, DC 20201. Requests may be also be sent by FAX: 202-619-7870 or by e-mail: HHS.SOC@hhs.gov.

(B) Exportation may not proceed until FDA has authorized exportation of the investigational new drug. FDA may deny authorization if the statements provided under paragraphs (b)(5)(i)(A)(1) or (b)(5)(i)(A)(2) of this section are inadequate or if exportation is contrary to public health.

(ii) *Situations where the investigational new drug is to be used for a sudden and immediate national emergency.* There may be instances where exportation of an investigational new drug is needed so that the drug may be used in a sudden and immediate national emergency that has developed or is developing. In such cases:

(A) A person may export an investigational new drug under paragraph (b)(4) of this section without making an affirmation with respect to any one or more of paragraphs (b)(4)(i), (b)(4)(iv), (b)(4)(v), (b)(4)(vi), (b)(4)(vii), (b)(4)(viii), (b)(4)(ix), and/or (b)(4)(xi), provided that he or she:

(1) Provides a written statement explaining why compliance with each such paragraph is not feasible or is contrary to the best interests of the individuals who are expected to receive the investigational new drug and

(2) Provides sufficient information from an authorized official of the importing country's government to enable the Secretary, or his or her designee, to decide whether a national emergency has developed or is developing in the importing country, whether the investigational new drug will be used solely for that national emergency, and whether prompt exportation of the investigational new drug is necessary. Persons who wish to obtain a determination from the Secretary should direct their requests to Secretary's Operations Center, Office of Emergency Operations and Security Programs, Office of Public Health Emergency Preparedness, Office of the Secretary, Department of Health and Human Services, 200 Independence Ave. SW., Washington, DC 20201. Requests may be also be sent by FAX: 202-619-7870 or by e-mail: HHS.SOC@hhs.gov.

(B) Exportation may proceed without prior FDA authorization.

(c) *Limitations.* Exportation under paragraph (b) of this section may not occur if:

(1) For drugs exported under paragraph (b)(1) of this section, the IND pertaining to the clinical investigation is no longer in effect;

(2) For drugs exported under paragraph (b)(2) of this section, the requirements in section 802(b)(1), (f), or (g) of the act are no longer met;

(3) For drugs exported under paragraph (b)(3) of this section, the requirements in section 802(c), (f), or (g) of the act are no longer met;

(4) For drugs exported under paragraph (b)(4) of this section, the conditions underlying the certification or the statements submitted under paragraph (b)(5) of this section are no longer met; or

(5) For any investigational new drugs under this section, the drug no longer complies with the laws of the importing country.

(d) *Insulin and antibiotics.* New insulin and antibiotic drug products may be exported for investigational use in accordance with section 801(e)(1) of the act without complying with this section.

[52 FR 8831, Mar. 19, 1987, as amended at 52 FR 23031, June 17, 1987; 64 FR 401, Jan. 5, 1999; 67 FR 9586, Mar. 4, 2002; 70 FR 70729, Nov. 23, 2005]

§ 312.120 Foreign clinical studies not conducted under an IND.

(a) *Acceptance of studies.* (1) FDA will accept as support for an IND or application for marketing approval (an application under section 505 of the act or section 351 of the Public Health Service Act (the PHS Act) (42 U.S.C. 262)) a well-designed and well-conducted foreign clinical study not conducted under an IND, if the following conditions are met:

(i) The study was conducted in accordance with good clinical practice (GCP). For the purposes of this section, GCP is defined as a standard for the design, conduct, performance, monitoring, auditing, recording, analysis, and reporting of clinical trials in a way that provides assurance that the data and reported results are credible and accurate and that the rights, safety, and well-being of trial subjects are protected. GCP includes review and approval (or provision of a favorable opinion) by an independent ethics committee (IEC) before initiating a study, continuing review of an ongoing study by an IEC, and obtaining and documenting the freely given informed consent of the subject (or a subject's legally authorized representative, if the subject is unable to provide informed consent) before initiating a study. GCP does not require informed consent in life-threatening situations when the IEC reviewing the study finds, before initiation of the study, that informed consent is not feasible and either that the conditions present are consistent with those described in § 50.23 or § 50.24(a) of this chapter, or that the measures described in the study protocol or elsewhere will protect the rights, safety, and well-being of subjects; and

(ii) FDA is able to validate the data from the study through an onsite inspection if the agency deems it necessary.

(2) Although FDA will not accept as support for an IND or application for marketing approval a study that does not meet the conditions of paragraph (a)(1) of this section, FDA will examine data from such a study.

(3) Marketing approval of a new drug based solely on foreign clinical data is governed by § 314.106 of this chapter.

(b) *Supporting information.* A sponsor or applicant who submits data from a foreign clinical study not conducted under an IND as support for an IND or application for marketing approval must submit to FDA, in addition to information required elsewhere in parts 312, 314, or 601 of this chapter, a description of the actions the sponsor or applicant took to ensure that the research conformed to GCP as described in paragraph (a)(1)(i) of this section. The description is not required to duplicate information already submitted in the IND or application for marketing approval. Instead, the description must provide either the following information or a cross-reference to another section of the submission where the information is located:

(1) The investigator's qualifications;

(2) A description of the research facilities;

(3) A detailed summary of the protocol and results of the study and, should FDA request, case records maintained by the investigator or additional background data such as hospital or other institutional records;

(4) A description of the drug substance and drug product used in the study, including a description of the components, formulation, specifications, and, if available, bioavailability of the specific drug product used in the clinical study;

(5) If the study is intended to support the effectiveness of a drug product, information showing that the study is adequate and well controlled under §314.126 of this chapter;

(6) The name and address of the IEC that reviewed the study and a statement that the IEC meets the definition in §312.3 of this chapter. The sponsor or applicant must maintain records supporting such statement, including records of the names and qualifications of IEC members, and make these records available for agency review upon request;

(7) A summary of the IEC's decision to approve or modify and approve the study, or to provide a favorable opinion;

(8) A description of how informed consent was obtained;

(9) A description of what incentives, if any, were provided to subjects to participate in the study;

(10) A description of how the sponsor(s) monitored the study and ensured that the study was carried out consistently with the study protocol; and

(11) A description of how investigators were trained to comply with GCP (as described in paragraph (a)(1)(i) of this section) and to conduct the study in accordance with the study protocol, and a statement on whether written commitments by investigators to comply with GCP and the protocol were obtained. Any signed written commitments by investigators must be maintained by the sponsor or applicant and made available for agency review upon request.

(c) Waivers. (1) A sponsor or applicant may ask FDA to waive any applicable requirements under paragraphs (a)(1) and (b) of this section. A waiver request may be submitted in an IND or in an information amendment to an IND, or in an application or in an amendment or supplement to an application submitted under part 314 or 601 of this chapter. A waiver request is required to contain at least one of the following:

(i) An explanation why the sponsor's or applicant's compliance with the requirement is unnecessary or cannot be achieved;

(ii) A description of an alternative submission or course of action that satisfies the purpose of the requirement; or

(iii) Other information justifying a waiver.

(2) FDA may grant a waiver if it finds that doing so would be in the interest of the public health.

(d) *Records.* A sponsor or applicant must retain the records required by this section for a foreign clinical study not conducted under an IND as follows:

(1) If the study is submitted in support of an application for marketing approval, for 2 years after an agency decision on that application;

(2) If the study is submitted in support of an IND but not an application for marketing approval, for 2 years after the submission of the IND.

[73 FR 22815, Apr. 28, 2008]

§312.130 Availability for public disclosure of data and information in an IND.

(a) The existence of an investigational new drug application will not be disclosed by FDA unless it has previously been publicly disclosed or acknowledged.

(b) The availability for public disclosure of all data and information in an investigational new drug application for a new drug will be handled in accordance with the provisions established in §314.430 for the confidentiality of data and information in applications submitted in part 314. The availability for public disclosure of all data and information in an investigational new drug application for a biological product will be governed by the provisions of §§601.50 and 601.51.

(c) Notwithstanding the provisions of §314.430, FDA shall disclose upon request to an individual to whom an investigational new drug has been given a copy of any IND safety report relating to the use in the individual.

(d) The availability of information required to be publicly disclosed for investigations involving an exception from informed consent under §50.24 of this chapter will be handled as follows: Persons wishing to request the publicly disclosable information in the IND that was required to be filed in Docket Number 95S-0158 in the Division of Dockets Management (HFA-305), Food and Drug Administration, 5630 Fishers Lane, rm. 1061, Rockville, MD 20852, shall submit a request under the Freedom of Information Act.

[52 FR 8831, Mar. 19, 1987. Redesignated at 53 FR 41523, Oct. 21, 1988, as amended at 61 FR 51530, Oct. 2, 1996; 64 FR 401, Jan. 5, 1999; 68 FR 24879, May 9, 2003]

§312.140 Address for correspondence.

(a) A sponsor must send an initial IND submission to the Center for Drug Evaluation and Research (CDER) or to the Center for Biologics Evaluation and Research (CBER), depending on the Center responsible for regulating the product as follows:

(1) *For drug products regulated by CDER.* Send the IND submission to the Central Document Room, Center for Drug Evaluation and Research, Food and Drug Administration, 5901-B Ammendale Rd., Beltsville, MD 20705-1266; except send an IND submission for an in vivo bioavailability or bioequivalence study in humans to support an abbreviated new drug application to the Office of Generic Drugs (HFD-600), Center for Drug Evaluation and Research, Food and Drug Administration, Metro Park North VII, 7620 Standish Pl., Rockville, MD 20855.

(2) *For biological products regulated by CDER.* Send the IND submission to the Central Document Room, Center for Drug Evaluation and Research, Food and Drug Administration, 5901-B Ammendale Rd., Beltsville, MD 20705-1266.

(3) *For biological products regulated by CBER.* Send the IND submission to the Food and Drug Administration, Center for Biologics Evaluation and Research, Document Control Center, 10903 New Hampshire Ave., Bldg. 71, Rm. G112, Silver Spring, MD 20993-0002.

(b) On receiving the IND, the responsible Center will inform the sponsor which one of the divisions in CDER or CBER is responsible for the IND. Amendments, reports, and other correspondence relating to matters covered by the IND should be sent to the appropriate center at the address indicated in this section and marked to the attention of the responsible division. The outside wrapper of each submission shall state what is contained in the submission, for example, "IND Application", "Protocol Amendment", etc.

(c) All correspondence relating to export of an investigational drug under §312.110(b)(2) shall be submitted to the International Affairs Staff (HFY-50), Office of Health Affairs, Food and Drug Administration, 5600 Fishers Lane, Rockville, MD 20857.

[70 FR 14981, Mar. 24, 2005, as amended at 74 FR 13113, Mar. 26, 2009; 74 FR 55771, Oct. 29, 2009; 75 FR 37295, June 29, 2010; 80 FR 18091, Apr. 3, 2015; 81 FR 17066, Mar. 28, 2016]

§312.145 Guidance documents.

(a) FDA has made available guidance documents under §10.115 of this chapter to help you to comply with certain requirements of this part.

(b) The Center for Drug Evaluation and Research (CDER) and the Center for Biologics Evaluation and Research (CBER) maintain lists of guidance documents that apply to the centers' regulations. The lists are maintained on the Internet and are published annually in the Federal Register. A request for a copy of the CDER list should be directed to the Office of Training and Communications, Division of Drug Information, Center for Drug Evaluation and Research, Food and Drug Administration, 10903 New Hampshire Ave., Silver Spring, MD 20993-0002. A request for a copy of the CBER list should be directed to the Food and Drug Administration, Center for Biologics Evaluation and Research, Office of Communication, Outreach and Development, 10903 New Hampshire Ave., Bldg. 71, Rm. 3103, Silver Spring, MD 20993-0002.

[65 FR 56479, Sept. 19, 2000, as amended at 74 FR 13113, Mar. 26, 2009; 80 FR 18091, Apr. 3, 2015]

Subpart G—Drugs for Investigational Use in Laboratory Research Animals or In Vitro Tests

§ 312.160 Drugs for investigational use in laboratory research animals or in vitro tests.

(a) *Authorization to ship.* (1)(i) A person may ship a drug intended solely for tests in vitro or in animals used only for laboratory research purposes if it is labeled as follows:

CAUTION: Contains a new drug for investigational use only in laboratory research animals, or for tests in vitro. Not for use in humans.

(ii) A person may ship a biological product for investigational in vitro diagnostic use that is listed in § 312.2(b)(2)(ii) if it is labeled as follows:

CAUTION: Contains a biological product for investigational in vitro diagnostic tests only.

(2) A person shipping a drug under paragraph (a) of this section shall use due diligence to assure that the consignee is regularly engaged in conducting such tests and that the shipment of the new drug will actually be used for tests in vitro or in animals used only for laboratory research.

(3) A person who ships a drug under paragraph (a) of this section shall maintain adequate records showing the name and post office address of the expert to whom the drug is shipped and the date, quantity, and batch or code mark of each shipment and delivery. Records of shipments under paragraph (a)(1)(i) of this section are to be maintained for a period of 2 years after the shipment. Records and reports of data and shipments under paragraph (a)(1)(ii) of this section are to be maintained in accordance with § 312.57(b). The person who ships the drug shall upon request from any properly authorized officer or employee of the Food and Drug Administration, at reasonable times, permit such officer or employee to have access to and copy and verify records required to be maintained under this section.

(b) *Termination of authorization to ship.* FDA may terminate authorization to ship a drug under this section if it finds that:

(1) The sponsor of the investigation has failed to comply with any of the conditions for shipment established under this section; or

(2) The continuance of the investigation is unsafe or otherwise contrary to the public interest or the drug is used for purposes other than bona fide scientific investigation. FDA will notify the person shipping the drug of its finding and invite immediate correction. If correction is not immediately made, the person shall have an opportunity for a regulatory hearing before FDA pursuant to part 16.

(c) *Disposition of unused drug.* The person who ships the drug under paragraph (a) of this section shall assure the return of all unused supplies of the drug from individual investigators whenever the investigation discontinues or the investigation is terminated. The person who ships the drug may authorize in writing alternative disposition of unused supplies of the drug provided this alternative disposition does not expose humans to risks from the drug, either directly or indirectly (e.g., through food-producing animals). The shipper shall maintain records of any alternative disposition.

[52 FR 8831, Mar. 19, 1987, as amended at 52 FR 23031, June 17, 1987. Redesignated at 53 FR 41523, Oct. 21, 1988; 67 FR 9586, Mar. 4, 2002]

Source: 74 FR 40942, Aug. 13, 2009, unless otherwise noted.

(a) *Scope.* This subpart contains the requirements for the use of investigational new drugs and approved drugs where availability is limited by a risk evaluation and mitigation strategy (REMS) when the primary purpose is to diagnose, monitor, or treat a patient's disease or condition. The aim of this subpart is to facilitate the availability of such drugs to patients with serious diseases or conditions when there is no comparable or satisfactory alternative therapy to diagnose, monitor, or treat the patient's disease or condition.

(b) *Definitions.* The following definitions of terms apply to this subpart:

Immediately life-threatening disease or condition means a stage of disease in which there is reasonable likelihood that death will occur within a matter of months or in which premature death is likely without early treatment.

Serious disease or condition means a disease or condition associated with morbidity that has substantial impact on day-to-day functioning. Short-lived and self-limiting morbidity will usually not be sufficient, but the morbidity need not be irreversible, provided it is persistent or recurrent. Whether a disease or condition is serious is a matter of clinical judgment, based on its impact on such factors as survival, day-to-day functioning, or the likelihood that the disease, if left untreated, will progress from a less severe condition to a more serious one.

§ 312.305 Requirements for all expanded access uses.

The criteria, submission requirements, safeguards, and beginning treatment information set out in this section apply to all expanded access uses described in this subpart. Additional criteria, submission requirements, and safeguards that apply to specific types of expanded access are described in §§ 312.310 through 312.320.

(a) *Criteria.* FDA must determine that:

(1) The patient or patients to be treated have a serious or immediately life-threatening disease or condition, and there is no comparable or satisfactory alternative therapy to diagnose, monitor, or treat the disease or condition;

(2) The potential patient benefit justifies the potential risks of the treatment use and those potential risks are not unreasonable in the context of the disease or condition to be treated; and

(3) Providing the investigational drug for the requested use will not interfere with the initiation, conduct, or completion of clinical investigations that could support marketing approval of the expanded access use or otherwise compromise the potential development of the expanded access use.

(b) *Submission.* (1) An expanded access submission is required for each type of expanded access described in this subpart. The submission may be a new IND or a protocol amendment to an existing IND. Information required for a submission may be supplied by referring to pertinent information contained in an existing IND if the sponsor of the existing IND grants a right of reference to the IND.

(2) The expanded access submission must include:

(i) A cover sheet (Form FDA 1571) meeting the requirements of § 312.23(a);

(ii) The rationale for the intended use of the drug, including a list of available therapeutic options that would ordinarily be tried before resorting to the investigational drug or an explanation of why the use of the investigational drug is preferable to the use of available therapeutic options;

(iii) The criteria for patient selection or, for an individual patient, a description of the patient's disease or condition, including recent medical history and previous treatments of the disease or condition;

(iv) The method of administration of the drug, dose, and duration of therapy;

(v) A description of the facility where the drug will be manufactured;

(vi) Chemistry, manufacturing, and controls information adequate to ensure the proper identification, quality, purity, and strength of the investigational drug;

(vii) Pharmacology and toxicology information adequate to conclude that the drug is reasonably safe at the dose and duration proposed for expanded access use (ordinarily, information that would be adequate to permit clinical testing of the drug in a population of the size expected to be treated); and

(viii) A description of clinical procedures, laboratory tests, or other monitoring necessary to evaluate the effects of the drug and minimize its risks.

(3) The expanded access submission and its mailing cover must be plainly marked "EXPANDED ACCESS SUBMISSION." If the expanded access submission is for a treatment IND or treatment protocol, the applicable box on Form FDA 1571 must be checked.

(c) *Safeguards.* The responsibilities of sponsors and investigators set forth in subpart D of this part are applicable to expanded access use under this subpart as described in this paragraph.

(1) A licensed physician under whose immediate direction an investigational drug is administered or dispensed for an expanded access use under this subpart is considered an investigator, for purposes of this part, and must comply with the responsibilities for investigators set forth in subpart D of this part to the extent they are applicable to the expanded access use.

(2) An individual or entity that submits an expanded access IND or protocol under this subpart is considered a sponsor, for purposes of this part, and must comply with the responsibilities for sponsors set forth in subpart D of this part to the extent they are applicable to the expanded access use.

(3) A licensed physician under whose immediate direction an investigational drug is administered or dispensed, and who submits an IND for expanded access use under this subpart is considered a sponsor-investigator, for purposes of this part, and must comply with the responsibilities for sponsors and investigators set forth in subpart D of this part to the extent they are applicable to the expanded access use.

(4) *Investigators.* In all cases of expanded access, investigators are responsible for reporting adverse drug events to the sponsor, ensuring that the informed consent requirements of part 50 of this chapter are met, ensuring that IRB review of the expanded access use is obtained in a manner consistent with the requirements of part 56 of this chapter, and maintaining accurate case histories and drug disposition records and retaining records in a manner consistent with the requirements of § 312.62. Depending on the type of expanded access, other investigator responsibilities under subpart D may also apply.

(5) *Sponsors.* In all cases of expanded access, sponsors are responsible for submitting IND safety reports and annual reports (when the IND or protocol continues for 1 year or longer) to FDA as required by §§ 312.32 and 312.33, ensuring that licensed physicians are qualified to administer the investigational drug for the expanded access use, providing licensed physicians with the information needed to minimize the risk and maximize the potential benefits of the investigational drug (the investigator's brochure must be provided if one exists for the drug), maintaining an effective IND for the expanded access use, and maintaining adequate drug disposition records and retaining records in a manner consistent with the requirements of § 312.57. Depending on the type of expanded access, other sponsor responsibilities under subpart D may also apply.

(d) *Beginning treatment*—(1) *INDs.* An expanded access IND goes into effect 30 days after FDA receives the IND or on earlier notification by FDA that the expanded access use may begin.

(2) *Protocols.* With the following exceptions, expanded access use under a protocol submitted under an existing IND may begin as described in § 312.30(a).

(i) Expanded access use under the emergency procedures described in § 312.310(d) may begin when the use is authorized by the FDA reviewing official.

(ii) Expanded access use under § 312.320 may begin 30 days after FDA receives the protocol or upon earlier notification by FDA that use may begin.

(3) *Clinical holds*. FDA may place any expanded access IND or protocol on clinical hold as described in § 312.42.

§ 312.310 Individual patients, including for emergency use.

Under this section, FDA may permit an investigational drug to be used for the treatment of an individual patient by a licensed physician.

(a) *Criteria*. The criteria in § 312.305(a) must be met; and the following determinations must be made:

(1) The physician must determine that the probable risk to the person from the investigational drug is not greater than the probable risk from the disease or condition; and

(2) FDA must determine that the patient cannot obtain the drug under another IND or protocol.

(b) *Submission*. The expanded access submission must include information adequate to demonstrate that the criteria in § 312.305(a) and paragraph (a) of this section have been met. The expanded access submission must meet the requirements of § 312.305(b).

(1) If the drug is the subject of an existing IND, the expanded access submission may be made by the sponsor or by a licensed physician.

(2) A sponsor may satisfy the submission requirements by amending its existing IND to include a protocol for individual patient expanded access.

(3) A licensed physician may satisfy the submission requirements by obtaining from the sponsor permission for FDA to refer to any information in the IND that would be needed to support the expanded access request (right of reference) and by providing any other required information not contained in the IND (usually only the information specific to the individual patient).

(c) *Safeguards*. (1) Treatment is generally limited to a single course of therapy for a specified duration unless FDA expressly authorizes multiple courses or chronic therapy.

(2) At the conclusion of treatment, the licensed physician or sponsor must provide FDA with a written summary of the results of the expanded access use, including adverse effects.

(3) FDA may require sponsors to monitor an individual patient expanded access use if the use is for an extended duration.

(4) When a significant number of similar individual patient expanded access requests have been submitted, FDA may ask the sponsor to submit an IND or protocol for the use under § 312.315 or § 312.320.

(d) *Emergency procedures*. If there is an emergency that requires the patient to be treated before a written submission can be made, FDA may authorize the expanded access use to begin without a written submission. The FDA reviewing official may authorize the emergency use by telephone.

(1) Emergency expanded access use may be requested by telephone, facsimile, or other means of electronic communications. For investigational biological drug products regulated by the Center for Biologics Evaluation and Research, the request should be directed to the Office of Communication, Outreach and Development, Center for Biologics Evaluation and Research, 240-402-8010 or 1-800-835-4709, e-mail: *ocod@fda.hhs.gov*. For all other investigational drugs, the request for authorization should be directed to the Division of Drug Information, Center for Drug Evaluation and Research, 301-796-3400, e-mail: *druginfo@fda.hhs.gov*. After normal working hours (8 a.m. to 4:30 p.m.), the request should be directed to the FDA Emergency Call Center, 866-300-4374, e-mail: emergency.operations@fda.hhs.gov.

(2) The licensed physician or sponsor must explain how the expanded access use will meet the requirements of §§ 312.305 and 312.310 and must agree to submit an expanded access submission within 15 working days of FDA's authorization of the use.

[74 FR 40942, Aug. 13, 2009, as amended at 75 FR 32659, June 9, 2010; 80 FR 18091, Apr. 3, 2015]

§ 312.315 Intermediate-size patient populations.

Under this section, FDA may permit an investigational drug to be used for the treatment of a patient population smaller than that typical of a treatment IND or treatment protocol. FDA may ask a sponsor to consolidate expanded access under this section when the agency has received a significant number of requests for individual patient expanded access to an investigational drug for the same use.

(a) *Need for expanded access.* Expanded access under this section may be needed in the following situations:

(1) *Drug not being developed.* The drug is not being developed, for example, because the disease or condition is so rare that the sponsor is unable to recruit patients for a clinical trial.

(2) *Drug being developed.* The drug is being studied in a clinical trial, but patients requesting the drug for expanded access use are unable to participate in the trial. For example, patients may not be able to participate in the trial because they have a different disease or stage of disease than the one being studied or otherwise do not meet the enrollment criteria, because enrollment in the trial is closed, or because the trial site is not geographically accessible.

(3) *Approved or related drug.* (i) The drug is an approved drug product that is no longer marketed for safety reasons or is unavailable through marketing due to failure to meet the conditions of the approved application, or

(ii) The drug contains the same active moiety as an approved drug product that is unavailable through marketing due to failure to meet the conditions of the approved application or a drug shortage.

(b) *Criteria.* The criteria in § 312.305(a) must be met; and FDA must determine that:

(1) There is enough evidence that the drug is safe at the dose and duration proposed for expanded access use to justify a clinical trial of the drug in the approximate number of patients expected to receive the drug under expanded access; and

(2) There is at least preliminary clinical evidence of effectiveness of the drug, or of a plausible pharmacologic effect of the drug to make expanded access use a reasonable therapeutic option in the anticipated patient population.

(c) *Submission.* The expanded access submission must include information adequate to satisfy FDA that the criteria in § 312.305(a) and paragraph (b) of this section have been met. The expanded access submission must meet the requirements of § 312.305(b). In addition:

(1) The expanded access submission must state whether the drug is being developed or is not being developed and describe the patient population to be treated.

(2) If the drug is not being actively developed, the sponsor must explain why the drug cannot currently be developed for the expanded access use and under what circumstances the drug could be developed.

(3) If the drug is being studied in a clinical trial, the sponsor must explain why the patients to be treated cannot be enrolled in the clinical trial and under what circumstances the sponsor would conduct a clinical trial in these patients.

(d) *Safeguards.* (1) Upon review of the IND annual report, FDA will determine whether it is appropriate for the expanded access to continue under this section.

(i) If the drug is not being actively developed or if the expanded access use is not being developed (but another use is being developed), FDA will consider whether it is possible to conduct a clinical study of the expanded access use.

(ii) If the drug is being actively developed, FDA will consider whether providing the investigational drug for expanded access use is interfering with the clinical development of the drug.

(iii) As the number of patients enrolled increases, FDA may ask the sponsor to submit an IND or protocol for the use under § 312.320.

(2) The sponsor is responsible for monitoring the expanded access protocol to ensure that licensed physicians comply with the protocol and the regulations applicable to investigators.

§ 312.320 Treatment IND or treatment protocol.

Under this section, FDA may permit an investigational drug to be used for widespread treatment use.

(a) *Criteria*. The criteria in § 312.305(a) must be met, and FDA must determine that:

(1) *Trial status*. (i) The drug is being investigated in a controlled clinical trial under an IND designed to support a marketing application for the expanded access use, or

(ii) All clinical trials of the drug have been completed; and

(2) *Marketing status*. The sponsor is actively pursuing marketing approval of the drug for the expanded access use with due diligence; and

(3) *Evidence*. (i) When the expanded access use is for a serious disease or condition, there is sufficient clinical evidence of safety and effectiveness to support the expanded access use. Such evidence would ordinarily consist of data from phase 3 trials, but could consist of compelling data from completed phase 2 trials; or

(ii) When the expanded access use is for an immediately life-threatening disease or condition, the available scientific evidence, taken as a whole, provides a reasonable basis to conclude that the investigational drug may be effective for the expanded access use and would not expose patients to an unreasonable and significant risk of illness or injury. This evidence would ordinarily consist of clinical data from phase 3 or phase 2 trials, but could be based on more preliminary clinical evidence.

(b) *Submission*. The expanded access submission must include information adequate to satisfy FDA that the criteria in § 312.305(a) and paragraph (a) of this section have been met. The expanded access submission must meet the requirements of § 312.305(b).

(c) *Safeguard*. The sponsor is responsible for monitoring the treatment protocol to ensure that licensed physicians comply with the protocol and the regulations applicable to investigators.

• • •

PART 314—APPLICATIONS FOR FDA APPROVAL TO MARKET A NEW DRUG

Authority: 21 U.S.C. 321, 331, 351, 352, 353, 355, 355a, 355f, 356, 356a, 356b, 356c, 356e, 360cc, 371, 374, 379e, 379k-1.
Source: 50 FR 7493, Feb. 22, 1985, unless otherwise noted.
Editorial note: Nomenclature changes to part 314 appear at 69 FR 13717, Mar. 24, 2004; 81 FR 69639, Oct. 6, 2016.

Subpart A—General Provisions

§ 314.1 Scope of this part.

(a) This part sets forth procedures and requirements for the submission to, and the review by, the Food and Drug Administration of applications and abbreviated applications to market a new drug under section 505 of the Federal Food, Drug, and Cosmetic Act, as well as amendments, supplements, and postmarketing reports to them.

(b) This part does not apply to drug products subject to licensing by FDA under the Public Health Service Act (58 Stat. 632 as amended (42 U.S.C. 201 et seq.)) and subchapter F of chapter I of title 21 of the Code of Federal Regulations.

(c) References in this part to regulations in the Code of Federal Regulations are to chapter I of title 21, unless otherwise noted.

[50 FR 7493, Feb. 22, 1985, as amended at 57 FR 17981, Apr. 28, 1992; 64 FR 401, Jan. 5, 1999]

§ 314.2 Purpose.

The purpose of this part is to establish an efficient and thorough drug review process in order to: (a) Facilitate the approval of drugs shown to be safe and effective; and (b) ensure the disapproval of drugs not shown to be safe and effective. These regulations are also intended to establish an effective system for FDA's surveillance of marketed drugs. These regulations shall be construed in light of these objectives.

§ 314.3 Definitions.

(a) The definitions and interpretations contained in section 201 of the Federal Food, Drug, and Cosmetic Act apply to those terms when used in this part and part 320 of this chapter.

(b) The following definitions of terms apply to this part and part 320 of this chapter:

180-day exclusivity period is the 180-day period beginning on the date of the first commercial marketing of the drug (including the commercial marketing of the reference listed drug) by any first applicant. The 180-day period ends on the day before the date on which an ANDA submitted by an applicant other than a first applicant could be approved.

505(b)(2) application is an NDA submitted under section 505(b)(1) of the Federal Food, Drug, and Cosmetic Act for a drug for which at least some of the investigations described in section 505(b)(1)(A) of the Federal Food, Drug, and Cosmetic Act and relied upon by the applicant for approval of the NDA were not conducted by or for the applicant and for which the applicant has not obtained a right of reference or use from the person by or for whom the investigations were conducted.

Abbreviated application, abbreviated new drug application, or ANDA is the application described under § 314.94, including all amendments and supplements to the application.

Acknowledgment letter is a written, postmarked communication from FDA to an applicant stating that the Agency has determined that an ANDA is sufficiently complete to permit a substantive review. An acknowledgment letter indicates that the ANDA is regarded as received.

Act is the Federal Food, Drug, and Cosmetic Act (section 201 et seq. (21 U.S.C. 301 et seq.)).

Active ingredient is any component that is intended to furnish pharmacological activity or other direct effect in the diagnosis, cure, mitigation, treatment, or prevention of disease, or to affect the structure or any function of the body of man or other animals. The term includes those components that may undergo chemical change in the manufacture of the drug product and be present in the drug product in a modified form intended to furnish the specified activity or effect.

Active moiety is the molecule or ion, excluding those appended portions of the molecule that cause the drug to be an ester, salt (including a salt with hydrogen or coordination bonds), or other noncovalent derivative (such as a complex, chelate, or clathrate) of the molecule, responsible for the physiological or pharmacological action of the drug substance.

ANDA holder is the applicant that owns an approved ANDA.

Applicant is any person who submits an NDA (including a 505(b)(2) application) or ANDA or an amendment or supplement to an NDA or ANDA under this part to obtain FDA approval of a new drug and any person who owns an approved NDA (including a 505(b)(2) application) or ANDA.

Application, new drug application, or NDA is the application described under § 314.50, including all amendments and supplements to the application. An NDA refers to "stand-alone" applications submitted under section 505(b)(1) of the Federal Food, Drug, and Cosmetic Act and to 505(b)(2) applications.

Approval letter is a written communication to an applicant from FDA approving an NDA or an ANDA.

Assess the effects of the change is to evaluate the effects of a manufacturing change on the identity, strength, quality, purity, and potency of a drug product as these factors may relate to the safety or effectiveness of the drug product.

Authorized generic drug is a listed drug, as defined in this section, that has been approved under section 505(c) of the Federal Food, Drug, and Cosmetic Act and is marketed, sold, or distributed directly or indirectly to the retail class of trade with labeling, packaging (other than repackaging as the listed drug in blister packs, unit doses, or similar packaging for use in institutions), product code, labeler code, trade name, or trademark that differs from that of the listed drug.

Bioavailability is the rate and extent to which the active ingredient or active moiety is absorbed from a drug product and becomes available at the site of drug action. For drug products that are not intended to be absorbed into the bloodstream, bioavailability may be assessed by scientifically valid measurements intended to reflect the rate and extent to which the active ingredient or active moiety becomes available at the site of drug action.

Bioequivalence is the absence of a significant difference in the rate and extent to which the active ingredient or active moiety in pharmaceutical equivalents or pharmaceutical alternatives becomes available at the site of drug action when administered at the same molar dose under similar conditions in an appropriately designed study. Where there is an intentional difference in rate (e.g., in certain extended-release dosage forms), certain pharmaceutical equivalents or alternatives may be considered bioequivalent if there is no significant difference in the extent to which the active ingredient or moiety from each product becomes available at the site of drug action. This applies only if the difference in the rate at which the active ingredient or moiety becomes available at the site of drug action is intentional and is reflected in the proposed labeling, is not essential to the attainment of effective body drug concentrations on chronic use, and is considered medically insignificant for the drug. For drug products that are not intended to be absorbed into the bloodstream, bioequivalence may be assessed by scientifically valid measurements intended to reflect the rate and extent to which the active ingredient or active moiety becomes available at the site of drug action.

Bioequivalence requirement is a requirement imposed by FDA for in vitro and/or in vivo testing of specified drug products that must be satisfied as a condition of marketing.

Class 1 resubmission is the resubmission of an NDA or efficacy supplement, following receipt of a complete response letter, that contains one or more of the following: Final printed labeling, draft labeling, certain safety updates, stability updates to support provisional or final dating periods, commitments to perform postmarketing studies (including proposals for such studies), assay validation data, final release testing on the last lots used to support approval, minor reanalyses of previously submitted data, and other comparatively minor information.

Class 2 resubmission is the resubmission of an NDA or efficacy supplement, following receipt of a complete response letter, that includes any item not specified in the definition of "Class 1 resubmission," including any item that would require presentation to an advisory committee.

Commercial marketing is the introduction or delivery for introduction into interstate commerce of a drug product described in an ANDA, outside the control of the ANDA applicant, except that the term does not include transfer of the drug product for investigational use under part 312 of this chapter or transfer of the drug product to parties identified in the ANDA for reasons other than sale. Commercial marketing includes the introduction or delivery for introduction into interstate commerce of the reference listed drug by the ANDA applicant.

Complete response letter is a written communication to an applicant from FDA usually describing all of the deficiencies that the Agency has identified in an NDA or ANDA that must be satisfactorily addressed before it can be approved.

Component is any ingredient intended for use in the manufacture of a drug product, including those that may not appear in such drug product.

Date of approval is the date on the approval letter from FDA stating that the NDA or ANDA is approved, except that the date of approval for an NDA described in section 505(x)(1) of the Federal Food, Drug, and Cosmetic Act is determined as described in section 505(x)(2) of the Federal Food, Drug, and Cosmetic Act. "Date of approval" refers only to a final approval and not to a tentative approval.

Dosage form is the physical manifestation containing the active and inactive ingredients that delivers a dose of the drug product. This includes such factors as:

(1) The physical appearance of the drug product;

(2) The physical form of the drug product prior to dispensing to the patient;

(3) The way the product is administered; and

(4) The design features that affect frequency of dosing.

Drug product is a finished dosage form, e.g., tablet, capsule, or solution, that contains a drug substance, generally, but not necessarily, in association with one or more other ingredients.

Drug substance is an active ingredient that is intended to furnish pharmacological activity or other direct effect in the diagnosis, cure, mitigation, treatment, or prevention of disease or to affect the structure or any function of the human body, but does not include intermediates used in the synthesis of such ingredient.

Efficacy supplement is a supplement to an approved NDA proposing to make one or more related changes from among the following changes to product labeling:

(1) Add or modify an indication or claim;

(2) Revise the dose or dose regimen;

(3) Provide for a new route of administration;

(4) Make a comparative efficacy claim naming another drug product;

(5) Significantly alter the intended patient population;

(6) Change the marketing status from prescription to over-the-counter use;

(7) Provide for, or provide evidence of effectiveness necessary for, the traditional approval of a product originally approved under subpart H of this part; or

(8) Incorporate other information based on at least one adequate and well-controlled clinical study.

FDA or Agency is the Food and Drug Administration.

First applicant is an ANDA applicant that, on the first day on which a substantially complete application containing a paragraph IV certification is submitted for approval of a drug, submits a substantially complete application that contains, and for which the applicant lawfully maintains, a paragraph IV certification for the drug.

Inactive ingredient is any component other than an active ingredient.

Listed drug is a new drug product that has been approved under section 505(c) of the Federal Food, Drug, and Cosmetic Act for safety and effectiveness or under section 505(j) of the Federal Food, Drug, and Cosmetic Act, which has not been withdrawn or suspended under section 505(e)(1) through (5) or section 505(j)(6) of the Federal Food, Drug, and Cosmetic Act, and which has not been withdrawn from sale for what FDA has determined are reasons of safety or effectiveness. Listed drug status is evidenced by the drug product's identification in the current edition of FDA's "Approved Drug Products With Therapeutic Equivalence Evaluations" (the list) as an approved drug. A drug product is deemed to be a listed drug on the date of approval for the NDA or ANDA for that drug product.

NDA holder is the applicant that owns an approved NDA.

Newly acquired information is data, analyses, or other information not previously submitted to the Agency, which may include (but is not limited to) data derived from new clinical studies, reports of adverse events, or new analyses of previously submitted data (e.g., meta-analyses) if the studies, events, or analyses reveal risks of a different type or greater severity or frequency than previously included in submissions to FDA.

Original application or original NDA is a pending NDA for which FDA has never issued a complete response letter or approval letter, or an NDA that was submitted again after FDA had refused to file it or after it was withdrawn without being approved.

Paragraph IV acknowledgment letter is a written, postmarked communication from FDA to an applicant stating that the Agency has determined that a 505(b)(2) application or ANDA containing a paragraph IV certification is sufficiently complete to permit a substantive review. A paragraph IV acknowledgment letter indicates that the 505(b)(2) application is regarded as filed or the ANDA is regarded as received.

Paragraph IV certification is a patent certification of invalidity, unenforceability, or noninfringement described in § 314.50(i)(1)(i)(A)(4) or § 314.94(a)(12)(i)(A)(4).

Patent owner is the owner of the patent for which information is submitted for an NDA.

Pharmaceutical alternatives are drug products that contain the identical therapeutic moiety, or its precursor, but not necessarily in the same amount or dosage form or as the same salt or ester. Each such drug product individually meets either the identical or its own respective compendial or other applicable standard of identity, strength, quality, and purity, including potency and, where applicable, content uniformity, disintegration times, and/or dissolution rates.

Pharmaceutical equivalents are drug products in identical dosage forms and route(s) of administration that contain identical amounts of the identical active drug ingredient, i.e., the same salt or ester of the same therapeutic moiety, or, in the case of modified-release dosage forms that require a reservoir or overage or such forms as prefilled syringes where residual volume may vary, that deliver identical amounts of the active drug ingredient over the identical dosing period; do not necessarily contain the same inactive ingredients; and meet the identical compendial or other applicable standard of identity, strength, quality, and purity, including potency and, where applicable, content uniformity, disintegration times, and/or dissolution rates.

Postmark is an independently verifiable evidentiary record of the date on which a document is transmitted, in an unmodifiable format, to another party. For postmarks made by the U.S. Postal Service or a designated delivery service, the date of transmission is the date on which the document is received by the domestic mail service of the U.S. Postal Service or by a designated delivery service. For postmarks documenting an electronic event, the date of transmission is the date (in a particular time zone) that FDA sends the electronic transmission on its host system as evidenced by a verifiable record. If the sender and the intended recipient are located in different time zones, it is the sender's time zone that provides the controlling date of electronic transmission.

Reference listed drug is the listed drug identified by FDA as the drug product upon which an applicant relies in seeking approval of its ANDA.

Reference standard is the drug product selected by FDA that an applicant seeking approval of an ANDA must use in conducting an in vivo bioequivalence study required for approval.

Resubmission, in the context of a complete response letter, is submission by the applicant of all materials needed to fully address all deficiencies identified in the complete response letter. An NDA or ANDA for which FDA issued a complete response letter, but which was withdrawn before approval and later submitted again, is not a resubmission.

Right of reference or use is the authority to rely upon, and otherwise use, an investigation for the purpose of obtaining approval of an NDA, including the ability to make available the underlying raw data from the investigation for FDA audit, if necessary.

Same drug product formulation is the formulation of the drug product submitted for approval and any formulations that have minor differences in composition or method of manufacture from the formulation submitted for approval, but are similar enough to be relevant to the Agency's determination of bioequivalence.

Specification is the quality standard (i.e., tests, analytical procedures, and acceptance criteria) provided in an approved NDA or ANDA to confirm the quality of drug substances, drug products, intermediates, raw materials, reagents, components, in-process materials, container closure systems, and other materials used in the production of a drug substance or drug product. For the purpose of this definition, acceptance criteria means numerical limits, ranges, or other criteria for the tests described.

Strength is the amount of drug substance contained in, delivered, or deliverable from a drug product, which includes:

(1)(i) The total quantity of drug substance in mass or units of activity in a dosage unit or container closure (e.g., weight/unit dose, weight/volume or weight/weight in a container closure, or units/volume or units/weight in a container closure); and/or, as applicable.

(ii) The concentration of the drug substance in mass or units of activity per unit volume or mass (e.g., weight/weight, weight/volume, or units/volume); or

(2) Such other criteria the Agency establishes for determining the amount of drug substance contained in, delivered, or deliverable from a drug product if the weights and measures described in paragraph (i) of this definition do not apply (e.g., certain drug-device combination products for which the amount of drug substance is emitted per use or unit time).

Substantially complete application is an ANDA that on its face is sufficiently complete to permit a substantive review. Sufficiently complete means that the ANDA contains all the information required under section 505(j)(2)(A) of the Federal Food, Drug, and Cosmetic Act and does not contain a deficiency described in § 314.101(d) and (e).

Tentative approval is notification that an NDA or ANDA otherwise meets the requirements for approval under the Federal Food, Drug, and Cosmetic Act, but cannot be approved because there is a 7-year period of orphan exclusivity for a listed drug under section 527 of the Federal Food, Drug, and Cosmetic Act and § 316.31 of this chapter, or that a 505(b)(2) application or ANDA otherwise meets the requirements for approval under the Federal Food, Drug, and Cosmetic Act, but cannot be approved until the conditions in § 314.107(b)(1)(iii), (b)(3), or (c) are met; because there is a period of exclusivity for the listed drug under § 314.108; because there is a period of pediatric exclusivity for the listed drug under section 505A of the Federal Food, Drug, and Cosmetic Act; because there is a period of exclusivity for the listed drug under section 505E of the Federal Food, Drug, and Cosmetic Act; or because a court order pursuant to 35 U.S.C. 271(e)(4)(A) orders that the NDA or ANDA may be approved no earlier than the date specified. A drug product that is granted tentative approval is not an approved drug and will not be approved until FDA issues an approval letter after any necessary additional review of the NDA or ANDA.

The list is the list of approved drug products published in FDA's current "Approved Drug Products With Therapeutic Equivalence Evaluations," available electronically on FDA's Web site at *http://www.fda.gov/cder.*

Therapeutic equivalents are approved drug products that are pharmaceutical equivalents for which bioequivalence has been demonstrated, and that can be expected to have the same clinical effect and safety profile when administered to patients under the conditions specified in the labeling.

[81 FR 69636, Oct. 6, 2016]

Subpart B—Applications

§ 314.50 Content and format of an NDA.

NDAs and supplements to approved NDAs are required to be submitted in the form and contain the information, as appropriate for the particular submission, required under this section. Three copies of the NDA are required: An archival copy, a review copy, and a field copy. An NDA for a new chemical entity will generally contain an application form, an index, a summary, five or six technical sections, case report tabulations of patient data, case report forms, drug samples, and labeling, including, if applicable, any Medication Guide required under part 208 of this chapter. Other NDAs will generally contain only some of those items, and information will be limited to that needed to support the particular submission. These include an NDA of the type described in section 505(b)(2) of the Federal Food, Drug, and Cosmetic Act, an amendment, and a supplement. The NDA is required to contain reports of all investigations of the drug product sponsored by the applicant, and all other information about the drug pertinent to an evaluation of the NDA that is received or otherwise obtained by the applicant from any source. FDA will maintain guidance documents on the format and content of NDAs to assist applicants in their preparation.

(a) *Application form.* The applicant must submit a completed and signed application form that contains the following:

(1) The name and address of the applicant; the date of the NDA; the NDA number if previously issued (for example, if the NDA is a resubmission or an amendment or supplement); the name of the drug product, including its established, proprietary, code, and chemical names; the dosage form and strength; the route of administration; the identification numbers of all INDs (as defined in § 312.3(b) of this chapter) that are referenced in the NDA; the identification numbers of all drug master files and other applications under this part that are referenced in the NDA; and the drug product's proposed indications for use.

(2) A statement whether the submission is an original submission, a 505(b)(2) application, a resubmission, or a supplement to an application under § 314.70.

(3) A statement whether the applicant proposes to market the drug product as a prescription or an over-the-counter product.

(4) A check-list identifying what enclosures required under this section the applicant is submitting.

(5) The applicant, or the applicant's attorney, agent, or other authorized official must sign the NDA. If the person signing the NDA does not reside or have a place of business within the United States, the NDA is required to contain the name and address of, and be countersigned by, an attorney, agent, or other authorized official who resides or maintains a place of business within the United States.

(b) *Index*. The archival copy of the NDA is required to contain a comprehensive index by volume number and page number to the summary under paragraph (c) of this section, the technical sections under paragraph (d) of this section, and the supporting information under paragraph (f) of this section.

(c) *Summary*. (1) An NDA is required to contain a summary of the NDA in enough detail that the reader may gain a good general understanding of the data and information in the NDA, including an understanding of the quantitative aspects of the data. The summary is not required for supplements under § 314.70. Resubmissions of an NDA should contain an updated summary, as appropriate. The summary should discuss all aspects of the NDA, and synthesize the information into a well-structured and unified document. The summary should be written at approximately the level of detail required for publication in, and meet the editorial standards generally applied by, refereed scientific and medical journals. In addition to the agency personnel reviewing the summary in the context of their review of the NDA, FDA may furnish the summary to FDA advisory committee members and agency officials whose duties require an understanding of the NDA. To the extent possible, data in the summary should be presented in tabular and graphic forms. FDA has prepared a guideline under § 10.90(b) that provides information about how to prepare a summary. The summary required under this paragraph may be used by FDA or the applicant to prepare the Summary Basis of Approval document for public disclosure (under § 314.430(e)(2)(ii)) when the NDA is approved.

(2) The summary is required to contain the following information:

(i) The proposed text of the labeling, including, if applicable, any Medication Guide required under part 208 of this chapter, for the drug, with annotations to the information in the summary and technical sections of the NDA that support the inclusion of each statement in the labeling, and, if the NDA is for a prescription drug, statements describing the reasons for omitting a section or subsection of the labeling format in § 201.57 of this chapter.

(ii) A statement identifying the pharmacologic class of the drug and a discussion of the scientific rationale for the drug, its intended use, and the potential clinical benefits of the drug product.

(iii) A brief description of the marketing history, if any, of the drug outside the United States, including a list of the countries in which the drug has been marketed, a list of any countries in which the drug has been withdrawn from marketing for any reason related to safety or effectiveness, and a list of countries in which applications for marketing are pending. The description is required to describe both marketing by the applicant and, if known, the marketing history of other persons.

(iv) A summary of the chemistry, manufacturing, and controls section of the NDA.

(v) A summary of the nonclinical pharmacology and toxicology section of the NDA.

(vi) A summary of the human pharmacokinetics and bioavailability section of the NDA.

(vii) A summary of the microbiology section of the NDA (for anti-infective drugs only).

(viii) A summary of the clinical data section of the NDA, including the results of statistical analyses of the clinical trials.

(ix) A concluding discussion that presents the benefit and risk considerations related to the drug, including a discussion of any proposed additional studies or surveillance the applicant intends to conduct postmarketing.

(d) *Technical sections*. The NDA is required to contain the technical sections described below. Each technical section is required to contain data and information in sufficient detail to permit the agency to make a knowledgeable judgment about whether to approve the NDA or whether grounds exist under section 505(d) of the Federal Food, Drug, and Cosmetic Act to refuse to approve the NDA. The required technical sections are as follows:

(1) *Chemistry, manufacturing, and controls section.* A section describing the composition, manufacture, and specification of the drug substance and the drug product, including the following:

(i) *Drug substance.* A full description of the drug substance including its physical and chemical characteristics and stability; the name and address of its manufacturer; the method of synthesis (or isolation) and purification of the drug substance; the process controls used during manufacture and packaging; and the specifications necessary to ensure the identity, strength, quality, and purity of the drug substance and the bioavailability of the drug products made from the substance, including, for example, tests, analytical procedures, and acceptance criteria relating to stability, sterility, particle size, and crystalline form. The NDA may provide additionally for the use of alternatives to meet any of these requirements, including alternative sources, process controls, and analytical procedures. Reference to the current edition of the U.S. Pharmacopeia and the National Formulary may satisfy relevant requirements in this paragraph.

(ii)((a)) *Drug product.* A list of all components used in the manufacture of the drug product (regardless of whether they appear in the drug product) and a statement of the composition of the drug product; the specifications for each component; the name and address of each manufacturer of the drug product; a description of the manufacturing and packaging procedures and in-process controls for the drug product; the specifications necessary to ensure the identity, strength, quality, purity, potency, and bioavailability of the drug product, including, for example, tests, analytical procedures, and acceptance criteria relating to sterility, dissolution rate, container closure systems; and stability data with proposed expiration dating. The NDA may provide additionally for the use of alternatives to meet any of these requirements, including alternative components, manufacturing and packaging procedures, in-process controls, and analytical procedures. Reference to the current edition of the U.S. Pharmacopeia and the National Formulary may satisfy relevant requirements in this paragraph.

(b) Unless provided by paragraph (d)(1)(ii)(a) of this section, for each batch of the drug product used to conduct a bioavailability or bioequivalence study described in § 320.38 or § 320.63 of this chapter or used to conduct a primary stability study: The batch production record; the specification for each component and for the drug product; the names and addresses of the sources of the active and noncompendial inactive components and of the container and closure system for the drug product; the name and address of each contract facility involved in the manufacture, processing, packaging, or testing of the drug product and identification of the operation performed by each contract facility; and the results of any test performed on the components used in the manufacture of the drug product as required by § 211.84(d) of this chapter and on the drug product as required by § 211.165 of this chapter.

(c) The proposed or actual master production record, including a description of the equipment, to be used for the manufacture of a commercial lot of the drug product or a comparably detailed description of the production process for a representative batch of the drug product.

(iii) *Environmental impact.* The NDA is required to contain either a claim for categorical exclusion under § 25.30 or 25.31 of this chapter or an environmental assessment under § 25.40 of this chapter.

(iv) The applicant may, at its option, submit a complete chemistry, manufacturing, and controls section 90 to 120 days before the anticipated submission of the remainder of the NDA. FDA will review such early submissions as resources permit.

(v) The applicant must include a statement certifying that the field copy of the NDA has been provided to the applicant's home FDA district office.

(2) Nonclinical pharmacology and toxicology section. A section describing, with the aid of graphs and tables, animal and in vitro studies with drug, including the following:

(i) Studies of the pharmacological actions of the drug in relation to its proposed therapeutic indication and studies that otherwise define the pharmacologic properties of the drug or are pertinent to possible adverse effects.

(ii) Studies of the toxicological effects of the drug as they relate to the drug's intended clinical uses, including, as appropriate, studies assessing the drug's acute, subacute, and chronic toxicity; carcinogenicity; and studies of toxicities related to the drug's particular mode of administration or conditions of use.

(iii) Studies, as appropriate, of the effects of the drug on reproduction and on the developing fetus.

(iv) Any studies of the absorption, distribution, metabolism, and excretion of the drug in animals.

(v) For each nonclinical laboratory study subject to the good laboratory practice regulations under part 58 a statement that it was conducted in compliance with the good laboratory practice regulations in part 58, or, if the study was not conducted in compliance with those regulations, a brief statement of the reason for the noncompliance.

(3) *Human pharmacokinetics and bioavailability section.* A section describing the human pharmacokinetic data and human bioavailability data, or information supporting a waiver of the submission of in vivo bioavailability data under subpart B of part 320, including the following:

(i) A description of each of the bioavailability and pharmacokinetic studies of the drug in humans performed by or on behalf of the applicant that includes a description of the analytical procedures and statistical methods used in each study and a statement with respect to each study that it either was conducted in compliance with the institutional review board regulations in part 56, or was not subject to the regulations under § 56.104 or § 56.105, and that it was conducted in compliance with the informed consent regulations in part 50.

(ii) If the NDA describes in the chemistry, manufacturing, and controls section tests, analytical procedures, and acceptance criteria needed to assure the bioavailability of the drug product or drug substance, or both, a statement in this section of the rationale for establishing the tests, analytical procedures, and acceptance criteria, including data and information supporting the rationale.

(iii) A summarizing discussion and analysis of the pharmacokinetics and metabolism of the active ingredients and the bioavailability or bioequivalence, or both, of the drug product.

(4) *Microbiology section.* If the drug is an anti-infective drug, a section describing the microbiology data, including the following:

(i) A description of the biochemical basis of the drug's action on microbial physiology.

(ii) A description of the antimicrobial spectra of the drug, including results of in vitro preclinical studies to demonstrate concentrations of the drug required for effective use.

(iii) A description of any known mechanisms of resistance to the drug, including results of any known epidemiologic studies to demonstrate prevalence of resistance factors.

(iv) A description of clinical microbiology laboratory procedures (for example, in vitro sensitivity discs) needed for effective use of the drug.

(5) *Clinical data section.* A section describing the clinical investigations of the drug, including the following:

(i) A description and analysis of each clinical pharmacology study of the drug, including a brief comparison of the results of the human studies with the animal pharmacology and toxicology data.

(ii) A description and analysis of each controlled clinical study pertinent to a proposed use of the drug, including the protocol and a description of the statistical analyses used to evaluate the study. If the study report is an interim analysis, this is to be noted and a projected completion date provided. Controlled clinical studies that have not been analyzed in detail for any reason (e.g., because they have been discontinued or are incomplete) are to be included in this section, including a copy of the protocol and a brief description of the results and status of the study.

(iii) A description of each uncontrolled clinical study, a summary of the results, and a brief statement explaining why the study is classified as uncontrolled.

(iv) A description and analysis of any other data or information relevant to an evaluation of the safety and effectiveness of the drug product obtained or otherwise received by the applicant from any source, foreign or domestic, including information derived from clinical investigations, including controlled and uncontrolled studies of uses of the drug other than those proposed in the NDA, commercial marketing experience, reports in the scientific literature, and unpublished scientific papers.

(v) An integrated summary of the data demonstrating substantial evidence of effectiveness for the claimed indications. Evidence is also required to support the dosage and administration section of the labeling, including support for the dosage and dose interval recommended. The effectiveness data must be presented by gender, age, and racial subgroups and must identify any modifications of dose or dose interval needed for specific subgroups. Effectiveness data from other subgroups of the population of patients treated, when appropriate, such as patients with renal failure or patients with different levels of severity of the disease, also must be presented.

(vi) A summary and updates of safety information, as follows:

(a) The applicant must submit an integrated summary of all available information about the safety of the drug product, including pertinent animal data, demonstrated or potential adverse effects of the drug, clinically significant drug/drug interactions, and other safety considerations, such as data from epidemiological studies of related drugs. The safety data must be presented by gender, age, and racial subgroups. When appropriate, safety data from other subgroups of the population of patients treated also must be presented, such as for patients with renal failure or patients with different levels of severity of the disease. A description of any statistical analyses performed in analyzing safety data should also be included, unless already included under paragraph (d)(5)(ii) of this section.

(b) The applicant must, under section 505(i) of the Federal Food, Drug, and Cosmetic Act, update periodically its pending NDA with new safety information learned about the drug that may reasonably affect the statement of contraindications, warnings, precautions, and adverse reactions in the draft labeling and, if applicable, any Medication Guide required under part 208 of this chapter. These "safety update reports" must include the same kinds of information (from clinical studies, animal studies, and other sources) and must be submitted in the same format as the integrated summary in paragraph (d)(5)(vi)(a) of this section. In addition, the reports must include the case report forms for each patient who died during a clinical study or who did not complete the study because of an adverse event (unless this requirement is waived). The applicant must submit these reports (1) 4 months after the initial submission; (2) in a resubmission following receipt of a complete response letter; and (3) at other times as requested by FDA. Before submitting the first such report, applicants are encouraged to consult with FDA regarding further details on its form and content.

(vii) If the drug has a potential for abuse, a description and analysis of studies or information related to abuse of the drug, including a proposal for scheduling under the Controlled Substances Act. A description of any studies related to overdosage is also required, including information on dialysis, antidotes, or other treatments, if known.

(viii) An integrated summary of the benefits and risks of the drug, including a discussion of why the benefits exceed the risks under the conditions stated in the labeling.

(ix) A statement with respect to each clinical study involving human subjects that it either was conducted in compliance with the institutional review board regulations in part 56, or was not subject to the regulations under § 56.104 or § 56.105, and that it was conducted in compliance with the informed consent regulations in part 50.

(x) If a sponsor has transferred any obligations for the conduct of any clinical study to a contract research organization, a statement containing the name and address of the contract research organization, identification of the clinical study, and a listing of the obligations transferred. If all obligations governing the conduct of the study have been transferred, a general statement of this transfer—in lieu of a listing of the specific obligations transferred—may be submitted.

(xi) If original subject records were audited or reviewed by the sponsor in the course of monitoring any clinical study to verify the accuracy of the case reports submitted to the sponsor, a list identifying each clinical study so audited or reviewed.

(6) *Statistical section*. A section describing the statistical evaluation of clinical data, including the following:

(i) A copy of the information submitted under paragraph (d)(5)(ii) of this section concerning the description and analysis of each controlled clinical study, and the documentation and supporting statistical analyses used in evaluating the controlled clinical studies.

(ii) A copy of the information submitted under paragraph (d)(5)(vi)(a) of this section concerning a summary of information about the safety of the drug product, and the documentation and supporting statistical analyses used in evaluating the safety information.

(7) *Pediatric use section.* A section describing the investigation of the drug for use in pediatric populations, including an integrated summary of the information (the clinical pharmacology studies, controlled clinical studies, or uncontrolled clinical studies, or other data or information) that is relevant to the safety and effectiveness and benefits and risks of the drug in pediatric populations for the claimed indications, a reference to the full descriptions of such studies provided under paragraphs (d)(3) and (d)(5) of this section, and information required to be submitted under § 314.55.

(e) *Samples and labeling.* (1) Upon request from FDA, the applicant must submit the samples described below to the places identified in the Agency's request. FDA generally will ask applicants to submit samples directly to two or more Agency laboratories that will perform all necessary tests on the samples and validate the applicant's analytical procedures.

(i) Four representative samples of the following, each sample in sufficient quantity to permit FDA to perform three times each test described in the NDA to determine whether the drug substance and the drug product meet the specifications given in the NDA:

(a) The drug product proposed for marketing;

(b) The drug substance used in the drug product from which the samples of the drug product were taken; and

(c) Reference standards and blanks (except that reference standards recognized in an official compendium need not be submitted).

(ii) Samples of the finished market package, if requested by FDA.

(2) The applicant must submit the following in the archival copy of the NDA:

(i) Three copies of the analytical procedures and related descriptive information contained in the chemistry, manufacturing, and controls section under paragraph (d)(1) of this section for the drug substance and the drug product that are necessary for FDA's laboratories to perform all necessary tests on the samples and to validate the applicant's analytical procedures. The related descriptive information includes a description of each sample; the proposed regulatory specifications for the drug; a detailed description of the methods of analysis; supporting data for accuracy, specificity, precision and ruggedness; and complete results of the applicant's tests on each sample.

(ii) Copies of the label and all labeling for the drug product (including, if applicable, any Medication Guide required under part 208 of this chapter) for the drug product (4 copies of draft labeling or 12 copies of final printed labeling).

(f) *Case report forms and tabulations.* The archival copy of the NDA is required to contain the following case report tabulations and case report forms:

(1) *Case report tabulations.* The NDA is required to contain tabulations of the data from each adequate and well-controlled study under § 314.126 (Phase 2 and Phase 3 studies as described in §§ 312.21 (b) and (c) of this chapter), tabulations of the data from the earliest clinical pharmacology studies (Phase 1 studies as described in § 312.21(a) of this chapter), and tabulations of the safety data from other clinical studies. Routine submission of other patient data from uncontrolled studies is not required. The tabulations are required to include the data on each patient in each study, except that the applicant may delete those tabulations which the agency agrees, in advance, are not pertinent to a review of the drug's safety or effectiveness. Upon request, FDA will discuss with the applicant in a "pre-NDA" conference those tabulations that may be appropriate for such deletion. Barring unforeseen circumstances, tabulations agreed to be deleted at such a conference will not be requested during the conduct of FDA's review of the NDA. If such unforeseen circumstances do occur, any request for deleted tabulations will be made by the director of the FDA division responsible for reviewing the NDA, in accordance with paragraph (f)(3) of this section.

(2) *Case report forms.* The NDA is required to contain copies of individual case report forms for each patient who died during a clinical study or who did not complete the study because of an adverse event, whether believed to be drug related or not, including patients receiving reference drugs or placebo. This requirement may be waived by FDA for specific studies if the case report forms are unnecessary for a proper review of the study.

(3) *Additional data.* The applicant must submit to FDA additional case report forms and tabulations needed to conduct a proper review of the NDA, as requested by the director of the FDA division responsible for reviewing the NDA. The applicant's failure to submit information requested by FDA within 30 days after receipt of the request may result in the agency viewing any eventual submission as a major amendment under § 314.60 and extending the review period as necessary. If desired by the applicant, the FDA division director will verify in writing any request for additional data that was made orally.

(4) *Presentation and format.* Applicants are invited to meet with FDA before submitting an NDA to discuss the presentation and format of supporting information. If the applicant and FDA agree, the applicant may submit tabulations of patient data and case report forms in an alternate form.

(g) *Other.* The following general requirements apply to the submission of information within the summary under paragraph (c) of this section and within the technical sections under paragraph (d) of this section.

(1) The applicant ordinarily is not required to resubmit information previously submitted, but may incorporate the information by reference. A reference to information submitted previously is required to identify the file by name, reference number, volume, and page number in the agency's records where the information can be found. A reference to information submitted to the agency by a person other than the applicant is required to contain a written statement that authorizes the reference and that is signed by the person who submitted the information.

(2) The applicant must submit an accurate and complete English translation of each part of the NDA that is not in English. The applicant must submit a copy of each original literature publication for which an English translation is submitted.

(3) If an applicant who submits an NDA under section 505(b) of the Federal Food, Drug, and Cosmetic Act obtains a "right of reference or use," as defined under § 314.3(b), to an investigation described in clause (A) of section 505(b)(1) of the Federal Food, Drug, and Cosmetic Act, the applicant must include in its NDA a written statement signed by the owner of the data from each such investigation that the applicant may rely on in support of the approval of its NDA, and provide FDA access to, the underlying raw data that provide the basis for the report of the investigation submitted in its NDA.

(h) *Patent information.* The NDA is required to contain the patent information described under § 314.53.

(i) *Patent certification*—(1) *Contents.* A 505(b)(2) application is required to contain the following:

(i) *Patents claiming drug substance, drug product, or method of use.* (A) An appropriate patent certification or statement with respect to each patent issued by the U.S. Patent and Trademark Office that, in the opinion of the applicant and to the best of its knowledge, claims the drug substance or drug product on which investigations that are relied upon by the applicant for approval of its 505(b)(2) application were conducted or that claims an approved use for such drug and for which information is required to be filed under section 505(b) and (c) of the Federal Food, Drug, and Cosmetic Act and § 314.53. For each such patent, the applicant must provide the patent number and certify, in its opinion and to the best of its knowledge, one of the following circumstances:

(1) That the patent information has not been submitted to FDA. The applicant must entitle such a certification "Paragraph I Certification";

(2) That the patent has expired. The applicant must entitle such a certification "Paragraph II Certification";

(3) The date on which the patent will expire. The applicant must entitle such a certification "Paragraph III Certification"; or

(4)(i) That the patent is invalid, unenforceable, or will not be infringed by the manufacture, use, or sale of the drug product for which the 505(b)(2) application is submitted. The applicant must entitle such a certification "Paragraph IV Certification". This certification must be submitted in the following form:

> I, (name of applicant), certify that Patent No. ____ (*is invalid, unenforceable, or will not be infringed by the manufacture, use, or sale of*) (*name of proposed drug product*) for which this 505(b)(2) application is submitted.

(ii) The certification must be accompanied by a statement that the applicant will comply with the requirements under § 314.52(a) with respect to providing a notice to each owner of the patent or its representative and to the NDA holder (or, if the NDA holder does not reside or maintain a place of business within the United States, its attorney, agent, or other authorized official) for the drug product that is claimed by the patent or a use of which is claimed by the patent and with the requirements under § 314.52(b) with respect to sending the notice and under § 314.52(c) with respect to the content of the notice.

(B) If the drug on which investigations that are relied upon by the applicant were conducted is itself a licensed generic drug of a patented drug first approved under section 505(b) of the Federal Food, Drug, and Cosmetic Act, an appropriate patent certification or statement under this section with respect to each patent that claims the first-approved patented drug or that claims an approved use for such a drug.

(C) If, before the date of submission of an original 505(b)(2) application, there is a drug product approved in an NDA that is pharmaceutically equivalent to the drug product for which the original 505(b)(2) application is submitted, an appropriate patent certification or statement under this section with respect to each patent that claims the drug substance or drug product or that claims an approved use for one such drug product.

(ii) *No relevant patents.* If, in the opinion of the applicant and to the best of its knowledge, there are no patents described in paragraph (i)(1)(i) of this section, a certification in the following form:

> In the opinion and to the best knowledge of (name of applicant), there are no patents that claim the drug or drugs on which investigations that are relied upon in this 505(b)(2) application were conducted or that claim a use of such drug or drugs.

(iii) *Method-of-use patent.* (A) If information that is submitted under section 505(b) or (c) of the Federal Food, Drug, and Cosmetic Act and § 314.53 is for a method-of-use patent, and the labeling for the drug product for which the applicant is seeking approval does not include an indication or other condition of use that is covered by the method-of-use patent, a statement explaining that the method-of-use patent does not claim a proposed indication or other condition of use.

(B) If the labeling of the drug product for which the applicant is seeking approval includes an indication or other condition of use that, according to the patent information submitted under section 505(b) or (c) of the Federal Food, Drug, and Cosmetic Act and § 314.53 or in the opinion of the applicant, is claimed by a method-of-use patent, the applicant must submit an applicable certification under paragraph (i)(1)(i) of this section.

(2) [Reserved]

(3) *Licensing agreements.* If a 505(b)(2) application is submitted for a drug or method of using a drug claimed by a patent and the applicant has a licensing agreement with the patent owner, the applicant must submit a paragraph IV certification as to that patent and a statement that the applicant has been granted a patent license. If the patent owner consents to approval of the 505(b)(2) application (if otherwise eligible for approval) as of a specific date, the 505(b)(2) application must contain a written statement from the patent owner that it has a licensing agreement with the applicant and that it consents to approval of the 505(b)(2) application as of a specific date.

(4) *Untimely filing of patent information.* (i) If a patent described in paragraph (i)(1)(i)(A) of this section is issued and the holder of the approved NDA for the patented drug does not file with FDA the required information on the patent within 30 days of issuance of the patent, an applicant who submitted a 505(b)(2) application that, before the submission of the patent information, contained an appropriate patent certification or statement is not required to submit a patent certification or statement to address the patent or patent information that is late-listed with respect to the pending 505(b)(2) application. Except as provided in § 314.53(f)(1), an NDA holder's amendment to the description of the approved method(s) of use claimed by the patent will be considered untimely filing of patent information unless:

(A) The amendment to the description of the approved method(s) of use claimed by the patent is submitted within 30 days of patent issuance;

(B) The amendment to the description of the approved method(s) of use claimed by the patent is submitted within 30 days of approval of a corresponding change to product labeling; or

(C) The amendment to the description of the approved method(s) of use claimed by the patent is submitted within 30 days of a decision by the U.S. Patent and Trademark Office or by a Federal district court, the Court of Appeals for the Federal Circuit, or the U.S. Supreme Court that is specific to the patent and alters the construction of a method-of-use claim(s) of the patent, and the amendment contains a copy of the decision.

(ii) An applicant whose 505(b)(2) application is submitted after the NDA holder's untimely filing of patent information or whose 505(b)(2) application was previously filed but did not contain an appropriate patent certification or statement at the time of the patent submission must submit a certification under paragraph (i)(1)(i) of this section and/or a statement under paragraph (i)(1)(iii) of this section as to that patent.

(5) *Disputed patent information.* If an applicant disputes the accuracy or relevance of patent information submitted to FDA, the applicant may seek a confirmation of the correctness of the patent information in accordance with the procedures under § 314.53(f). Unless the patent information is withdrawn, the applicant must submit an appropriate certification or statement for each listed patent.

(6) *Amended certifications.* A patent certification or statement submitted under paragraphs (i)(1)(i) through (iii) of this section may be amended at any time before the approval of the 505(b)(2) application. An applicant must submit an amended certification as an amendment to a pending 505(b)(2) application. If an applicant with a pending 505(b)(2) application voluntarily makes a patent certification for an untimely filed patent, the applicant may withdraw the patent certification for the untimely filed patent. Once an amendment is submitted to change the certification, the 505(b)(2) application will no longer be considered to contain the prior certification.

(i) *After finding of infringement.* An applicant who has submitted a paragraph IV certification and is sued for patent infringement must submit an amendment to change its certification if a court enters a final decision from which no appeal has been or can be taken, or signs and enters a settlement order or consent decree in the action that includes a finding that the patent is infringed, unless the final decision, settlement order, or consent decree also finds the patent to be invalid. In its amendment, the applicant must certify under paragraph (i)(1)(i)(A)(3) of this section that the patent will expire on a specific date or, with respect to a patent claiming a method of use, the applicant may instead provide a statement under paragraph (i)(1)(iii) of this section if the applicant amends its 505(b)(2) application such that the applicant is no longer seeking approval for a method of use claimed by the patent. Once an amendment for the change has been submitted, the 505(b)(2) application will no longer be considered to contain a paragraph IV certification to the patent. If a final decision finds the patent to be invalid and infringed, an amended certification is not required.

(ii) *After request to remove a patent or patent information from the list.* If the list reflects that an NDA holder has requested that a patent or patent information be removed from the list and no ANDA applicant is eligible for 180-day exclusivity based on a paragraph IV certification to that patent, the patent or patent information will be removed and any applicant with a pending 505(b)(2) application (including a tentatively approved 505(b)(2) application) who has made a certification with respect to such patent must submit an amendment to withdraw its certification. In the amendment, the applicant must state the reason for withdrawing the certification or statement (that the patent has been removed from the list). If the list reflects that an NDA holder has requested that a patent or patent information be removed from the list and one or more first applicants are eligible for 180-day exclusivity based on a paragraph IV certification to that patent, the patent will remain listed until any 180-day exclusivity based on that patent has expired or has been extinguished. A 505(b)(2) applicant is not required to provide or maintain a certification to a patent or patent information that remains listed only for purposes of a first applicant's 180-day exclusivity for its ANDA. Once an amendment to withdraw the certification has been submitted, the 505(b)(2) application will no longer be considered to contain a paragraph IV certification to the patent. If removal of a patent from the list results in there being no patents listed for the listed drug(s) identified in the 505(b)(2) application, the applicant must submit an amended certification reflecting that there are no listed patents.

(iii) *Other amendments.* (A) Except as provided in paragraphs (i)(4) and (i)(6)(iii)(B) of this section:

(1) An applicant must amend a submitted certification or statement if, at any time before the approval of the 505(b)(2) application, the applicant learns that the submitted certification or statement is no longer accurate; and

(2) An applicant must submit an appropriate patent certification or statement under paragraph (i)(1) of this section if, after submission of the 505(b)(2) application, a new patent is issued by the U.S. Patent and Trademark Office that, in the opinion of the applicant and to the best of its knowledge, claims a listed drug relied upon or that claims an approved use for such listed drug for which information is required to be filed under section 505(b) and (c) of the Federal Food, Drug, and Cosmetic Act and § 314.53.

(B) An applicant is not required to submit a supplement to change a submitted certification when information on an otherwise applicable patent is submitted after the approval of the 505(b)(2) application.

(j) *Claimed exclusivity.* A new drug product, upon approval, may be entitled to a period of marketing exclusivity under the provisions of § 314.108. If an applicant believes its drug product is entitled to a period of exclusivity, it must submit with the NDA prior to approval the following information:

(1) A statement that the applicant is claiming exclusivity.

(2) A reference to the appropriate paragraph under § 314.108 that supports its claim.

(3) If the applicant claims exclusivity under § 314.108(b)(2), information to show that, to the best of its knowledge or belief, a drug has not previously been approved under section 505(b) of the Federal Food, Drug, and Cosmetic Act containing any active moiety in the drug for which the applicant is seeking approval.

(4) If the applicant claims exclusivity under § 314.108(b)(4) or (b)(5), the following information to show that the NDA contains "new clinical investigations" that are "essential to approval of the NDA or supplement" and were "conducted or sponsored by the applicant:"

(i) *"New clinical investigations."* A certification that to the best of the applicant's knowledge each of the clinical investigations included in the NDA meets the definition of "new clinical investigation" set forth in § 314.108(a).

(ii) *"Essential to approval."* A list of all published studies or publicly available reports of clinical investigations known to the applicant through a literature search that are relevant to the conditions for which the applicant is seeking approval, a certification that the applicant has thoroughly searched the scientific literature and, to the best of the applicant's knowledge, the list is complete and accurate and, in the applicant's opinion, such published studies or publicly available reports do not provide a sufficient basis for the approval of the conditions for which the applicant is seeking approval without reference to the new clinical investigation(s) in the NDA, and an explanation as to why the studies or reports are insufficient.

(iii) *"Conducted or sponsored by."* If the applicant was the sponsor named in the Form FDA 1571 for an IND under which the new clinical investigation(s) that is essential to the approval of its NDA was conducted, identification of the IND by number. If the applicant was not the sponsor of the IND under which the clinical investigation(s) was conducted, a certification that the applicant or its predecessor in interest provided substantial support for the clinical investigation(s) that is essential to the approval of its NDA, and information supporting the certification.To demonstrate "substantial support," an applicant must either provide a certified statement from a certified public accountant that the applicant provided 50 percent or more of the cost of conducting the study or provide an explanation of why FDA should consider the applicant to have conducted or sponsored the study if the applicant's financial contribution to the study is less than 50 percent or the applicant did not sponsor the investigational new drug. A predecessor in interest is an entity, e.g., a corporation, that the applicant has taken over, merged with, or purchased, or from which the applicant has purchased all rights to the drug. Purchase of nonexclusive rights to a clinical investigation after it is completed is not sufficient to satisfy this definition.

(k) *Financial certification or disclosure statement.* The NDA must contain a financial certification or disclosure statement or both as required by part 54 of this chapter.

(l) *Format of an original NDA*—(1) *Archival copy.* The applicant must submit a complete archival copy of the NDA that contains the information required under paragraphs (a) through (f) of this section. FDA will maintain the archival copy during the review of the NDA to permit individual reviewers to refer to information that is not contained in their particular technical sections of the NDA, to give other agency personnel access to the NDA for official business, and to maintain in one place a complete copy of the NDA. Except as required by paragraph (l)(1)(i) of this section, applicants may submit the archival copy on paper or in electronic format provided that electronic submissions are made in accordance with part 11 of this chapter.

(i) *Labeling.* The content of labeling required under § 201.100(d)(3) of this chapter (commonly referred to as the package insert or professional labeling), including all text, tables, and figures, must be submitted to the agency in electronic format as described in paragraph (l)(5) of this section. This requirement is in addition to the requirements of paragraph (e)(2)(ii) of this section that copies of the formatted label and all labeling be submitted. Submissions under this paragraph must be made in accordance with part 11 of this chapter, except for the requirements of § 11.10(a), (c) through (h), and (k), and the corresponding requirements of § 11.30.

(ii) [Reserved]

(2) *Review copy.* The applicant must submit a review copy of the NDA. Each of the technical sections, described in paragraphs (d)(1) through (6) of this section, in the review copy is required to be separately bound with a copy of the application form required under paragraph (a) of this section and a copy of the summary required under paragraph (c) of this section.

(3) *Field copy.* The applicant must submit a field copy of the NDA that contains the technical section described in paragraph (d)(1) of this section, a copy of the application form required under paragraph (a) of this section, a copy of the summary required under paragraph (c) of this section, and a certification that the field copy is a true copy of the technical section described in paragraph (d)(1) of this section contained in the archival and review copies of the NDA.

(4) *Binding folders.* The applicant may obtain from FDA sufficient folders to bind the archival, the review, and the field copies of the NDA.

(5) *Electronic format submissions.* Electronic format submissions must be in a form that FDA can process, review, and archive. FDA will periodically issue guidance on how to provide the electronic submission (e.g., method of transmission, media, file formats, preparation and organization of files).

[50 FR 7493, Feb. 22, 1985]

Editorial note: For Federal Register citations affecting § 314.50, see the List of CFR Sections Affected, which appears in the Finding Aids section of the printed volume and at *www.fdsys.gov*.

§ 314.52 Notice of certification of invalidity, unenforceability, or noninfringement of a patent.

(a) Notice of certification. For each patent that claims the listed drug or drugs relied upon or that claims a use for such listed drug or drugs and for which the 505(b)(2) applicant submits a paragraph IV certification, the applicant must send notice of such certification by registered or certified mail, return receipt requested, or by a designated delivery service, as defined in paragraph (g) of this section, to each of the following persons:

(1) Each owner of the patent that is the subject of the certification or the representative designated by the owner to receive the notice. The name and address of the patent owner or its representative may be obtained from the U.S. Patent and Trademark Office; and

(2) The holder of the approved NDA under section 505(b) of the Federal Food, Drug, and Cosmetic Act for each drug product which is claimed by the patent or a use of which is claimed by the patent and for which the applicant is seeking approval, or, if the NDA holder does not reside or maintain a place of business within the United States, the NDA holder's attorney, agent, or other authorized official. The name and address of the NDA holder or its attorney, agent, or authorized official may be obtained by sending a written or electronic communication to the Orange Book Staff, Office of Generic Drugs, 7620 Standish Pl., Rockville, MD 20855, or to the Orange Book Staff at the email address listed on the Agency's Web site at *http://www.fda.gov.*

(3) This paragraph (a) does not apply to a method-of-use patent that does not claim a use for which the applicant is seeking approval.

(4) An applicant may send notice by an alternative method only if FDA has agreed in advance that the method will produce an acceptable form of documentation.

(b) *Sending the notice.* (1) Except as provided under paragraph (d) of this section, the applicant must send the notice required by paragraph (a) of this section on or after the date of filing described in § 314.101(a)(2) or (3), as applicable, but not later than 20 days after the date of the postmark on the paragraph IV acknowledgment letter. The 20-day clock described in this paragraph (b) begins on the day after the date of the postmark on the paragraph IV acknowledgment letter. When the 20th day falls on Saturday, Sunday, or a Federal holiday, the 20th day will be the next day that is not a Saturday, Sunday, or Federal holiday.

(2) Any notice required by paragraph (a) of this section is invalid if it is sent before the date of filing described in § 314.101(a)(2) or, if FDA notifies the applicant that FDA has refused to file the 505(b)(2) application, before the date described in § 314.101(a)(3) on which the 505(b)(2) application is filed. The applicant will not have complied with this paragraph (b) until it sends valid notice.

(3) The applicant must submit to FDA an amendment to its 505(b)(2) application that includes a statement certifying that the notice has been provided to each person identified under paragraph (a) of this section and that the notice met the content requirement under paragraph (c) of this section. A copy of the notice itself need not be submitted to the Agency.

(c) *Content of a notice.* In the notice, the applicant must cite section 505(b)(3)(D) of the Federal Food, Drug, and Cosmetic Act and the notice must include, but is not limited to, the following information:

(1) A statement that a 505(b)(2) application that contains any required bioavailability or bioequivalence studies has been submitted by the applicant and filed by FDA.

(2) The NDA number.

(3) The established name, if any, as defined in section 502(e)(3) of the Federal Food, Drug, and Cosmetic Act, of the proposed drug product.

(4) The active ingredient, strength, and dosage form of the proposed drug product.

(5) The patent number and expiration date of each patent on the list alleged to be invalid, unenforceable, or not infringed.

(6) A detailed statement of the factual and legal basis of the applicant's opinion that the patent is not valid, unenforceable, or will not be infringed. The applicant must include in the detailed statement:

(i) For each claim of a patent alleged not to be infringed, a full and detailed explanation of why the claim is not infringed.

(ii) For each claim of a patent alleged to be invalid or unenforceable, a full and detailed explanation of the grounds supporting the allegation.

(7) If the applicant alleges that the patent will not be infringed and the applicant seeks to preserve the option to later file a civil action for declaratory judgment in accordance with section 505(c)(3)(D) of the Federal Food, Drug, and Cosmetic Act, then the notice must be accompanied by an offer of confidential access to the 505(b)(2) application for the sole and limited purpose of evaluating possible infringement of the patent that is the subject of the paragraph IV certification.

(8) If the applicant does not reside or have a place of business in the United States, the name and address of an agent in the United States authorized to accept service of process for the applicant.

(d) *Amendment or supplement to a 505(b)(2) application.* (1) If, after the date of filing described in §314.101(a)(2) or (3), as applicable, an applicant submits an amendment or supplement to its 505(b)(2) application that includes a paragraph IV certification, the applicant must send the notice required by paragraph (a) of this section at the same time that the amendment or supplement to the 505(b)(2) application is submitted to FDA, regardless of whether the applicant has already given notice with respect to another such certification contained in the 505(b)(2) application or in an amendment or supplement to the 505(b)(2) application.

(2) If, before the date of filing described in §314.101(a)(2) or (3), as applicable, an applicant submits a paragraph IV certification in an amendment, the applicant must send the notice required by paragraph (a) of this section in accordance with the procedures in paragraph (b) of this section.

(3) An applicant that submits an amendment or supplement to seek approval of a different strength must provide notice of any paragraph IV certification in accordance with paragraph (d)(1) or (2) of this section, as applicable.

(e) *Documentation of timely sending and receipt of notice.* The applicant must amend its 505(b)(2) application to provide documentation of the date of receipt of the notice required under paragraph (a) of this section by each person provided the notice. The amendment must be submitted to FDA within 30 days after the last date on which notice was received by a person described in paragraph (a) of this section. The applicant's amendment also must include documentation that its notice was sent on a date that complies with the timeframe required by paragraph (b) or (d) of this section, as applicable. FDA will accept, as adequate documentation of the date the notice was sent, a copy of the registered mail receipt, certified mail receipt, or receipt from a designated delivery service, as defined in paragraph (g) of this section. FDA will accept as adequate documentation of the date of receipt a return receipt, a signature proof of delivery by a designated delivery service, or a letter acknowledging receipt by the person provided the notice. An applicant may rely on another form of documentation only if FDA has agreed to such documentation in advance. A copy of the notice itself need not be submitted to the Agency.

(f) *Forty-five day period after receipt of notice.* If the requirements of this section are met, the Agency will presume the notice to be complete and sufficient and will count the day following the date of receipt of the notice by the patent owner or its representative and by the approved NDA holder or its attorney, agent, or other authorized official as the first day of the 45-day period provided for in section 505(c)(3)(C) of the Federal Food, Drug, and Cosmetic Act. FDA may, if the applicant amends its 505(b)(2) application with a written statement that a later date should be used, count from such later date.

(g) *Designated delivery services.* (1) For purposes of this section, the term "designated delivery service" is any delivery service provided by a trade or business that the Agency determines:

(i) Is available to the general public throughout the United States;

(ii) Records electronically to its database, kept in the regular course of its business, or marks on the cover in which any item referred to in this section is to be delivered, the date on which such item was given to such trade or business for delivery; and

(iii) Provides overnight or 2-day delivery service throughout the United States.

(2) FDA may periodically issue guidance regarding designated delivery services.

[81 FR 69641, Oct. 6, 2016]

§ 314.53 Submission of patent information.

(a) *Who must submit patent information.* This section applies to any applicant who submits to FDA an NDA or an amendment to it under section 505(b) of the Federal Food, Drug, and Cosmetic Act and § 314.50 or a supplement to an approved NDA under § 314.70, except as provided in paragraph (d)(2) of this section.

(b) *Patents for which information must be submitted and patents for which information must not be submitted—*(1) *General requirements.* An applicant described in paragraph (a) of this section must submit to its NDA the required information, on the required FDA declaration form, set forth in paragraph (c) of this section for each patent that claims the drug or a method of using the drug that is the subject of the NDA or amendment or supplement to it and with respect to which a claim of patent infringement could reasonably be asserted if a person not licensed by the owner of the patent engaged in the manufacture, use, or sale of the drug product. For purposes of this part, such patents consist of drug substance (active ingredient) patents, drug product (formulation and composition) patents, and method-of-use patents. For patents that claim the drug substance, the applicant must submit information only on those patents that claim the drug substance that is the subject of the pending or approved NDA or that claim a drug substance that is the same as the active ingredient that is the subject of the approved or pending NDA. For patents that claim only a polymorph that is the same as the active ingredient described in the approved or pending NDA, the applicant must certify in the required FDA declaration form that the applicant has test data, as set forth in paragraph (b)(2) of this section, demonstrating that a drug product containing the polymorph will perform the same as the drug product described in the NDA. For patents that claim a drug product, the applicant must submit information only on those patents that claim the drug product, as is defined in § 314.3, that is described in the pending or approved NDA. For patents that claim a method of use, the applicant must submit information only on those patents that claim indications or other conditions of use for which approval is sought or has been granted in the NDA. The applicant must separately identify each pending or approved method of use and related patent claim(s). For approved NDAs, the NDA holder's description of the patented method of use required by paragraph (c)(2)(ii)(P)(3) of this section must describe only the approved method(s) of use claimed by the patent for which a claim of patent infringement could reasonably be asserted if a person not licensed by the owner of the patent engaged in the manufacture, use, or sale of the drug product. If the method(s) of use claimed by the patent does not cover an indication or other approved condition of use in its entirety, the applicant must describe only the specific approved method of use claimed by the patent for which a claim of patent infringement could reasonably be asserted if a person not licensed by the owner of the patent engaged in the manufacture, use, or sale of the drug product. For approved NDAs, the NDA holder submitting information on the method-of-use patent must identify with specificity the section(s) and subsection(s) of the approved labeling that describes the method(s) of use claimed by the patent submitted. Process patents, patents claiming packaging, patents claiming metabolites, and patents claiming intermediates are not covered by this section, and information on these patents must not be submitted to FDA.

(2) *Test data for submission of patent information for patents that claim only a polymorph.* The test data, referenced in paragraph (b)(1) of this section, must include the following:

(i) A full description of the polymorphic form of the drug substance, including its physical and chemical characteristics and stability; the method of synthesis (or isolation) and purification of the drug substance; the process controls used during manufacture and packaging; and such specifications and analytical methods as are necessary to assure the identity, strength, quality, and purity of the polymorphic form of the drug substance;

(ii) The executed batch record for a drug product containing the polymorphic form of the drug substance and documentation that the batch was manufactured under current good manufacturing practice requirements;

(iii) Demonstration of bioequivalence between the executed batch of the drug product that contains the polymorphic form of the drug substance and the drug product as described in the NDA;

(iv) A list of all components used in the manufacture of the drug product containing the polymorphic form and a statement of the composition of the drug product; a statement of the specifications and analytical methods for each component; a description of the manufacturing and packaging procedures and in-process controls for the drug product; such specifications and analytical methods as are necessary to assure the identity, strength, quality, purity, and bioavailability of the drug product, including release and stability data complying with the approved product specifications to demonstrate pharmaceutical equivalence and comparable product stability; and

(v) Comparative in vitro dissolution testing on 12 dosage units each of the executed test batch and the NDA product.

(c) *Reporting requirements*—(1) *General requirements.* An applicant described in paragraph (a) of this section must submit the required patent information described in paragraph (c)(2) of this section for each patent that meets the requirements described in paragraph (b) of this section. We will not accept the patent information unless it is submitted on the appropriate form, Form FDA 3542 or 3542a, and contains the information required in paragraph (c)(2) of this section. These forms may be obtained on the Internet at *http://www.fda.gov* by searching for "forms".

(2) *Drug substance (active ingredient), drug product (formulation or composition), and method-of-use patents*—(i) *Original declaration.* For each patent that claims a drug substance (active ingredient), drug product (formulation and composition), or method of use, the applicant must submit Form FDA 3542a. The following information and verification is required, subject to the exceptions listed in paragraph (c)(2)(i)(S) of this section:

(A) NDA number;

(B) The NDA applicant's name, full address, phone number and, if available, fax number and email address;

(C) Trade name (or proposed trade name) of new drug;

(D) Active ingredient(s) of new drug;

(E) Strength(s) of new drug;

(F) Dosage form(s) and route(s) of administration of new drug, and whether the applicant proposes to market the new drug for prescription use or over-the-counter use;

(G) U.S. patent number, issue date, and expiration date of patent submitted;

(H) The patent owner's name, full address, phone number and, if available, fax number and email address;

(I) The name, full address, phone number and, if available, fax number and email address of an agent or representative who resides or maintains a place of business within the United States authorized to receive notice of patent certification under section 505(b)(3) and (j)(2)(B) of the Federal Food, Drug, and Cosmetic Act and §§ 314.52 and 314.95 (if patent owner or NDA applicant or holder does not reside or have a place of business within the United States);

(J) Information on whether the patent has been submitted previously for the NDA or supplement;

(K) If the patent has been submitted previously for listing, identify all change(s) from the previously submitted patent information and specify whether the change is related to the patent or related to an FDA action or procedure;

(L) Information on whether the patent is a product-by-process patent in which the product claimed is novel;

(M) Information on the drug substance (active ingredient) patent, including the following:

(1) Whether the patent claims a drug substance that is an active ingredient in the drug product described in the NDA or supplement;

(2) Whether the patent claims only a polymorph that is the same active ingredient that is described in the pending NDA or supplement;

(3) Whether the applicant has test data, described in paragraph (b)(2) of this section, demonstrating that a drug product containing only the polymorph will perform the same as the drug product described in the NDA or supplement, and a description of the polymorphic form(s) claimed by the patent for which such test data exist;

(4) Whether the patent claims only a metabolite of the active ingredient; and

(5) Whether the patent claims only an intermediate;

(N) Information on the drug product (composition/formulation) patent, including the following:

(1) Whether the patent claims the drug product for which approval is being sought, as defined in § 314.3; and

(2) Whether the patent claims only an intermediate;

(O) Information on each method-of-use patent, including the following:

(1) Whether the patent claims one or more methods of using the drug product for which approval is being sought and a description of each pending method of use and related patent claim of the patent being submitted;

(2) Identification of the specific section(s) and subsection(s) of the proposed labeling for the drug product that describes the method of use claimed by the patent submitted; and

(3) An applicant that submits information for a patent that claims one or more methods of using the drug product must also submit information described in either paragraph (c)(2)(i)(M) or (N) of this section, regarding whether that patent also claims either the drug substance (active ingredient) or the drug product (composition/formulation).

(P) Whether there are no relevant patents that claim the drug substance (active ingredient), drug product (formulation or composition), or method(s) of use, for which the applicant is seeking approval and with respect to which a claim of patent infringement could reasonably be asserted if a person not licensed by the owner of the patent engaged in the manufacture, use, or sale of the drug product;

(Q) A signed verification that states:

The undersigned declares that this is an accurate and complete submission of patent information for the NDA, amendment, or supplement pending under section 505 of the Federal Food, Drug, and Cosmetic Act. This time-sensitive patent information is submitted pursuant to 21 CFR 314.53. I attest that I am familiar with 21 CFR 314.53 and this submission complies with the requirements of the regulation. I verify under penalty of perjury that the foregoing is true and correct.

(R) Information on whether the applicant, patent owner or attorney, agent, representative, or other authorized official signed the form; the name of the person; and the full address, phone number and, if available, the fax number and email address; and

(S) Exceptions to required submission of patent information:

(1) If an applicant submits the information described in paragraph (c)(2)(i)(M) of this section for a patent that claims the drug substance (active ingredient) and meets the requirements for listing on that basis, then the applicant is not required to provide the information described in paragraph (c)

(2)(i)(N) of this section on whether that patent also claims the drug product (composition/formulation);

(2) If an applicant submits the information described in paragraph (c)(2)(i)(N) of this section for a patent that claims the drug product (composition/formulation) and meets the requirements for listing on that basis, then the applicant is not required to provide the information described in paragraph (c)(2)(i)(M) of this section on whether that patent also claims the drug substance (active ingredient);

(3) If the applicant submits a supplement for a change other than one of the changes listed under paragraph (d)(2)(i) of this section, then the patent information submission requirements of paragraph (d)(2)(ii) of this section apply.

(ii) *Submission of patent information upon and after approval.* Within 30 days after the date of approval of its NDA or supplement, the applicant must submit Form FDA 3542 for each patent that claims the drug substance (active ingredient), drug product (formulation and composition), or approved method of use. FDA will not list or publish patent information if it is not provided on this form or if the patent declaration does not contain the required information or indicates the patent is not eligible for listing. Patent information must also be submitted for patents issued after the date of approval of the NDA as required in paragraph (c)(2)(ii) of this section. As described in paragraph (d)(3) of this section, to be timely filed, patent information for patents issued after the date of approval of the NDA must be submitted to FDA within 30 days of the date of issuance of the patent. If the applicant submits the required patent information within the 30 days, but we notify an applicant that a declaration form is incomplete or shows that the patent is not eligible for listing, the applicant must submit an acceptable declaration form within 15 days of FDA notification to be considered timely filed. The following information and verification statement is required, subject to the exceptions listed in paragraph (c)(2)(ii)(T) of this section:

(A) NDA number;

(B) The NDA holder's name, full address, phone number and, if available, fax number and email address;

(C) Trade name of new drug;

(D) Active ingredient(s) of new drug;

(E) Strength(s) of new drug;

(F) Dosage form(s) and route(s) of administration of new drug, and whether the new drug is approved for prescription use or over-the-counter use;

(G) Approval date of NDA or supplement;

(H) U.S. patent number, issue date, and expiration date of patent submitted;

(I) The patent owner's name, full address, phone number and, if available, fax number and email address;

(J) The name, full address, phone number and, if available, fax number and email address of an agent or representative who resides or maintains a place of business within the United States authorized to receive notice of patent certification under section 505(b)(3) and (j)(2)(B) of the Federal Food, Drug, and Cosmetic Act and §§ 314.52 and 314.95 (if patent owner or NDA applicant or holder does not reside or have a place of business within the United States);

(K) Information on whether the patent has been submitted previously for the NDA or supplement;

(L) If the patent has been submitted previously for listing, identify all change(s) from the previously submitted patent information and specify whether the change is related to the patent or related to an FDA action or procedure;

(M) Information on whether the patent is a product-by-process patent in which the product claimed is novel;

(N) Information on the drug substance (active ingredient) patent, including the following:

(1) Whether the patent claims a drug substance that is an active ingredient in the drug product described in the approved NDA;

(2) Whether the patent claims only a polymorph that is the same as the active ingredient that is described in the approved NDA;

(3) Whether the applicant has test data, described in paragraph (b)(2) of this section, demonstrating that a drug product containing only the polymorph will perform the same as the drug product described in the approved NDA and a description of the polymorphic form(s) claimed by the patent for which such test data exist;

(4) Whether the patent claims only a metabolite of the active ingredient; and

(5) Whether the patent claims only an intermediate;

(O) Information on the drug product (composition/formulation) patent, including the following:

(1) Whether the patent claims the approved drug product as defined in § 314.3; and

(2) Whether the patent claims only an intermediate;

(P) Information on each method-of-use patent, including the following:

(1) Whether the patent claims one or more approved methods of using the approved drug product and a description of each approved method of use and related patent claim of the patent being submitted;

(2) Identification of the specific section(s) and subsection(s) of the approved labeling for the drug product that describes the method of use claimed by the patent submitted;

(3) The description of the patented method of use as required for publication, which must contain adequate information to assist 505(b)(2) and ANDA applicants in determining whether a listed method-of-use patent claims a use for which the 505(b)(2) or ANDA applicant is not seeking approval (for example, if the method(s) of use claimed by the patent does not cover an indication or other approved condition of use in its entirety, then the applicant must describe only the specific approved method of use claimed by the patent for which a claim of patent infringement could reasonably be asserted if a person not licensed by the owner of the patent engaged in the manufacture, use, or sale of the drug product); and

(4) An applicant that submits information for a patent that claims one or more methods of using the drug product must also submit information described in either paragraph (c)(2)(ii)(N) or (O) of this section, regarding whether that patent also claims either the drug substance (active ingredient) or the drug product (composition/formulation).

(Q) Whether there are no relevant patents that claim the approved drug substance (active ingredient), the approved drug product (formulation or composition), or approved method(s) of use and with respect to which a claim of patent infringement could reasonably be asserted if a person not licensed by the owner of the patent engaged in the manufacture, use, or sale of the drug product;

(R) A signed verification that states:

The undersigned declares that this is an accurate and complete submission of patent information for the NDA, amendment, or supplement approved under section 505 of the Federal Food, Drug, and Cosmetic Act. This time-sensitive patent information or response to a request under 21 CFR 314.53(f)(1) is submitted pursuant to 21 CFR 314.53. I attest that I am familiar with 21 CFR 314.53 and this submission complies with the requirements of the regulation. I verify under penalty of perjury that the foregoing is true and correct.

(S) Information on whether the applicant, patent owner or attorney, agent, representative, or other authorized official signed the form; the name of the person; and the full address, phone number and, if available, the fax number and email address; and

(T) Exceptions to required submission of patent information:

(1) If an applicant submits the information described in paragraph (c)(2)(ii)(N) of this section for a patent that claims the drug substance (active ingredient) and meets the requirements for listing on that basis, then the applicant is not required to provide the information described in paragraph (c)(2)(ii)(O) of this section on whether that patent also claims the drug product (composition/formulation).

(2) If an applicant submits the information described in paragraph (c)(2)(ii)(O) of this section for a patent that claims the drug product (composition/formulation) and meets the requirements for listing on that basis, then the applicant is not required to provide the information described in paragraph (c)(2)(ii)(N) of this section on whether that patent also claims the drug substance (active ingredient).

(3) If the applicant submits a supplement for a change other than one of the changes listed under paragraph (d)(2)(i) of this section, then the patent information submission requirements of paragraph (d)(2)(ii) of this section apply.

(3) *No relevant patents.* If the applicant believes that there are no relevant patents that claim the drug substance (active ingredient), drug product (formulation or composition), or the method(s) of use for which the applicant has received approval, and with respect to which a claim of patent infringement could reasonably be asserted if a person not licensed by the owner of the patent engaged in the manufacture, use, or sale of the drug product, the applicant will verify this information in the appropriate form, Form FDA 3542 or 3542a.

(4) *Authorized signature.* The declarations required by this section must be signed by the applicant or patent owner, or the applicant's or patent owner's attorney, agent (representative), or other authorized official.

(d) *When and where to submit patent information*—(1) *Original NDA.* An applicant must submit with its original NDA submitted under this part, the information described in paragraph (c) of this section on each drug substance (active ingredient), drug product (formulation and composition), and method-of-use patent issued before the NDA is filed with FDA and for which patent information is required to be submitted under this section. If a patent is issued after the NDA is filed with FDA but before the NDA is approved, the applicant must, within 30 days of the date of issuance of the patent, submit the required patent information in an amendment to the NDA under § 314.60.

(2) *Supplements.* (i) An applicant must submit patent information required under paragraph (c) of this section for a patent that claims the drug substance, drug product, or method of use for which approval is sought in any of the following supplements:

(A) To add or change the dosage form or route of administration;

(B) To add or change the strength; or

(C) To change the drug product from prescription use to over-the-counter use.

(ii) If the applicant submits a supplement for a change other than one of the changes listed under paragraph (d)(2)(i) of this section (for example, to change the formulation, to add a new indication or other condition of use, or to make any other patented change regarding the drug substance, drug product, or any method of use), the following patent information submission requirements apply:

(A) If existing patents for which information required by paragraph (c) of this section has already been submitted to FDA for the product approved in the original NDA claim the changed product, the applicant is not required to resubmit this patent information pursuant to paragraph (c) of this section unless the published description of the patented method of use would change upon approval of the supplement, and FDA will continue to list this patent information for the product;

(B) If one or more existing patents for which information has already been submitted to FDA no longer claim the changed product, the applicant must submit a request under paragraph (f)(2)(iv) of this section to remove that patent information from the list at the time of approval of the supplement;

(C) If one or more existing drug substance (active ingredient), drug product (formulation and composition), or method-of-use patents claim the changed product for which approval is sought in the supplement and such patent information has not been submitted to FDA, the applicant must submit the patent information required under paragraph (c) of this section.

(3) *Newly issued patents.* If a patent is issued for a drug substance, drug product, or method of use after an NDA is approved, the applicant must submit to FDA, as described in paragraph (d)(4) of this section, the required patent information within 30 days of the date of issuance of the patent. If the required patent information is not submitted within 30 days of the issuance of the patent, FDA will list the patent, but patent certifications or statements will be governed by the provisions regarding untimely filed patent information at §§ 314.50(i)(4) and (6) and 314.94(a)(12)(vi) and (viii).

(4) *Submission of Forms FDA 3542a and 3542—*(i) *Patent information submitted with the filing of an NDA, amendment, or supplement.* The applicant must submit patent information required by paragraphs (c)(1) and (c)(2)(i) of this section and § 314.50(h) or § 314.70(f) on Form FDA 3542a to the Central Document Room, Center for Drug Evaluation and Research, Food and Drug Administration, 5901-B Ammendale Rd., Beltsville, MD 20705-1266, or to FDA in an electronic format submission that complies with § 314.50(l)(5). Form FDA 3542a should not be submitted to the Orange Book Staff in the Office of Generic Drugs.

(ii) *Patent information submitted upon and after approval of an NDA or supplement.* The applicant must submit patent information required by paragraphs (c)(1) and (c)(2)(ii) of this section on Form FDA 3542 to the Central Document Room, Center for Drug Evaluation and Research, Food and Drug Administration, 5901-B Ammendale Rd., Beltsville, MD 20705-1266, or to FDA in an electronic format submission that complies with § 314.50(l)(5). Form FDA 3542 should not be submitted to the Orange Book Staff in the Office of Generic Drugs.

(5) *Submission date.* Patent information will be considered to be submitted to FDA for purposes of paragraph (d)(3) of this section as of the earlier of the date the information submitted on Form FDA 3542 is date-stamped by the Central Document Room, or officially received by FDA in an electronic format submission that complies with § 314.50(l)(5).

(6) *Identification.* Each submission of patent information, except information submitted with an original NDA, must bear prominent identification as to its contents, i.e., "Patent Information," or, if submitted after approval of an NDA, "Time Sensitive Patent Information."

(e) *Public disclosure of patent information.* FDA will publish in the list the patent number and expiration date of each patent that is required to be, and is, submitted to FDA by an applicant, and for each method-of-use patent, the description of the method of use claimed by the patent as required by § 314.53(c)(2)(ii)(P)(3). FDA will publish such patent information upon approval of the NDA, or, if the patent information is submitted by the applicant after approval of an NDA as provided under paragraph (d)(2) of this section, as soon as possible after the submission to the Agency of the patent information. A request for copies of the submitted patent information must be sent in writing to the Freedom of Information Staff at the address listed on the Agency's Web site at *http://www.fda.gov.* The submitted patent information, and requests to remove a patent or patent information from the list, may be subject to public disclosure.

(f) *Correction of patent information errors—*(1) *Requests by persons other than the NDA holder.* If any person disputes the accuracy or relevance of patent information submitted to the Agency under this section and published by FDA in the list, or believes that an NDA holder has failed to submit required patent information, that person must first notify the Agency in a written or electronic communication titled "314.53(f) Patent Listing Dispute." The patent listing dispute communication must include a statement of dispute that describes the specific grounds for disagreement regarding the accuracy or relevance of patent information for FDA to send to the applicable NDA holder. For a dispute regarding the accuracy or relevance of patent information regarding an approved method of using the drug product, this statement of dispute must be only a narrative description (no more than 250 words) of the person's interpretation of the scope of the patent. This statement of dispute must only contain information for which the person consents to disclosure because FDA will send the text of the statement to the applicable NDA holder without review or redaction. The patent listing dispute communication should be directed to the Office of Generic Drugs, OGD Document Room, Attention: Orange Book Staff, 7620 Standish Pl., Rockville, MD 20855, or to the Orange Book Staff at the email address listed on the Agency's Web site at *http://www.fda.gov.*

(i) *Communication with the NDA holder*—(A) *Drug substance or drug product claim.* For requests submitted under this paragraph (f)(1) that are directed to the accuracy or relevance of submitted patent information regarding a drug substance or drug product claim, the Agency will send the statement of dispute to the applicable NDA holder. The NDA holder must confirm the correctness of the patent information and include the signed verification required by paragraph (c)(2)(ii)(R) of this section or withdraw or amend the patent information in accordance with paragraph (f)(2) of this section within 30 days of the date on which the Agency sends the statement of dispute. Unless the NDA holder withdraws or amends its patent information in response to the patent listing dispute, the Agency will not change the patent information in the Orange Book.

(B) *Method-of-use claim.* For requests submitted under this paragraph (f)(1) that are directed to the accuracy or relevance of submitted patent information regarding an approved method of using the drug product, FDA will send the statement of dispute to the NDA holder. The NDA holder must confirm the correctness of its description of the approved method of use claimed by the patent that has been included as the "Use Code" in the Orange Book, or withdraw or amend the patent information in accordance with paragraph (f)(2) of this section, provide a narrative description (no more than 250 words) of the NDA holder's interpretation of the scope of the patent that explains why the existing or amended "Use Code" describes only the specific approved method of use claimed by the patent for which a claim of patent infringement could reasonably be asserted if a person not licensed by the owner of the patent engaged in the manufacture, use, or sale of the drug product, and include the signed verification required by paragraph (c)(2)(ii)(R) of this section within 30 days of the date on which the Agency sends the statement of dispute. The narrative description must only contain information for which the NDA holder consents to disclosure because FDA will send the text of the statement to the person who submitted the patent listing dispute without review or redaction.

(1) If the NDA holder confirms the correctness of the patent information, provides the narrative description required by paragraph (f)(1)(i)(B) of this section, and includes the signed verification required by paragraph (c)(2)(ii)(R) of this section within 30 days of the date on which the Agency sends the statement of dispute, the Agency will not change the patent information in the Orange Book.

(2) If the NDA holder responds to the patent listing dispute with amended patent information in accordance with paragraph (f)(2) of this section, provides the narrative description required by paragraph (f)(1)(i)(B) of this section, and includes the signed verification required by paragraph (c)(2)(ii)(R) of this section within 30 days of the date on which the Agency sends the statement of dispute, FDA will update the Orange Book to reflect the amended patent information.

(ii) *Patent certification or statement during and after patent listing dispute.* A 505(b)(2) application or ANDA must contain an appropriate certification or statement for each listed patent, including the disputed patent, during and after the patent listing dispute.

(iii) *Information on patent listing disputes.* FDA will promptly post information on its Web site regarding whether a patent listing dispute has been submitted for a published description of a patented method of use for a drug product and whether the NDA holder has timely responded to the patent listing dispute.

(2) *Requests by the NDA holder*—(i) *Patents or patent claims that no longer meet the statutory requirements for listing.* If the NDA holder determines that a patent or patent claim no longer meets the requirements for listing in section 505(b)(1) or (c)(2) of the Federal Food, Drug, and Cosmetic Act (including if there has been a judicial finding of invalidity for a listed patent, from which no appeal has been or can be taken), the NDA holder is required to promptly notify FDA to amend the patent information or withdraw the patent or patent information and request that the patent or patent information be removed from the list. If the NDA holder is required by court order to amend patent information or withdraw a patent from the list, it must submit an amendment to its NDA that includes a copy of the order, within 14 days of the date the order was entered, to the Central Document Room, Center for Drug Evaluation and Research, Food and Drug Administration, 5901-B Ammendale Rd., Beltsville, MD 20705-1266. The amendment to the NDA must bear the identification described in paragraph (d)(6) of this section. FDA will remove a patent or patent information from the list if there is no first applicant eligible for 180-day exclusivity based on a paragraph IV certification to that patent or after the 180-day exclusivity period of a first applicant based on that patent has expired or has been extinguished.

(ii) Patent term restoration. If the term of a listed patent is extended pursuant to 35 U.S.C. 156(e), the NDA holder must submit on Form FDA 3542 a correction to the expiration date of the patent. This correction must be submitted within 30 days of receipt of a certificate of extension as described in 35 U.S.C. 156(e)(1) or documentation of an extension of the term of the patent as described in 35 U.S.C. 156(e)(2).

(iii) *Submission of corrections or changes to patent information.* Corrections or changes to previously submitted patent information, other than withdrawal of a patent and requests to remove a patent from the list, must be submitted on Form FDA 3542 or 3542a, as appropriate, in an amendment or supplement to the NDA. The amendment or supplement to the NDA must bear the identification described in paragraph (d)(6) of this section. We will not accept the corrections or changes unless they are submitted on the appropriate forms.

(iv) *Submission of patent withdrawals and requests to remove a patent from the list.* Withdrawal of a patent and requests to remove a patent from the list must be submitted to the same addresses described in paragraph (d)(4)(ii) of this section, except that the withdrawal or request to remove a patent from the list is not required to be submitted on Form FDA 3542 and may be submitted by letter. Withdrawal of a patent and a request to remove a patent from the list must contain the following information:

(A) The NDA number to which the request applies;

(B) Each product(s) approved in the NDA to which the request applies; and

(C) The patent number.

[81 FR 69643, Oct. 6, 2016]

§ 314.54 Procedure for submission of a 505(b)(2) application requiring investigations for approval of a new indication for, or other change from, a listed drug.

(a) The Federal Food, Drug, and Cosmetic Act does not permit approval of an ANDA for a new indication, nor does it permit approval of other changes in a listed drug if investigations, other than bioavailability or bioequivalence studies, are essential to the approval of the change. Any person seeking approval of a drug product that represents a modification of a listed drug (e.g., a new indication or new dosage form) and for which investigations, other than bioavailability or bioequivalence studies, are essential to the approval of the changes may, except as provided in paragraph (b) of this section, submit a 505(b)(2) application. This 505(b)(2) application need contain only that information needed to support the modification(s) of the listed drug.

(1) The applicant must submit a complete archival copy of the application that contains the following:

(i) The information required under § 314.50(a), (b), (c), (d)(1), (d)(3), (e), and (g), except that § 314.50(d)(1)(ii)(c) must contain the proposed or actual master production record, including a description of the equipment, to be used for the manufacture of a commercial lot of the drug product.

(ii) The information required under § 314.50 (d)(2), (d)(4) (if an anti-infective drug), (d)(5), (d)(6), and (f) as needed to support the safety and effectiveness of the drug product.

(iii) Identification of each listed drug for which FDA has made a finding of safety and effectiveness and on which finding the applicant relies in seeking approval of its proposed drug product by established name, if any, proprietary name, dosage form, strength, route of administration, name of listed drug's application holder, and listed drug's approved NDA number. The listed drug(s) identified as relied upon must include a drug product approved in an NDA that:

(A) Is pharmaceutically equivalent to the drug product for which the original 505(b)(2) application is submitted; and

(B) Was approved before the original 505(b)(2) application was submitted.

(iv) If the applicant is seeking approval only for a new indication and not for the indications approved for the listed drug on which the applicant relies, a certification so stating.

(v) Any patent information required under section 505(b)(1) of the Federal Food, Drug, and Cosmetic Act with respect to any patent which claims the drug for which approval is sought or a method of using such drug and to which a claim of patent infringement could reasonably be asserted if a person not licensed by the owner of the patent engaged in the manufacture, use, or sale of the drug product.

(vi) Any patent certification or statement required under section 505(b)(2) of the Federal Food, Drug, and Cosmetic Act with respect to any relevant patents that claim the listed drug(s) on which investigations relied on by the applicant for approval of the application were conducted, or that claim a use for the listed drug(s). A 505(b)(2) applicant seeking approval of a drug that is pharmaceutically equivalent to a listed drug approved in an NDA implicitly relies upon one such pharmaceutically equivalent listed drug.

(vii) If the applicant believes the change for which it is seeking approval is entitled to a period of exclusivity, the information required under § 314.50(j).

(2) The applicant must submit a review copy that contains the technical sections described in § 314.50(d)(1), except that the section described in § 314.50(d)(1)(ii)(c) must contain the proposed or actual master production record, including a description of the equipment, to be used for the manufacture of a commercial lot of the drug product, and § 314.50(d)(3), and the technical sections described in § 314.50(d)(2), (d)(4) through (6), and (f) when needed to support the modification. Each of the technical sections in the review copy is required to be separately bound with a copy of the information required under § 314.50(a), (b), and (c) and a copy of the proposed labeling.

(3) The information required by § 314.50 (d)(2), (d)(4) (if an anti-infective drug), (d)(5), (d)(6), and (f) for the listed drug on which the applicant relies must be satisfied by reference to the listed drug under paragraph (a)(1)(iii) of this section.

(4) The applicant must submit a field copy of the 505(b)(2) application that contains the technical section described in § 314.50(d)(1), a copy of the information required under § 314.50(a) and (c), and certification that the field copy is a true copy of the technical section described in § 314.50(d)(1) contained in the archival and review copies of the 505(b)(2) application.

(b) A 505(b)(2) application may not be submitted under this section for a drug product whose only difference from a listed drug is that:

(1) The extent to which its active ingredient(s) is absorbed or otherwise made available to the site of action is less than that of the listed drug; or

(2) The rate at which its active ingredient(s) is absorbed or otherwise made available to the site of action is unintentionally less than that of the listed drug.

[57 FR 17982, Apr. 28, 1992; 57 FR 61612, Dec. 28, 1992, as amended at 58 FR 47351, Sept. 8, 1993; 59 FR 50364, Oct. 3, 1994; 81 FR 69647, Oct. 6, 2016]

§ 314.55 Pediatric use information.

(a) *Required assessment.* Except as provided in paragraphs (b), (c), and (d) of this section, each application for a new active ingredient, new indication, new dosage form, new dosing regimen, or new route of administration shall contain data that are adequate to assess the safety and effectiveness of the drug product for the claimed indications in all relevant pediatric subpopulations, and to support dosing and administration for each pediatric subpopulation for which the drug is safe and effective. Where the course of the disease and the effects of the drug are sufficiently similar in adults and pediatric patients, FDA may conclude that pediatric effectiveness can be extrapolated from adequate and well-controlled studies in adults usually supplemented with other information obtained in pediatric patients, such as pharmacokinetic studies. Studies may not be needed in each pediatric age group, if data from one age group can be extrapolated to another. Assessments of safety and effectiveness required under this section for a drug product that represents a meaningful therapeutic benefit over existing treatments for pediatric patients must be carried out using appropriate formulations for each age group(s) for which the assessment is required.

(b) *Deferred submission.* (1) FDA may, on its own initiative or at the request of an applicant, defer submission of some or all assessments of safety and effectiveness described in paragraph (a) of this section until after approval of the drug product for use in adults. Deferral may be granted if, among other reasons, the drug is ready for approval in adults before studies in pediatric patients are complete, or pediatric studies should be delayed until additional safety or effectiveness data have been collected. If an applicant requests deferred submission, the request must provide a certification from the applicant of the grounds for delaying pediatric studies, a description of the planned or ongoing studies, and evidence that the studies are being or will be conducted with due diligence and at the earliest possible time.

(2) If FDA determines that there is an adequate justification for temporarily delaying the submission of assessments of pediatric safety and effectiveness, the drug product may be approved for use in adults subject to the requirement that the applicant submit the required assessments within a specified time.

(c) *Waivers*—(1) *General.* FDA may grant a full or partial waiver of the requirements of paragraph (a) of this section on its own initiative or at the request of an applicant. A request for a waiver must provide an adequate justification.

(2) *Full waiver.* An applicant may request a waiver of the requirements of paragraph (a) of this section if the applicant certifies that:

(i) The drug product does not represent a meaningful therapeutic benefit over existing treatments for pediatric patients and is not likely to be used in a substantial number of pediatric patients;

(ii) Necessary studies are impossible or highly impractical because, e.g., the number of such patients is so small or geographically dispersed; or

(iii) There is evidence strongly suggesting that the drug product would be ineffective or unsafe in all pediatric age groups.

(3) *Partial waiver.* An applicant may request a waiver of the requirements of paragraph (a) of this section with respect to a specified pediatric age group, if the applicant certifies that:

(i) The drug product does not represent a meaningful therapeutic benefit over existing treatments for pediatric patients in that age group, and is not likely to be used in a substantial number of patients in that age group;

(ii) Necessary studies are impossible or highly impractical because, e.g., the number of patients in that age group is so small or geographically dispersed;

(iii) There is evidence strongly suggesting that the drug product would be ineffective or unsafe in that age group; or

(iv) The applicant can demonstrate that reasonable attempts to produce a pediatric formulation necessary for that age group have failed.

(4) *FDA action on waiver.* FDA shall grant a full or partial waiver, as appropriate, if the agency finds that there is a reasonable basis on which to conclude that one or more of the grounds for waiver specified in paragraphs (c)(2) or (c)(3) of this section have been met. If a waiver is granted on the ground that it is not possible to develop a pediatric formulation, the waiver will cover only those pediatric age groups requiring that formulation. If a waiver is granted because there is evidence that the product would be ineffective or unsafe in pediatric populations, this information will be included in the product's labeling.

(5) *Definition of "meaningful therapeutic benefit".* For purposes of this section and § 201.23 of this chapter, a drug will be considered to offer a meaningful therapeutic benefit over existing therapies if FDA estimates that:

(i) If approved, the drug would represent a significant improvement in the treatment, diagnosis, or prevention of a disease, compared to marketed products adequately labeled for that use in the relevant pediatric population. Examples of how improvement might be demonstrated include, for example, evidence of increased effectiveness in treatment, prevention, or diagnosis of disease, elimination or substantial reduction of a treatment-limiting drug reaction, documented enhancement of compliance, or evidence of safety and effectiveness in a new subpopulation; or

(ii) The drug is in a class of drugs or for an indication for which there is a need for additional therapeutic options.

(d) Exemption for orphan drugs. This section does not apply to any drug for an indication or indications for which orphan designation has been granted under part 316, subpart C, of this chapter.

[63 FR 66670, Dec. 2, 1998]

§ 314.60 Amendments to an unapproved NDA, supplement, or resubmission.

(a) *Submission of NDA.* FDA generally assumes that when an original NDA, supplement to an approved NDA, or resubmission of an NDA or supplement is submitted to the Agency for review, the applicant believes that the Agency can approve the NDA, supplement, or resubmission as submitted. However, the applicant may submit an amendment to an NDA, supplement, or resubmission that has been filed under § 314.101 but is not yet approved.

(b) Submission of major amendment. (1) Submission of a major amendment to an original NDA, efficacy supplement, or resubmission of an NDA or efficacy supplement within 3 months of the end of the initial review cycle constitutes an agreement by the applicant under section 505(c) of the Federal Food, Drug, and Cosmetic Act to extend the initial review cycle by 3 months. (For references to a resubmission of an NDA or efficacy supplement in paragraph (b) of this section, the timeframe for reviewing the resubmission is the "review cycle" rather than the "initial review cycle.") FDA may instead defer review of the amendment until the subsequent review cycle. If the agency extends the initial review cycle for an original NDA, efficacy supplement, or resubmission under this paragraph, the division responsible for reviewing the NDA, supplement, or resubmission will notify the applicant of the extension. The initial review cycle for an original NDA, efficacy supplement, or resubmission of an NDA or efficacy supplement may be extended only once due to submission of a major amendment. FDA may, at its discretion, review any subsequent major amendment during the initial review cycle (as extended) or defer review until the subsequent review cycle.

(2) Submission of a major amendment to an original NDA, efficacy supplement, or resubmission of an NDA or efficacy supplement more than 3 months before the end of the initial review cycle will not extend the cycle. FDA may, at its discretion, review such an amendment during the initial review cycle or defer review until the subsequent review cycle.

(3) Submission of an amendment to an original NDA, efficacy supplement, or resubmission of an NDA or efficacy supplement that is not a major amendment will not extend the initial review cycle. FDA may, at its discretion, review such an amendment during the initial review cycle or defer review until the subsequent review cycle.

(4) Submission of a major amendment to a manufacturing supplement within 2 months of the end of the initial review cycle constitutes an agreement by the applicant under section 505(c) of the Federal Food, Drug, and Cosmetic Act to extend the initial review cycle by 2 months. FDA may instead defer review of the amendment until the subsequent review cycle. If the agency extends the initial review cycle for a manufacturing supplement under this paragraph, the division responsible for reviewing the supplement will notify the applicant of the extension. The initial review cycle for a manufacturing supplement may be extended only once due to submission of a major amendment. FDA may, at its discretion, review any subsequent major amendment during the initial review cycle (as extended) or defer review until the subsequent review cycle.

(5) Submission of an amendment to a supplement other than an efficacy or manufacturing supplement will not extend the initial review cycle. FDA may, at its discretion, review such an amendment during the initial review cycle or defer review until the subsequent review cycle.

(6) A major amendment may not include data to support an indication or claim that was not included in the original NDA, supplement, or resubmission, but it may include data to support a minor modification of an indication or claim that was included in the original NDA, supplement, or resubmission.

(7) When FDA defers review of an amendment until the subsequent review cycle, the agency will notify the applicant of the deferral in the complete response letter sent to the applicant under § 314.110 of this part.

(c) *Limitation on certain amendments.* (1) An unapproved NDA may not be amended if all of the following conditions apply:

(i) The unapproved NDA is for a drug for which a previous NDA has been approved and granted a period of exclusivity in accordance with section 505(c)(3)(E)(ii) of the Federal Food, Drug, and Cosmetic Act that has not expired;

(ii) The applicant seeks to amend the unapproved NDA to include a published report of an investigation that was conducted or sponsored by the applicant entitled to exclusivity for the drug;

(iii) The applicant has not obtained a right of reference or use to the investigation described in paragraph (c)(1)(ii) of this section; and

(iv) The report of the investigation described in paragraph (c)(1)(ii) of this section would be essential to the approval of the unapproved NDA.

(2) The submission of an amendment described in paragraph (c)(1) of this section will cause the unapproved NDA to be deemed to be withdrawn by the applicant under § 314.65 on the date of receipt by FDA of the amendment. The amendment will be considered a resubmission of the NDA,

which may not be accepted except as provided in accordance with section 505(c)(3)(E)(ii) of the Federal Food, Drug, and Cosmetic Act.

(d) *Field copy.* The applicant must submit a field copy of each amendment to a section of the NDA described in § 314.50(d)(1). The applicant must include in its submission of each such amendment to FDA a statement certifying that a field copy of the amendment has been sent to the applicant's home FDA district office.

(e) Different drug. An applicant may not amend a 505(b)(2) application to seek approval of a drug that is a different drug from the drug in the original submission of the 505(b)(2) application. For purposes of this paragraph (e), a drug is a different drug if it has been modified to have a different active ingredient, different route of administration, different dosage form, or difference in excipients that requires either a separate clinical study to establish safety or effectiveness or, for topical products, that requires a separate in vivo demonstration of bioequivalence. However, notwithstanding the limitation described in this paragraph (e), an applicant may amend the 505(b)(2) application to seek approval of a different strength.

(f) *Patent certification requirements.* (1) An amendment to a 505(b)(2) application is required to contain an appropriate patent certification or statement described in § 314.50(i) or a recertification for a previously submitted paragraph IV certification if approval is sought for any of the following types of amendments:

(i) To add a new indication or other condition of use;

(ii) To add a new strength;

(iii) To make other than minor changes in product formulation; or

(iv) To change the physical form or crystalline structure of the active ingredient.

(2) If the amendment to the 505(b)(2) application does not contain a patent certification or statement, the applicant must verify that the proposed change described in the amendment is not one of the types of amendments described in paragraph (f)(1) of this section.

[50 FR 7493, Feb. 22, 1985, as amended at 57 FR 17983, Apr. 28, 1992; 58 FR 47352, Sept. 8, 1993; 63 FR 5252, Feb. 2, 1998; 69 FR 18764, Apr. 8, 2004; 73 FR 39608, July 10, 2008; 81 FR 69648, Oct. 6, 2016]

§ 314.65 Withdrawal by the applicant of an unapproved application.

An applicant may at any time withdraw an application that is not yet approved by notifying the Food and Drug Administration in writing. If, by the time it receives such notice, the agency has identified any deficiencies in the application, we will list such deficiencies in the letter we send the applicant acknowledging the withdrawal. A decision to withdraw the application is without prejudice to refiling. The agency will retain the application and will provide a copy to the applicant on request under the fee schedule in § 20.45 of FDA's public information regulations.

[50 FR 7493, Feb. 22, 1985, as amended at 68 FR 25287, May 12, 2003; 73 FR 39609, July 10, 2008]

§ 314.70 Supplements and other changes to an approved NDA.

(a) *Changes to an approved NDA.* (1)(i) Except as provided in paragraph (a)(1)(ii) of this section, the applicant must notify FDA about each change in each condition established in an approved NDA beyond the variations already provided for in the NDA. The notice is required to describe the change fully. Depending on the type of change, the applicant must notify FDA about the change in a supplement under paragraph (b) or (c) of this section or by inclusion of the information in the annual report to the NDA under paragraph (d) of this section.

(ii) The submission and grant of a written request for an exception or alternative under § 201.26 of this chapter satisfies the applicable requirements in paragraphs (a) through (c) of this section.

However, any grant of a request for an exception or alternative under § 201.26 of this chapter must be reported as part of the annual report to the NDA under paragraph (d) of this section.

(2) The NDA holder must assess the effects of the change before distributing a drug product made with a manufacturing change.

(3) Notwithstanding the requirements of paragraphs (b) and (c) of this section, an applicant must make a change provided for in those paragraphs in accordance with a regulation or guidance that provides for a less burdensome notification of the change (for example, by submission of a supplement that does not require approval prior to distribution of the product or in an annual report).

(4) The applicant must promptly revise all promotional labeling and advertising to make it consistent with any labeling change implemented in accordance with paragraphs (b) and (c) of this section.

(5) Except for a supplement providing for a change in the labeling, the applicant must include in each supplement and amendment to a supplement providing for a change under paragraph (b) or (c) of this section a statement certifying that a field copy has been provided in accordance with § 314.440(a)(4).

(6) A supplement or annual report must include a list of all changes contained in the supplement or annual report. For supplements, this list must be provided in the submission.

(b) *Changes requiring supplement submission and approval prior to distribution of the product made using the change (major changes).* (1) A supplement must be submitted for any change in the drug substance, drug product, production process, quality controls, equipment, or facilities that has a substantial potential to have an adverse effect on the identity, strength, quality, purity, or potency of the drug product as these factors may relate to the safety or effectiveness of the drug product.

(2) These changes include, but are not limited to:

(i) Except those described in paragraphs (c) and (d) of this section, changes in the qualitative or quantitative formulation of the drug product, including inactive ingredients, or in the specifications provided in the approved NDA;

(ii) Changes requiring completion of studies in accordance with part 320 of this chapter to demonstrate the equivalence of the drug product to the drug product as manufactured without the change or to the reference listed drug;

(iii) Changes that may affect drug substance or drug product sterility assurance, such as changes in drug substance, drug product, or component sterilization method(s) or an addition, deletion, or substitution of steps in an aseptic processing operation;

(iv) Changes in the synthesis or manufacture of the drug substance that may affect the impurity profile and/or the physical, chemical, or biological properties of the drug substance;

(v) The following labeling changes:

(A) Changes in labeling, except those described in paragraphs (c)(6)(iii), (d)(2)(ix), or (d)(2)(x) of this section;

(B) If applicable, any change to a Medication Guide required under part 208 of this chapter, except for changes in the information specified in § 208.20(b)(8)(iii) and (b)(8)(iv) of this chapter; and

(C) Any change to the information required by § 201.57(a) of this chapter, with the following exceptions that may be reported in an annual report under paragraph (d)(2)(x) of this section:

(1) Removal of a listed section(s) specified in § 201.57(a)(5) of this chapter; and

(2) Changes to the most recent revision date of the labeling as specified in § 201.57(a)(15) of this chapter.

(vi) Changes in a drug product container closure system that controls the drug product delivered to a patient or changes in the type (e.g., glass to high density polyethylene (HDPE), HDPE to polyvinyl chloride, vial to syringe) or composition (e.g., one HDPE resin to another HDPE resin) of a packaging component that may affect the impurity profile of the drug product.

(vii) Changes solely affecting a natural product, a recombinant DNA-derived protein/polypeptide, or a complex or conjugate of a drug substance with a monoclonal antibody for the following:

(A) Changes in the virus or adventitious agent removal or inactivation method(s);

(B) Changes in the source material or cell line; and

(C) Establishment of a new master cell bank or seed.

(viii) Changes to a drug product under an NDA that is subject to a validity assessment because of significant questions regarding the integrity of the data supporting that NDA.

(3) The applicant must obtain approval of a supplement from FDA prior to distribution of a drug product made using a change under paragraph (b) of this section. Except for submissions under paragraph (e) of this section, the following information must be contained in the supplement:

(i) A detailed description of the proposed change;

(ii) The drug product(s) involved;

(iii) The manufacturing site(s) or area(s) affected;

(iv) A description of the methods used and studies performed to assess the effects of the change;

(v) The data derived from such studies;

(vi) For a natural product, a recombinant DNA-derived protein/polypeptide, or a complex or conjugate of a drug substance with a monoclonal antibody, relevant validation protocols and a list of relevant standard operating procedures must be provided in addition to the requirements in paragraphs (b)(3)(iv) and (b)(3)(v) of this section; and

(vii) For sterilization process and test methodologies related to sterilization process validation, relevant validation protocols and a list of relevant standard operating procedures must be provided in addition to the requirements in paragraphs (b)(3)(iv) and (b)(3)(v) of this section.

(4) An applicant may ask FDA to expedite its review of a supplement for public health reasons or if a delay in making the change described in it would impose an extraordinary hardship on the applicant. Such a supplement should be plainly marked: "Prior Approval Supplement-Expedited Review Requested."

(c) *Changes requiring supplement submission at least 30 days prior to distribution of the drug product made using the change (moderate changes).* (1) A supplement must be submitted for any change in the drug substance, drug product, production process, quality controls, equipment, or facilities that has a moderate potential to have an adverse effect on the identity, strength, quality, purity, or potency of the drug product as these factors may relate to the safety or effectiveness of the drug product. If the supplement provides for a labeling change under paragraph (c)(6)(iii) of this section, 12 copies of the final printed labeling must be included.

(2) These changes include, but are not limited to:

(i) A change in the container closure system that does not affect the quality of the drug product, except those described in paragraphs (b) and (d) of this section; and

(ii) Changes solely affecting a natural protein, a recombinant DNA-derived protein/polypeptide or a complex or conjugate of a drug substance with a monoclonal antibody, including:

(A) An increase or decrease in production scale during finishing steps that involves different equipment; and

(B) Replacement of equipment with that of a different design that does not affect the process methodology or process operating parameters.

(iii) Relaxation of an acceptance criterion or deletion of a test to comply with an official compendium that is consistent with FDA statutory and regulatory requirements.

(3) A supplement submitted under paragraph (c)(1) of this section is required to give a full explanation of the basis for the change and identify the date on which the change is to be made. The supplement must be labeled "Supplement—Changes Being Effected in 30 Days" or, if applicable under paragraph (c)(6) of this section, "Supplement—Changes Being Effected."

(4) Pending approval of the supplement by FDA, except as provided in paragraph (c)(6) of this section, distribution of the drug product made using the change may begin not less than 30 days after receipt of the supplement by FDA. The information listed in paragraphs (b)(3)(i) through (b)(3)(vii) of this section must be contained in the supplement.

(5) The applicant must not distribute the drug product made using the change if within 30 days following FDA's receipt of the supplement, FDA informs the applicant that either:

(i) The change requires approval prior to distribution of the drug product in accordance with paragraph (b) of this section; or

(ii) Any of the information required under paragraph (c)(4) of this section is missing; the applicant must not distribute the drug product made using the change until the supplement has been amended to provide the missing information.

(6) The agency may designate a category of changes for the purpose of providing that, in the case of a change in such category, the holder of an approved NDA may commence distribution of the drug product involved upon receipt by the agency of a supplement for the change. These changes include, but are not limited to:

(i) Addition to a specification or changes in the methods or controls to provide increased assurance that the drug substance or drug product will have the characteristics of identity, strength, quality, purity, or potency that it purports or is represented to possess;

(ii) A change in the size and/or shape of a container for a nonsterile drug product, except for solid dosage forms, without a change in the labeled amount of drug product or from one container closure system to another;

(iii) Changes in the labeling to reflect newly acquired information, except for changes to the information required in § 201.57(a) of this chapter (which must be made under paragraph (b)(2)(v)(C) of this section), to accomplish any of the following:

(A) To add or strengthen a contraindication, warning, precaution, or adverse reaction for which the evidence of a causal association satisfies the standard for inclusion in the labeling under § 201.57(c) of this chapter;

(B) To add or strengthen a statement about drug abuse, dependence, psychological effect, or overdosage;

(C) To add or strengthen an instruction about dosage and administration that is intended to increase the safe use of the drug product;

(D) To delete false, misleading, or unsupported indications for use or claims for effectiveness; or

(E) Any labeling change normally requiring a supplement submission and approval prior to distribution of the drug product that FDA specifically requests be submitted under this provision.

(7) If the agency disapproves the supplemental NDA, it may order the manufacturer to cease distribution of the drug product(s) made with the manufacturing change.

(d) *Changes to be described in an annual report (minor changes).* (1) Changes in the drug substance, drug product, production process, quality controls, equipment, or facilities that have a minimal potential to have an adverse effect on the identity, strength, quality, purity, or potency of the drug product as these factors may relate to the safety or effectiveness of the drug product must be documented by the applicant in the next annual report in accordance with § 314.81(b)(2).

(2) These changes include, but are not limited to:

(i) Any change made to comply with a change to an official compendium, except a change described in paragraph (c)(2)(iii) of this section, that is consistent with FDA statutory and regulatory requirements.

(ii) The deletion or reduction of an ingredient intended to affect only the color of the drug product;

(iii) Replacement of equipment with that of the same design and operating principles except those equipment changes described in paragraph (c) of this section;

(iv) A change in the size and/or shape of a container containing the same number of dosage units for a nonsterile solid dosage form drug product, without a change from one container closure system to another;

(v) A change within the container closure system for a nonsterile drug product, based upon a showing of equivalency to the approved system under a protocol approved in the NDA or published in an official compendium;

(vi) An extension of an expiration dating period based upon full shelf life data on production batches obtained from a protocol approved in the NDA;

(vii) The addition or revision of an alternative analytical procedure that provides the same or increased assurance of the identity, strength, quality, purity, or potency of the material being tested as the analytical procedure described in the approved NDA, or deletion of an alternative analytical procedure;

(viii) The addition by embossing, debossing, or engraving of a code imprint to a solid oral dosage form drug product other than a modified release dosage form, or a minor change in an existing code imprint;

(ix) A change in the labeling concerning the description of the drug product or in the information about how the drug product is supplied, that does not involve a change in the dosage strength or dosage form; and

(x) An editorial or similar minor change in labeling, including a change to the information allowed by paragraphs (b)(2)(v)(C)(1) and (2) of this section.

(3) For changes under this category, the applicant is required to submit in the annual report:

(i) A statement by the holder of the approved NDA that the effects of the change have been assessed;

(ii) A full description of the manufacturing and controls changes, including the manufacturing site(s) or area(s) involved;

(iii) The date each change was implemented;

(iv) Data from studies and tests performed to assess the effects of the change; and,

(v) For a natural product, recombinant DNA-derived protein/polypeptide, complex or conjugate of a drug substance with a monoclonal antibody, sterilization process or test methodology related to sterilization process validation, a cross-reference to relevant validation protocols and/or standard operating procedures.

(e) *Protocols.* An applicant may submit one or more protocols describing the specific tests and studies and acceptance criteria to be achieved to demonstrate the lack of adverse effect for specified types of manufacturing changes on the identity, strength, quality, purity, and potency of the drug product as these factors may relate to the safety or effectiveness of the drug product. Any such protocols, if not included in the approved NDA, or changes to an approved protocol, must be submitted as a supplement requiring approval from FDA prior to distribution of a drug product produced with the manufacturing change. The supplement, if approved, may subsequently justify a reduced reporting category for the particular change because the use of the protocol for that type of change reduces the potential risk of an adverse effect.

(f) *Patent information.* The applicant must comply with the patent information requirements under section 505(c)(2) of the Federal Food, Drug, and Cosmetic Act and § 314.53.

(g) *Claimed exclusivity.* If an applicant claims exclusivity under § 314.108 upon approval of a supplement for change to its previously approved drug product, the applicant must include with its supplement the information required under § 314.50(j).

(h) *Different drug.* An applicant may not supplement a 505(b)(2) application to seek approval of a drug that is a different drug from the drug in the approved 505(b)(2) application. For purposes of this paragraph (h), a drug is a different drug if it has been modified to have a different active ingredient, different route of administration, different dosage form, or difference in excipients that requires either a separate clinical study to establish safety or effectiveness or, for topical products, that requires a separate in vivo demonstration of bioequivalence. However, notwithstanding the limitation described in this paragraph (h), an applicant may supplement the 505(b)(2) application to seek approval of a different strength.

[69 FR 18764, Apr. 8, 2004, as amended at 71 FR 3997, Jan. 24, 2006; 72 FR 73600, Dec. 28, 2007; 73 FR 49609, Aug. 22, 2008; 81 FR 69648, Oct. 6, 2016]

§ 314.71 Procedures for submission of a supplement to an approved application.

(a) Only the applicant may submit a supplement to an application.

(b) All procedures and actions that apply to an application under § 314.50 also apply to supplements, except that the information required in the supplement is limited to that needed to support the change. A supplement is required to contain an archival copy and a review copy that include an application form and appropriate technical sections, samples, and labeling; except that a supplement for a change other than a change in labeling is required also to contain a field copy.

(c) All procedures and actions that apply to applications under this part, including actions by applicants and the Food and Drug Administration, also apply to supplements except as specified otherwise in this part.

[50 FR 7493, Feb. 22, 1985, as amended at 50 FR 21238, May 23, 1985; 58 FR 47352, Sept. 8, 1993; 67 FR 9586, Mar. 4, 2002; 73 FR 39609, July 10, 2008]

§ 314.72 Change in ownership of an application.

(a) An applicant may transfer ownership of its application. At the time of transfer the new and former owners are required to submit information to the Food and Drug Administration as follows:

(1) The former owner shall submit a letter or other document that states that all rights to the application have been transferred to the new owner.

(2) The new owner shall submit an application form signed by the new owner and a letter or other document containing the following:

(i) The new owner's commitment to agreements, promises, and conditions made by the former owner and contained in the application;

(ii) The date that the change in ownership is effective; and

(iii) Either a statement that the new owner has a complete copy of the approved application, including supplements and records that are required to be kept under § 314.81, or a request for a copy of the application from FDA's files. FDA will provide a copy of the application to the new owner under the fee schedule in § 20.45 of FDA's public information regulations.

(b) The new owner shall advise FDA about any change in the conditions in the approved application under § 314.70, except the new owner may advise FDA in the next annual report about a change in the drug product's label or labeling to change the product's brand or the name of its manufacturer, packer, or distributor.

[50 FR 7493, Feb. 22, 1985; 50 FR 14212, Apr. 11, 1985, as amended at 50 FR 21238, May 23, 1985; 67 FR 9586, Mar. 4, 2002; 68 FR 25287, May 12, 2003]

§ 314.80 Postmarketing reporting of adverse drug experiences.

(a) *Definitions.* The following definitions of terms apply to this section:

Adverse drug experience. Any adverse event associated with the use of a drug in humans, whether or not considered drug related, including the following: An adverse event occurring in the course of the use of a drug product in professional practice; an adverse event occurring from drug overdose whether accidental or intentional; an adverse event occurring from drug abuse; an adverse event occurring from drug withdrawal; and any failure of expected pharmacological action.

Individual case safety report (ICSR). A description of an adverse drug experience related to an individual patient or subject.

ICSR attachments. Documents related to the adverse drug experience described in an ICSR, such as medical records, hospital discharge summaries, or other documentation.

Disability. A substantial disruption of a person's ability to conduct normal life functions.

Life-threatening adverse drug experience. Any adverse drug experience that places the patient, in the view of the initial reporter, at immediate risk of death from the adverse drug experience as it occurred, i.e., it does not include an adverse drug experience that, had it occurred in a more severe form, might have caused death.

Serious adverse drug experience. Any adverse drug experience occurring at any dose that results in any of the following outcomes: Death, a life-threatening adverse drug experience, inpatient hospitalization or prolongation of existing hospitalization, a persistent or significant disability/incapacity, or a congenital anomaly/birth defect. Important medical events that may not result in death, be life-threatening, or require hospitalization may be considered a serious adverse drug experience when, based upon appropriate medical judgment, they may jeopardize the patient or subject and may require medical or surgical intervention to prevent one of the outcomes listed in this definition. Examples of such medical events include allergic bronchospasm requiring intensive treatment in an emergency room or at home, blood dyscrasias or convulsions that do not result in inpatient hospitalization, or the development of drug dependency or drug abuse.

Unexpected adverse drug experience. Any adverse drug experience that is not listed in the current labeling for the drug product. This includes events that may be symptomatically and pathophysiologically related to an event listed in the labeling, but differ from the event because of greater severity or specificity. For example, under this definition, hepatic necrosis would be unexpected (by virtue of greater severity) if the labeling only referred to elevated hepatic enzymes or hepatitis. Similarly, cerebral thromboembolism and cerebral vasculitis would be unexpected (by virtue of greater specificity) if the labeling only listed cerebral vascular accidents. "Unexpected," as used in this definition, refers to an adverse drug experience that has not been previously observed (i.e., included in the labeling) rather than from the perspective of such experience not being anticipated from the pharmacological properties of the pharmaceutical product.

(b) Review of adverse drug experiences. Each applicant having an approved application under § 314.50 or, in the case of a 505(b)(2) application, an effective approved application, must promptly review all adverse drug experience information obtained or otherwise received by the applicant from any source, foreign or domestic, including information derived from commercial marketing experience, postmarketing clinical investigations, postmarketing epidemiological/surveillance studies, reports in the scientific literature, and unpublished scientific papers. Applicants are not required to resubmit to FDA adverse drug experience reports forwarded to the applicant by FDA; however, applicants must submit all followup information on such reports to FDA. Any person subject to the reporting requirements under paragraph (c) of this section must also develop written procedures for the surveillance, receipt, evaluation, and reporting of postmarketing adverse drug experiences to FDA.

(c) Reporting requirements. The applicant must submit to FDA adverse drug experience information as described in this section. Except as provided in paragraph (g)(2) of this section, these reports must be submitted to the Agency in electronic format as described in paragraph (g)(1) of this section.

(1)(i) Postmarketing 15-day "Alert reports". The applicant must report each adverse drug experience that is both serious and unexpected, whether foreign or domestic, as soon as possible but no later than 15 calendar days from initial receipt of the information by the applicant.

(ii) Postmarketing 15-day "Alert reports"—followup. The applicant must promptly investigate all adverse drug experiences that are the subject of these postmarketing 15-day Alert reports and must submit followup reports within 15 calendar days of receipt of new information or as requested by FDA. If additional information is not obtainable, records should be maintained of the unsuccessful steps taken to seek additional information.

(iii) Submission of reports. The requirements of paragraphs (c)(1)(i) and (c)(1)(ii) of this section, concerning the submission of postmarketing 15-day Alert reports, also apply to any person other than the applicant whose name appears on the label of an approved drug product as a manufacturer, packer, or distributor (nonapplicant). To avoid unnecessary duplication in the submission to FDA of reports required by paragraphs (c)(1)(i) and (c)(1)(ii) of this section, obligations of a nonapplicant may be met by submission of all reports of serious adverse drug experiences to the applicant. If a nonapplicant elects to submit adverse drug experience reports to the applicant rather than to FDA, the nonapplicant must submit, by any appropriate means, each report to the applicant within 5 calendar days of initial receipt of the information by the nonapplicant, and the applicant must then comply with the requirements of this section. Under this circumstance, the nonapplicant must maintain a record of this action which must include:

(A) A copy of each adverse drug experience report;

(B) The date the report was received by the nonapplicant;

(C) The date the report was submitted to the applicant; and

(D) The name and address of the applicant.

(2) Periodic adverse drug experience reports. (i) The applicant must report each adverse drug experience not reported under paragraph (c)(1)(i) of this section at quarterly intervals, for 3 years from the date of approval of the application, and then at annual intervals. The applicant must submit each quarterly report within 30 days of the close of the quarter (the first quarter beginning on the date of approval of the application) and each annual report within 60 days of the anniversary date of approval of the application. Upon written notice, FDA may extend or reestablish the requirement that an applicant submit quarterly reports, or require that the applicant submit reports under this section at different times than those stated. For example, the agency may reestablish a quarterly reporting requirement following the approval of a major supplement. Followup information to adverse drug experiences submitted in a periodic report may be submitted in the next periodic report.

(ii) Each periodic report is required to contain:

(A) Descriptive information. (1) A narrative summary and analysis of the information in the report;

(2) An analysis of the 15-day Alert reports submitted during the reporting interval (all 15-day Alert reports being appropriately referenced by the applicant's patient identification code, adverse reaction term(s), and date of submission to FDA);

(3) A history of actions taken since the last report because of adverse drug experiences (for example, labeling changes or studies initiated); and

(4) An index consisting of a line listing of the applicant's patient identification code, and adverse reaction term(s) for all ICSRs submitted under paragraph (c)(2)(ii)(B) of this section.

(B) ICSRs for serious, expected, and nonserious adverse drug experiences. An ICSR for each adverse drug experience not reported under paragraph (c)(1)(i) of this section (all serious, expected and nonserious adverse drug experiences). All such ICSRs must be submitted to FDA (either individually or in one or more batches) within the timeframe specified in paragraph (c)(2)(i) of this section. ICSRs must only be submitted to FDA once.

(iii) Periodic reporting, except for information regarding 15-day Alert reports, does not apply to adverse drug experience information obtained from postmarketing studies (whether or not conducted under an investigational new drug application), from reports in the scientific literature, and from foreign marketing experience.

(d) Scientific literature. A 15-day Alert report based on information in the scientific literature must be accompanied by a copy of the published article. The 15-day reporting requirements in paragraph (c)(1)(i) of this section (i.e., serious, unexpected adverse drug experiences) apply only to reports found in scientific and medical journals either as case reports or as the result of a formal clinical trial.

(e) Postmarketing studies. An applicant is not required to submit a 15-day Alert report under paragraph (c) of this section for an adverse drug experience obtained from a postmarketing study (whether or not conducted under an investigational new drug application) unless the applicant concludes that there is a reasonable possibility that the drug caused the adverse experience.

(f) Information reported on ICSRs. ICSRs include the following information:

(1) Patient information.

(i) Patient identification code;

(ii) Patient age at the time of adverse drug experience, or date of birth;

(iii) Patient gender; and

(iv) Patient weight.

(2) Adverse drug experience.

(i) Outcome attributed to adverse drug experience;

(ii) Date of adverse drug experience;

(iii) Date of ICSR submission;

(iv) Description of adverse drug experience (including a concise medical narrative);

(v) Adverse drug experience term(s);

(vi) Description of relevant tests, including dates and laboratory data; and

(vii) Other relevant patient history, including preexisting medical conditions.

(3) Suspect medical product(s).

(i) Name;

(ii) Dose, frequency, and route of administration used;

(iii) Therapy dates;

(iv) Diagnosis for use (indication);

(v) Whether the product is a prescription or nonprescription product;

(vi) Whether the product is a combination product as defined in § 3.2(e) of this chapter;

(vii) Whether adverse drug experience abated after drug use stopped or dose reduced;

(viii) Whether adverse drug experience reappeared after reintroduction of drug;

(ix) Lot number;

(x) Expiration date;

(xi) National Drug Code (NDC) number; and

(xii) Concomitant medical products and therapy dates.

(4) Initial reporter information.

(i) Name, address, and telephone number;

(ii) Whether the initial reporter is a health care professional; and

(iii) Occupation, if a health care professional.

(5) Applicant information.

(i) Applicant name and contact office address;

(ii) Telephone number;

(iii) Report source, such as spontaneous, literature, or study;

(iv) Date the report was received by applicant;

(v) Application number and type;

(vi) Whether the ICSR is a 15-day "Alert report";

(vii) Whether the ICSR is an initial report or followup report; and

(viii) Unique case identification number, which must be the same in the initial report and any subsequent followup report(s).

(g) Electronic format for submissions. (1) Safety report submissions, including ICSRs, ICSR attachments, and the descriptive information in periodic reports, must be in an electronic format that FDA can process, review, and archive. FDA will issue guidance on how to provide the electronic submission (e.g., method of transmission, media, file formats, preparation and organization of files).

(2) An applicant or nonapplicant may request, in writing, a temporary waiver of the requirements in paragraph (g)(1) of this section. These waivers will be granted on a limited basis for good cause shown. FDA will issue guidance on requesting a waiver of the requirements in paragraph (g)(1) of this section.

(h) Multiple reports. An applicant should not include in reports under this section any adverse drug experiences that occurred in clinical trials if they were previously submitted as part of the approved application. If a report applies to a drug for which an applicant holds more than one approved application, the applicant should submit the report to the application that was first approved. If a report refers to more than one drug marketed by an applicant, the applicant should submit the report to the application for the drug listed first in the report.

(i) Patient privacy. An applicant should not include in reports under this section the names and addresses of individual patients; instead, the applicant should assign a unique code for identification of the patient. The applicant should include the name of the reporter from whom the information was received as part of the initial reporter information, even when the reporter is the patient. The names of patients, health care professionals, hospitals, and geographical identifiers in adverse drug

experience reports are not releasable to the public under FDA's public information regulations in part 20 of this chapter.

(j) Recordkeeping. The applicant must maintain for a period of 10 years records of all adverse drug experiences known to the applicant, including raw data and any correspondence relating to adverse drug experiences.

(k) Withdrawal of approval. If an applicant fails to establish and maintain records and make reports required under this section, FDA may withdraw approval of the application and, thus, prohibit continued marketing of the drug product that is the subject of the application.

(l) Disclaimer. A report or information submitted by an applicant under this section (and any release by FDA of that report or information) does not necessarily reflect a conclusion by the applicant or FDA that the report or information constitutes an admission that the drug caused or contributed to an adverse effect. An applicant need not admit, and may deny, that the report or information submitted under this section constitutes an admission that the drug caused or contributed to an adverse effect. For purposes of this provision, the term "applicant" also includes any person reporting under paragraph (c)(1)(iii) of this section.

[50 FR 7493, Feb. 22, 1985; 50 FR 14212, Apr. 11, 1985, as amended at 50 FR 21238, May 23, 1985; 51 FR 24481, July 3, 1986; 52 FR 37936, Oct. 13, 1987; 55 FR 11580, Mar. 29, 1990; 57 FR 17983, Apr. 28, 1992; 62 FR 34168, June 25, 1997; 62 FR 52251, Oct. 7, 1997; 63 FR 14611, Mar. 26, 1998; 67 FR 9586, Mar. 4, 2002; 69 FR 13473, Mar. 23, 2004; 74 FR 13113, Mar. 26, 2009; 79 FR 33088, June 10, 2014]

§ 314.81 Other postmarketing reports.

(a) *Applicability*. Each applicant shall make the reports for each of its approved applications and abbreviated applications required under this section and section 505(k) of the act.

(b) *Reporting requirements.* The applicant shall submit to the Food and Drug Administration at the specified times two copies of the following reports:

(1) *NDA—Field alert report.* The applicant shall submit information of the following kinds about distributed drug products and articles to the FDA district office that is responsible for the facility involved within 3 working days of receipt by the applicant. The information may be provided by telephone or other rapid communication means, with prompt written followup. The report and its mailing cover should be plainly marked: "NDA—Field Alert Report."

(i) Information concerning any incident that causes the drug product or its labeling to be mistaken for, or applied to, another article.

(ii) Information concerning any bacteriological contamination, or any significant chemical, physical, or other change or deterioration in the distributed drug product, or any failure of one or more distributed batches of the drug product to meet the specification established for it in the application.

(2) *Annual report.* The applicant shall submit each year within 60 days of the anniversary date of U.S. approval of the application, two copies of the report to the FDA division responsible for reviewing the application. Each annual report is required to be accompanied by a completed transmittal Form FDA 2252 (Transmittal of Periodic Reports for Drugs for Human Use), and must include all the information required under this section that the applicant received or otherwise obtained during the annual reporting interval that ends on the U.S. anniversary date. The report is required to contain in the order listed:

(i) *Summary*. A brief summary of significant new information from the previous year that might affect the safety, effectiveness, or labeling of the drug product. The report is also required to contain a brief description of actions the applicant has taken or intends to take as a result of this new information, for example, submit a labeling supplement, add a warning to the labeling, or initiate a new study. The summary shall briefly state whether labeling supplements for pediatric use have been submitted and whether new studies in the pediatric population to support appropriate labeling for the pediatric population have been initiated. Where possible, an estimate of patient exposure to the drug product, with special reference to the pediatric population (neonates, infants, children, and adolescents) shall be provided, including dosage form.

(ii)(a) *Distribution data.* Information about the quantity of the drug product distributed under the approved application, including that distributed to distributors. The information is required to include the National Drug Code (NDC) number, the total number of dosage units of each strength or potency distributed (e.g., 100,000/5 milligram tablets, 50,000/10 milliliter vials), and the quantities distributed for domestic use and the quantities distributed for foreign use. Disclosure of financial or pricing data is not required.

(b) *Authorized generic drugs.* If applicable, the date each authorized generic drug (as defined in § 314.3) entered the market, the date each authorized generic drug ceased being distributed, and the corresponding trade or brand name. Each dosage form and/or strength is a different authorized generic drug and should be listed separately. The first annual report submitted on or after January 25, 2010 must include the information listed in this paragraph for any authorized generic drug that was marketed during the time period covered by an annual report submitted after January 1, 1999. If information is included in the annual report with respect to any authorized generic drug, a copy of that portion of the annual report must be sent to the Food and Drug Administration, Center for Drug Evaluation and Research, Office of New Drug Quality Assessment, Bldg. 21, rm. 2562, 10903 New Hampshire Ave., Silver Spring, MD 20993-0002, and marked "Authorized Generic Submission" or, by e-mail, to the Authorized Generics electronic mailbox at AuthorizedGenerics@fda.hhs.gov with "Authorized Generic Submission" indicated in the subject line. However, at such time that FDA has required that annual reports be submitted in an electronic format, the information required by this paragraph must be submitted as part of the annual report, in the electronic format specified for submission of annual reports at that time, and not as a separate submission under the preceding sentence in this paragraph.

(iii) *Labeling.* (a) Currently used professional labeling, patient brochures or package inserts (if any), and a representative sample of the package labels.

(b) The content of labeling required under § 201.100(d)(3) of this chapter (i.e., the package insert or professional labeling), including all text, tables, and figures, must be submitted in electronic format. Electronic format submissions must be in a form that FDA can process, review, and archive. FDA will periodically issue guidance on how to provide the electronic submission (e.g., method of transmission, media, file formats, preparation and organization of files). Submissions under this paragraph must be made in accordance with part 11 of this chapter, except for the requirements of § 11.10(a), (c) through (h), and (k), and the corresponding requirements of § 11.30.

(c) A summary of any changes in labeling that have been made since the last report listed by date in the order in which they were implemented, or if no changes, a statement of that fact.

(iv) *Chemistry, manufacturing, and controls changes.* (a) Reports of experiences, investigations, studies, or tests involving chemical or physical properties, or any other properties of the drug (such as the drug's behavior or properties in relation to microorganisms, including both the effects of the drug on microorganisms and the effects of microorganisms on the drug). These reports are only required for new information that may affect FDA's previous conclusions about the safety or effectiveness of the drug product.

(b) A full description of the manufacturing and controls changes not requiring a supplemental application under § 314.70 (b) and (c), listed by date in the order in which they were implemented.

(v) *Nonclinical laboratory studies.* Copies of unpublished reports and summaries of published reports of new toxicological findings in animal studies and in vitro studies (e.g., mutagenicity) conducted by, or otherwise obtained by, the applicant concerning the ingredients in the drug product. The applicant shall submit a copy of a published report if requested by FDA.

(vi) *Clinical data.* (a) Published clinical trials of the drug (or abstracts of them), including clinical trials on safety and effectiveness; clinical trials on new uses; biopharmaceutic, pharmacokinetic, and clinical pharmacology studies; and reports of clinical experience pertinent to safety (for example, epidemiologic studies or analyses of experience in a monitored series of patients) conducted by or otherwise obtained by the applicant. Review articles, papers describing the use of the drug product in medical practice, papers and abstracts in which the drug is used as a research tool, promotional articles, press clippings, and papers that do not contain tabulations or summaries of original data should not be reported.

(b) Summaries of completed unpublished clinical trials, or prepublication manuscripts if available, conducted by, or otherwise obtained by, the applicant. Supporting information should not be reported. (A study is considered completed 1 year after it is concluded.)

(c) Analysis of available safety and efficacy data in the pediatric population and changes proposed in the labeling based on this information. An assessment of data needed to ensure appropriate labeling for the pediatric population shall be included.

(vii) *Status reports of postmarketing study commitments.* A status report of each postmarketing study of the drug product concerning clinical safety, clinical efficacy, clinical pharmacology, and nonclinical toxicology that is required by FDA (e.g., accelerated approval clinical benefit studies, pediatric studies) or that the applicant has committed, in writing, to conduct either at the time of approval of an application for the drug product or a supplement to an application, or after approval of the application or a supplement. For pediatric studies, the status report shall include a statement indicating whether postmarketing clinical studies in pediatric populations were required by FDA under § 201.23 of this chapter. The status of these postmarketing studies shall be reported annually until FDA notifies the applicant, in writing, that the agency concurs with the applicant's determination that the study commitment has been fulfilled or that the study is either no longer feasible or would no longer provide useful information.

(a) *Content of status report.* The following information must be provided for each postmarketing study reported under this paragraph:

(1) *Applicant's name.*

(2) *Product name.* Include the approved drug product's established name and proprietary name, if any.

(3) *NDA, ANDA, and supplement number.*

(4) *Date of U.S. approval of NDA or ANDA.*

(5) *Date of postmarketing study commitment.*

(6) *Description of postmarketing study commitment.* The description must include sufficient information to uniquely describe the study. This information may include the purpose of the study, the type of study, the patient population addressed by the study and the indication(s) and dosage(s) that are to be studied.

(7) *Schedule for completion and reporting of the postmarketing study commitment.* The schedule should include the actual or projected dates for submission of the study protocol to FDA, completion of patient accrual or initiation of an animal study, completion of the study, submission of the final study report to FDA, and any additional milestones or submissions for which projected dates were specified as part of the commitment. In addition, it should include a revised schedule, as appropriate. If the schedule has been previously revised, provide both the original schedule and the most recent, previously submitted revision.

(8) *Current status of the postmarketing study commitment.* The status of each postmarketing study should be categorized using one of the following terms that describes the study's status on the anniversary date of U.S. approval of the application or other agreed upon date:

(i) *Pending.* The study has not been initiated, but does not meet the criterion for delayed.

(ii) *Ongoing.* The study is proceeding according to or ahead of the original schedule described under paragraph (b)(2)(vii)(a)(7) of this section.

(iii) *Delayed.* The study is behind the original schedule described under paragraph (b)(2)(vii)(a)(7) of this section.

(iv) *Terminated.* The study was ended before completion but a final study report has not been submitted to FDA.

(v) *Submitted.* The study has been completed or terminated and a final study report has been submitted to FDA.

(9) *Explanation of the study's status.* Provide a brief description of the status of the study, including the patient accrual rate (expressed by providing the number of patients or subjects enrolled to date, and the total planned enrollment), and an explanation of the study's status identified under paragraph (b)(2)(vii)(a)(8) of this section. If the study has been completed, include the date the study was completed and the date the final study report was submitted to FDA, as applicable. Provide a revised schedule, as well as the reason(s) for the revision, if the schedule under paragraph (b)(2)(vii)(a)(7) of this section has changed since the last report.

(b) *Public disclosure of information.* Except for the information described in this paragraph, FDA may publicly disclose any information described in paragraph (b)(2)(vii) of this section, concerning a postmarketing study, if the agency determines that the information is necessary to identify the applicant or to establish the status of the study, including the reasons, if any, for failure to conduct, complete, and report the study. Under this section, FDA will not publicly disclose trade secrets, as defined in § 20.61 of this chapter, or information, described in § 20.63 of this chapter, the disclosure of which would constitute an unwarranted invasion of personal privacy.

(viii) Status of other postmarketing studies. A status report of any postmarketing study not included under paragraph (b)(2)(vii) of this section that is being performed by, or on behalf of, the applicant. A status report is to be included for any chemistry, manufacturing, and controls studies that the applicant has agreed to perform and for all product stability studies.

(ix) *Log of outstanding regulatory business.* To facilitate communications between FDA and the applicant, the report may, at the applicant's discretion, also contain a list of any open regulatory business with FDA concerning the drug product subject to the application (e.g., a list of the applicant's unanswered correspondence with the agency, a list of the agency's unanswered correspondence with the applicant).

(3) *Other reporting*—(i) *Advertisements and promotional labeling.* The applicant shall submit specimens of mailing pieces and any other labeling or advertising devised for promotion of the drug product at the time of initial dissemination of the labeling and at the time of initial publication of the advertisement for a prescription drug product. Mailing pieces and labeling that are designed to contain samples of a drug product are required to be complete, except the sample of the drug product may be omitted. Each submission is required to be accompanied by a completed transmittal Form FDA-2253 (Transmittal of Advertisements and Promotional Labeling for Drugs for Human Use) and is required to include a copy of the product's current professional labeling. Form FDA-2253 is available on the Internet at *http://www.fda.gov/opacom/morechoices/fdaforms/cder.html.*

(ii) *Special reports.* Upon written request the agency may require that the applicant submit the reports under this section at different times than those stated.

(iii) *Notification of a permanent discontinuance or an interruption in manufacturing.* (a) An applicant of a prescription drug product must notify FDA in writing of a permanent discontinuance of manufacture of the drug product or an interruption in manufacturing of the drug product that is likely to lead to a meaningful disruption in supply of that drug in the United States if:

(1) The drug product is life supporting, life sustaining, or intended for use in the prevention or treatment of a debilitating disease or condition, including any such drug used in emergency medical care or during surgery; and

(2) The drug product is not a radiopharmaceutical drug product.

(b) Notifications required by paragraph (b)(3)(iii)(a) of this section must be submitted to FDA electronically in a format that FDA can process, review, and archive:

(1) At least 6 months prior to the date of the permanent discontinuance or interruption in manufacturing; or

(2) If 6 months' advance notice is not possible because the permanent discontinuance or interruption in manufacturing was not reasonably anticipated 6 months in advance, as soon as practicable thereafter, but in no case later than 5 business days after the permanent discontinuance or interruption in manufacturing occurs.

(c) Notifications required by paragraph (b)(3)(iii)(a) of this section must include the following information:

(1) The name of the drug subject to the notification, including the NDC for such drug;

(2) The name of the applicant;

(3) Whether the notification relates to a permanent discontinuance of the drug or an interruption in manufacturing of the drug;

(4) A description of the reason for the permanent discontinuance or interruption in manufacturing; and

(5) The estimated duration of the interruption in manufacturing.

(d)(1) FDA will maintain a publicly available list of drugs that are determined by FDA to be in shortage. This drug shortages list will include the following information:

(i) The names and NDC(s) for such drugs;

(ii) The name of each applicant for such drugs;

(iii) The reason for the shortage, as determined by FDA from the following categories: Requirements related to complying with good manufacturing practices; regulatory delay; shortage of an active ingredient; shortage of an inactive ingredient component; discontinuation of the manufacture of the drug; delay in shipping of the drug; demand increase for the drug; or other reason; and

(iv) The estimated duration of the shortage.

(2) FDA may choose not to make information collected to implement this paragraph available on the drug shortages list or available under section 506C(c) of the Federal Food, Drug, and Cosmetic Act (21 U.S.C. 356c(c)) if FDA determines that disclosure of such information would adversely affect the public health (such as by increasing the possibility of hoarding or other disruption of the availability of the drug to patients). FDA will also not provide information on the public drug shortages list or under section 506C(c) of the Federal Food, Drug, and Cosmetic Act that is protected by 18 U.S.C. 1905 or 5 U.S.C. 552(b)(4), including trade secrets and commercial or financial information that is considered confidential or privileged under § 20.61 of this chapter.

(e) If an applicant fails to submit a notification as required under paragraph (b)(3)(iii)(a) of this section and in accordance with paragraph (b)(3)(iii)(b) of this section, FDA will issue a letter to the applicant informing it of such failure.

(1) Not later than 30 calendar days after the issuance of such a letter, the applicant must submit to FDA a written response setting forth the basis for noncompliance and providing the required notification under paragraph (b)(3)(iii)(a) of this section and including the information required under paragraph (b)(3)(iii)(c) of this section; and

(2) Not later than 45 calendar days after the issuance of a letter under paragraph (b)(3)(iii)(e) of this section, FDA will make the letter and the applicant's response to the letter public, unless, after review of the applicant's response, FDA determines that the applicant had a reasonable basis for not notifying FDA as required under paragraph (b)(3)(iii)(a) of this section.

(f) The following definitions of terms apply to paragraph (b)(3)(iii) of this section:

Drug shortage or shortage means a period of time when the demand or projected demand for the drug within the United States exceeds the supply of the drug.

Intended for use in the prevention or treatment of a debilitating disease or condition means a drug product intended for use in the prevention or treatment of a disease or condition associated with mortality or morbidity that has a substantial impact on day-to-day functioning.

Life supporting or life sustaining means a drug product that is essential to, or that yields information that is essential to, the restoration or continuation of a bodily function important to the continuation of human life.

Meaningful disruption means a change in production that is reasonably likely to lead to a reduction in the supply of a drug by a manufacturer that is more than negligible and affects the ability of the manufacturer to fill orders or meet expected demand for its product, and does not include interruptions in manufacturing due to matters such as routine maintenance or insignificant changes in manufacturing so long as the manufacturer expects to resume operations in a short period of time.

(iv) Withdrawal of approved drug product from sale. (a) Within 30 calendar days of the withdrawal of an approved drug from sale, applicants who are manufacturers, repackers, or relabelers subject to part 207 of this chapter must submit the following information about the drug, in accordance with the applicable requirements described in §§ 207.61 and 207.65:

(1) The National Drug Code (NDC);

(2) The identity of the drug by established name and by proprietary name, if any;

(3) The new drug application number or abbreviated application number;

(4) The date on which the drug is expected to be no longer in commercial distribution. FDA requests that the reason for withdrawal of the drug from sale be included with the information.

(b) Within 30 calendar days of the withdrawal of an approved drug from sale, applicants who are not subject to part 207 of this chapter must submit the information listed in paragraphs (b)(3)(iv)(a)(1) through (4) of this section. The information must be submitted either electronically or in writing to the Drug Registration and Listing Office, Food and Drug Administration, Center for Drug Evaluation and Research.

(c) Reporting under paragraph (b)(3)(iv)(a) of this section constitutes compliance with the requirements of § 207.57 of this chapter to update drug listing information with respect to the withdrawal from sale.

(c) General requirements—(1) *Multiple applications.* For all reports required by this section, the applicant shall submit the information common to more than one application only to the application first approved, and shall not report separately on each application. The submission is required to identify all the applications to which the report applies.

(2) Patient identification. Applicants should not include in reports under this section the names and addresses of individual patients; instead, the applicant should code the patient names whenever possible and retain the code in the applicant's files. The applicant shall maintain sufficient pa-

tient identification information to permit FDA, by using that information alone or along with records maintained by the investigator of a study, to identify the name and address of individual patients; this will ordinarily occur only when the agency needs to investigate the reports further or when there is reason to believe that the reports do not represent actual results obtained.

(d) Withdrawal of approval. If an applicant fails to make reports required under this section, FDA may withdraw approval of the application and, thus, prohibit continued marketing of the drug product that is the subject of the application.

(Collection of information requirements approved by the Office of Management and Budget under control number 0910-0001)

[50 FR 7493, Feb. 22, 1985; 50 FR 14212, Apr. 11, 1985, as amended at 50 FR 21238, May 23, 1985; 55 FR 11580, Mar. 29, 1990; 57 FR 17983, Apr. 28, 1992; 63 FR 66670, Dec. 2, 1998; 64 FR 401, Jan. 5, 1999; 65 FR 64617, Oct. 30, 2000; 66 FR 10815, Feb. 20, 2001; 68 FR 69019, Dec. 11, 2003; 69 FR 18766, Apr. 8, 2004; 69 FR 48775, Aug. 11, 2004; 72 FR 58999, Oct. 18, 2007; 74 FR 13113, Mar. 26, 2009; 74 FR 37167, July 28, 2009; 76 FR 78539, Dec. 19, 2011; 80 FR 38938, July 8, 2015; 81 FR 60221, Aug. 31, 2016]

§ 314.90 Waivers.

(a) An applicant may ask the Food and Drug Administration to waive under this section any requirement that applies to the applicant under §§ 314.50 through 314.81. An applicant may ask FDA to waive under § 314.126(c) any criteria of an adequate and well-controlled study described in § 314.126(b). A waiver request under this section is required to be submitted with supporting documentation in an NDA, or in an amendment or supplement to an NDA. The waiver request is required to contain one of the following:

(1) An explanation why the applicant's compliance with the requirement is unnecessary or cannot be achieved;

(2) A description of an alternative submission that satisfies the purpose of the requirement; or

(3) Other information justifying a waiver.

(b) FDA may grant a waiver if it finds one of the following:

(1) The applicant's compliance with the requirement is unnecessary for the agency to evaluate the NDA or compliance cannot be achieved;

(2) The applicant's alternative submission satisfies the requirement; or

(3) The applicant's submission otherwise justifies a waiver.

(c) If FDA grants the applicant's waiver request with respect to a requirement under §§ 314.50 through 314.81, the waived requirement will not constitute a basis for refusal to approve an NDA under § 314.125.

[50 FR 7493, Feb. 22, 1985, as amended at 50 FR 21238, May 23, 1985; 67 FR 9586, Mar. 4, 2002; 81 FR 69649, Oct. 6, 2016]

Subpart C—Abbreviated Applications

Source: 57 FR 17983, Apr. 28, 1992, unless otherwise noted.

§ 314.92 Drug products for which abbreviated applications may be submitted.

(a) Abbreviated applications are suitable for the following drug products within the limits set forth under § 314.93:

(1) Drug products that are the same as a listed drug. A "listed drug" is defined in § 314.3. For determining the suitability of an abbreviated new drug application, the term "same as" means identical in active ingredient(s), dosage form, strength, route of administration, and conditions of use, except

that conditions of use for which approval cannot be granted because of exclusivity or an existing patent may be omitted. If a listed drug has been voluntarily withdrawn from or not offered for sale by its manufacturer, a person who wishes to submit an abbreviated new drug application for the drug shall comply with § 314.122.

(2) [Reserved]

(3) Drug products that have been declared suitable for an abbreviated new drug application submission by FDA through the petition procedures set forth under § 10.30 of this chapter and § 314.93.

(b) FDA will publish in the list listed drugs for which abbreviated applications may be submitted. The list is available from the Superintendent of Documents, U.S. Government Printing Office, Washington, DC 20402, 202-783-3238.

[57 FR 17983, Apr. 28, 1992, as amended at 64 FR 401, Jan. 5, 1999]

§ 314.93 Petition to request a change from a listed drug.

(a) The only changes from a listed drug for which the agency will accept a petition under this section are those changes described in paragraph (b) of this section. Petitions to submit ANDAs for other changes from a listed drug will not be approved.

(b) A person who wants to submit an ANDA for a drug product which is not identical to a listed drug in route of administration, dosage form, and strength, or in which one active ingredient is substituted for one of the active ingredients in a listed combination drug, must first obtain permission from FDA to submit such an ANDA.

(c) To obtain permission to submit an ANDA for a change described in paragraph (b) of this section, a person must submit and obtain approval of a petition requesting the change. A person seeking permission to request such a change from a reference listed drug shall submit a petition in accordance with § 10.20 of this chapter and in the format specified in § 10.30 of this chapter. The petition shall contain the information specified in § 10.30 of this chapter and any additional information required by this section. If any provision of § 10.20 or § 10.30 of this chapter is inconsistent with any provision of this section, the provisions of this section apply.

(d) The petitioner shall identify a listed drug and include a copy of the proposed labeling for the drug product that is the subject of the petition and a copy of the approved labeling for the listed drug. The petitioner may, under limited circumstances, identify more than one listed drug, for example, when the proposed drug product is a combination product that differs from the combination reference listed drug with regard to an active ingredient, and the different active ingredient is an active ingredient of a listed drug. The petitioner shall also include information to show that:

(1) The active ingredients of the proposed drug product are of the same pharmacological or therapeutic class as those of the reference listed drug.

(2) The drug product can be expected to have the same therapeutic effect as the reference listed drug when administered to patients for each condition of use in the reference listed drug's labeling for which the applicant seeks approval.

(3) If the proposed drug product is a combination product with one different active ingredient, including a different ester or salt, from the reference listed drug, that the different active ingredient has previously been approved in a listed drug or is a drug that does not meet the definition of "new drug" in section 201(p) of the Federal Food, Drug, and Cosmetic Act.

(e) No later than 90 days after the date a petition that is permitted under paragraph (a) of this section is submitted, FDA will approve or disapprove the petition.

(1) FDA will approve a petition properly submited under this section unless it finds that:

(i) Investigations must be conducted to show the safety and effectiveness of the drug product or of any of its active ingredients, its route of administration, dosage form, or strength which differs from the reference listed drug; or

(ii) For a petition that seeks to change an active ingredient, the drug product that is the subject of the petition is not a combination drug; or

(iii) For a combination drug product that is the subject of the petition and has an active ingredient different from the reference listed drug:

(A) The drug product may not be adequately evaluated for approval as safe and effective on the basis of the information required to be submitted under § 314.94; or

(B) The petition does not contain information to show that the different active ingredient of the drug product is of the same pharmacological or therapeutic class as the ingredient of the reference listed drug that is to be changed and that the drug product can be expected to have the same therapeutic effect as the reference listed drug when administered to patients for each condition of use in the listed drug's labeling for which the applicant seeks approval; or

(C) The different active ingredient is not an active ingredient in a listed drug or a drug that meets the requirements of section 201(p) of the Federal Food, Drug, and Cosmetic Act; or

(D) The remaining active ingredients are not identical to those of the listed combination drug; or

(iv) Any of the proposed changes from the listed drug would jeopardize the safe or effective use of the product so as to necessitate significant labeling changes to address the newly introduced safety or effectiveness problem; or

(v) FDA has determined that the reference listed drug has been withdrawn from sale for safety or effectiveness reasons under § 314.161, or the reference listed drug has been voluntarily withdrawn from sale and the agency has not determined whether the withdrawal is for safety or effectiveness reasons; or

(vi) A drug product is approved in an NDA for the change described in the petition.

(2) For purposes of this paragraph, "investigations must be conducted" means that information derived from animal or clinical studies is necessary to show that the drug product is safe or effective. Such information may be contained in published or unpublished reports.

(3) If FDA approves a petition submitted under this section, the agency's response may describe what additional information, if any, will be required to support an ANDA for the drug product. FDA may, at any time during the course of its review of an ANDA, request additional information required to evaluate the change approved under the petition.

(f)(1) FDA may withdraw approval of a petition if the agency receives any information demonstrating that the petition no longer satisfies the conditions under paragraph (e) of this section.

(2) If, after approval of a petition and before approval of an ANDA submitted pursuant to the approved petition, a drug product is approved in an NDA for the change described in the petition, the petition and the listed drug identified in the petition can no longer be the basis for ANDA submission, irrespective of whether FDA has withdrawn approval of the petition. A person seeking approval for such drug product must submit a new ANDA that identifies the pharmaceutically equivalent reference listed drug as the basis for ANDA submission and comply with applicable regulatory requirements.

[57 FR 17983, Apr. 28, 1992, as amended at 81 FR 69649, Oct. 6, 2016]

§ 314.94 Content and format of an ANDA.

ANDAs are required to be submitted in the form and contain the information required under this section. Three copies of the ANDA are required, an archival copy, a review copy, and a field copy. FDA will maintain guidance documents on the format and content of ANDAs to assist applicants in their preparation.

(a) *ANDAs.* Except as provided in paragraph (b) of this section, the applicant must submit a complete archival copy of the abbreviated new drug application that includes the following:

(1) *Application form.* The applicant must submit a completed and signed application form that contains the information described under § 314.50(a)(1), (a)(3), (a)(4), and (a)(5). The applicant must state whether the submission is an ANDA under this section or a supplement to an ANDA under § 314.97.

(2) *Table of contents.* The archival copy of the ANDA is required to contain a table of contents that shows the volume number and page number of the contents of the submission.

(3) *Basis for ANDA submission.* An ANDA must refer to a listed drug. Ordinarily, that listed drug will be the drug product selected by the Agency as the reference standard for conducting bioequivalence testing. The ANDA must contain:

(i) The name of the reference listed drug, including its dosage form and strength. For an ANDA based on an approved petition under § 10.30 of this chapter and § 314.93, the reference listed drug must be the same as the listed drug referenced in the approved petition.

(ii) A statement as to whether, according to the information published in the list, the reference listed drug is entitled to a period of marketing exclusivity under section 505(j)(5)(F) of the Federal Food, Drug, and Cosmetic Act.

(iii) For an ANDA based on an approved petition under § 10.30 of this chapter and § 314.93, a reference to the FDA-assigned docket number for the petition and a copy of FDA's correspondence approving the petition.

(4) *Conditions of use.* (i) A statement that the conditions of use prescribed, recommended, or suggested in the labeling proposed for the drug product have been previously approved for the reference listed drug.

(ii) A reference to the applicant's annotated proposed labeling and to the currently approved labeling for the reference listed drug provided under paragraph (a)(8) of this section.

(5) *Active ingredients.* (i) For a single-active-ingredient drug product, information to show that the active ingredient is the same as that of the reference single-active-ingredient listed drug, as follows:

(A) A statement that the active ingredient of the proposed drug product is the same as that of the reference listed drug.

(B) A reference to the applicant's annotated proposed labeling and to the currently approved labeling for the reference listed drug provided under paragraph (a)(8) of this section.

(ii) For a combination drug product, information to show that the active ingredients are the same as those of the reference listed drug except for any different active ingredient that has been the subject of an approved petition, as follows:

(A) A statement that the active ingredients of the proposed drug product are the same as those of the reference listed drug, or if one of the active ingredients differs from one of the active ingredients of the reference listed drug and the ANDA is submitted under the approval of a petition under § 314.93 to vary such active ingredient, information to show that the other active ingredients of the drug product are the same as the other active ingredients of the reference listed drug, information to show that the different active ingredient is an active ingredient of another listed drug or of a drug that does not meet the definition of "new drug" in section 201(p) of the Federal Food, Drug, and Cosmetic Act, and such other information about the different active ingredient that FDA may require.

(B) A reference to the applicant's annotated proposed labeling and to the currently approved labeling for the reference listed drug provided under paragraph (a)(8) of this section.

(6) *Route of administration, dosage form, and strength.* (i) Information to show that the route of administration, dosage form, and strength of the drug product are the same as those of the reference listed drug except for any differences that have been the subject of an approved petition, as follows:

(A) A statement that the route of administration, dosage form, and strength of the proposed drug product are the same as those of the reference listed drug.

(B) A reference to the applicant's annotated proposed labeling and to the currently approved labeling for the reference listed drug provided under paragraph (a)(8) of this section.

(ii) If the route of administration, dosage form, or strength of the drug product differs from the reference listed drug and the ANDA is submitted under an approved petition under § 314.93, such information about the different route of administration, dosage form, or strength that FDA may require.

(7) *Bioequivalence*. (i) Information that shows that the drug product is bioequivalent to the reference listed drug upon which the applicant relies. A complete study report must be submitted for the bioequivalence study upon which the applicant relies for approval. For all other bioequivalence studies conducted on the same drug product formulation as defined in § 314.3(b), the applicant must submit either a complete or summary report. If a summary report of a bioequivalence study is submitted and FDA determines that there may be bioequivalence issues or concerns with the product, FDA may require that the applicant submit a complete report of the bioequivalence study to FDA; or

(ii) If the ANDA is submitted pursuant to a petition approved under § 314.93, the results of any bioavailability or bioequivalence testing required by the Agency, or any other information required by the Agency to show that the active ingredients of the proposed drug product are of the same pharmacological or therapeutic class as those in the reference listed drug and that the proposed drug product can be expected to have the same therapeutic effect as the reference listed drug. If the proposed drug product contains a different active ingredient than the reference listed drug, FDA will consider the proposed drug product to have the same therapeutic effect as the reference listed drug if the applicant provides information demonstrating that:

(A) There is an adequate scientific basis for determining that substitution of the specific proposed dose of the different active ingredient for the dose of the member of the same pharmacological or therapeutic class in the reference listed drug will yield a resulting drug product whose safety and effectiveness have not been adversely affected.

(B) The unchanged active ingredients in the proposed drug product are bioequivalent to those in the reference listed drug.

(C) The different active ingredient in the proposed drug product is bioequivalent to an approved dosage form containing that ingredient and approved for the same indication as the proposed drug product or is bioequivalent to a drug product offered for that indication which does not meet the definition of "new drug" under section 201(p) of the Federal Food, Drug, and Cosmetic Act.

(iii) For each in vivo or in vitro bioequivalence study contained in the ANDA:

(A) A description of the analytical and statistical methods used in each study; and

(B) With respect to each study involving human subjects, a statement that the study either was conducted in compliance with the institutional review board regulations in part 56 of this chapter, or was not subject to the regulations under § 56.104 or § 56.105 of this chapter, and that it was conducted in compliance with the informed consent regulations in part 50 of this chapter.

(8) *Labeling*—(i) *Listed drug labeling.* A copy of the currently approved labeling (including, if applicable, any Medication Guide required under part 208 of this chapter) for the listed drug referred to in the ANDA, if the ANDA relies on a reference listed drug.

(ii) *Copies of proposed labeling.* Copies of the label and all labeling for the drug product including, if applicable, any Medication Guide required under part 208 of this chapter (4 copies of draft labeling or 12 copies of final printed labeling).

(iii) *Statement on proposed labeling.* A statement that the applicant's proposed labeling including, if applicable, any Medication Guide required under part 208 of this chapter is the same as the labeling of the reference listed drug except for differences annotated and explained under paragraph (a)(8)(iv) of this section.

(iv) *Comparison of approved and proposed labeling.* A side-by-side comparison of the applicant's proposed labeling including, if applicable, any Medication Guide required under part 208 of this chapter with the approved labeling for the reference listed drug with all differences annotated and explained. Labeling (including the container label, package insert, and, if applicable, Medication Guide) proposed for the drug product must be the same as the labeling approved for the reference listed drug, except for changes required because of differences approved under a petition filed under § 314.93 or because the drug product and the reference listed drug are produced or distributed by different manufacturers. Such differences between the applicant's proposed labeling and labeling approved for the reference listed drug may include differences in expiration date, formulation, bioavailability, or pharmacokinetics, labeling revisions made to comply with current FDA labeling guidelines or other guidance, or omission of an indication or other aspect of labeling protected by patent or accorded exclusivity under section 505(j)(5)(F) of the Federal Food, Drug, and Cosmetic Act.

(9) *Chemistry, manufacturing, and controls.* (i) The information required under § 314.50(d)(1), except that the information required under § 314.50(d)(1)(ii)(c) must contain the proposed or actual master production record, including a description of the equipment, to be used for the manufacture of a commercial lot of the drug product.

(ii) *Inactive ingredients.* Unless otherwise stated in paragraphs (a)(9)(iii) through (a)(9)(v) of this section, an applicant must identify and characterize the inactive ingredients in the proposed drug product and provide information demonstrating that such inactive ingredients do not affect the safety or efficacy of the proposed drug product.

(iii) *Inactive ingredient changes permitted in drug products intended for parenteral use.* Generally, a drug product intended for parenteral use must contain the same inactive ingredients and in the same concentration as the reference listed drug identified by the applicant under paragraph (a)(3) of this section. However, an applicant may seek approval of a drug product that differs from the reference listed drug in preservative, buffer, or antioxidant provided that the applicant identifies and characterizes the differences and provides information demonstrating that the differences do not affect the safety or efficacy of the proposed drug product.

(iv) *Inactive ingredient changes permitted in drug products intended for ophthalmic or otic use.* Generally, a drug product intended for ophthalmic or otic use must contain the same inactive ingredients and in the same concentration as the reference listed drug identified by the applicant under paragraph (a)(3) of this section. However, an applicant may seek approval of a drug product that differs from the reference listed drug in preservative, buffer, substance to adjust tonicity, or thickening agent provided that the applicant identifies and characterizes the differences and provides information demonstrating that the differences do not affect the safety or efficacy of the proposed drug product, except that, in a product intended for ophthalmic use, an applicant may not change a buffer or substance to adjust tonicity for the purpose of claiming a therapeutic advantage over or difference from the listed drug, e.g., by using a balanced salt solution as a diluent as opposed to an isotonic saline solution, or by making a significant change in the pH or other change that may raise questions of irritability.

(v) *Inactive ingredient changes permitted in drug products intended for topical use.* Generally, a drug product intended for topical use, solutions for aerosolization or nebulization, and nasal solutions shall contain the same inactive ingredients as the reference listed drug identified by the applicant under paragraph (a)(3) of this section. However, an ANDA may include different inactive ingredients provided that the applicant identifies and characterizes the differences and provides information demonstrating that the differences do not affect the safety or efficacy of the proposed drug product.

(10) *Samples.* The information required under § 314.50(e)(1) and (e)(2)(i). Samples need not be submitted until requested by FDA.

(11) *Other.* The information required under § 314.50(g).

(12) *Patent certification*—(i) *Patents claiming drug substance, drug product, or method of use.* (A) An appropriate patent certification or statement with respect to each patent issued by the U.S. Patent and Trademark Office that, in the opinion of the applicant and to the best of its knowledge, claims the reference listed drug or that claims a use of such listed drug for which the applicant is seeking approval under section 505(j) of the Federal Food, Drug, and Cosmetic Act and for which information is required to be filed under section 505(b) and (c) of the Federal Food, Drug, and Cosmetic Act and § 314.53. For each such patent, the applicant must provide the patent number and certify, in its opinion and to the best of its knowledge, one of the following circumstances:

(1) That the patent information has not been submitted to FDA. The applicant must entitle such a certification "Paragraph I Certification";

(2) That the patent has expired. The applicant must entitle such a certification "Paragraph II Certification";

(3) The date on which the patent will expire. The applicant must entitle such a certification "Paragraph III Certification"; or

(4)(i) That the patent is invalid, unenforceable, or will not be infringed by the manufacture, use, or sale of the drug product for which the ANDA is submitted. The applicant must entitle such a certification "Paragraph IV Certification". This certification must be submitted in the following form:

> I, *(name of applicant)*, certify that Patent No. ______ *(is invalid, unenforceable, or will not be infringed by the manufacture, use, or sale of) (name of proposed drug product)* for which this ANDA is submitted.

(ii) The certification must be accompanied by a statement that the applicant will comply with the requirements under § 314.95(a) with respect to providing a notice to each owner of the patent or its representative and to the NDA holder (or, if the NDA holder does not reside or maintain a place of business within the United States, its attorney, agent, or other authorized official) for the listed drug, with the requirements under § 314.95(b) with respect to sending the notice, and with the requirements under § 314.95(c) with respect to the content of the notice.

(B) If the ANDA refers to a listed drug that is itself a licensed generic product of a patented drug first approved under section 505(b) of the Federal Food, Drug, and Cosmetic Act, an appropriate patent certification or statement under paragraph (a)(12)(i) and/or (iii) of this section with respect to each patent that claims the first-approved patented drug or that claims a use for such drug.

(ii) *No relevant patents.* If, in the opinion of the applicant and to the best of its knowledge, there are no patents described in paragraph (a)(12)(i) of this section, a certification in the following form:

> In the opinion and to the best knowledge of (name of applicant), there are no patents that claim the listed drug referred to in this ANDA or that claim a use of the listed drug.

(iii) *Method-of-use patent.* (A) If patent information is submitted under section 505(b) or (c) of the Federal Food, Drug, and Cosmetic Act and § 314.53 for a patent claiming a method of using the listed drug, and the labeling for the drug product for which the applicant is seeking approval does not include an indication or other condition of use that is covered by the method-of-use patent, a statement explaining that the method-of-use patent does not claim a proposed indication or other condition of use.

(B) If the labeling of the drug product for which the applicant is seeking approval includes an indication or other condition of use that, according to the patent information submitted under section 505(b) or (c) of the Federal Food, Drug, and Cosmetic Act and § 314.53 or in the opinion of the applicant, is claimed by a method-of-use patent, an applicable certification under paragraph (a)(12)(i) of this section.

(iv) [Reserved]

(v) *Licensing agreements.* If the ANDA is for a drug or method of using a drug claimed by a patent and the applicant has a licensing agreement with the patent owner, the applicant must submit a paragraph IV certification as to that patent and a statement that the applicant has been granted a patent license. If the patent owner consents to approval of the ANDA (if otherwise eligible for approval) as of a specific date, the ANDA must contain a written statement from the patent owner that it has a licensing agreement with the applicant and that it consents to approval of the ANDA as of a specific date.

(vi) *Untimely filing of patent information.* (A) If a patent on the listed drug is issued and the holder of the approved NDA for the listed drug does not file with FDA the required information on the patent within 30 days of issuance of the patent, an applicant who submitted an ANDA for that drug that contained an appropriate patent certification or statement before the submission of the patent information is not required to submit a patent certification or statement to address the patent or patent information that is late-listed with respect to the pending ANDA. Except as provided in § 314.53(f)(1), an NDA holder's amendment to the description of the approved method(s) of use claimed by the patent will be considered untimely filing of patent information unless:

(1) The amendment to the description of the approved method(s) of use claimed by the patent is submitted within 30 days of patent issuance;

(2) The amendment to the description of the approved method(s) of use claimed by the patent is submitted within 30 days of approval of a corresponding change to product labeling; or

(3) The amendment to the description of the approved method(s) of use claimed by the patent is submitted within 30 days of a decision by the U.S. Patent and Trademark Office or by a Federal district court, the Court of Appeals for the Federal Circuit, or the U.S. Supreme Court that is specific to the patent and alters the construction of a method-of-use claim(s) of the patent, and the amendment contains a copy of the decision.

(B) An applicant whose ANDA is submitted after the NDA holder's untimely filing of patent information, or whose pending ANDA was previously submitted but did not contain an appropriate patent certification or statement at the time of the patent submission, must submit a certification under paragraph (a)(12)(i) of this section and/or a statement under paragraph (a)(12)(iii) of this section as to that patent.

(vii) *Disputed patent information.* If an applicant disputes the accuracy or relevance of patent information submitted to FDA, the applicant may seek a confirmation of the correctness of the patent information in accordance with the procedures under § 314.53(f). Unless the patent information is withdrawn, the applicant must submit an appropriate certification or statement for each listed patent.

(viii) *Amended certifications.* A patent certification or statement submitted under paragraphs (a)(12)(i) through (iii) of this section may be amended at any time before the approval of the ANDA. If an applicant with a pending ANDA voluntarily makes a patent certification for an untimely filed patent, the applicant may withdraw the patent certification for the untimely filed patent. An applicant must submit an amended certification as an amendment to a pending ANDA. Once an amendment is submitted to change a certification, the ANDA will no longer be considered to contain the prior certification.

(A) *After finding of infringement.* An applicant who has submitted a paragraph IV certification and is sued for patent infringement must submit an amendment to change its certification if a court enters a final decision from which no appeal has been or can be taken, or signs and enters a settlement order or consent decree in the action that includes a finding that the patent is infringed, unless the final decision, settlement order, or consent decree also finds the patent to be invalid. In its amendment, the applicant must certify under paragraph (a)(12)(i)(A)(3) of this section that the patent will expire on a specific date or, with respect to a patent claiming a method of use, the applicant may instead provide a statement under paragraph (a)(12)(iii) of this section if the applicant amends its ANDA such that the applicant is no longer seeking approval for a method of use claimed by the patent. Once an amendment for the change has been submitted, the ANDA will no longer be considered to contain a paragraph IV certification to the patent. If a final judgment finds the patent to be invalid and infringed, an amended certification is not required.

(B) *After request to remove a patent or patent information from the list.* If the list reflects that an NDA holder has requested that a patent or patent information be removed from the list and no ANDA applicant is eligible for 180-day exclusivity based on a paragraph IV certification to that patent, the patent or patent information will be removed and any applicant with a pending ANDA (including a tentatively approved ANDA) who has made a certification with respect to such patent must submit an amendment to withdraw its certification. In the amendment, the applicant must state the reason for withdrawing the certification or statement (that the patent has been removed from the list). If the list reflects that an NDA holder has requested that a patent or patent information be removed from the list and one or more first applicants are eligible for 180-day exclusivity based on a paragraph IV certification to that patent, the patent will remain listed until any 180-day exclusivity based on that patent has expired or has been extinguished. After any applicable 180-day exclusivity has expired or has been extinguished, the patent or patent information will be removed and any applicant with a pending ANDA (including a tentatively approved ANDA) who has made a certification with respect to such patent must submit an amendment to withdraw its certification. Once an amendment to withdraw the certification has been submitted, the ANDA will no longer be considered to contain a paragraph IV certification to the patent. If removal of a patent from the list results in there being no patents listed for the listed drug identified in the ANDA, the applicant must submit an amended certification reflecting that there are no relevant patents.

(C) *Other amendments.* (1) Except as provided in paragraphs (a)(12)(vi) and (a)(12)(viii)(C)(2) of this section:

(i) An applicant must amend a submitted certification or statement if, at any time before the date of approval of the ANDA, the applicant learns that the submitted certification or statement is no longer accurate; and

(ii) An applicant must submit an appropriate patent certification or statement under paragraph (a)(12)(i) and/or (iii) of this section if, after submission of the ANDA, a new patent is issued by the U.S. Patent and Trademark Office that, in the opinion of the applicant and to the best of its knowledge, claims the reference listed drug or that claims an approved use for such reference listed drug and for which information is required to be filed under section 505(b) and (c) of the Federal Food, Drug, and Cosmetic Act and § 314.53. For a paragraph IV certification, the certification must not be submitted earlier than the first working day after the day the patent is published in the list.

(2) An applicant is not required to submit a supplement to change a submitted certification when information on a patent on the listed drug is submitted after the approval of the ANDA.

(13) *Financial certification or disclosure statement.* An ANDA must contain a financial certification or disclosure statement as required by part 54 of this chapter.

(b) *Drug products subject to the Drug Efficacy Study Implementation (DESI) review.* If the ANDA is for a duplicate of a drug product that is subject to FDA's DESI review (a review of drug products approved as safe between 1938 and 1962) or other DESI-like review and the drug product evaluated in the review is a listed drug, the applicant must comply with the provisions of paragraph (a) of this section.

(c) [Reserved]

(d) *Format of an ANDA.* (1) The applicant must submit a complete archival copy of the ANDA as required under paragraphs (a) and (c) of this section. FDA will maintain the archival copy during the review of the ANDA to permit individual reviewers to refer to information that is not contained in their particular technical sections of the ANDA, to give other Agency personnel access to the ANDA for official business, and to maintain in one place a complete copy of the ANDA.

(i) *Format of submission.* An applicant may submit portions of the archival copy of the ANDA in any form that the applicant and FDA agree is acceptable, except as provided in paragraph (d)(1)(ii) of this section.

(ii) *Labeling.* The content of labeling required under § 201.100(d)(3) of this chapter (commonly referred to as the package insert or professional labeling), including all text, tables, and figures, must be submitted to the agency in electronic format as described in paragraph (d)(1)(iii) of this section. This requirement applies to the content of labeling for the proposed drug product only and is in addition to the requirements of paragraph (a)(8)(ii) of this section that copies of the formatted label and all proposed labeling be submitted. Submissions under this paragraph must be made in accordance with part 11 of this chapter, except for the requirements of § 11.10(a), (c) through (h), and (k), and the corresponding requirements of § 11.30.

(iii) *Electronic format submissions.* Electronic format submissions must be in a form that FDA can process, review, and archive. FDA will periodically issue guidance on how to provide the electronic submission (e.g., method of transmission, media, file formats, preparation and organization of files).

(2) For ANDAs, the applicant must submit a review copy of the ANDA that contains two separate sections. One section must contain the information described under paragraphs (a)(2) through (6) and (8) and (9) of this section and section 505(j)(2)(A)(vii) of the Federal Food, Drug, and Cosmetic Act and a copy of the analytical procedures and descriptive information needed by FDA's laboratories to perform tests on samples of the proposed drug product and to validate the applicant's analytical procedures. The other section must contain the information described under paragraphs (a)(3), (7), and (8) of this section. Each of the sections in the review copy is required to contain a copy of the application form described under paragraph (a) of this section.

(3) [Reserved]

(4) The applicant may obtain from FDA sufficient folders to bind the archival, the review, and the field copies of the ANDA.

(5) The applicant must submit a field copy of the ANDA that contains the technical section described in paragraph (a)(9) of this section, a copy of the application form required under paragraph (a)(1) of this section, and a certification that the field copy is a true copy of the technical section described in paragraph (a)(9) of this section contained in the archival and review copies of the ANDA.

[57 FR 17983, Apr. 28, 1992; 57 FR 29353, July 1, 1992, as amended at 58 FR 47352, Sept. 8, 1993; 59 FR 50364, Oct. 3, 1994; 63 FR 5252, Feb. 2, 1998; 63 FR 66399, Dec. 1, 1998; 64 FR 401, Jan. 5, 1999; 65 FR

56479, Sept. 19, 2000; 67 FR 77672, Dec. 19, 2002; 68 FR 69019, Dec. 11, 2003; 69 FR 18766, Apr. 8, 2004; 74 FR 2861, Jan. 16, 2009; 76 FR 13880, Mar. 15, 2011; 81 FR 69649, Oct. 6, 2016]

§ 314.95 Notice of certification of invalidity, unenforceability, or noninfringement of a patent.

(a) *Notice of certification.* For each patent that claims the listed drug or that claims a use for such listed drug for which the applicant is seeking approval and for which the applicant submits a paragraph IV certification, the applicant must send notice of such certification by registered or certified mail, return receipt requested, or by a designated delivery service, as defined in paragraph (g) of this section to each of the following persons:

(1) Each owner of the patent that is the subject of the certification or the representative designated by the owner to receive the notice. The name and address of the patent owner or its representative may be obtained from the U.S. Patent and Trademark Office; and

(2) The holder of the approved NDA under section 505(b) of the Federal Food, Drug, and Cosmetic Act for the listed drug that is claimed by the patent and for which the applicant is seeking approval, or, if the NDA holder does not reside or maintain a place of business within the United States, the NDA holder's attorney, agent, or other authorized official. The name and address of the NDA holder or its attorney, agent, or authorized official may be obtained by sending a written or electronic communication to the Orange Book Staff, Office of Generic Drugs, 7620 Standish Pl., Rockville, MD 20855 or to the Orange Book Staff at the email address listed on the Agency's Web site at *http://www.fda.gov.*

(3) This paragraph (a) does not apply to a method-of-use patent that does not claim a use for which the applicant is seeking approval.

(4) An applicant may send notice by an alternative method only if FDA has agreed in advance that the method will produce an acceptable form of documentation.

(b) *Sending the notice.* (1) Except as provided under paragraph (d) of this section, the applicant must send the notice required by paragraph (a) of this section on or after the date it receives a paragraph IV acknowledgment letter from FDA, but not later than 20 days after the date of the postmark on the paragraph IV acknowledgment letter. The 20-day clock described in this paragraph (b) begins on the day after the date of the postmark on the paragraph IV acknowledgment letter. When the 20th day falls on Saturday, Sunday, or a Federal holiday, the 20th day will be the next day that is not a Saturday, Sunday, or Federal holiday.

(2) Any notice required by paragraph (a) of this section is invalid if it is sent before the applicant's receipt of a paragraph IV acknowledgment letter, or before the first working day after the day the patent is published in the list. The applicant will not have complied with this paragraph (b) until it sends valid notice.

(3) The applicant must submit to FDA an amendment to its ANDA that includes a statement certifying that the notice has been provided to each person identified under paragraph (a) of this section and that the notice met the content requirements under paragraph (c) of this section. A copy of the notice itself need not be submitted to the Agency.

(c) *Contents of a notice.* In the notice, the applicant must cite section 505(j)(2)(B)(iv) of the Federal Food, Drug, and Cosmetic Act and the notice must include, but is not limited to, the following information:

(1) A statement that FDA has received an ANDA submitted by the applicant containing any required bioavailability or bioequivalence data or information.

(2) The ANDA number.

(3) A statement that the applicant has received the paragraph IV acknowledgment letter for the ANDA.

(4) The established name, if any, as defined in section 502(e)(3) of the Federal Food, Drug, and Cosmetic Act, of the proposed drug product.

(5) The active ingredient, strength, and dosage form of the proposed drug product.

(6) The patent number and expiration date of each listed patent for the reference listed drug alleged to be invalid, unenforceable, or not infringed.

(7) A detailed statement of the factual and legal basis of the applicant's opinion that the patent is not valid, unenforceable, or will not be infringed. The applicant must include in the detailed statement:

(i) For each claim of a patent alleged not to be infringed, a full and detailed explanation of why the claim is not infringed.

(ii) For each claim of a patent alleged to be invalid or unenforceable, a full and detailed explanation of the grounds supporting the allegation.

(8) If the applicant alleges that the patent will not be infringed and the applicant seeks to preserve the option to later file a civil action for declaratory judgment in accordance with section 505(j)(5)(C) of the Federal Food, Drug, and Cosmetic Act, then the notice must be accompanied by an offer of confidential access to the ANDA for the sole and limited purpose of evaluating possible infringement of the patent that is the subject of the paragraph IV certification.

(9) If the applicant does not reside or have a place of business in the United States, the name and address of an agent in the United States authorized to accept service of process for the applicant.

(d) *Amendment or supplement to an ANDA.* (1) If, after receipt of a paragraph IV acknowledgment letter or acknowledgment letter, an applicant submits an amendment or supplement to its ANDA that includes a paragraph IV certification, the applicant must send the notice required by paragraph (a) of this section at the same time that the amendment or supplement to the ANDA is submitted to FDA, regardless of whether the applicant has already given notice with respect to another such certification contained in the ANDA or in an amendment or supplement to the ANDA.

(2) If, before receipt of a paragraph IV acknowledgment letter, an applicant submits an amendment to its ANDA that includes a paragraph IV certification, the applicant must send the notice required by paragraph (a) of this section in accordance with the procedures in paragraph (b) of this section. If an ANDA applicant's notice of its paragraph IV certification is timely provided in accordance with paragraph (b) of this section and the applicant has not submitted a previous paragraph IV certification, FDA will base its determination of whether the applicant is a first applicant on the date of submission of the amendment containing the paragraph IV certification.

(3) An applicant that submits an amendment or supplement to seek approval of a different strength must provide notice of any paragraph IV certification in accordance with paragraph (d)(1) or (2) of this section, as applicable.

(e) *Documentation of timely sending and receipt of notice.* The applicant must amend its ANDA to provide documentation of the date of receipt of the notice required under paragraph (a) of this section by each person provided the notice. The amendment must be submitted to FDA within 30 days after the last date on which notice was received by a person described in paragraph (a) of this section. The applicant's amendment also must include documentation that its notice was sent on a date that complies with the timeframe required by paragraph (b) or (d) of this section, as applicable, and a dated printout of the entry for the reference listed drug in FDA's "Approved Drug Products With Therapeutic Equivalence Evaluations" (the list) that includes the patent that is the subject of the paragraph IV certification. FDA will accept, as adequate documentation of the date the notice was sent, a copy of the registered mail receipt, certified mail receipt, or receipt from a designated delivery service as defined in paragraph (g) of this section. FDA will accept as adequate documentation of the date of receipt a return receipt, signature proof of delivery by a designated delivery service, or a letter acknowledging receipt by the person provided the notice. An applicant may rely on another form of documentation only if FDA has agreed to such documentation in advance. A copy of the notice itself need not be submitted to the Agency.

(f) *Forty-five day period after receipt of notice.* If the requirements of this section are met, FDA will presume the notice to be complete and sufficient, and it will count the day following the date of receipt of the notice by the patent owner or its representative and by the approved NDA holder or its attorney, agent, or other authorized official as the first day of the 45-day period provided for in section 505(j)(5)(B)(iii) of the Federal Food, Drug, and Cosmetic Act. FDA may, if the applicant provides a written statement to FDA that a later date should be used, count from such later date.

(g) *Designated delivery services.* (1) For purposes of this section, the term "designated delivery service" means any delivery service provided by a trade or business that the Agency determines:

(i) Is available to the general public throughout the United States;

(ii) Records electronically to its database, kept in the regular course of its business, or marks on the cover in which any item referred to in this section is to be delivered, the date on which such item was given to such trade or business for delivery; and

(iii) Provides overnight or 2-day delivery service throughout the United States.

(2) FDA may periodically issue guidance regarding designated delivery services.

[81 FR 69651, Oct. 6, 2016]

§ 314.96 Amendments to an unapproved ANDA.

(a) *ANDA.* (1) An applicant may amend an ANDA that is submitted under § 314.94, but not yet approved, to revise existing information or provide additional information. Amendments containing bioequivalence studies must contain reports of all bioequivalence studies conducted by the applicant on the same drug product formulation, unless the information has previously been submitted to FDA in the ANDA. A complete study report must be submitted for any bioequivalence study upon which the applicant relies for approval. For all other bioequivalence studies conducted on the same drug product formulation as defined in § 314.3 of this chapter, the applicant must submit either a complete or summary report. If a summary report of a bioequivalence study is submitted and FDA determines that there may be bioequivalence issues or concerns with the product, FDA may require that the applicant submit a complete report of the bioequivalence study to FDA.

(2) Submission of an amendment containing significant data or information before the end of the initial review cycle constitutes an agreement between FDA and the applicant to extend the initial review cycle only for the time necessary to review the significant data or information and for no more than 180 days.

(b) *Field copy.* The applicant must submit a field copy of each amendment under § 314.94(a)(9). The applicant, other than a foreign applicant, must include in its submission of each such amendment to FDA a statement certifying that a field copy of the amendment has been sent to the applicant's home FDA district office.

(c) *Different listed drug.* An applicant may not amend an ANDA to seek approval of a drug referring to a listed drug that is different from the reference listed drug identified in the ANDA. This paragraph (c) applies if, at any time before the approval of the ANDA, a different listed drug is approved that is the pharmaceutical equivalent to the product in the ANDA and is designated as a reference listed drug. This paragraph (c) also applies if changes are proposed in an amendment to the ANDA such that the proposed product is a pharmaceutical equivalent to a different listed drug than the reference listed drug identified in the ANDA. A change of the reference listed drug must be submitted in a new ANDA. However, notwithstanding the limitation described in this paragraph (c), an applicant may amend the ANDA to seek approval of a different strength.

(d)(1) *Patent certification requirements.* An amendment to an ANDA is required to contain an appropriate patent certification or statement described in § 314.94(a)(12) or a recertification for a previously submitted paragraph IV certification if approval is sought for any of the following types of amendments:

(i) To add a new indication or other condition of use;

(ii) To add a new strength;

(iii) To make other than minor changes in product formulation; or

(iv) To change the physical form or crystalline structure of the active ingredient.

(2) If the amendment to the ANDA does not contain a patent certification or statement, the applicant must verify that the proposed change described in the amendment is not one of the types of amendments described in paragraph (d)(1) of this section.

[57 FR 17983, Apr. 28, 1992, as amended at 58 FR 47352, Sept. 8, 1993; 64 FR 401, Jan. 5, 1999; 73 FR 39609, July 10, 2008; 74 FR 2861, Jan. 16, 2009; 81 FR 69652, Oct. 6, 2016]

§ 314.97 Supplements and other changes to an approved ANDA.

(a) *General requirements.* The applicant must comply with the requirements of §§ 314.70 and 314.71 regarding the submission of supplemental ANDAs and other changes to an approved ANDA.

(b) *Different listed drug.* An applicant may not supplement an ANDA to seek approval of a drug referring to a listed drug that is different from the current reference listed drug identified in the ANDA. This paragraph (b) applies if changes are proposed in a supplement to the ANDA such that the proposed product is a pharmaceutical equivalent to a different listed drug than the reference listed drug identified in the ANDA. A change of reference listed drug must be submitted in a new ANDA. However, notwithstanding the limitation described in this paragraph (b), an applicant may supplement the ANDA to seek approval of a different strength.

[81 FR 69653, Oct. 6, 2016]

§ 314.98 Postmarketing reports.

(a) Each applicant having an approved abbreviated new drug application under § 314.94 that is effective must comply with the requirements of § 314.80 regarding the reporting and recordkeeping of adverse drug experiences.

(b) Each applicant must make the reports required under § 314.81 and section 505(k) of the Federal Food, Drug, and Cosmetic Act for each of its approved abbreviated applications.

[79 FR 33089, June 10, 2014]

§ 314.99 Other responsibilities of an applicant of an ANDA.

(a) An applicant must comply with the requirements of § 314.65 regarding withdrawal by the applicant of an unapproved ANDA and § 314.72 regarding a change in ownership of an ANDA.

(b) An applicant may ask FDA to waive under this section any requirement that applies to the applicant under §§ 314.92 through 314.99. The applicant must comply with the requirements for a waiver under § 314.90. If FDA grants the applicant's waiver request with respect to a requirement under §§ 314.92 through 314.99, the waived requirement will not constitute a basis for refusal to approve an ANDA under § 314.127.

81 FR 69653, Oct. 6, 2016]

Subpart D—FDA Action on Applications and Abbreviated Applications

Source: 50 FR 7493, Feb. 22, 1985, unless otherwise noted. Redesignated at 57 FR 17983, Apr. 28, 1992.

§ 314.100 Timeframes for reviewing applications and abbreviated applications.

(a) Except as provided in paragraph (c) of this section, within 180 days of receipt of an application for a new drug under section 505(b) of the act or an abbreviated application for a new drug under section 505(j) of the act, FDA will review it and send the applicant either an approval letter under § 314.105 or a complete response letter under § 314.110. This 180-day period is called the "initial review cycle."

(b) At any time before approval, an applicant may withdraw an application under § 314.65 or an abbreviated application under § 314.99 and later submit it again for consideration.

(c) The initial review cycle may be adjusted by mutual agreement between FDA and an applicant or as provided in §§ 314.60 and 314.96, as the result of a major amendment.

[73 FR 39609, July 10, 2008]

§ 314.101 Filing an NDA and receiving an ANDA.

(a) *Filing an NDA.* (1) Within 60 days after FDA receives an NDA, the Agency will determine whether the NDA may be filed. The filing of an NDA means that FDA has made a threshold determination that the NDA is sufficiently complete to permit a substantive review.

(2) If FDA finds that none of the reasons in paragraphs (d) and (e) of this section for refusing to file the NDA apply, the Agency will file the NDA and notify the applicant in writing. In the case of a 505(b)(2) application that contains a paragraph IV certification, the applicant will be notified via a paragraph IV acknowledgment letter. The date of filing will be the date 60 days after the date FDA received the NDA. The date of filing begins the 180-day period described in section 505(c) of the Federal Food, Drug, and Cosmetic Act. This 180-day period is called the "filing clock."

(3) If FDA refuses to file the NDA, the Agency will notify the applicant in writing and state the reason under paragraph (d) or (e) of this section for the refusal. If FDA refuses to file the NDA under paragraph (d) of this section, the applicant may request in writing within 30 days of the date of the Agency's notification an informal conference with the Agency about whether the Agency should file the NDA. If, following the informal conference, the applicant requests that FDA file the NDA (with or without amendments to correct the deficiencies), the Agency will file the NDA over protest under paragraph (a)(2) of this section, notify the applicant in writing, and review it as filed. If the NDA is filed over protest, the date of filing will be the date 60 days after the date the applicant requested the informal conference. The applicant need not resubmit a copy of an NDA that is filed over protest. If FDA refuses to file the NDA under paragraph (e) of this section, the applicant may amend the NDA and resubmit it, and the Agency will make a determination under this section whether it may be filed.

(b)(1) *Receiving an ANDA.* An ANDA will be evaluated after it is submitted to determine whether the ANDA may be received. Receipt of an ANDA means that FDA has made a threshold determination that the abbreviated application is substantially complete.

(2) If FDA finds that none of the reasons in paragraphs (d) and (e) of this section for considering the ANDA not to have been received applies, the ANDA is substantially complete and the Agency will receive the ANDA and notify the applicant in writing. If FDA determines, upon evaluation, that an ANDA was substantially complete as of the date it was submitted to FDA, FDA will consider the ANDA to have been received as of the date of submission. In the case of an ANDA that contains a paragraph IV certification, the applicant will be notified via a paragraph IV acknowledgment letter.

(3) If FDA considers the ANDA not to have been received under paragraph (d) or (e) of this section, FDA will notify the applicant of the refuse-to-receive decision. The applicant may then:

(i) Withdraw the ANDA under § 314.99; or

(ii) Correct the deficiencies and resubmit the ANDA; or

(iii) Take no action, in which case FDA may consider the ANDA withdrawn after 1 year.

(c) [Reserved]

(d) *NDA or ANDA deficiencies.* FDA may refuse to file an NDA or may not consider an ANDA to be received if any of the following applies:

(1) The NDA or ANDA does not contain a completed application form.

(2) The NDA or ANDA is not submitted in the form required under § 314.50 or § 314.94.

(3) The NDA or ANDA is incomplete because it does not on its face contain information required under section 505(b) or section 505(j) of the Federal Food, Drug, and Cosmetic Act and § 314.50 or § 314.94. In determining whether an ANDA is incomplete on its face, FDA will consider the nature (e.g., major or minor) of the deficiencies, including the number of deficiencies in the ANDA.

(4) The applicant fails to submit a complete environmental assessment, which addresses each of the items specified in the applicable format under § 25.40 of this chapter or fails to provide sufficient information to establish that the requested action is subject to categorical exclusion under § 25.30 or § 25.31 of this chapter.

(5) The NDA or ANDA does not contain an accurate and complete English translation of each part of the NDA or ANDA that is not in English.

(6) The NDA or ANDA does not contain a statement for each nonclinical laboratory study that the study was conducted in compliance with the requirements set forth in part 58 of this chapter, or, for each study not conducted in compliance with part 58 of this chapter, a brief statement of the reason for the noncompliance.

(7) The NDA or ANDA does not contain a statement for each clinical study that the study was conducted in compliance with the institutional review board regulations in part 56 of this chapter, or was not subject to those regulations, and that it was conducted in compliance with the informed consent regulations in part 50 of this chapter, or, if the study was subject to but was not conducted in compliance with those regulations, the NDA or ANDA does not contain a brief statement of the reason for the noncompliance.

(8) The drug product that is the subject of the submission is already covered by an approved NDA or ANDA and the applicant of the submission:

(i) Has an approved NDA or ANDA for the same drug product; or

(ii) Is merely a distributor and/or repackager of the already approved drug product.

(9) The NDA is submitted as a 505(b)(2) application for a drug that is a duplicate of a listed drug and is eligible for approval under section 505(j) of the Federal Food, Drug, and Cosmetic Act.

(e) *Regulatory deficiencies.* The Agency will refuse to file an NDA or will consider an ANDA not to have been received if any of the following applies:

(1) The drug product is subject to licensing by FDA under the Public Health Service Act (42 U.S.C. 201 et seq.) and subchapter F of this chapter.

(2) Submission of a 505(b)(2) application or an ANDA is not permitted under section 505(c)(3)(E)(ii), 505(j)(5)(F)(ii), 505A(b)(1)(A)(i)(I), 505A(c)(1)(A)(i)(I), or 505E(a) of the Federal Food, Drug, and Cosmetic Act.

(f) Outcome of FDA review. (1) Within 180 days after the date of filing, plus the period of time the review period was extended (if any), FDA will either:

(i) Approve the NDA; or

(ii) Issue a notice of opportunity for a hearing if the applicant asked FDA to provide it an opportunity for a hearing on an NDA in response to a complete response letter.

(2) Within 180 days after the date of receipt, plus the period of time the review clock was extended (if any), FDA will either approve or disapprove the ANDA. If FDA disapproves the ANDA, FDA will issue a notice of opportunity for hearing if the applicant asked FDA to provide it an opportunity for a hearing on an ANDA in response to a complete response letter.

(3) This paragraph (f) does not apply to NDAs or ANDAs that have been withdrawn from FDA review by the applicant.

[81 FR 69653, Oct. 6, 2016]

§ 314.102 Communications between FDA and applicants.

(a) *General principles.* During the course of reviewing an application or an abbreviated application, FDA shall communicate with applicants about scientific, medical, and procedural issues that arise during the review process. Such communication may take the form of telephone conversations, letters, or meetings, whichever is most appropriate to discuss the particular issue at hand. Communications shall be appropriately documented in the application in accordance with § 10.65 of this chapter. Further details on the procedures for communication between FDA and applicants are contained in a staff manual guide that is publicly available.

(b) *Notification of easily correctable deficiencies.* FDA reviewers shall make every reasonable effort to communicate promptly to applicants easily correctable deficiencies found in an application or an abbreviated application when those deficiencies are discovered, particularly deficiencies concerning chemistry, manufacturing, and controls issues. The agency will also inform applicants promptly of its need for more data or information or for technical changes in the application or the abbreviated application needed to facilitate the agency's review. This early communication is intended to permit applicants to correct such readily identified deficiencies relatively early in the review process and to submit an amendment before the review period has elapsed. Such early communication would not ordinarily apply to major scientific issues, which require consideration of the entire pending application or abbreviated application by agency managers as well as reviewing staff. Instead, major scientific issues will ordinarily be addressed in a complete response letter.

(c) *Ninety-day conference.* Approximately 90 days after the agency receives the application, FDA will provide applicants with an opportunity to meet with agency reviewing officials. The purpose of the meeting will be to inform applicants of the general progress and status of their applications, and to advise applicants of deficiencies that have been identified by that time and that have not already been communicated. This meeting will be available on applications for all new chemical entities and major new indications of marketed drugs. Such meetings will be held at the applicant's option, and may be held by telephone if mutually agreed upon. Such meetings would not ordinarily be held on abbreviated applications because they are not submitted for new chemical entities or new indications.

(d) *End-of-review conference.* At the conclusion of FDA's review of an NDA as designated by the issuance of a complete response letter, FDA will provide the applicant with an opportunity to meet with agency reviewing officials. The purpose of the meeting will be to discuss what further steps need to be taken by the applicant before the application can be approved. Requests for such meetings must be directed to the director of the division responsible for reviewing the application.

(e) *Other meetings.* Other meetings between FDA and applicants may be held, with advance notice, to discuss scientific, medical, and other issues that arise during the review process. Requests for meetings shall be directed to the director of the division responsible for reviewing the application or abbreviated application. FDA will make every attempt to grant requests for meetings that involve important issues and that can be scheduled at mutually convenient times. However, "drop-in" visits (i.e., an unannounced and unscheduled visit by a company representative) are discouraged except for urgent matters, such as to discuss an important new safety issue.

[57 FR 17988, Apr. 28, 1992; 57 FR 29353, July 1, 1992, as amended at 73 FR 39609, July 10, 2008]

§ 314.103 Dispute resolution.

(a) *General.* FDA is committed to resolving differences between applicants and FDA reviewing divisions with respect to technical requirements for applications or abbreviated applications as quickly and amicably as possible through the cooperative exchange of information and views.

(b) *Administrative and procedural issues.* When administrative or procedural disputes arise, the applicant should first attempt to resolve the matter with the division responsible for reviewing the application or abbreviated application, beginning with the consumer safety officer assigned to the application or abbreviated application. If resolution is not achieved, the applicant may raise the matter with the person designated as ombudsman, whose function shall be to investigate what has happened and to facilitate a timely and equitable resolution. Appropriate issues to raise with the ombudsman include resolving difficulties in scheduling meetings, obtaining timely replies to inquiries, and obtaining timely completion of pending reviews. Further details on this procedure are contained in a staff manual guide that is publicly available under FDA's public information regulations in part 20.

(c) *Scientific and medical disputes.* (1) Because major scientific issues are ordinarily communicated to applicants in a complete response letter pursuant to § 314.110, the "end-of-review conference" described in § 314.102(d) will provide a timely forum for discussing and resolving, if possible, scientific and medical issues on which the applicant disagrees with the agency. In addition, the "ninety-day conference" described in § 314.102(c) will provide a timely forum for discussing and resolving, if possible, issues identified by that date.

(2) When scientific or medical disputes arise at other times during the review process, applicants should discuss the matter directly with the responsible reviewing officials. If necessary, applicants may request a meeting with the appropriate reviewing officials and management representatives in order to seek a resolution. Ordinarily, such meetings would be held first with the Division Director, then with the Office Director, and finally with the Center Director if the matter is still unresolved. Requests for such meetings shall be directed to the director of the division responsible for reviewing the application or abrreviated application. FDA will make every attempt to grant requests for meetings that involve important issues and that can be scheduled at mutually convenient times.

(3) In requesting a meeting designed to resolve a scientific or medical dispute, applicants may suggest that FDA seek the advice of outside experts, in which case FDA may, in its discretion, invite to the meeting one or more of its advisory committee members or other consultants, as designated by the agency. Applicants may also bring their own consultants. For major scientific and medical policy issues not resolved by informal meetings, FDA may refer the matter to one of its standing advisory committees for its consideration and recommendations.

[50 FR 7493, Feb. 22, 1985; 50 FR 14212, Apr. 11, 1985, as amended at 57 FR 17989, Apr. 28, 1992; 73 FR 39609, July 10, 2008]

§ 314.104 Drugs with potential for abuse.

The Food and Drug Administration will inform the Drug Enforcement Administration under section 201(f) of the Controlled Substances Act (21 U.S.C. 801) when an application or abbreviated application is submitted for a drug that appears to have an abuse potential.

[57 FR 17989, Apr. 28, 1992]

§ 314.105 Approval of an NDA and an ANDA.

(a) FDA will approve an NDA and send the applicant an approval letter if none of the reasons in § 314.125 for refusing to approve the NDA applies. FDA will issue a tentative approval letter if an NDA otherwise meets the requirements for approval under the Federal Food, Drug, and Cosmetic Act, but cannot be approved because there is a 7-year period of orphan exclusivity for the listed drug under section 527 of the Federal Food, Drug, and Cosmetic Act and § 316.31 of this chapter, or if a 505(b)(2) application otherwise meets the requirements for approval under the Federal Food, Drug, and Cosmetic Act, but cannot be approved until the conditions in § 314.107(b)(3) are met; because there is a period of exclusivity for the listed drug under § 314.108; because there is a period of pediatric exclusivity for the listed drug under section 505A of the Federal Food, Drug, and Cosmetic Act; or because there is a period of exclusivity for the listed drug under section 505E of the Federal Food, Drug, and Cosmetic Act. A drug product that is granted tentative approval is not an approved drug and will not be approved until FDA issues an approval after any necessary additional review of the NDA. FDA's tentative approval of a drug product is based on information available to FDA at the time of the tentative approval letter (i.e., information in the 505(b)(2) application and the status of current good manufacturing practices of the facilities used in the manufacturing and testing of the drug product) and is therefore subject to change on the basis of new information that may come to FDA's attention. A new drug product may not be marketed until the date of approval.

(b) FDA will approve an NDA and issue the applicant an approval letter on the basis of draft labeling if the only deficiencies in the NDA concern editorial or similar minor deficiencies in the draft labeling. Such approval will be conditioned upon the applicant incorporating the specified labeling changes exactly as directed, and upon the applicant submitting to FDA a copy of the final printed labeling prior to marketing.

(c) FDA will approve an NDA after it determines that the drug meets the statutory standards for safety and effectiveness, manufacturing and controls, and labeling, and an ANDA after it determines that the drug meets the statutory standards for manufacturing and controls, labeling, and, where applicable, bioequivalence. While the statutory standards apply to all drugs, the many kinds of drugs that are subject to the statutory standards and the wide range of uses for those drugs demand flexibility in applying the standards. Thus FDA is required to exercise its scientific judgment to determine the kind and quantity of data and information an applicant is required to provide for a particular drug to meet the statutory standards. FDA makes its views on drug products and classes of drugs available through guidance documents, recommendations, and other statements of policy.

(d) FDA will approve an ANDA and send the applicant an approval letter if none of the reasons in § 314.127 for refusing to approve the ANDA applies. FDA will issue a tentative approval letter if an ANDA otherwise meets the requirements for approval under the Federal Food, Drug, and Cosmetic Act, but cannot be approved because there is a 7-year period of orphan exclusivity for the listed drug under section 527 of the Federal Food, Drug, and Cosmetic Act and § 316.31 of this chapter, or cannot be approved until the conditions in § 314.107(b)(3) or (c) are met; because there is a period of exclusivity for the listed drug under § 314.108; because there is a period of pediatric exclusivity for the listed drug under section 505A of the Federal Food, Drug, and Cosmetic Act; or because there is a period of exclusivity for the listed drug under section 505E of the Federal Food, Drug, and Cosmetic Act. A drug product that is granted tentative approval is not an approved drug and will not be approved until FDA issues an approval after any necessary additional review of the ANDA. FDA's tentative approval of a drug product is based on information available to FDA at the time of the tentative approval letter (i.e., information in the ANDA and the status of current good manufacturing practices of the facilities used in the manufacturing and testing of the drug product) and is therefore subject to change on the basis of new information that may come to FDA's attention. A new drug product may not be marketed until the date of approval.

[81 FR 69654, Oct. 6, 2016]

§ 314.106 Foreign data.

(a) *General.* The acceptance of foreign data in an application generally is governed by § 312.120 of this chapter.

(b) *As sole basis for marketing approval.* An application based solely on foreign clinical data meeting U.S. criteria for marketing approval may be approved if: (1) The foreign data are applicable to the U.S. population and U.S. medical practice; (2) the studies have been performed by clinical investigators of recognized competence; and (3) the data may be considered valid without the need for an on-site inspection by FDA or, if FDA considers such an inspection to be necessary, FDA is able to validate the data through an on-site inspection or other appropriate means. Failure of an application to meet any of these criteria will result in the application not being approvable based on the foreign data alone. FDA will apply this policy in a flexible manner according to the nature of the drug and the data being considered.

(c) *Consultation between FDA and applicants.* Applicants are encouraged to meet with agency officials in a "presubmission" meeting when approval based solely on foreign data will be sought.

[50 FR 7493, Feb. 22, 1985, as amended at 55 FR 11580, Mar. 29, 1990]

§ 314.107 Date of approval of a 505(b)(2) application or ANDA.

(a) *General.* A drug product may be introduced or delivered for introduction into interstate commerce when the 505(b)(2) application or ANDA for the drug product is approved. A 505(b)(2) application or ANDA for a drug product is approved on the date FDA issues an approval letter under § 314.105 for the 505(b)(2) application or ANDA.

(b) *Effect of patent(s) on the listed drug.* As described in paragraphs (b)(1) and (2) of this section, the status of patents listed for the listed drug(s) relied upon or reference listed drug, as applicable, must be considered in determining the first possible date on which a 505(b)(2) application or ANDA can be approved. The criteria in paragraphs (b)(1) and (2) of this section will be used to determine, for each relevant patent, the date that patent will no longer prevent approval. The first possible date on which the 505(b)(2) application or ANDA can be approved will be calculated for each patent, and the 505(b)(2) application or ANDA may be approved on the last applicable date.

(1) *Timing of approval based on patent certification or statement.* If none of the reasons in § 314.125 or § 314.127, as applicable, for refusing to approve the 505(b)(2) application or ANDA applies, and none of the reasons in paragraph (d) of this section for delaying approval applies, the 505(b)(2) application or ANDA may be approved as follows:

(i) Immediately, if the applicant certifies under § 314.50(i) or § 314.94(a)(12) that:

(A) The applicant is aware of a relevant patent but the patent information required under section 505(b) or (c) of the Federal Food, Drug, and Cosmetic Act has not been submitted to FDA; or

(B) The relevant patent has expired; or

(C) The relevant patent is invalid, unenforceable, or will not be infringed, except as provided in paragraphs (b)(3) and (c) of this section, and the 45-day period provided for in section 505(c)(3)(C) and (j)(5)(B)(iii) of the Federal Food, Drug, and Cosmetic Act has expired; or

(D) There are no relevant patents.

(ii) Immediately, if the applicant submits an appropriate statement under § 314.50(i) or § 314.94(a)(12) explaining that a method-of-use patent does not claim an indication or other condition of use for which the applicant is seeking approval, except that if the applicant also submits a paragraph IV certification to the patent, then the 505(b)(2) application or ANDA may be approved as provided in paragraph (b)(1)(i)(C) of this section.

(iii) On the date specified, if the applicant certifies under § 314.50(i) or § 314.94(a)(12) that the relevant patent will expire on a specified date.

(2) *Patent information filed after submission of 505(b)(2) application or ANDA.* If the holder of the approved NDA for the listed drug submits patent information required under § 314.53 after the date on which the 505(b)(2) application or ANDA was submitted to FDA, the 505(b)(2) applicant or ANDA applicant must comply with the requirements of § 314.50(i)(4) and (6) and § 314.94(a)(12)(vi) and (viii) regarding submission of an appropriate patent certification or statement. If the applicant submits an amendment certifying under § 314.50(i)(1)(i)(A)(4) or § 314.94(a)(12)(i)(A)(4) that the relevant patent is invalid, unenforceable, or will not be infringed, and complies with the requirements of § 314.52 or § 314.95, the 505(b)(2) application or ANDA may be approved immediately upon submission of documentation of receipt of notice of paragraph IV certification under § 314.52(e) or § 314.95(e). The 45-day period provided for in section 505(c)(3)(C) and (j)(5)(B)(iii) of the Federal Food, Drug, and Cosmetic Act does not apply in these circumstances.

(3) *Disposition of patent litigation*—(i) *Approval upon expiration of 30-month period or 71/2 years from date of listed drug approval.* (A) Except as provided in paragraphs (b)(3)(ii) through (viii) of this section, if, with respect to patents for which required information was submitted under § 314.53 before the date on which the 505(b)(2) application or ANDA was submitted to FDA (excluding an amendment or supplement to the 505(b)(2) application or ANDA), the applicant certifies under § 314.50(i) or § 314.94(a)(12) that the relevant patent is invalid, unenforceable, or will not be infringed, and the patent owner or its representative or the exclusive patent licensee brings suit for patent infringement within 45 days of receipt of the notice of certification from the applicant under § 314.52 or § 314.95, the 505(b)(2) application or ANDA may be approved 30 months after the later of the date of the receipt of the notice of certification by any owner of the listed patent or by the NDA holder (or its representative(s)) unless the court has extended or reduced the period because of a failure of either the plaintiff or defendant to cooperate reasonably in expediting the action; or

(B) If the patented drug product qualifies for 5 years of exclusive marketing under § 314.108(b)(2) and the patent owner or its representative or the exclusive patent licensee brings suit for patent infringement during the 1-year period beginning 4 years after the date of approval of the patented drug and within 45 days of receipt of the notice of certification from the applicant under § 314.52 or § 314.95, the 505(b)(2) application or ANDA may be approved at the expiration of the 71/2 years from the date of approval of the NDA for the patented drug product.

(ii) *Federal district court decision of invalidity, unenforceability, or non-infringement.* If before the expiration of the 30-month period, or 71/2 years where applicable, the district court decides that the patent is invalid, unenforceable, or not infringed (including any substantive determination that there is no cause of action for patent infringement or invalidity), the 505(b)(2) application or ANDA may be approved on:

(A) The date on which the court enters judgment reflecting the decision; or

(B) The date of a settlement order or consent decree signed and entered by the court stating that the patent that is the subject of the certification is invalid, unenforceable, or not infringed.

(iii) Appeal of Federal district court judgment of infringement. If before the expiration of the 30-month period, or 71/2 years where applicable, the district court decides that the patent has been infringed, and if the judgment of the district court is appealed, the 505(b)(2) application or ANDA may be approved on:

(A) The date on which the mandate is issued by the court of appeals entering judgment that the patent is invalid, unenforceable, or not infringed (including any substantive determination that there is no cause of action for patent infringement or invalidity); or

(B) The date of a settlement order or consent decree signed and entered by the court of appeals stating that the patent that is the subject of the certification is invalid, unenforceable, or not infringed.

(iv) *Affirmation or non-appeal of Federal district court judgment of infringement.* If before the expiration of the 30-month period, or 71/2 years where applicable, the district court decides that the patent has been infringed, and if the judgment of the district court is not appealed or is affirmed, the 505(b)(2) application or ANDA may be approved no earlier than the date specified by the district court in an order under 35 U.S.C. 271(e)(4)(A).

(v) *Grant of preliminary injunction by Federal district court.* If before the expiration of the 30-month period, or 71/2 years where applicable, the district court grants a preliminary injunction prohibiting the applicant from engaging in the commercial manufacture or sale of the drug product until the court decides the issues of patent validity and infringement, and if the court later decides that:

(A) The patent is invalid, unenforceable, or not infringed, the 505(b)(2) application or ANDA may be approved as provided in paragraph (b)(3)(ii) of this section; or

(B) The patent is infringed, the 505(b)(2) application or ANDA may be approved as provided in paragraph (b)(3)(iii) or (iv) of this section, whichever is applicable.

(vi) *Written consent to approval by patent owner or exclusive patent licensee.* If before the expiration of the 30-month period, or 71/2 years where applicable, the patent owner or the exclusive patent licensee (or their representatives) agrees in writing that the 505(b)(2) application or ANDA may be approved any time on or after the date of the consent, approval may be granted on or after that date.

(vii) *Court order terminating 30-month or 71/2-year period.* If before the expiration of the 30-month period, or 71/2 years where applicable, the court enters an order requiring the 30-month or 71/2-year period to be terminated, the 505(b)(2) application or ANDA may be approved in accordance with the court's order.

(viii) *Court order of dismissal without a finding of infringement.* If before the expiration of the 30-month period, or 71/2 years where applicable, the court(s) enter(s) an order of dismissal, with or without prejudice, without a finding of infringement in each pending suit for patent infringement brought within 45 days of receipt of the notice of paragraph IV certification sent by the 505(b)(2) or ANDA applicant, the 505(b)(2) application or ANDA may be approved on or after the date of the order.

(4) *Tentative approval.* FDA will issue a tentative approval letter when tentative approval is appropriate in accordance with this section. In order for a 505(b)(2) application or ANDA to be approved under paragraph (b)(3) of this section, the applicant must receive an approval letter from the Agency. Tentative approval of an NDA or ANDA does not constitute "approval" of an NDA or ANDA and cannot, absent an approval letter from the Agency, result in an approval under paragraph (b)(3) of this section.

(c) *Timing of approval of subsequent ANDA.* (1) If an ANDA contains a paragraph IV certification for a relevant patent and the ANDA is not that of a first applicant, the ANDA is regarded as the ANDA of a subsequent applicant. The ANDA of a subsequent applicant will not be approved during the period when any first applicant is eligible for 180-day exclusivity or during the 180-day exclusivity period of a first applicant. Any applicable 180-day exclusivity period cannot extend beyond the expiration of the patent upon which the 180-day exclusivity period was based.

(2) A first applicant must submit correspondence to its ANDA notifying FDA within 30 days of the date of its first commercial marketing of its drug product or the reference listed drug. If an applicant does not notify FDA, as required in this paragraph (c)(2), of this date, the date of first commercial marketing will be deemed to be the date of the drug product's approval.

(3) If FDA concludes that a first applicant is not actively pursuing approval of its ANDA, FDA may immediately approve an ANDA(s) of a subsequent applicant(s) if the ANDA(s) is otherwise eligible for approval.

(d) *Delay due to exclusivity.* The Agency will also delay the approval of a 505(b)(2) application or ANDA if delay is required by the exclusivity provisions in § 314.108; section 527 of the Federal Food, Drug, and Cosmetic Act and § 316.31 of this chapter; section 505A of the Federal Food, Drug, and Cosmetic Act; or section 505E of the Federal Food, Drug, and Cosmetic Act. When the approval of a 505(b)(2) application or ANDA is delayed under this section and § 314.108; section 527 of the Federal Food, Drug, and Cosmetic Act and § 316.31 of this chapter; section 505A of the Federal Food, Drug, and Cosmetic Act; or section 505E of the Federal Food, Drug, and Cosmetic Act, the 505(b)(2) application or ANDA will be approved on the latest of the days specified under this section and § 314.108; section 527 of the Federal Food, Drug, and Cosmetic Act and § 316.31 of this chapter; section 505A of the Federal Food, Drug, and Cosmetic Act; or section 505E of the Federal Food, Drug, and Cosmetic Act, as applicable.

(e) *Notification of court actions or written consent to approval.* (1) The applicant must submit the following information to FDA, as applicable:

(i) A copy of any judgment by the court (district court or mandate of the court of appeals) or settlement order or consent decree signed and entered by the court (district court or court of appeals) finding a patent described in paragraph (b)(3) of this section invalid, unenforceable, or not infringed, or finding the patent valid and infringed;

(ii) Written notification of whether or not any action by the court described in paragraph (e)(1)(i) of this section has been appealed within the time permitted for an appeal;

(iii) A copy of any order entered by the court terminating the 30-month or 71/2-year period as described in paragraph (b)(3)(i), (ii), (vii), or (viii) of this section;

(iv) A copy of any written consent to approval by the patent owner or exclusive patent licensee described in paragraph (b)(3)(vi) of this section;

(v) A copy of any preliminary injunction described in paragraph (b)(3)(v) of this section, and a copy of any subsequent court order lifting the injunction; and

(vi) A copy of any court order pursuant to 35 U.S.C. 271(e)(4)(A) ordering that a 505(b)(2) application or ANDA may be approved no earlier than the date specified (irrespective of whether the injunction relates to a patent described in paragraph (b)(3) of this section).

(2) All information required by paragraph (e)(1) of this section must be sent to the applicant's NDA or ANDA, as appropriate, within 14 days of the date of entry by the court, the date of appeal or expiration of the time for appeal, or the date of written consent to approval, as applicable.

(f) *Forty-five day period after receipt of notice of paragraph IV certification*—(1) *Computation of 45-day time clock.* The 45-day clock described in paragraph (b)(3) of this section as to each recipient required to receive notice of paragraph IV certification under § 314.52 or § 314.95 begins on the day after the date of receipt of the applicant's notice of paragraph IV certification by the recipient. When the 45th day falls on Saturday, Sunday, or a Federal holiday, the 45th day will be the next day that is not a Saturday, Sunday, or a Federal holiday.

(2) *Notification of filing of legal action.* (i) The 505(b)(2) or ANDA applicant must notify FDA in writing within 14 days of the filing of any legal action filed within 45 days of receipt of the notice of paragraph IV certification by any recipient. A 505(b)(2) applicant must send the notification to its NDA. An ANDA applicant must send the notification to its ANDA. The notification to FDA of the legal action must include:

(A) The 505(b)(2) application or ANDA number.

(B) The name of the 505(b)(2) or ANDA applicant.

(C) The established name of the drug product or, if no established name exists, the name(s) of the active ingredient(s), the drug product's strength, and dosage form.

(D) A statement that an action for patent infringement, identified by court, case number, and the patent number(s) of the patent(s) at issue in the action, has been filed in an appropriate court on a specified date.

(ii) A patent owner or NDA holder (or its representative(s)) may also notify FDA of the filing of any legal action for patent infringement. The notice should contain the information and be sent to the offices or divisions described in paragraph (f)(2)(i) of this section.

(iii) If the 505(b)(2) or ANDA applicant, the patent owner(s), the NDA holder, or its representative(s) does not notify FDA in writing before the expiration of the 45-day time period or the completion of the Agency's review of the 505(b)(2) application or ANDA, whichever occurs later, that a legal action for patent infringement was filed within 45 days of receipt of the notice of paragraph IV certification, the 505(b)(2) application or ANDA may be approved upon expiration of the 45-day period (if the 505(b)(2) or ANDA applicant confirms that a legal action for patent infringement has not been filed) or upon completion of the Agency's review of the 505(b)(2) application or ANDA, whichever is later.

(3) Waiver. If the patent owner or NDA holder who is an exclusive patent licensee (or its representative(s)) waives its opportunity to file a legal action for patent infringement within 45 days of a receipt of the notice of certification and the patent owner or NDA holder who is an exclusive patent licensee (or its representative(s)) submits to FDA a valid waiver before the 45 days elapse, the 505(b)(2) application or ANDA may be approved upon completion of the Agency's review of the NDA or ANDA. FDA will only accept a waiver in the following form:

> (Name of patent owner or NDA holder who is an exclusive patent licensee or its representative(s)) has received notice from *(name of applicant) under (section 505(b)(3) or 505(j)(2)(B) of the Federal Food, Drug, and Cosmetic Act)* and does not intend to file an action for patent infringement against *(name of applicant)* concerning the drug *(name of drug)* before *(date on which 45 days elapse). (Name of patent owner or NDA holder who is an exclusive patent licensee)* waives the opportunity provided by *(section 505(c)(3)(C) or 505(j)(5)(B)(iii) of the Federal Food, Drug, and Cosmetic Act)* and does not object to FDA's approval of *(name of applicant)'s (505(b)(2) application or ANDA)* for *(name of drug)* with an approval date on or after the date of this submission.

(g) Conversion of approval to tentative approval. If FDA issues an approval letter in error or a court enters an order requiring, in the case of an already approved 505(b)(2) application or ANDA, that the date of approval be delayed, FDA will convert the approval to a tentative approval if appropriate.

[81 FR 69655, Oct. 6, 2016]

§ 314.108 New drug product exclusivity.

(a) *Definitions.* The definitions in § 314.3 and the following definitions of terms apply to this section:

Approved under section 505(b) means an NDA submitted under section 505(b) and approved on or after October 10, 1962, or an application that was "deemed approved" under section 107(c)(2) of Public Law 87-781.

Bioavailability study means a study to determine the bioavailability or the pharmacokinetics of a drug.

Clinical investigation means any experiment other than a bioavailability study in which a drug is administered or dispensed to, or used on, human subjects.

Conducted or sponsored by the applicant with regard to an investigation means that before or during the investigation, the applicant was named in Form FDA-1571 filed with FDA as the sponsor of the investigational new drug application under which the investigation was conducted, or the applicant or the applicant's predecessor in interest, provided substantial support for the investigation. To demonstrate "substantial support," an applicant must either provide a certified statement from a certified public accountant that the applicant provided 50 percent or more of the cost of conducting the study or provide an explanation why FDA should consider the applicant to have conducted or sponsored the study if the applicant's financial contribution to the study is less than 50 percent or the applicant did not sponsor the investigational new drug. A predecessor in interest is an entity, e.g., a corporation, that the applicant has taken over, merged with, or purchased, or from which the applicant has purchased all rights to the drug. Purchase of nonexclusive rights to a clinical investigation after it is completed is not sufficient to satisfy this definition.

Essential to approval means, with regard to an investigation, that there are no other data available that could support approval of the NDA.

New chemical entity means a drug that contains no active moiety that has been approved by FDA in any other NDA submitted under section 505(b) of the Federal Food, Drug, and Cosmetic Act.

New clinical investigation means an investigation in humans the results of which have not been relied on by FDA to demonstrate substantial evidence of effectiveness of a previously approved drug product for any indication or of safety for a new patient population and do not duplicate the results of another investigation that was relied on by the agency to demonstrate the effectiveness or safety in a new patient population of a previously approved drug product. For purposes of this section, data from a clinical investigation previously submitted for use in the comprehensive evaluation of the safety of a drug product but not to support the effectiveness of the drug product would be considered new.

(b) Submission of and timing of approval of a 505(b)(2) application or ANDA. (1) [Reserved]

(2) If a drug product that contains a new chemical entity was approved after September 24, 1984, in an NDA submitted under section 505(b) of the Federal Food, Drug, and Cosmetic Act, no person may submit a 505(b)(2) application or ANDA under section 505(j) of the Federal Food, Drug, and Cosmetic Act for a drug product that contains the same active moiety as in the new chemical entity for a period of 5 years from the date of approval of the first approved NDA, except that the 505(b)(2) application or ANDA may be submitted after 4 years if it contains a certification of patent invalidity or noninfringement described in § 314.50(i)(1)(i)(A)(4) or § 314.94(a)(12)(i)(A)(4).

(3) The approval of a 505(b)(2) application or ANDA described in paragraph (b)(2) of this section will occur as provided in § 314.107(b)(1) or (2), unless the owner of a patent that claims the drug, the patent owner's representative, or exclusive licensee brings suit for patent infringement against the applicant during the 1-year period beginning 48 months after the date of approval of the NDA for the new chemical entity and within 45 days after receipt of the notice described at § 314.52 or § 314.95, in which case, approval of the 505(b)(2) application or ANDA will occur as provided in § 314.107(b)(3).

(4) If an NDA:

(i) Was submitted under section 505(b) of the Federal Food, Drug, and Cosmetic Act;

(ii) Was approved after September 24, 1984;

(iii) Was for a drug product that contains an active moiety that has been previously approved in another NDA under section 505(b) of the Federal Food, Drug, and Cosmetic Act; and

(iv) Contained reports of new clinical investigations (other than bioavailability studies) conducted or sponsored by the applicant that were essential to approval of the application, for a period of 3 years after the date of approval of the application, the Agency will not approve a 505(b)(2) application or an ANDA for the conditions of approval of the NDA, or an ANDA submitted pursuant to an approved petition under section 505(j)(2)(C) of the Federal Food, Drug, and Cosmetic Act that relies on the information supporting the conditions of approval of an original NDA.

(5) If a supplemental NDA:

(i) Was approved after September 24, 1984; and

(ii) Contained reports of new clinical investigations (other than bioavailability studies) that were conducted or sponsored by the applicant that were essential to approval of the supplemental NDA, for a period of 3 years after the date of approval of the supplemental application, the Agency will not approve a 505(b)(2) application or an ANDA for a change, or an ANDA submitted pursuant to an approved petition under section 505(j)(2)(C) of the Federal Food, Drug, and Cosmetic Act that relies on the information supporting a change approved in the supplemental NDA.

[59 FR 50368, Oct. 3, 1994, as amended at 81 FR 69657, Oct. 6, 2016]

§ 314.110 Complete response letter to the applicant.

(a) *Complete response letter.* FDA will send the applicant a complete response letter if the agency determines that we will not approve the application or abbreviated application in its present form for one or more of the reasons given in § 314.125 or § 314.127, respectively.

(1) *Description of specific deficiencies.* A complete response letter will describe all of the specific deficiencies that the agency has identified in an application or abbreviated application, except as stated in paragraph (a)(3) of this section.

(2) *Complete review of data.* A complete response letter reflects FDA's complete review of the data submitted in an original application or abbreviated application (or, where appropriate, a resubmission) and any amendments that the agency has reviewed. The complete response letter will identify any amendments that the agency has not yet reviewed.

(3) *Inadequate data.* If FDA determines, after an application is filed or an abbreviated application is received, that the data submitted are inadequate to support approval, the agency might issue a complete response letter without first conducting required inspections and/or reviewing proposed product labeling.

(4) *Recommendation of actions for approval.* When possible, a complete response letter will recommend actions that the applicant might take to place the application or abbreviated application in condition for approval.

(b) *Applicant actions.* After receiving a complete response letter, the applicant must take one of following actions:

(1) *Resubmission.* Resubmit the application or abbreviated application, addressing all deficiencies identified in the complete response letter.

(i) A resubmission of an application or efficacy supplement that FDA classifies as a Class 1 resubmission constitutes an agreement by the applicant to start a new 2-month review cycle beginning on the date FDA receives the resubmission.

(ii) A resubmission of an application or efficacy supplement that FDA classifies as a Class 2 resubmission constitutes an agreement by the applicant to start a new 6-month review cycle beginning on the date FDA receives the resubmission.

(iii) A resubmission of an NDA supplement other than an efficacy supplement constitutes an agreement by the applicant to start a new review cycle the same length as the initial review cycle for the supplement (excluding any extension due to a major amendment of the initial supplement), beginning on the date FDA receives the resubmission.

(iv) A major resubmission of an abbreviated application constitutes an agreement by the applicant to start a new 6-month review cycle beginning on the date FDA receives the resubmission.

(v) A minor resubmission of an abbreviated application constitutes an agreement by the applicant to start a new review cycle beginning on the date FDA receives the resubmission.

(2) *Withdrawal.* Withdraw the application or abbreviated application. A decision to withdraw an application or abbreviated application is without prejudice to a subsequent submission.

(3) *Request opportunity for hearing.* Ask the agency to provide the applicant an opportunity for a hearing on the question of whether there are grounds for denying approval of the application or abbreviated application under section 505(d) or (j)(4) of the act, respectively. The applicant must submit the request to the Associate Director for Policy, Center for Drug Evaluation and Research, Food and Drug Administration, 10903 New Hampshire Ave., Silver Spring, MD 20993. Within 60 days of the date of the request for an opportunity for a hearing, or within a different time period to which FDA and the applicant agree, the agency will either approve the application or abbreviated application under § 314.105, or refuse to approve the application under § 314.125 or abbreviated application under § 314.127 and give the applicant written notice of an opportunity for a hearing under § 314.200 and section 505(c)(1)(B) or (j)(5)(c) of the act on the question of whether there are grounds for denying approval of the application or abbreviated application under section 505(d) or (j)(4) of the act, respectively.

(c) *Failure to take action.* (1) An applicant agrees to extend the review period under section 505(c)(1) or (j)(5)(A) of the act until it takes any of the actions listed in paragraph (b) of this section. For an application or abbreviated application, FDA may consider an applicant's failure to take any of such actions within 1 year after issuance of a complete response letter to be a request by the applicant to withdraw the application, unless the applicant has requested an extension of time in which to resubmit the application. FDA will grant any reasonable request for such an extension. FDA may consider an applicant's failure to resubmit the application within the extended time period or to request an additional extension to be a request by the applicant to withdraw the application.

(2) If FDA considers an applicant's failure to take action in accordance with paragraph (c)(1) of this section to be a request to withdraw the application, the agency will notify the applicant in writing. The applicant will have 30 days from the date of the notification to explain why the application should not be withdrawn and to request an extension of time in which to resubmit the application. FDA will grant any reasonable request for an extension. If the applicant does not respond to the notification within 30 days, the application will be deemed to be withdrawn.

[73 FR 39609, July 10, 2008]

§ 314.120 [Reserved]

§ 314.122 Submitting an abbreviated application for, or a 505(j)(2)(C) petition that relies on, a listed drug that is no longer marketed.

(a) An abbreviated new drug application that refers to, or a petition under section 505(j)(2)(C) of the act and § 314.93 that relies on, a listed drug that has been voluntarily withdrawn from sale in the United States must be accompanied by a petition seeking a determination whether the listed drug was withdrawn for safety or effectiveness reasons. The petition must be submitted under §§ 10.25(a) and 10.30 of this chapter and must contain all evidence available to the petitioner concerning the reasons for the withdrawal from sale.

(b) When a petition described in paragraph (a) of this section is submitted, the agency will consider the evidence in the petition and any other evidence before the agency, and determine whether the listed drug is withdrawn from sale for safety or effectiveness reasons, in accordance with the procedures in § 314.161.

(c) An abbreviated new drug application described in paragraph (a) of this section will be disapproved, under § 314.127(a)(11), and a 505(j)(2)(C) petition described in paragraph (a) of this section will be disapproved, under § 314.93(e)(1)(iv), unless the agency determines that the withdrawal of the listed drug was not for safety or effectiveness reasons.

(d) Certain drug products approved for safety and effectiveness that were no longer marketed on September 24, 1984, are not included in the list. Any person who wishes to obtain marketing approval for such a drug product under an abbreviated new drug application must petition FDA for a determination whether the drug product was withdrawn from the market for safety or effectiveness reasons and request that the list be amended to include the drug product. A person seeking such a determination shall use the petition procedures established in § 10.30 of this chapter. The petitioner shall include in the petition information to show that the drug product was approved for safety and effectiveness and all evidence available to the petitioner concerning the reason that marketing of the drug product ceased.

[57 FR 17990, Apr. 28, 1992; 57 FR 29353, July 1, 1992]

§ 314.125 Refusal to approve an NDA.

(a) The Food and Drug Administration will refuse to approve the NDA and for a new drug give the applicant written notice of an opportunity for a hearing under § 314.200 on the question of whether there are grounds for denying approval of the NDA under section 505(d) of the Federal Food, Drug, and Cosmetic Act, if:

(1) FDA sends the applicant a complete response letter under § 314.110;

(2) The applicant requests an opportunity for hearing for a new drug on the question of whether the NDA is approvable; and

(3) FDA finds that any of the reasons given in paragraph (b) of this section apply.

(b) FDA may refuse to approve an NDA for any of the following reasons, unless the requirement has been waived under § 314.90:

(1) The methods to be used in, and the facilities and controls used for, the manufacture, processing, packing, or holding of the drug substance or the drug product are inadequate to preserve its identity, strength, quality, purity, stability, and bioavailability.

(2) The investigations required under section 505(b) of the Federal Food, Drug, and Cosmetic Act do not include adequate tests by all methods reasonably applicable to show whether or not the drug is safe for use under the conditions prescribed, recommended, or suggested in its proposed labeling.

(3) The results of the tests show that the drug is unsafe for use under the conditions prescribed, recommended, or suggested in its proposed labeling or the results do not show that the drug product is safe for use under those conditions.

(4) There is insufficient information about the drug to determine whether the product is safe for use under the conditions prescribed, recommended, or suggested in its proposed labeling.

(5) There is a lack of substantial evidence consisting of adequate and well-controlled investigations, as defined in § 314.126, that the drug product will have the effect it purports or is represented to have under the conditions of use prescribed, recommended, or suggested in its proposed labeling.

(6) The proposed labeling is false or misleading in any particular.

(7) The NDA contains an untrue statement of a material fact.

(8) The drug product's proposed labeling does not comply with the requirements for labels and labeling in part 201.

(9) The NDA does not contain bioavailability or bioequivalence data required under part 320 of this chapter.

(10) A reason given in a letter refusing to file the NDA under § 314.101(d), if the deficiency is not corrected.

(11) The drug will be manufactured in whole or in part in an establishment that is not registered and not exempt from registration under section 510 of the Federal Food, Drug, and Cosmetic Act and part 207.

(12) The applicant does not permit a properly authorized officer or employee of the Department of Health and Human Services an adequate opportunity to inspect the facilities, controls, and any records relevant to the NDA.

(13) The methods to be used in, and the facilities and controls used for, the manufacture, processing, packing, or holding of the drug substance or the drug product do not comply with the current good manufacturing practice regulations in parts 210 and 211.

(14) The NDA does not contain an explanation of the omission of a report of any investigation of the drug product sponsored by the applicant, or an explanation of the omission of other information about the drug pertinent to an evaluation of the NDA that is received or otherwise obtained by the applicant from any source.

(15) A nonclinical laboratory study that is described in the NDA and that is essential to show that the drug is safe for use under the conditions prescribed, recommended, or suggested in its proposed labeling was not conducted in compliance with the good laboratory practice regulations in part 58 of this chapter and no reason for the noncompliance is provided or, if it is, the differences between the practices used in conducting the study and the good laboratory practice regulations do not support the validity of the study.

(16) Any clinical investigation involving human subjects described in the NDA, subject to the institutional review board regulations in part 56 of this chapter or informed consent regulations in part 50 of this chapter, was not conducted in compliance with those regulations such that the rights or safety of human subjects were not adequately protected.

(17) The applicant or contract research organization that conducted a bioavailability or bioequivalence study described in § 320.38 or § 320.63 of this chapter that is contained in the NDA refuses to permit an inspection of facilities or records relevant to the study by a properly authorized officer or employee of the Department of Health and Human Services or refuses to submit reserve samples of the drug products used in the study when requested by FDA.

(18) For a new drug, the NDA failed to contain the patent information required by section 505(b)(1) of the Federal Food, Drug, and Cosmetic Act.

(19) The 505(b)(2) application failed to contain a patent certification or statement with respect to each listed patent for a drug product approved in an NDA that:

(i) Is pharmaceutically equivalent to the drug product for which the original 505(b)(2) application is submitted; and

(ii) Was approved before the original 505(b)(2) application was submitted.

(c) For drugs intended to treat life-threatening or severely-debilitating illnesses that are developed in accordance with §§ 312.80 through 312.88 of this chapter, the criteria contained in paragraphs (b) (3), (4), and (5) of this section shall be applied according to the considerations contained in § 312.84 of this chapter.

[50 FR 7493, Feb. 22, 1985, as amended at 53 FR 41524, Oct. 21, 1988; 57 FR 17991, Apr. 28, 1992; 58 FR 25926, Apr. 28, 1993; 64 FR 402, Jan. 5, 1999; 73 FR 39610, July 10, 2008; 74 FR 9766, Mar. 6, 2009; 81 FR 60221, Aug. 31, 2016; 81 FR 69658, Oct. 6, 2016]

§ 314.126 Adequate and well-controlled studies.

(a) The purpose of conducting clinical investigations of a drug is to distinguish the effect of a drug from other influences, such as spontaneous change in the course of the disease, placebo effect, or biased observation. The characteristics described in paragraph (b) of this section have been developed over a period of years and are recognized by the scientific community as the essentials of an adequate and well-controlled clinical investigation. The Food and Drug Administration considers these characteristics in determining whether an investigation is adequate and well-controlled for purposes of section 505 of the act. Reports of adequate and well-controlled investigations provide the primary basis for determining whether there is "substantial evidence" to support the claims of effectiveness for new drugs. Therefore, the study report should provide sufficient details of study design, conduct, and analysis to allow critical evaluation and a determination of whether the characteristics of an adequate and well-controlled study are present.

(b) An adequate and well-controlled study has the following characteristics:

(1) There is a clear statement of the objectives of the investigation and a summary of the proposed or actual methods of analysis in the protocol for the study and in the report of its results. In addition, the protocol should contain a description of the proposed methods of analysis, and the study report should contain a description of the methods of analysis ultimately used. If the protocol does not contain a description of the proposed methods of analysis, the study report should describe how the methods used were selected.

(2) The study uses a design that permits a valid comparison with a control to provide a quantitative assessment of drug effect. The protocol for the study and report of results should describe the study design precisely; for example, duration of treatment periods, whether treatments are parallel, sequential, or crossover, and whether the sample size is predetermined or based upon some interim analysis. Generally, the following types of control are recognized:

(i) *Placebo concurrent control.* The test drug is compared with an inactive preparation designed to resemble the test drug as far as possible. A placebo-controlled study may include additional treatment groups, such as an active treatment control or a dose-comparison control, and usually includes randomization and blinding of patients or investigators, or both.

(ii) *Dose-comparison concurrent control.* At least two doses of the drug are compared. A dose-comparison study may include additional treatment groups, such as placebo control or active control. Dose-comparison trials usually include randomization and blinding of patients or investigators, or both.

(iii) *No treatment concurrent control.* Where objective measurements of effectiveness are available and placebo effect is negligible, the test drug is compared with no treatment. No treatment concurrent control trials usually include randomization.

(iv) *Active treatment concurrent control.* The test drug is compared with known effective therapy; for example, where the condition treated is such that administration of placebo or no treatment would be contrary to the interest of the patient. An active treatment study may include additional treatment groups, however, such as a placebo control or a dose-comparison control. Active treatment trials usually include randomization and blinding of patients or investigators, or both. If the intent of the trial is to show similarity of the test and control drugs, the report of the study should assess the ability of the study to have detected a difference between treatments. Similarity of test drug and active control can mean either that both drugs were effective or that neither was effective. The analysis of the study should explain why the drugs should be considered effective in the study, for example, by reference to results in previous placebo-controlled studies of the active control drug.

(v) *Historical control.* The results of treatment with the test drug are compared with experience historically derived from the adequately documented natural history of the disease or condition, or from the results of active treatment, in comparable patients or populations. Because historical control populations usually cannot be as well assessed with respect to pertinent variables as can concurrent control populations, historical control designs are usually reserved for special circumstances. Examples include studies of diseases with high and predictable mortality (for example, certain malignancies) and studies in which the effect of the drug is self-evident (general anesthetics, drug metabolism).

(3) The method of selection of subjects provides adequate assurance that they have the disease or condition being studied, or evidence of susceptibility and exposure to the condition against which prophylaxis is directed.

(4) The method of assigning patients to treatment and control groups minimizes bias and is intended to assure comparability of the groups with respect to pertinent variables such as age, sex, severity of disease, duration of disease, and use of drugs or therapy other than the test drug. The protocol for the study and the report of its results should describe how subjects were assigned to groups. Ordinarily, in a concurrently controlled study, assignment is by randomization, with or without stratification.

(5) Adequate measures are taken to minimize bias on the part of the subjects, observers, and analysts of the data. The protocol and report of the study should describe the procedures used to accomplish this, such as blinding.

(6) The methods of assessment of subjects' response are well-defined and reliable. The protocol for the study and the report of results should explain the variables measured, the methods of observation, and criteria used to assess response.

(7) There is an analysis of the results of the study adequate to assess the effects of the drug. The report of the study should describe the results and the analytic methods used to evaluate them, including any appropriate statistical methods. The analysis should assess, among other things, the comparability of test and control groups with respect to pertinent variables, and the effects of any interim data analyses performed.

(c) The Director of the Center for Drug Evaluation and Research may, on the Director's own initiative or on the petition of an interested person, waive in whole or in part any of the criteria in paragraph (b) of this section with respect to a specific clinical investigation, either prior to the investigation or in the evaluation of a completed study. A petition for a waiver is required to set forth clearly and concisely the specific criteria from which waiver is sought, why the criteria are not reasonably applicable to the particular clinical investigation, what alternative procedures, if any, are to be, or have been employed, and what results have been obtained. The petition is also required to state why the clinical investigations so conducted will yield, or have yielded, substantial evidence of effectiveness, notwithstanding nonconformance with the criteria for which waiver is requested.

(d) For an investigation to be considered adequate for approval of a new drug, it is required that the test drug be standardized as to identity, strength, quality, purity, and dosage form to give significance to the results of the investigation.

(e) Uncontrolled studies or partially controlled studies are not acceptable as the sole basis for the approval of claims of effectiveness. Such studies carefully conducted and documented, may provide corroborative support of well-controlled studies regarding efficacy and may yield valuable data regarding safety of the test drug. Such studies will be considered on their merits in the light of the principles listed here, with the exception of the requirement for the comparison of the treated subjects with controls. Isolated case reports, random experience, and reports lacking the details which permit scientific evaluation will not be considered.

[50 FR 7493, Feb. 22, 1985, as amended at 50 FR 21238, May 23, 1985; 55 FR 11580, Mar. 29, 1990; 64 FR 402, Jan. 5, 1999; 67 FR 9586, Mar. 4, 2002]

§ 314.127 Refusal to approve an ANDA.

(a) FDA will refuse to approve an ANDA for a new drug under section 505(j) of the Federal Food, Drug, and Cosmetic Act for any of the following reasons, unless the requirement has been waived under § 314.99:

(1) The methods used in, or the facilities and controls used for, the manufacture, processing, and packing of the drug product are inadequate to ensure and preserve its identity, strength, quality, and purity.

(2) Information submitted with the ANDA is insufficient to show that each of the proposed conditions of use has been previously approved for the listed drug referred to in the ANDA.

(3)(i) If the reference listed drug has only one active ingredient, information submitted with the ANDA is insufficient to show that the active ingredient is the same as that of the reference listed drug;

(ii) If the reference listed drug has more than one active ingredient, information submitted with the ANDA is insufficient to show that the active ingredients are the same as the active ingredients of the reference listed drug; or

(iii) If the reference listed drug has more than one active ingredient and if the ANDAis for a drug product that has an active ingredient different from the reference listed drug:

(A) Information submitted with the ANDA is insufficient to show:

(1) That the other active ingredients are the same as the active ingredients of the reference listed drug; or

(2) That the different active ingredient is an active ingredient of a listed drug or a drug that does not meet the requirements of section 201(p) of the Federal Food, Drug, and Cosmetic Act; or

(B) No petition to submit an ANDA for the drug product with the different active ingredient was approved under § 314.93.

(4)(i) If the ANDA is for a drug product whose route of administration, dosage form, or strength purports to be the same as that of the listed drug referred to in the ANDA, information submitted in the abbreviated new drug application is insufficient to show that the route of administration, dosage form, or strength is the same as that of the reference listed drug; or

(ii) If the ANDA is for a drug product whose route of administration, dosage form, or strength is different from that of the listed drug referred to in the application, no petition to submit an ANDA for the drug product with the different route of administration, dosage form, or strength was approved under § 314.93.

(5) If the ANDA was submitted under the approval of a petition under § 314.93, the ANDA did not contain the information required by FDA with respect to the active ingredient, route of administration, dosage form, or strength that is not the same as that of the reference listed drug.

(6)(i) Information submitted in the ANDA is insufficient to show that the drug product is bioequivalent to the listed drug referred to in the ANDA; or

(ii) If the ANDA was submitted under a petition approved under § 314.93, information submitted in the ANDA is insufficient to show that the active ingredients of the drug product are of the same pharmacological or therapeutic class as those of the reference listed drug and that the drug product can be expected to have the same therapeutic effect as the reference listed drug when administered to patients for each condition of use approved for the reference listed drug.

(7) Information submitted in the ANDA is insufficient to show that the labeling proposed for the drug is the same as the labeling approved for the listed drug referred to in the ANDA except for changes required because of differences approved in a petition under § 314.93 or because the drug product and the reference listed drug are produced or distributed by different manufacturers or because aspects of the listed drug's labeling are protected by patent, or by exclusivity, and such differences do not render the proposed drug product less safe or effective than the listed drug for all remaining, nonprotected conditions of use.

(8)(i) Information submitted in the ANDA or any other information available to FDA shows that:

(A) The inactive ingredients of the drug product are unsafe for use, as described in paragraph (a)(8)(ii) of this section, under the conditions prescribed, recommended, or suggested in the labeling proposed for the drug product; or

(B) The composition of the drug product is unsafe, as described in paragraph (a)(8)(ii) of this section, under the conditions prescribed, recommended, or suggested in the proposed labeling because of the type or quantity of inactive ingredients included or the manner in which the inactive ingredients are included.

(ii)(A) FDA will consider the inactive ingredients or composition of a drug product unsafe and refuse to approve an ANDA under paragraph (a)(8)(i) of this section if, on the basis of information available to the agency, there is a reasonable basis to conclude that one or more of the inactive ingredients of the proposed drug or its composition raises serious questions of safety or efficacy. From its experience with reviewing inactive ingredients, and from other information available to it, FDA may identify changes in inactive ingredients or composition that may adversely affect a drug product's safety or efficacy. The inactive ingredients or composition of a proposed drug product will be considered to raise serious questions of safety or efficacy if the product incorporates one or more of these changes. Examples of the changes that may raise serious questions of safety or efficacy include, but are not limited to, the following:

(1) A change in an inactive ingredient so that the product does not comply with an official compendium.

(2) A change in composition to include an inactive ingredient that has not been previously approved in a drug product for human use by the same route of administration.

(3) A change in the composition of a parenteral drug product to include an inactive ingredient that has not been previously approved in a parenteral drug product.

(4) A change in composition of a drug product for ophthalmic use to include an inactive ingredient that has not been previously approved in a drug for ophthalmic use.

(5) The use of a delivery or a modified release mechanism never before approved for the drug.

(6) A change in composition to include a significantly greater content of one or more inactive ingredients than previously used in the drug product.

(7) If the drug product is intended for topical administration, a change in the properties of the vehicle or base that might increase absorption of certain potentially toxic active ingredients thereby affecting the safety of the drug product, or a change in the lipophilic properties of a vehicle or base, e.g., a change from an oleaginous to a water soluble vehicle or base.

(B) FDA will consider an inactive ingredient in, or the composition of, a drug product intended for parenteral use to be unsafe and will refuse to approve the ANDA unless it contains the same inactive ingredients, other than preservatives, buffers, and antioxidants, in the same concentration as the listed drug, and, if it differs from the listed drug in a preservative, buffer, or antioxidant, the ANDA contains sufficient information to demonstrate that the difference does not affect the safety or efficacy of the drug product.

(C) FDA will consider an inactive ingredient in, or the composition of, a drug product intended for ophthalmic or otic use unsafe and will refuse to approve the ANDA unless it contains the same inactive ingredients, other than preservatives, buffers, substances to adjust tonicity, or thickening agents, in the same concentration as the listed drug, and if it differs from the listed drug in a preservative, buffer, substance to adjust tonicity, or thickening agent, the ANDA contains sufficient information to demonstrate that the difference does not affect the safety or efficacy of the drug product and the labeling does not claim any therapeutic advantage over or difference from the listed drug.

(9) Approval of the listed drug referred to in the ANDA has been withdrawn or suspended for grounds described in § 314.150(a) or FDA has published a notice of opportunity for hearing to withdraw approval of the reference listed drug under § 314.150(a).

(10) Approval of the listed drug referred to in the ANDA has been withdrawn under § 314.151 or FDA has proposed to withdraw approval of the reference listed drug under § 314.151(a).

(11) FDA has determined that the reference listed drug has been withdrawn from sale for safety or effectiveness reasons under § 314.161, or the reference listed drug has been voluntarily withdrawn from sale and the agency has not determined whether the withdrawal is for safety or effectiveness reasons, or approval of the reference listed drug has been suspended under § 314.153, or the agency has issued an initial decision proposing to suspend the reference listed drug under § 314.153(a)(1).

(12) The abbreviated new drug application does not meet any other requirement under section 505(j)(2)(A) of the Federal Food, Drug, and Cosmetic Act.

(13) The abbreviated new drug application contains an untrue statement of material fact.

(14) For an ANDA submitted pursuant to an approved petition under § 10.30 of this chapter and § 314.93, an NDA subsequently has been approved for the change described in the approved petition.

(b) FDA may refuse to approve an ANDA for a new drug if the applicant or contract research organization that conducted a bioavailability or bioequivalence study described in § 320.63 of this chapter that is contained in the ANDA refuses to permit an inspection of facilities or records relevant to the study by a properly authorized officer or employee of the Department of Health and Human Services or refuses to submit reserve samples of the drug products used in the study when requested by FDA.

[57 FR 17991, Apr. 28, 1992; 57 FR 29353, July 1, 1992, as amended at 58 FR 25927, Apr. 28, 1993; 67 FR 77672, Dec. 19, 2002; 81 FR 69658, Oct. 6, 2016]

§ 314.150 Withdrawal of approval of an application or abbreviated application.

(a) The Food and Drug Administration will notify the applicant, and, if appropriate, all other persons who manufacture or distribute identical, related, or similar drug products as defined in §§ 310.6 and 314.151(a) of this chapter and for a new drug afford an opportunity for a hearing on a proposal to withdraw approval of the application or abbreviated new drug application under section 505(e) of the act and under the procedure in § 314.200, if any of the following apply:

(1) The Secretary of Health and Human Services has suspended the approval of the application or abbreviated application for a new drug on a finding that there is an imminent hazard to the public health. FDA will promptly afford the applicant an expedited hearing following summary suspension on a finding of imminent hazard to health.

(2) FDA finds:

(i) That clinical or other experience, tests, or other scientific data show that the drug is unsafe for use under the conditions of use upon the basis of which the application or abbreviated application was approved; or

(ii) That new evidence of clinical experience, not contained in the application or not available to FDA until after the application or abbreviated application was approved, or tests by new methods, or tests by methods not deemed reasonably applicable when the application or abbreviated application was approved, evaluated together with the evidence available when the application or abbreviated application was approved, reveal that the drug is not shown to be safe for use under the conditions of use upon the basis of which the application or abbreviated application was approved; or

(iii) Upon the basis of new information before FDA with respect to the drug, evaluated together with the evidence available when the application or abbreviated application was approved, that there is a lack of substantial evidence from adequate and well-controlled investigations as defined in § 314.126, that the drug will have the effect it is purported or represented to have under the conditions of use prescribed, recommended, or suggested in its labeling; or

(iv) That the application or abbreviated application contains any untrue statement of a material fact; or

(v) That the patent information prescribed by section 505(c) of the act was not submitted within 30 days after the receipt of written notice from FDA specifying the failure to submit such information; or

(b) FDA may notify the applicant, and, if appropriate, all other persons who manufacture or distribute identical, related, or similar drug products as defined in § 310.6, and for a new drug afford an opportunity for a hearing on a proposal to withdraw approval of the application or abbreviated new drug application under section 505(e) of the act and under the procedure in § 314.200, if the agency finds:

(1) That the applicant has failed to establish a system for maintaining required records, or has repeatedly or deliberately failed to maintain required records or to make required reports under section 505(k) or 507(g) of the act and § 314.80, § 314.81, or § 314.98, or that the applicant has refused to permit access to, or copying or verification of, its records.

(2) That on the basis of new information before FDA, evaluated together with the evidence available when the application or abbreviated application was approved, the methods used in, or the facilities and controls used for, the manufacture, processing, and packing of the drug are inadequate to ensure and preserve its identity, strength, quality, and purity and were not made adequate within a reasonable time after receipt of written notice from the agency.

(3) That on the basis of new information before FDA, evaluated together with the evidence available when the application or abbreviated application was approved, the labeling of the drug, based on a fair evaluation of all material facts, is false or misleading in any particular, and the labeling was not corrected by the applicant within a reasonable time after receipt of written notice from the agency.

(4) That the applicant has failed to comply with the notice requirements of section 510(j)(2) of the act.

(5) That the applicant has failed to submit bioavailability or bioequivalence data required under part 320 of this chapter.

(6) The application or abbreviated application does not contain an explanation of the omission of a report of any investigation of the drug product sponsored by the applicant, or an explanation of the omission of other information about the drug pertinent to an evaluation of the application or abbreviated application that is received or otherwise obtained by the applicant from any source.

(7) That any nonclinical laboratory study that is described in the application or abbreviated application and that is essential to show that the drug is safe for use under the conditions prescribed, recommended, or suggested in its labeling was not conducted in compliance with the good laboratory practice regulations in part 58 of this chapter and no reason for the noncompliance was provided or, if it was, the differences between the practices used in conducting the study and the good laboratory practice regulations do not support the validity of the study.

(8) Any clinical investigation involving human subjects described in the application or abbreviated application, subject to the institutional review board regulations in part 56 of this chapter or informed consent regulations in part 50 of this chapter, was not conducted in compliance with those regulations such that the rights or safety of human subjects were not adequately protected.

(9) That the applicant or contract research organization that conducted a bioavailability or bioequivalence study described in § 320.38 or § 320.63 of this chapter that is contained in the application or abbreviated application refuses to permit an inspection of facilities or records relevant to the study by a properly authorized officer or employee of the Department of Health and Human Services or refuses to submit reserve samples of the drug products used in the study when requested by FDA.

(10) That the labeling for the drug product that is the subject of the abbreviated new drug application is no longer consistent with that for the listed drug referred to in the abbreviated new drug application, except for differences approved in the abbreviated new drug application or those differences resulting from:

(i) A patent on the listed drug issued after approval of the abbreviated new drug application; or

(ii) Exclusivity accorded to the listed drug after approval of the abbreviated new drug application that do not render the drug product less safe or effective than the listed drug for any remaining, nonprotected condition(s) of use.

(c) FDA will withdraw approval of an application or abbreviated application if the applicant requests its withdrawal because the drug subject to the application or abbreviated application is no longer being marketed, provided none of the conditions listed in paragraphs (a) and (b) of this section applies to the drug. FDA will consider a written request for a withdrawal under this paragraph to be a waiver of an opportunity for hearing otherwise provided for in this section. Withdrawal of approval of an application or abbreviated application under this paragraph is without prejudice to refiling.

(d) FDA may notify an applicant that it believes a potential problem associated with a drug is sufficiently serious that the drug should be removed from the market and may ask the applicant to waive the opportunity for hearing otherwise provided for under this section, to permit FDA to withdraw approval of the application or abbreviated application for the product, and to remove voluntarily the product from the market. If the applicant agrees, the agency will not make a finding under paragraph (b) of this section, but will withdraw approval of the application or abbreviated application in a notice published in the Federal Register that contains a brief summary of the agency's and the applicant's views of the reasons for withdrawal.

[57 FR 17993, Apr. 28, 1992, as amended at 58 FR 25927, Apr. 28, 1993; 64 FR 402, Jan. 5, 1999]

§ 314.151 Withdrawal of approval of an abbreviated new drug application under section 505(j)(5) of the act.

(a) Approval of an abbreviated new drug application approved under § 314.105(d) may be withdrawn when the agency withdraws approval, under § 314.150(a) or under this section, of the approved drug referred to in the abbreviated new drug application. If the agency proposed to withdraw approval of a listed drug under § 314.150(a), the holder of an approved application for the listed drug has a right to notice and opportunity for hearing. The published notice of opportunity for hearing will identify all drug products approved under § 314.105(d) whose applications are subject to withdrawal under this section if the listed drug is withdrawn, and will propose to withdraw such drugs. Holders of approved applications for the identified drug products will be provided notice and an opportunity to respond to the proposed withdrawal of their applications as described in paragraphs (b) and (c) of this section.

(b)(1) The published notice of opportunity for hearing on the withdrawal of the listed drug will serve as notice to holders of identified abbreviated new drug applications of the grounds for the proposed withdrawal.

(2) Holders of applications for drug products identified in the notice of opportunity for hearing may submit written comments on the notice of opportunity for hearing issued on the proposed

withdrawal of the listed drug. If an abbreviated new drug application holder submits comments on the notice of opportunity for hearing and a hearing is granted, the abbreviated new drug application holder may participate in the hearing as a nonparty participant as provided for in § 12.89 of this chapter.

(3) Except as provided in paragraphs (c) and (d) of this section, the approval of an abbreviated new drug application for a drug product identified in the notice of opportunity for hearing on the withdrawal of a listed drug will be withdrawn when the agency has completed the withdrawal of approval of the listed drug.

(c)(1) If the holder of an application for a drug identified in the notice of opportunity for hearing has submitted timely comments but does not have an opportunity to participate in a hearing because a hearing is not requested or is settled, the submitted comments will be considered by the agency, which will issue an initial decision. The initial decision will respond to the comments, and contain the agency's decision whether there are grounds to withdraw approval of the listed drug and of the abbreviated new drug applications on which timely comments were submitted. The initial decision will be sent to each abbreviated new drug application holder that has submitted comments.

(2) Abbreviated new drug application holders to whom the initial decision was sent may, within 30 days of the issuance of the initial decision, submit written objections.

(3) The agency may, at its discretion, hold a limited oral hearing to resolve dispositive factual issues that cannot be resolved on the basis of written submissions.

(4) If there are no timely objections to the initial decision, it will become final at the expiration of 30 days.

(5) If timely objections are submitted, they will be reviewed and responded to in a final decision.

(6) The written comments received, the initial decision, the evidence relied on in the comments and in the initial decision, the objections to the initial decision, and, if a limited oral hearing has been held, the transcript of that hearing and any documents submitted therein, shall form the record upon which the agency shall make a final decision.

(7) Except as provided in paragraph (d) of this section, any abbreviated new drug application whose holder submitted comments on the notice of opportunity for hearing shall be withdrawn upon the issuance of a final decision concluding that the listed drug should be withdrawn for grounds as described in § 314.150(a). The final decision shall be in writing and shall constitute final agency action, reviewable in a judicial proceeding.

(8) Documents in the record will be publicly available in accordance with § 10.20(j) of this chapter. Documents available for examination or copying will be placed on public display in the Division of Dockets Management (HFA-305), Food and Drug Administration, room. 1-23, 12420 Parklawn Dr., Rockville, MD 20857, promptly upon receipt in that office.

(d) If the agency determines, based upon information submitted by the holder of an abbreviated new drug application, that the grounds for withdrawal of the listed drug are not applicable to a drug identified in the notice of opportunity for hearing, the final decision will state that the approval of the abbreviated new drug application for such drug is not withdrawn.

[57 FR 17994, Apr. 28, 1992]

§ 314.152 Notice of withdrawal of approval of an application or abbreviated application for a new drug.

If the Food and Drug Administration withdraws approval of an application or abbreviated application for a new drug, FDA will publish a notice in the Federal Register announcing the withdrawal of approval. If the application or abbreviated application was withdrawn for grounds described in

§314.150(a) or §314.151, the notice will announce the removal of the drug from the list of approved drugs published under section 505(j)(6) of the act and shall satisfy the requirement of §314.162(b).

[57 FR 17994, Apr. 28, 1992]

§314.153 Suspension of approval of an abbreviated new drug application.

(a) *Suspension of approval.* The approval of an abbreviated new drug application approved under §314.105(d) shall be suspended for the period stated when:

(1) The Secretary of the Department of Health and Human Services, under the imminent hazard authority of section 505(e) of the act or the authority of this paragraph, suspends approval of a listed drug referred to in the abbreviated new drug application, for the period of the suspension;

(2) The agency, in the notice described in paragraph (b) of this section, or in any subsequent written notice given an abbreviated new drug application holder by the agency, concludes that the risk of continued marketing and use of the drug is inappropriate, pending completion of proceedings to withdraw or suspend approval under §314.151 or paragraph (b) of this section; or

(3) The agency, under the procedures set forth in paragraph (b) of this section, issues a final decision stating the determination that the abbreviated application is suspended because the listed drug on which the approval of the abbreviated new drug application depends has been withdrawn from sale for reasons of safety or effectiveness or has been suspended under paragraph (b) of this section. The suspension will take effect on the date stated in the decision and will remain in effect until the agency determines that the marketing of the drug has resumed or that the withdrawal is not for safety or effectiveness reasons.

(b) *Procedures for suspension of abbreviated new drug applications when a listed drug is voluntarily withdrawn for safety or effectiveness reasons.* (1) If a listed drug is voluntarily withdrawn from sale, and the agency determines that the withdrawal from sale was for reasons of safety or effectiveness, the agency will send each holder of an approved abbreviated new drug application that is subject to suspension as a result of this determination a copy of the agency's initial decision setting forth the reasons for the determination. The initial decision will also be placed on file with the Division of Dockets Management (HFA-305), Food and Drug Administration, room 1-23, 12420 Parklawn Dr., Rockville, MD 20857.

(2) Each abbreviated new drug application holder will have 30 days from the issuance of the initial decision to present, in writing, comments and information bearing on the initial decision. If no comments or information is received, the initial decision will become final at the expiration of 30 days.

(3) Comments and information received within 30 days of the issuance of the initial decision will be considered by the agency and responded to in a final decision.

(4) The agency may, in its discretion, hold a limited oral hearing to resolve dispositive factual issues that cannot be resolved on the basis of written submissions.

(5) If the final decision affirms the agency's initial decision that the listed drug was withdrawn for reasons of safety or effectiveness, the decision will be published in the Federal Register in compliance with §314.152, and will, except as provided in paragraph (b)(6) of this section, suspend approval of all abbreviated new drug applications identified under paragraph (b)(1) of this section and remove from the list the listed drug and any drug whose approval was suspended under this paragraph. The notice will satisfy the requirement of §314.162(b). The agency's final decision and copies of materials on which it relies will also be filed with the Division of Dockets Management (address in paragraph (b)(1) of this section).

(6) If the agency determines in its final decision that the listed drug was withdrawn for reasons of safety or effectiveness but, based upon information submitted by the holder of an abbreviated new drug application, also determines that the reasons for the withdrawal of the listed drug are not relevant to the safety and effectiveness of the drug subject to such abbreviated new drug applica-

tion, the final decision will state that the approval of such abbreviated new drug application is not suspended.

(7) Documents in the record will be publicly available in accordance with § 10.20(j) of this chapter. Documents available for examination or copying will be placed on public display in the Division of Dockets Management (address in paragraph (b)(1) of this section) promptly upon receipt in that office.

[57 FR 17995, Apr. 28, 1992]

§ 314.160 Approval of an application or abbreviated application for which approval was previously refused, suspended, or withdrawn.

Upon the Food and Drug Administration's own initiative or upon request of an applicant, FDA may, on the basis of new data, approve an application or abbreviated application which it had previously refused, suspended, or withdrawn approval. FDA will publish a notice in the Federal Register announcing the approval.

[57 FR 17995, Apr. 28, 1992]

§ 314.161 Determination of reasons for voluntary withdrawal of a listed drug.

(a) A determination whether a listed drug that has been voluntarily withdrawn from sale was withdrawn for safety or effectiveness reasons may be made by the agency at any time after the drug has been voluntarily withdrawn from sale, but must be made:

(1) Prior to approving an abbreviated new drug application that refers to the listed drug;

(2) Whenever a listed drug is voluntarily withdrawn from sale and abbreviated new drug applications that referred to the listed drug have been approved; and

(3) When a person petitions for such a determination under §§ 10.25(a) and 10.30 of this chapter.

(b) Any person may petition under §§ 10.25(a) and 10.30 of this chapter for a determination whether a listed drug has been voluntarily withdrawn for safety or effectiveness reasons. Any such petition must contain all evidence available to the petitioner concerning the reason that the drug is withdrawn from sale.

(c) If the agency determines that a listed drug is withdrawn from sale for safety or effectiveness reasons, the agency will, except as provided in paragraph (d) of this section, publish a notice of the determination in the Federal Register.

(d) If the agency determines under paragraph (a) of this section that a listed drug is withdrawn from sale for safety and effectiveness reasons and there are approved abbreviated new drug applications that are subject to suspension under section 505(j)(5) of the act, FDA will initiate a proceeding in accordance with § 314.153(b).

(e) A drug that the agency determines is withdrawn for safety or effectiveness reasons will be removed from the list, under § 314.162. The drug may be relisted if the agency has evidence that marketing of the drug has resumed or that the withdrawal is not for safety or effectiveness reasons. A determination that the drug is not withdrawn for safety or effectiveness reasons may be made at any time after its removal from the list, upon the agency's initiative, or upon the submission of a petition under §§ 10.25(a) and 10.30 of this chapter. If the agency determines that the drug is not withdrawn for safety or effectiveness reasons, the agency shall publish a notice of this determination in the Federal Register. The notice will also announce that the drug is relisted, under § 314.162(c). The notice will also serve to reinstate approval of all suspended abbreviated new drug applications that referred to the listed drug.

[57 FR 17995, Apr. 28, 1992]

§ 314.162 Removal of a drug product from the list.

(a) FDA will remove a previously approved new drug product from the list for the period stated when:

(1) The agency withdraws or suspends approval of a new drug application or an abbreviated new drug application under § 314.150(a) or § 314.151 or under the imminent hazard authority of section 505(e) of the act, for the same period as the withdrawal or suspension of the application; or

(2) The agency, in accordance with the procedures in § 314.153(b) or § 314.161, issues a final decision stating that the listed drug was withdrawn from sale for safety or effectiveness reasons, or suspended under § 314.153(b), until the agency determines that the withdrawal from the market has ceased or is not for safety or effectiveness reasons.

(b) FDA will publish in the Federal Register a notice announcing the removal of a drug from the list.

(c) At the end of the period specified in paragraph (a)(1) or (a)(2) of this section, FDA will relist a drug that has been removed from the list. The agency will publish in the Federal Register a notice announcing the relisting of the drug.

[57 FR 17996, Apr. 28, 1992]

§ 314.170 Adulteration and misbranding of an approved drug.

All drugs, including those the Food and Drug Administration approves under section 505 of the act and this part, are subject to the adulteration and misbranding provisions in sections 501, 502, and 503 of the act. FDA is authorized to regulate approved new drugs by regulations issued through informal rulemaking under sections 501, 502, and 503 of the act.

[50 FR 7493, Feb. 22, 1985. Redesignated at 57 FR 17983, Apr. 28, 1992, and amended at 64 FR 402, Jan. 5, 1999]

Subpart E—Hearing Procedures for New Drugs

Source: 50 FR 7493, Feb. 22, 1985, unless otherwise noted. Redesignated at 57 FR 17983, Apr. 28, 1992.

§ 314.200 Notice of opportunity for hearing; notice of participation and request for hearing; grant or denial of hearing.

(a) *Notice of opportunity for hearing.* The Director of the Center for Drug Evaluation and Research, Food and Drug Administration, will give the applicant, and all other persons who manufacture or distribute identical, related, or similar drug products as defined in § 310.6 of this chapter, notice and an opportunity for a hearing on the Center's proposal to refuse to approve an application or to withdraw the approval of an application or abbreviated application under section 505(e) of the act. The notice will state the reasons for the action and the proposed grounds for the order.

(1) The notice may be general (that is, simply summarizing in a general way the information resulting in the notice) or specific (that is, either referring to specific requirements in the statute and regulations with which there is a lack of compliance, or providing a detailed description and analysis of the specific facts resulting in the notice).

(2) FDA will publish the notice in the Federal Register and will state that the applicant, and other persons subject to the notice under § 310.6, who wishes to participate in a hearing, has 30 days after the date of publication of the notice to file a written notice of participation and request for hearing. The applicant, or other persons subject to the notice under § 310.6, who fails to file a written notice of participation and request for hearing within 30 days, waives the opportunity for a hearing.

(3) It is the responsibility of every manufacturer and distributor of a drug product to review every notice of opportunity for a hearing published in the Federal Register to determine whether it cov-

ers any drug product that person manufactures or distributes. Any person may request an opinion of the applicability of a notice to a specific product that may be identical, related, or similar to a product listed in a notice by writing to the Division of New Drugs and Labeling Compliance, Office of Compliance, Center for Drug Evaluation and Research, Food and Drug Administration, 10903 New Hampshire Ave., Silver Spring, MD 20993-0002. A person shall request an opinion within 30 days of the date of publication of the notice to be eligible for an opportunity for a hearing under the notice. If a person requests an opinion, that person's time for filing an appearance and request for a hearing and supporting studies and analyses begins on the date the person receives the opinion from FDA.

(b) FDA will provide the notice of opportunity for a hearing to applicants and to other persons subject to the notice under § 310.6, as follows:

(1) To any person who has submitted an application or abbreviated application, by delivering the notice in person or by sending it by registered or certified mail to the last address shown in the application or abbreviated application.

(2) To any person who has not submitted an application or abbreviated application but who is subject to the notice under § 310.6 of this chapter, by publication of the notice in the Federal Register.

(c)(1) *Notice of participation and request for a hearing, and submission of studies and comments.* The applicant, or any other person subject to the notice under § 310.6, who wishes to participate in a hearing, shall file with the Division of Dockets Management (HFA-305), Food and Drug Administration, 5630 Fishers Lane, rm. 1061, Rockville, MD 20852, (i) within 30 days after the date of the publication of the notice (or of the date of receipt of an opinion requested under paragraph (a)(3) of this section) a written notice of participation and request for a hearing and (ii) within 60 days after the date of publication of the notice, unless a different period of time is specified in the notice of opportunity for a hearing, the studies on which the person relies to justify a hearing as specified in paragraph (d) of this section. The applicant, or other person, may incorporate by reference the raw data underlying a study if the data were previously submitted to FDA as part of an application, abbreviated application, or other report.

(2) FDA will not consider data or analyses submitted after 60 days in determining whether a hearing is warranted unless they are derived from well-controlled studies begun before the date of the notice of opportunity for hearing and the results of the studies were not available within 60 days after the date of publication of the notice. Nevertheless, FDA may consider other studies on the basis of a showing by the person requesting a hearing of inadvertent omission and hardship. The person requesting a hearing shall list in the request for hearing all studies in progress, the results of which the person intends later to submit in support of the request for a hearing. The person shall submit under paragraph (c)(1)(ii) of this section a copy of the complete protocol, a list of the participating investigators, and a brief status report of the studies.

(3) Any other interested person who is not subject to the notice of opportunity for a hearing may also submit comments on the proposal to withdraw approval of the application or abbreviated application. The comments are requested to be submitted within the time and under the conditions specified in this section.

(d) The person requesting a hearing is required to submit under paragraph (c)(1)(ii) of this section the studies (including all protocols and underlying raw data) on which the person relies to justify a hearing with respect to the drug product. Except, a person who requests a hearing on the refusal to approve an application is not required to submit additional studies and analyses if the studies upon which the person relies have been submitted in the application and in the format and containing the summaries required under § 314.50.

(1) If the grounds for FDA's proposed action concern the effectiveness of the drug, each request for hearing is required to be supported only by adequate and well-controlled clinical studies meeting

all of the precise requirements of § 314.126 and, for combination drug products, § 300.50, or by other studies not meeting those requirements for which a waiver has been previously granted by FDA under § 314.126. Each person requesting a hearing shall submit all adequate and well-controlled clinical studies on the drug product, including any unfavorable analyses, views, or judgments with respect to the studies. No other data, information, or studies may be submitted.

(2) The submission is required to include a factual analysis of all the studies submitted. If the grounds for FDA's proposed action concern the effectiveness of the drug, the analysis is required to specify how each study accords, on a point-by-point basis, with each criterion required for an adequate well-controlled clinical investigation established under § 314.126 and, if the product is a combination drug product, with each of the requirements for a combination drug established in § 300.50, or the study is required to be accompanied by an appropriate waiver previously granted by FDA. If a study concerns a drug or dosage form or condition of use or mode of administration other than the one in question, that fact is required to be clearly stated. Any study conducted on the final marketed form of the drug product is required to be clearly identified.

(3) Each person requesting a hearing shall submit an analysis of the data upon which the person relies, except that the required information relating either to safety or to effectiveness may be omitted if the notice of opportunity for hearing does not raise any issue with respect to that aspect of the drug; information on compliance with § 300.50 may be omitted if the drug product is not a combination drug product. A financial certification or disclosure statement or both as required by part 54 of this chapter must accompany all clinical data submitted. FDA can most efficiently consider submissions made in the following format.

I. Safety data.

A. Animal safety data.

1. Individual active components.

a. Controlled studies.

b. Partially controlled or uncontrolled studies.

2. Combinations of the individual active components.

a. Controlled studies.

b. Partially controlled or uncontrolled studies.

B. Human safety data.

1. Individual active components.

a. Controlled studies.

b. Partially controlled or uncontrolled studies.

c. Documented case reports.

d. Pertinent marketing experiences that may influence a determination about the safety of each individual active component.

2. Combinations of the individual active components.

a. Controlled studies.

b. Partially controlled or uncontrolled studies.

c. Documented case reports.

d. Pertinent marketing experiences that may influence a determination about the safety of each individual active component.

II. Effectiveness data.

A. Individual active components: Controlled studies, with an analysis showing clearly how each study satisfies, on a point-by-point basis, each of the criteria required by § 314.126.

B. Combinations of individual active components.

1. Controlled studies with an analysis showing clearly how each study satisfies on a point-by-point basis, each of the criteria required by § 314.126.

2. An analysis showing clearly how each requirement of § 300.50 has been satisfied.

III. A summary of the data and views setting forth the medical rationale and purpose for the drug and its ingredients and the scientific basis for the conclusion that the drug and its ingredients have been proven safe and/or effective for the intended use. If there is an absence of controlled studies in the material submitted or the requirements of any element of § 300.50 or § 314.126 have not been fully met, that fact is required to be stated clearly and a waiver obtained under § 314.126 is required to be submitted.

IV. A statement signed by the person responsible for such submission that it includes in full (or incorporates by reference as permitted in § 314.200(c)(2)) all studies and information specified in § 314.200(d).

(WARNING: A willfully false statement is a criminal offense, 18 U.S.C. 1001.)

(e) *Contentions that a drug product is not subject to the new drug requirements.* A notice of opportunity for a hearing encompasses all issues relating to the legal status of each drug product subject to it, including identical, related, and similar drug products as defined in § 310.6. A notice of appearance and request for a hearing under paragraph (c)(1)(i) of this section is required to contain any contention that the product is not a new drug because it is generally recognized as safe and effective within the meaning of section 201(p) of the act, or because it is exempt from part or all of the new drug provisions of the act under the exemption for products marketed before June 25, 1938, contained in section 201(p) of the act or under section 107(c) of the Drug Amendments of 1962, or for any other reason. Each contention is required to be supported by a submission under paragraph (c)(1)(ii) of this section and the Commissioner of Food and Drugs will make an administrative determination on each contention. The failure of any person subject to a notice of opportunity for a hearing, including any person who manufactures or distributes an identical, related, or similar drug product as defined in § 310.6, to submit a notice of participation and request for hearing or to raise all such contentions constitutes a waiver of any contentions not raised.

(1) A contention that a drug product is generally recognized as safe and effective within the meaning of section 201(p) of the act is required to be supported by submission of the same quantity and quality of scientific evidence that is required to obtain approval of an application for the product, unless FDA has waived a requirement for effectiveness (under § 314.126) or safety, or both. The submission should be in the format and with the analyses required under paragraph (d) of this section. A person who fails to submit the required scientific evidence required under paragraph (d) waives the contention. General recognition of safety and effectiveness shall ordinarily be based upon published studies which may be corroborated by unpublished studies and other data and information.

(2) A contention that a drug product is exempt from part or all of the new drug provisions of the act under the exemption for products marketed before June 25, 1938, contained in section 201(p) of the act, or under section 107(c) of the Drug Amendments of 1962, is required to be supported by evidence of past and present quantitative formulas, labeling, and evidence of marketing. A person who makes such a contention should submit the formulas, labeling, and evidence of marketing in the following format.

I. Formulation.

A. A copy of each pertinent document or record to establish the exact quantitative formulation of the drug (both active and inactive ingredients) on the date of initial marketing of the drug.

B. A statement whether such formulation has at any subsequent time been changed in any manner. If any such change has been made, the exact date, nature, and rationale for each change in formulation, including any deletion or change in the concentration of any active ingredient and/or inactive ingredient, should be stated, together with a copy of each pertinent document or record to establish the date and nature of each such change, including, but not limited to, the formula which resulted from each such change. If no such change has been made, a copy of representative documents or records showing the formula at representative points in time should be submitted to support the statement.

II. Labeling.

A. A copy of each pertinent document or record to establish the identity of each item of written, printed, or graphic matter used as labeling on the date the drug was initially marketed.

B. A statement whether such labeling has at any subsequent time been discontinued or changed in any manner. If such discontinuance or change has been made, the exact date, nature, and rationale for each discontinuance or change and a copy of each pertinent document or record to establish each such discontinuance or change should be submitted, including, but not limited to, the labeling which resulted from each such discontinuance or change. If no such discontinuance or change has been made, a copy of representative documents or records showing labeling at representative points in time should be submitted to support the statement.

III. Marketing.

A. A copy of each pertinent document or record to establish the exact date the drug was initially marketed.

B. A statement whether such marketing has at any subsequent time been discontinued. If such marketing has been discontinued, the exact date of each such discontinuance should be submitted, together with a copy of each pertinent document or record to establish each such date.

IV. Verification.

A statement signed by the person responsible for such submission, that all appropriate records have been searched and to the best of that person's knowledge and belief it includes a true and accurate presentation of the facts.

(WARNING: A willfully false statement is a criminal offense, 18 U.S.C. 1001.)

(3) The Food and Drug Administration will not find a drug product, including any active ingredient, which is identical, related, or similar, as described in § 310.6, to a drug product, including any active ingredient for which an application is or at any time has been effective or deemed approved, or approved under section 505 of the act, to be exempt from part or all of the new drug provisions of the act.

(4) A contention that a drug product is not a new drug for any other reason is required to be supported by submission of the factual records, data, and information that are necessary and appropriate to support the contention.

(5) It is the responsibility of every person who manufactures or distributes a drug product in reliance upon a "grandfather" provision of the act to maintain files that contain the data and information necessary fully to document and support that status.

(f) *Separation of functions.* Separation of functions commences upon receipt of a request for hearing. The Director of the Center for Drug Evaluation and Research, Food and Drug Administration, will prepare an analysis of the request and a proposed order ruling on the matter. The analysis and proposed order, the request for hearing, and any proposed order denying a hearing and response under paragraph (g) (2) or (3) of this section will be submitted to the Office of the Commissioner of Food and Drugs for review and decision. When the Center for Drug Evaluation and Research recommends denial of a hearing on all issues on which a hearing is requested, no representative of the Center will participate or advise in the review and decision by the Commissioner. When the Center for Drug Evaluation and Research recommends that a hearing be granted on one or more issues on which a hearing is requested, separation of functions terminates as to those issues, and representatives of the Center may participate or advise in the review and decision by the Commissioner on those issues. The Commissioner may modify the text of the issues, but may not deny a hearing on those issues. Separation of functions continues with respect to issues on which the Center for Drug Evaluation and Research has recommended denial of a hearing. The Commissioner will neither evaluate nor rule on the Center's recommendation on such issues and such issues will not be included in the notice of hearing. Participants in the hearing may make a motion to the presiding officer for the inclusion of any such issue in the hearing. The ruling on such a motion is subject to review in accordance with § 12.35(b). Failure to so move constitutes a waiver of the right to a hearing on such an issue. Separation of functions on all issues resumes upon issuance of a notice of hearing. The Office of the General Counsel, Department of Health and Human Services, will observe the same separation of functions.

(g) *Summary judgment.* A person who requests a hearing may not rely upon allegations or denials but is required to set forth specific facts showing that there is a genuine and substantial issue of fact that requires a hearing with respect to a particular drug product specified in the request for hearing.

(1) Where a specific notice of opportunity for hearing (as defined in paragraph (a)(1) of this section) is used, the Commissioner will enter summary judgment against a person who requests a hearing, making findings and conclusions, denying a hearing, if it conclusively appears from the face of the data, information, and factual analyses in the request for the hearing that there is no genuine and substantial issue of fact which precludes the refusal to approve the application or abbreviated application or the withdrawal of approval of the application or abbreviated application; for example, no adequate and well-controlled clinical investigations meeting each of the precise elements of § 314.126 and, for a combination drug product, § 300.50 of this chapter, showing effectiveness have been identified. Any order entering summary judgment is required to set forth the Commissioner's findings and conclusions in detail and is required to specify why each study submitted fails to meet the requirements of the statute and regulations or why the request for hearing does not raise a genuine and substantial issue of fact.

(2) When following a general notice of opportunity for a hearing (as defined in paragraph (a)(1) of this section) the Director of the Center for Drug Evaluation and Research concludes that summary judgment against a person requesting a hearing should be considered, the Director will serve upon the person requesting a hearing by registered mail a proposed order denying a hearing. This person has 60 days after receipt of the proposed order to respond with sufficient data, information, and analyses to demonstrate that there is a genuine and substantial issue of fact which justifies a hearing.

(3) When following a general or specific notice of opportunity for a hearing a person requesting a hearing submits data or information of a type required by the statute and regulations, and the Director of the Center for Drug Evaluation and Research concludes that summary judgment against the person should be considered, the Director will serve upon the person by registered mail a proposed order denying a hearing. The person has 60 days after receipt of the proposed order to respond with

sufficient data, information, and analyses to demonstrate that there is a genuine and substantial issue of fact which justifies a hearing.

(4) If review of the data, information, and analyses submitted show that the grounds cited in the notice are not valid, for example, that substantial evidence of effectiveness exists, the Commissioner will enter summary judgment for the person requesting the hearing, and rescind the notice of opportunity for hearing.

(5) If the Commissioner grants a hearing, it will begin within 90 days after the expiration of the time for requesting the hearing unless the parties otherwise agree in the case of denial of approval, and as soon as practicable in the case of withdrawal of approval.

(6) The Commissioner will grant a hearing if there exists a genuine and substantial issue of fact or if the Commissioner concludes that a hearing would otherwise be in the public interest.

(7) If the manufacturer or distributor of an identical, related, or similar drug product requests and is granted a hearing, the hearing may consider whether the product is in fact identical, related, or similar to the drug product named in the notice of opportunity for a hearing.

(8) A request for a hearing, and any subsequent grant or denial of a hearing, applies only to the drug products named in such documents.

(h) FDA will issue a notice withdrawing approval and declaring all products unlawful for drug products subject to a notice of opportunity for a hearing, including any identical, related, or similar drug product under § 310.6, for which an opportunity for a hearing is waived or for which a hearing is denied. The Commissioner may defer or stay the action pending a ruling on any related request for a hearing or pending any related hearing or other administrative or judicial proceeding.

[50 FR 7493, Feb. 22, 1985; 50 FR 14212, Apr. 11, 1985, as amended at 50 FR 21238, May 23, 1985; 55 FR 11580, Mar. 29, 1990; 57 FR 17996, Apr. 28, 1992; 59 FR 14364, Mar. 28, 1994; 63 FR 5252, Feb. 2, 1998; 67 FR 9586, Mar. 4, 2002; 68 FR 24879, May 9, 2003; 69 FR 48775, Aug. 11, 2004; 74 FR 13113, Mar. 26, 2009]

§ 314.201 Procedure for hearings.

Parts 10 through 16 apply to hearings relating to new drugs under section 505 (d) and (e) of the act.

§ 314.235 Judicial review.

(a) The Commissioner of Food and Drugs will certify the transcript and record. In any case in which the Commissioner enters an order without a hearing under § 314.200(g), the record certified by the Commissioner is required to include the requests for hearing together with the data and information submitted and the Commissioner's findings and conclusion.

(b) A manufacturer or distributor of an identical, related, or similar drug product under § 310.6 may seek judicial review of an order withdrawing approval of a new drug application, whether or not a hearing has been held, in a United States court of appeals under section 505(h) of the act.

Subpart F—[Reserved]

Subpart G—Miscellaneous Provisions

Source: 50 FR 7493, Feb. 22, 1985, unless otherwise noted. Redesignated at 57 FR 17983, Apr. 28, 1992.

§ 314.410 Imports and exports of new drugs.

(a) *Imports.* (1) A new drug may be imported into the United States if: (i) It is the subject of an approved application under this part; or (ii) it complies with the regulations pertaining to investigational new drugs under part 312; and it complies with the general regulations pertaining to imports under subpart E of part 1.

(2) A drug substance intended for use in the manufacture, processing, or repacking of a new drug may be imported into the United States if it complies with the labeling exemption in § 201.122 pertaining to shipments of drug substances in domestic commerce.

(b) *Exports.* (1) A new drug may be exported if it is the subject of an approved application under this part or it complies with the regulations pertaining to investigational new drugs under part 312.

(2) A new drug substance that is covered by an application approved under this part for use in the manufacture of an approved drug product may be exported by the applicant or any person listed as a supplier in the approved application, provided the drug substance intended for export meets the specification of, and is shipped with a copy of the labeling required for, the approved drug product.

(3) Insulin or an antibiotic drug may be exported without regard to the requirements in section 802 of the act if the insulin or antibiotic drug meets the requirements of section 801(e)(1) of the act.

[50 FR 7493, Feb. 22, 1985. Redesignated at 57 FR 17983, Apr. 28, 1992, and amended at 64 FR 402, Jan. 5, 1999; 69 FR 18766, Apr. 8, 2004]

§ 314.420 Drug master files.

(a) A drug master file is a submission of information to the Food and Drug Administration by a person (the drug master file holder) who intends it to be used for one of the following purposes: To permit the holder to incorporate the information by reference when the holder submits an investigational new drug application under part 312 or submits an application or an abbreviated application or an amendment or supplement to them under this part, or to permit the holder to authorize other persons to rely on the information to support a submission to FDA without the holder having to disclose the information to the person. FDA ordinarily neither independently reviews drug master files nor approves or disapproves submissions to a drug master file. Instead, the agency customarily reviews the information only in the context of an application under part 312 or this part. A drug master file may contain information of the kind required for any submission to the agency, including information about the following:

(1) [Reserved]

(2) Drug substance, drug substance intermediate, and materials used in their preparation, or drug product;

(3) Packaging materials;

(4) Excipient, colorant, flavor, essence, or materials used in their preparation;

(5) FDA-accepted reference information. (A person wishing to submit information and supporting data in a drug master file (DMF) that is not covered by Types II through IV DMF's must first submit a letter of intent to the Drug Master File Staff, Food and Drug Administration, 5901-B Ammendale Rd., Beltsville, MD 20705-1266.) FDA will then contact the person to discuss the proposed submission.

(b) An investigational new drug application or an application, abbreviated application, amendment, or supplement may incorporate by reference all or part of the contents of any drug master file in support of the submission if the holder authorizes the incorporation in writing. Each incorporation by reference is required to describe the incorporated material by name, reference number, volume, and page number of the drug master file.

(c) A drug master file is required to be submitted in two copies. The agency has prepared guidance that provides information about how to prepare a well-organized drug master file. If the drug master file holder adds, changes, or deletes any information in the file, the holder shall notify in writing, each person authorized to reference that information. Any addition, change, or deletion of information in a drug master file (except the list required under paragraph (d) of this section) is required to be submitted in two copies and to describe by name, reference number, volume, and page number the information affected in the drug master file.

(d) The drug master file is required to contain a complete list of each person currently authorized to incorporate by reference any information in the file, identifying by name, reference number, volume, and page number the information that each person is authorized to incorporate. If the holder restricts the authorization to particular drug products, the list is required to include the name of each drug product and the application number, if known, to which the authorization applies.

(e) The public availability of data and information in a drug master file, including the availability of data and information in the file to a person authorized to reference the file, is determined under part 20 and § 314.430.

[50 FR 7493, Feb. 22, 1985, as amended at 50 FR 21238, May 23, 1985; 53 FR 33122, Aug. 30, 1988; 55 FR 28380, July 11, 1990; 65 FR 1780, Jan. 12, 2000; 65 FR 56479, Sept. 19, 2000; 67 FR 9586, Mar. 4, 2002; 69 FR 13473, Mar. 23, 2004]

§ 314.430 Availability for public disclosure of data and information in an application or abbreviated application.

(a) The Food and Drug Administration will determine the public availability of any part of an application or abbreviated application under this section and part 20 of this chapter. For purposes of this section, the application or abbreviated application includes all data and information submitted with or incorporated by reference in the application or abbreviated application, including investigational new drug applications, drug master files under § 314.420, supplements submitted under § 314.70 or § 314.97, reports under § 314.80 or § 314.98, and other submissions. For purposes of this section, safety and effectiveness data include all studies and tests of a drug on animals and humans and all studies and tests of the drug for identity, stability, purity, potency, and bioavailability.

(b) FDA will not publicly disclose the existence of an application or abbreviated application before an approval letter is sent to the applicant under § 314.105 or tentative approval letter is sent to the applicant under § 314.107, unless the existence of the application or abbreviated application has been previously publicly disclosed or acknowledged.

(c) If the existence of an unapproved application or abbreviated application has not been publicly disclosed or acknowledged, no data or information in the application or abbreviated application is available for public disclosure.

(d)(1) If the existence of an application or abbreviated application has been publicly disclosed or acknowledged before the agency sends an approval letter to the applicant, no data or information contained in the application or abbreviated application is available for public disclosure before the agency sends an approval letter, but the Commissioner may, in his or her discretion, disclose a summary of selected portions of the safety and effectiveness data that are appropriate for public consideration of a specific pending issue; for example, for consideration of an open session of an FDA advisory committee.

(2) Notwithstanding paragraph (d)(1) of this section, FDA will make available to the public upon request the information in the investigational new drug application that was required to be filed in Docket Number 95S-0158 in the Division of Dockets Management (HFA-305), Food and Drug Administration, 5630 Fishers Lane, rm. 1061, Rockville, MD 20852, for investigations involving an exception from informed consent under § 50.24 of this chapter. Persons wishing to request this information shall submit a request under the Freedom of Information Act.

(e) After FDA sends an approval letter to the applicant, the following data and information in the application or abbreviated application are immediately available for public disclosure, unless the applicant shows that extraordinary circumstances exist. A list of approved applications and abbreviated applications, entitled "Approved Drug Products with Therapeutic Equivalence Evaluations," is available from the Government Printing Office, Washington, DC 20402. This list is updated monthly.

(1) [Reserved]

(2) If the application applies to a new drug, all safety and effectiveness data previously disclosed to the public as set forth in § 20.81 and a summary or summaries of the safety and effectiveness data and information submitted with or incorporated by reference in the application. The summaries do not constitute the full reports of investigations under section 505(b)(1) of the act (21 U.S.C. 355(b)(1)) on which the safety or effectiveness of the drug may be approved. The summaries consist of the following:

(i) For an application approved before July 1, 1975, internal agency records that describe safety and effectiveness data and information, for example, a summary of the basis for approval or internal reviews of the data and information, after deletion of the following:

(a) Names and any information that would identify patients or test subjects or investigators.

(b) Any inappropriate gratuitous comments unnecessary to an objective analysis of the data and information.

(ii) For an application approved on or after July 1, 1975, a Summary Basis of Approval (SBA) document that contains a summary of the safety and effectiveness data and information evaluated by FDA during the drug approval process. The SBA is prepared in one of the following ways:

(a) Before approval of the application, the applicant may prepare a draft SBA which the Center for Drug Evaluation and Research will review and may revise. The draft may be submitted with the application or as an amendment.

(b) The Center for Drug Evaluation and Research may prepare the SBA.

(3) A protocol for a test or study, unless it is shown to fall within the exemption established for trade secrets and confidential commercial information in § 20.61.

(4) Adverse reaction reports, product experience reports, consumer complaints, and other similar data and information after deletion of the following:

(i) Names and any information that would identify the person using the product.

(ii) Names and any information that would identify any third party involved with the report, such as a physician or hospital or other institution.

(5) A list of all active ingredients and any inactive ingredients previously disclosed to the public as set forth in § 20.81.

(6) An assay procedure or other analytical procedure, unless it serves no regulatory or compliance purpose and is shown to fall within the exemption established for trade secrets and confidential commercial information in § 20.61.

(7) All correspondence and written summaries of oral discussions between FDA and the applicant relating to the application, under the provisions of part 20.

(f) All safety and effectiveness data and information which have been submitted in an application and which have not previously been disclosed to the public are available to the public, upon request, at the time any one of the following events occurs unless extraordinary circumstances are shown:

(1) No work is being or will be undertaken to have the application approved.

(2) A final determination is made that the application is not approvable and all legal appeals have been exhausted.

(3) Approval of the application is withdrawn and all legal appeals have been exhausted.

(4) A final determination has been made that the drug is not a new drug.

(5) For applications submitted under section 505(b) of the act, the effective date of the approval of the first abbreviated application submitted under section 505(j) of the act which refers to such

drug, or the date on which the approval of an abbreviated application under section 505(j) of the act which refers to such drug could be made effective if such an abbreviated application had been submitted.

(6) For abbreviated applications submitted under section 505(j) of the act, when FDA sends an approval letter to the applicant.

(g) The following data and information in an application or abbreviated application are not available for public disclosure unless they have been previously disclosed to the public as set forth in § 20.81 of this chapter or they relate to a product or ingredient that has been abandoned and they do not represent a trade secret or confidential commercial or financial information under § 20.61 of this chapter:

(1) Manufacturing methods or processes, including quality control procedures.

(2) Production, sales distribution, and similar data and information, except that any compilation of that data and information aggregated and prepared in a way that does not reveal data or information which is not available for public disclosure under this provision is available for public disclosure.

(3) Quantitative or semiquantitative formulas.

(h) The compilations of information specified in § 20.117 are available for public disclosure.

[50 FR 7493, Feb. 22, 1985, as amended at 50 FR 21238, May 23, 1985; 55 FR 11580, Mar. 29, 1990; 57 FR 17996, Apr. 28, 1992; 61 FR 51530, Oct. 2, 1996; 64 FR 26698, May 13, 1998; 64 FR 402, Jan. 5, 1999; 66 FR 1832, Jan. 10, 2001; 68 FR 24879, May 9, 2003; 69 FR 18766, Apr. 8, 2004; 73 FR 39610, July 10, 2008]

§ 314.440 Addresses for applications and abbreviated applications.

(a) Applicants shall send applications, abbreviated applications, and other correspondence relating to matters covered by this part, except for products listed in paragraph (b) of this section, to the appropriate office identified below:

(1) Except as provided in paragraph (a)(4) of this section, an application under § 314.50 or § 314.54 submitted for filing should be directed to the Central Document Room, 5901-B Ammendale Rd., Beltsville, MD 20705-1266. Applicants may obtain information about folders for binding applications on the Internet at *http://www.fda.gov/cder/ddms/binders.htm.* After FDA has filed the application, the agency will inform the applicant which division is responsible for the application. Amendments, supplements, resubmissions, requests for waivers, and other correspondence about an application that has been filed should be addressed to 5901-B Ammendale Rd., Beltsville, MD 20705-1266, to the attention of the appropriate division.

(2) Except as provided in paragraph (a)(4) of this section, an abbreviated application under § 314.94, and amendments, supplements, and resubmissions should be directed to the Office of Generic Drugs (HFD-600), Center for Drug Evaluation and Research, Food and Drug Administration, Metro Park North VII, 7620 Standish Pl., Rockville, MD 20855. This includes items sent by parcel post or overnight courier service. Correspondence not associated with an abbreviated application should be addressed specifically to the intended office or division and to the person as follows: Office of Generic Drugs, Center for Drug Evaluation and Research, Food and Drug Administration, Attn: [insert name of person], Metro Park North II, HFD-[insert mail code of office or division], 7500 Standish Place, rm. 150, Rockville, MD 20855. The mail code for the Office of Generic Drugs is HFD-600, the mail codes for the Divisions of Chemistry I, II, and III are HFD-620, HFD-640, and HFD-630, respectively, and the mail code for the Division of Bioequivalence is HFD-650.

(3) A request for an opportunity for a hearing under § 314.110 on the question of whether there are grounds for denying approval of an application, except an application under paragraph (b) of this section, should be directed to the Associate Director for Policy (HFD-5).

(4) The field copy of an application, an abbreviated application, amendments, supplements, resubmissions, requests for waivers, and other correspondence about an application and an abbreviated application shall be sent to the applicant's home FDA district office, except that a foreign applicant shall send the field copy to the appropriate address identified in paragraphs (a)(1) and (a)(2) of this section.

(b) Applicants shall send applications and other correspondence relating to matters covered by this part for the drug products listed below to the Food and Drug Administration, Center for Biologics Evaluation and Research, Document Control Center, 10903 New Hampshire Ave., Bldg. 71, Rm. G112, Silver Spring, MD 20993-0002, except applicants shall send a request for an opportunity for a hearing under § 314.110 on the question of whether there are grounds for denying approval of an application to the Center for Biologics Evaluation and Research, ATTN: Director, at the same address.

(1) Ingredients packaged together with containers intended for the collection, processing, or storage of blood and blood components;

(2) Plasma volume expanders and hydroxyethyl starch for leukapheresis;

(3) Blood component processing solutions and shelf life extenders; and

(4) Oxygen carriers.

[50 FR 7493, Feb. 22, 1985, as amended at 50 FR 21238, May 23, 1985; 55 FR 11581, Mar. 29, 1990; 57 FR 17997, Apr. 28, 1992; 58 FR 47352, Sept. 8, 1993; 62 FR 43639, Aug. 15, 1997; 69 FR 13473, Mar. 23, 2004; 70 FR 14981, Mar. 24, 2005; 73 FR 39610, July 10, 2008; 74 FR 13113, Mar. 26, 2009; 75 FR 37295, June 29, 2010; 80 FR 18091, Apr. 3, 2015]

§ 314.445 Guidance documents.

(a) FDA has made available guidance documents under § 10.115 of this chapter to help you to comply with certain requirements of this part.

(b) The Center for Drug Evaluation and Research (CDER) maintains a list of guidance documents that apply to CDER's regulations. The list is maintained on the Internet and is published annually in the Federal Register. A request for a copy of the CDER list should be directed to the Office of Training and Communications, Division of Drug Information, Center for Drug Evaluation and Research, Food and Drug Administration, 10903 New Hampshire Ave., Silver Spring, MD 20993-0002.

[65 FR 56480, Sept. 19, 2000, as amended at 74 FR 13113, Mar. 26, 2009]

Subpart H—Accelerated Approval of New Drugs for Serious or Life-Threatening Illnesses

Source: 57 FR 58958, Dec. 11, 1992, unless otherwise noted.

§ 314.500 Scope.

This subpart applies to certain new drug products that have been studied for their safety and effectiveness in treating serious or life-threatening illnesses and that provide meaningful therapeutic benefit to patients over existing treatments (e.g., ability to treat patients unresponsive to, or intolerant of, available therapy, or improved patient response over available therapy).

[57 FR 58958, Dec. 11, 1992, as amended at 64 FR 402, Jan. 5, 1999]

§ 314.510 Approval based on a surrogate endpoint or on an effect on a clinical endpoint other than survival or irreversible morbidity.

FDA may grant marketing approval for a new drug product on the basis of adequate and well-controlled clinical trials establishing that the drug product has an effect on a surrogate endpoint that is reasonably likely, based on epidemiologic, therapeutic, pathophysiologic, or other evidence, to predict clinical benefit or on the basis of an effect on a clinical endpoint other than survival or irreversible morbidity. Approval under this section will be subject to the requirement that the applicant study the drug further, to verify and describe its clinical benefit, where there is uncertainty as to the relation of the surrogate endpoint to clinical benefit, or of the observed clinical benefit to ultimate outcome. Postmarketing studies would usually be studies already underway. When required to be conducted, such studies must also be adequate and well-controlled. The applicant shall carry out any such studies with due diligence.

§ 314.520 Approval with restrictions to assure safe use.

(a) If FDA concludes that a drug product shown to be effective can be safely used only if distribution or use is restricted, FDA will require such postmarketing restrictions as are needed to assure safe use of the drug product, such as:

(1) Distribution restricted to certain facilities or physicians with special training or experience; or

(2) Distribution conditioned on the performance of specified medical procedures.

(b) The limitations imposed will be commensurate with the specific safety concerns presented by the drug product.

§ 314.530 Withdrawal procedures.

(a) For new drugs approved under §§ 314.510 and 314.520, FDA may withdraw approval, following a hearing as provided in part 15 of this chapter, as modified by this section, if:

(1) A postmarketing clinical study fails to verify clinical benefit;

(2) The applicant fails to perform the required postmarketing study with due diligence;

(3) Use after marketing demonstrates that postmarketing restrictions are inadequate to assure safe use of the drug product;

(4) The applicant fails to adhere to the postmarketing restrictions agreed upon;

(5) The promotional materials are false or misleading; or

(6) Other evidence demonstrates that the drug product is not shown to be safe or effective under its conditions of use.

(b) Notice of opportunity for a hearing. The Director of the Center for Drug Evaluation and Research will give the applicant notice of an opportunity for a hearing on the Center's proposal to withdraw the approval of an application approved under § 314.510 or § 314.520. The notice, which will ordinarily be a letter, will state generally the reasons for the action and the proposed grounds for the order.

(c) *Submission of data and information.* (1) If the applicant fails to file a written request for a hearing within 15 days of receipt of the notice, the applicant waives the opportunity for a hearing.

(2) If the applicant files a timely request for a hearing, the agency will publish a notice of hearing in the Federal Register in accordance with §§ 12.32(e) and 15.20 of this chapter.

(3) An applicant who requests a hearing under this section must, within 30 days of receipt of the notice of opportunity for a hearing, submit the data and information upon which the applicant intends to rely at the hearing.

(d) *Separation of functions.* Separation of functions (as specified in § 10.55 of this chapter) will not apply at any point in withdrawal proceedings under this section.

(e) *Procedures for hearings.* Hearings held under this section will be conducted in accordance with the provisions of part 15 of this chapter, with the following modifications:

(1) An advisory committee duly constituted under part 14 of this chapter will be present at the hearing. The committee will be asked to review the issues involved and to provide advice and recommendations to the Commissioner of Food and Drugs.

(2) The presiding officer, the advisory committee members, up to three representatives of the applicant, and up to three representatives of the Center may question any person during or at the conclusion of the person's presentation. No other person attending the hearing may question a person making a presentation. The presiding officer may, as a matter of discretion, permit questions to be submitted to the presiding officer for response by a person making a presentation.

(f) *Judicial review.* The Commissioner's decision constitutes final agency action from which the applicant may petition for judicial review. Before requesting an order from a court for a stay of action pending review, an applicant must first submit a petition for a stay of action under § 10.35 of this chapter.

[57 FR 58958, Dec. 11, 1992, as amended at 64 FR 402, Jan. 5, 1999]

§ 314.540 Postmarketing safety reporting.

Drug products approved under this program are subject to the postmarketing recordkeeping and safety reporting applicable to all approved drug products, as provided in §§ 314.80 and 314.81.

§ 314.550 Promotional materials.

For drug products being considered for approval under this subpart, unless otherwise informed by the agency, applicants must submit to the agency for consideration during the preapproval review period copies of all promotional materials, including promotional labeling as well as advertisements, intended for dissemination or publication within 120 days following marketing approval. After 120 days following marketing approval, unless otherwise informed by the agency, the applicant must submit promotional materials at least 30 days prior to the intended time of initial dissemination of the labeling or initial publication of the advertisement.

§ 314.560 Termination of requirements.

If FDA determines after approval that the requirements established in § 314.520, § 314.530, or § 314.550 are no longer necessary for the safe and effective use of a drug product, it will so notify the applicant. Ordinarily, for drug products approved under § 314.510, these requirements will no longer apply when FDA determines that the required postmarketing study verifies and describes the drug product's clinical benefit and the drug product would be appropriate for approval under traditional procedures. For drug products approved under § 314.520, the restrictions would no longer apply when FDA determines that safe use of the drug product can be assured through appropriate labeling. FDA also retains the discretion to remove specific postapproval requirements upon review of a petition submitted by the sponsor in accordance with § 10.30.

Subpart I—Approval of New Drugs When Human Efficacy Studies Are Not Ethical or Feasible

Source: 67 FR 37995, May 31, 2002, unless otherwise noted.

§ 314.600 Scope.

This subpart applies to certain new drug products that have been studied for their safety and efficacy in ameliorating or preventing serious or life-threatening conditions caused by exposure to lethal or permanently disabling toxic biological, chemical, radiological, or nuclear substances. This subpart applies only to those new drug products for which: Definitive human efficacy studies cannot be conducted because it would be unethical to deliberately expose healthy human volunteers to a lethal or permanently disabling toxic biological, chemical, radiological, or nuclear substance; and field trials to study the product's effectiveness after an accidental or hostile exposure have not been feasible. This subpart does not apply to products that can be approved based on efficacy standards described elsewhere in FDA's regulations (e.g., accelerated approval based on surrogate markers or clinical endpoints other than survival or irreversible morbidity), nor does it address the safety evaluation for the products to which it does apply.

§314.610 Approval based on evidence of effectiveness from studies in animals.

(a) FDA may grant marketing approval for a new drug product for which safety has been established and for which the requirements of §314.600 are met based on adequate and well-controlled animal studies when the results of those animal studies establish that the drug product is reasonably likely to produce clinical benefit in humans. In assessing the sufficiency of animal data, the agency may take into account other data, including human data, available to the agency. FDA will rely on the evidence from studies in animals to provide substantial evidence of the effectiveness of these products only when:

(1) There is a reasonably well-understood pathophysiological mechanism of the toxicity of the substance and its prevention or substantial reduction by the product;

(2) The effect is demonstrated in more than one animal species expected to react with a response predictive for humans, unless the effect is demonstrated in a single animal species that represents a sufficiently well-characterized animal model for predicting the response in humans;

(3) The animal study endpoint is clearly related to the desired benefit in humans, generally the enhancement of survival or prevention of major morbidity; and

(4) The data or information on the kinetics and pharmacodynamics of the product or other relevant data or information, in animals and humans, allows selection of an effective dose in humans.

(b) Approval under this subpart will be subject to three requirements:

(1) *Postmarketing studies.* The applicant must conduct postmarketing studies, such as field studies, to verify and describe the drug's clinical benefit and to assess its safety when used as indicated when such studies are feasible and ethical. Such postmarketing studies would not be feasible until an exigency arises. When such studies are feasible, the applicant must conduct such studies with due diligence. Applicants must include as part of their application a plan or approach to postmarketing study commitments in the event such studies become ethical and feasible.

(2) *Approval with restrictions to ensure safe use.* If FDA concludes that a drug product shown to be effective under this subpart can be safely used only if distribution or use is restricted, FDA will require such postmarketing restrictions as are needed to ensure safe use of the drug product, commensurate with the specific safety concerns presented by the drug product, such as:

(i) Distribution restricted to certain facilities or health care practitioners with special training or experience;

(ii) Distribution conditioned on the performance of specified medical procedures, including medical followup; and

(iii) Distribution conditioned on specified recordkeeping requirements.

(3) Information to be provided to patient recipients. For drug products or specific indications approved under this subpart, applicants must prepare, as part of their proposed labeling, labeling to be provided to patient recipients. The patient labeling must explain that, for ethical or feasibility reasons, the drug's approval was based on efficacy studies conducted in animals alone and must give the drug's indication(s), directions for use (dosage and administration), contraindications, a description of any reasonably foreseeable risks, adverse reactions, anticipated benefits, drug interactions, and any other relevant information required by FDA at the time of approval. The patient labeling must be available with the product to be provided to patients prior to administration or dispensing of the drug product for the use approved under this subpart, if possible.

§ 314.620 Withdrawal procedures.

(a) *Reasons to withdraw approval.* For new drugs approved under this subpart, FDA may withdraw approval, following a hearing as provided in part 15 of this chapter, as modified by this section, if:

(1) A postmarketing clinical study fails to verify clinical benefit;

(2) The applicant fails to perform the postmarketing study with due diligence;

(3) Use after marketing demonstrates that postmarketing restrictions are inadequate to ensure safe use of the drug product;

(4) The applicant fails to adhere to the postmarketing restrictions applied at the time of approval under this subpart;

(5) The promotional materials are false or misleading; or

(6) Other evidence demonstrates that the drug product is not shown to be safe or effective under its conditions of use.

(b) *Notice of opportunity for a hearing.* The Director of the Center for Drug Evaluation and Research (CDER) will give the applicant notice of an opportunity for a hearing on CDER's proposal to withdraw the approval of an application approved under this subpart. The notice, which will ordinarily be a letter, will state generally the reasons for the action and the proposed grounds for the order.

(c) *Submission of data and information.* (1) If the applicant fails to file a written request for a hearing within 15 days of receipt of the notice, the applicant waives the opportunity for a hearing.

(2) If the applicant files a timely request for a hearing, the agency will publish a notice of hearing in the Federal Register in accordance with §§ 12.32(e) and 15.20 of this chapter.

(3) An applicant who requests a hearing under this section must, within 30 days of receipt of the notice of opportunity for a hearing, submit the data and information upon which the applicant intends to rely at the hearing.

(d) *Separation of functions.* Separation of functions (as specified in § 10.55 of this chapter) will not apply at any point in withdrawal proceedings under this section.

(e) *Procedures for hearings.* Hearings held under this section will be conducted in accordance with the provisions of part 15 of this chapter, with the following modifications:

(1) An advisory committee duly constituted under part 14 of this chapter will be present at the hearing. The committee will be asked to review the issues involved and to provide advice and recommendations to the Commissioner of Food and Drugs.

(2) The presiding officer, the advisory committee members, up to three representatives of the applicant, and up to three representatives of CDER may question any person during or at the conclusion of the person's presentation. No other person attending the hearing may question a person making a presentation. The presiding officer may, as a matter of discretion, permit questions to be submitted to the presiding officer for response by a person making a presentation.

(f) *Judicial review.* The Commissioner of Food and Drugs' decision constitutes final agency action from which the applicant may petition for judicial review. Before requesting an order from a court for a stay of action pending review, an applicant must first submit a petition for a stay of action under § 10.35 of this chapter.

§ 314.630 Postmarketing safety reporting.

Drug products approved under this subpart are subject to the postmarketing recordkeeping and safety reporting requirements applicable to all approved drug products, as provided in §§ 314.80 and 314.81.

§ 314.640 Promotional materials.

For drug products being considered for approval under this subpart, unless otherwise informed by the agency, applicants must submit to the agency for consideration during the preapproval review period copies of all promotional materials, including promotional labeling as well as advertisements, intended for dissemination or publication within 120 days following marketing approval. After 120 days following marketing approval, unless otherwise informed by the agency, the applicant must submit promotional materials at least 30 days prior to the intended time of initial dissemination of the labeling or initial publication of the advertisement.

§ 314.650 Termination of requirements.

If FDA determines after approval under this subpart that the requirements established in §§ 314.610(b)(2), 314.620, and 314.630 are no longer necessary for the safe and effective use of a drug product, FDA will so notify the applicant. Ordinarily, for drug products approved under § 314.610, these requirements will no longer apply when FDA determines that the postmarketing study verifies and describes the drug product's clinical benefit. For drug products approved under § 314.610, the restrictions would no longer apply when FDA determines that safe use of the drug product can be ensured through appropriate labeling. FDA also retains the discretion to remove specific postapproval requirements upon review of a petition submitted by the sponsor in accordance with § 10.30 of this chapter.

• • •

SUBCHAPTER F—BIOLOGICS

PART 600—BIOLOGICAL PRODUCTS: GENERAL

Authority: 21 U.S.C. 321, 351, 352, 353, 355, 356c, 356e, 360, 360i, 371, 374, 379k-1; 42 U.S.C. 216, 262, 263, 263a, 264, 300aa-25.

Cross references: For U.S. Customs Service regulations relating to viruses, serums, and toxins, see 19 CFR 12.21-12.23. For U.S. Postal Service regulations relating to the admissibility to the United States mails see parts 124 and 125 of the Domestic Mail Manual, that is incorporated by reference in 39 CFR part 111.

Subpart A—General Provisions

§ 600.2 Mailing addresses.

(a) *Licensed biological products regulated by the Center for Biologics Evaluation and Research (CBER).* Unless otherwise stated in paragraph (c) of this section, or as otherwise prescribed by FDA regulation, all submissions to CBER referenced in parts 600 through 680 of this chapter, as applicable, must be sent to: Food and Drug Administration, Center for Biologics Evaluation and Research, Document Control Center, 10903 New Hampshire Ave., Bldg. 71, Rm. G112, Silver Spring, MD 20993-0002. Examples of such submissions include: Biologics license applications (BLAs) and their amendments and supplements, biological product deviation reports, fatality reports, and other correspondence. Biological products samples must not be sent to this address but must be sent to the address in paragraph (c) of this section.

(b) *Licensed biological products regulated by the Center for Drug Evaluation and Research (CDER).* Unless otherwise stated in paragraphs (b)(1), (b)(2), or (c) of this section, or as otherwise prescribed by FDA regulation, all submissions to CDER referenced in parts 600, 601, and 610 of this chapter, as applicable, must be sent to: CDER Central Document Room, Center for Drug Evaluation and Research,

Food and Drug Administration, 5901B Ammendale Rd., Beltsville, MD 20705. Examples of such submissions include: BLAs and their amendments and supplements, and other correspondence.

(1) *Biological Product Deviation Reporting (CDER).* All biological product deviation reports required under §600.14 must be sent to: Division of Compliance Risk Management and Surveillance, Office of Compliance, Center for Drug Evaluation and Research, Food and Drug Administration, 10903 New Hampshire Ave., Silver Spring, MD 20993-0002.

(2) *Advertising and Promotional Labeling (CDER).* All advertising and promotional labeling supplements required under §601.12(f) of this chapter must be sent to: Division of Drug Marketing, Advertising and Communication, Center for Drug Evaluation and Research, Food and Drug Administration, 5901-B Ammendale Rd., Beltsville, MD 20705-1266.

(c) *Samples and Protocols for licensed biological products regulated by CBER or CDER.* (1) Biological product samples and/or protocols, other than radioactive biological product samples and protocols, required under §§600.13, 600.22, 601.15, 610.2, 660.6, 660.36, or 660.46 of this chapter must be sent by courier service to: Food and Drug Administration, Center for Biologics Evaluation and Research, ATTN: Sample Custodian, 10903 New Hampshire Ave., Bldg. 75, Rm. G707, Silver Spring, MD 20993-0002. The protocol(s) may be placed in the box used to ship the samples to CBER. A cover letter should not be included when submitting the protocol with the sample unless it contains pertinent information affecting the release of the lot.

(2) Radioactive biological products required under §610.2 of this chapter must be sent by courier service to: Food and Drug Administration, Center for Biologics Evaluation and Research, ATTN: Sample Custodian, c/o White Oak Radiation Safety Program, 10903 New Hampshire Ave., Bldg. 52-72, Rm. G406A, Silver Spring, MD 20993-0002.

(d) Address information for submissions to CBER and CDER other than those listed in parts 600 through 680 of this chapter are included directly in the applicable regulations.

(e) Obtain updated mailing address information for biological products regulated by CBER at *http://www.fda.gov/BiologicsBloodVaccines/default.htm*, or for biological products regulated by CDER at *http://www.fda.gov/Drugs/default.htm.*

[70 FR 14981, Mar. 24, 2005, as amended at 74 FR 13114, Mar. 26, 2009; 78 FR 19585, Apr. 2, 2013; 80 FR 18091, Apr. 3, 2015; 79 FR 33090, June 10, 2014]

§600.3 Definitions.

As used in this subchapter:

(a) *Act* means the Public Health Service Act (58 Stat. 682), approved July 1, 1944.

(b) *Secretary* means the Secretary of Health and Human Services and any other officer or employee of the Department of Health and Human Services to whom the authority involved has been delegated.

(c) *Commissioner of Food and Drugs* means the Commissioner of the Food and Drug Administration.

(d) *Center for Biologics Evaluation and Research* means Center for Biologics Evaluation and Research of the Food and Drug Administration.

(e) *State* means a State or the District of Columbia, Puerto Rico, or the Virgin Islands.

(f) *Possession* includes among other possessions, Puerto Rico and the Virgin Islands.

(g) *Products* includes biological products and trivalent organic arsenicals.

(h) *Biological product* means any virus, therapeutic serum, toxin, antitoxin, or analogous product applicable to the prevention, treatment or cure of diseases or injuries of man:

(1) A virus is interpreted to be a product containing the minute living cause of an infectious disease and includes but is not limited to filterable viruses, bacteria, rickettsia, fungi, and protozoa.

(2) A therapeutic serum is a product obtained from blood by removing the clot or clot components and the blood cells.

(3) A toxin is a product containing a soluble substance poisonous to laboratory animals or to man in doses of 1 milliliter or less (or equivalent in weight) of the product, and having the property, following the injection of non-fatal doses into an animal, of causing to be produced therein another soluble substance which specifically neutralizes the poisonous substance and which is demonstrable in the serum of the animal thus immunized.

(4) An antitoxin is a product containing the soluble substance in serum or other body fluid of an immunized animal which specifically neutralizes the toxin against which the animal is immune.

(5) A product is analogous:

(i) To a virus if prepared from or with a virus or agent actually or potentially infectious, without regard to the degree of virulence or toxicogenicity of the specific strain used.

(ii) To a therapeutic serum, if composed of whole blood or plasma or containing some organic constituent or product other than a hormone or an amino acid, derived from whole blood, plasma, or serum.

(iii) To a toxin or antitoxin, if intended, irrespective of its source of origin, to be applicable to the prevention, treatment, or cure of disease or injuries of man through a specific immune process.

(i) *Trivalent organic arsenicals* means arsphenamine and its derivatives (or any other trivalent organic arsenic compound) applicable to the prevention, treatment, or cure of diseases or injuries of man.

(j) A product is deemed applicable to the prevention, treatment, or cure of diseases or injuries of man irrespective of the mode of administration or application recommended, including use when intended through administration or application to a person as an aid in diagnosis, or in evaluating the degree of susceptibility or immunity possessed by a person, and including also any other use for purposes of diagnosis if the diagnostic substance so used is prepared from or with the aid of a biological product.

(k) Proper name, as applied to a product, means the name designated in the license for use upon each package of the product.

(l) *Dating period* means the period beyond which the product cannot be expected beyond reasonable doubt to yield its specific results.

(m) *Expiration date* means the calendar month and year, and where applicable, the day and hour, that the dating period ends.

(n) The word *standards* means specifications and procedures applicable to an establishment or to the manufacture or release of products, which are prescribed in this subchapter or established in the biologics license application designed to insure the continued safety, purity, and potency of such products.

(o) The word *continued* as applied to the safety, purity and potency of products is interpreted to apply to the dating period.

(p) The word *safety* means the relative freedom from harmful effect to persons affected, directly or indirectly, by a product when prudently administered, taking into consideration the character of the product in relation to the condition of the recipient at the time.

(q) The word *sterility* is interpreted to mean freedom from viable contaminating microorganisms, as determined by the tests conducted under § 610.12 of this chapter.

(r) *Purity* means relative freedom from extraneous matter in the finished product, whether or not harmful to the recipient or deleterious to the product. Purity includes but is not limited to relative freedom from residual moisture or other volatile substances and pyrogenic substances.

(s) The word *potency* is interpreted to mean the specific ability or capacity of the product, as indicated by appropriate laboratory tests or by adequately controlled clinical data obtained through the administration of the product in the manner intended, to effect a given result.

(t) *Manufacturer* means any legal person or entity engaged in the manufacture of a product subject to license under the act; "Manufacturer" also includes any legal person or entity who is an applicant for a license where the applicant assumes responsibility for compliance with the applicable product and establishment standards.

(u) *Manufacture* means all steps in propagation or manufacture and preparation of products and includes but is not limited to filling, testing, labeling, packaging, and storage by the manufacturer.

(v) *Location* includes all buildings, appurtenances, equipment and animals used, and personnel engaged by a manufacturer within a particular area designated by an address adequate for identification.

(w) *Establishment* has the same meaning as "facility" in section 351 of the Public Health Service Act and includes all locations.

(x) *Lot* means that quantity of uniform material identified by the manufacturer as having been thoroughly mixed in a single vessel.

(y) A *filling* refers to a group of final containers identical in all respects, which have been filled with the same product from the same bulk lot without any change that will affect the integrity of the filling assembly.

(z) *Process* refers to a manufacturing step that is performed on the product itself which may affect its safety, purity or potency, in contrast to such manufacturing steps which do not affect intrinsically the safety, purity or potency of the product.

(aa) *Selling agent or distributor* means any person engaged in the unrestricted distribution, other than by sale at retail, of products subject to license.

(bb) *Container* (referred to also as "final container") is the immediate unit, bottle, vial, ampule, tube, or other receptacle containing the product as distributed for sale, barter, or exchange.

(cc) *Package* means the immediate carton, receptacle, or wrapper, including all labeling matter therein and thereon, and the contents of the one or more enclosed containers. If no package, as defined in the preceding sentence, is used, the container shall be deemed to be the package.

(dd) *Label* means any written, printed, or graphic matter on the container or package or any such matter clearly visible through the immediate carton, receptacle, or wrapper.

(ee) *Radioactive biological product* means a biological product which is labeled with a radionuclide or intended solely to be labeled with a radionuclide.

(ff) *Amendment* is the submission of information to a pending license application or supplement, to revise or modify the application as originally submitted.

(gg) *Supplement* is a request to approve a change in an approved license application.

(hh) *Distributed* means the biological product has left the control of the licensed manufacturer.

(ii) *Control* means having responsibility for maintaining the continued safety, purity, and potency of the product and for compliance with applicable product and establishment standards, and for compliance with current good manufacturing practices.

(jj) *Assess the effects of the change*, as used in § 601.12 of this chapter, means to evaluate the effects of a manufacturing change on the identity, strength, quality, purity, and potency of a product as these factors may relate to the safety or effectiveness of the product.

(kk) *Specification*, as used in § 601.12 of this chapter, means the quality standard (i.e., tests, analytical procedures, and acceptance criteria) provided in an approved application to confirm the quality of products, intermediates, raw materials, reagents, components, in-process materials, container closure systems, and other materials used in the production of a product. For the purpose of this definition, acceptance criteria means numerical limits, ranges, or other criteria for the tests described.

(ll) *Complete response letter* means a written communication to an applicant from FDA usually describing all of the deficiencies that the agency has identified in a biologics license application or supplement that must be satisfactorily addressed before it can be approved.

(mm) *Resubmission* means a submission by the biologics license applicant or supplement applicant of all materials needed to fully address all deficiencies identified in the complete response letter. A biologics license application or supplement for which FDA issued a complete response letter, but which was withdrawn before approval and later submitted again, is not a resubmission.

[38 FR 32048, Nov. 20, 1973, as amended at 40 FR 31313, July 25, 1975; 55 FR 11014, Mar. 26, 1990; 61 FR 24232, May 14, 1996; 62 FR 39901, July 24, 1997; 64 FR 56449, Oct. 20, 1999; 65 FR 66634, Nov. 7, 2000; 69 FR 18766, Apr. 8, 2004; 70 FR 14982, Mar. 24, 2005; 73 FR 39610, July 10, 2008; 77 FR 26174, May 3, 2012]

Subpart B—Establishment Standards

§ 600.10 Personnel.

(a) [Reserved]

(b) *Personnel*. Personnel shall have capabilities commensurate with their assigned functions, a thorough understanding of the manufacturing operations which they perform, the necessary training and experience relating to individual products, and adequate information concerning the application of the pertinent provisions of this subchapter to their respective functions. Personnel shall include such professionally trained persons as are necessary to insure the competent performance of all manufacturing processes.

(c) *Restrictions on personnel*—(1) *Specific duties*. Persons whose presence can affect adversely the safety and purity of a product shall be excluded from the room where the manufacture of a product is in progress.

(2) *Sterile operations*. Personnel performing sterile operations shall wear clean or sterilized protective clothing and devices to the extent necessary to protect the product from contamination.

(3) *Pathogenic viruses and spore-forming organisms*. Persons working with viruses pathogenic for man or with spore-forming microorganisms, and persons engaged in the care of animals or animal quarters, shall be excluded from areas where other products are manufactured, or such persons shall change outer clothing, including shoes, or wear protective covering prior to entering such areas.

(4) *Live vaccine work areas*. Persons may not enter a live vaccine processing area after having worked with other infectious agents in any other laboratory during the same working day. Only persons actually concerned with propagation of the culture, production of the vaccine, and unit maintenance, shall be allowed in live vaccine processing areas when active work is in progress. Casual visitors shall be excluded from such units at all times and all others having business in such areas shall be admitted only under supervision. Street clothing, including shoes, shall be replaced or covered by suitable laboratory clothing before entering a live vaccine processing unit. Persons

caring for animals used in the manufacture of live vaccines shall be excluded from other animal quarters and from contact with other animals during the same working day.

[38 FR 32048, Nov. 20, 1973, as amended at 49 FR 23833, June 8, 1984; 55 FR 11014, Mar. 26, 1990; 62 FR 53538, Oct. 15, 1997; 68 FR 75119, Dec. 30, 2003]

§ 600.11 Physical establishment, equipment, animals, and care.

(a) *Work areas.* All rooms and work areas where products are manufactured or stored shall be kept orderly, clean, and free of dirt, dust, vermin and objects not required for manufacturing. Precautions shall be taken to avoid clogging and back-siphonage of drainage systems. Precautions shall be taken to exclude extraneous infectious agents from manufacturing areas. Work rooms shall be well lighted and ventilated. The ventilation system shall be arranged so as to prevent the dissemination of microorganisms from one manufacturing area to another and to avoid other conditions unfavorable to the safety of the product. Filling rooms, and other rooms where open, sterile operations are conducted, shall be adequate to meet manufacturing needs and such rooms shall be constructed and equipped to permit thorough cleaning and to keep air-borne contaminants at a minimum. If such rooms are used for other purposes, they shall be cleaned and prepared prior to use for sterile operations. Refrigerators, incubators and warm rooms shall be maintained at temperatures within applicable ranges and shall be free of extraneous material which might affect the safety of the product.

(b) *Equipment.* Apparatus for sterilizing equipment and the method of operation shall be such as to insure the destruction of contaminating microorganisms. The effectiveness of the sterilization procedure shall be no less than that achieved by an attained temperature of 121.5 °C maintained for 20 minutes by saturated steam or by an attained temperature of 170 °C maintained for 2 hours with dry heat. Processing and storage containers, filters, filling apparatus, and other pieces of apparatus and accessory equipment, including pipes and tubing, shall be designed and constructed to permit thorough cleaning and, where possible, inspection for cleanliness. All surfaces that come in contact with products shall be clean and free of surface solids, leachable contaminants, and other materials that will hasten the deterioration of the product or otherwise render it less suitable for the intended use. For products for which sterility is a factor, equipment shall be sterile, unless sterility of the product is assured by subsequent procedures.

(c) *Laboratory and bleeding rooms.* Rooms used for the processing of products, including bleeding rooms, shall be effectively fly-proofed and kept free of flies and vermin. Such rooms shall be so constructed as to insure freedom from dust, smoke and other deleterious substances and to permit thorough cleaning and disinfection. Rooms for animal injection and bleeding, and rooms for smallpox vaccine animals, shall be disinfected and be provided with the necessary water, electrical and other services.

(d) *Animal quarters and stables.* Animal quarters, stables and food storage areas shall be of appropriate construction, fly-proofed, adequately lighted and ventilated, and maintained in a clean, vermin-free and sanitary condition. No manure or refuse shall be stored as to permit the breeding of flies on the premises, nor shall the establishment be located in close proximity to off-property manure or refuse storage capable of engendering fly breeding.

(e) *Restrictions on building and equipment use*—(1) *Work of a diagnostic nature.* Laboratory procedures of a clinical diagnostic nature involving materials that may be contaminated, shall not be performed in space used for the manufacture of products except that manufacturing space which is used only occasionally may be used for diagnostic work provided spore-forming pathogenic microorganisms are not involved and provided the space is thoroughly cleaned and disinfected before the manufacture of products is resumed.

(2) *Spore-forming organisms for supplemental sterilization procedure control test.* Spore-forming organisms used as an additional control in sterilization procedures may be introduced into areas

used for the manufacture of products, only for the purposes of the test and only immediately before use for such purposes: Provided, That (i) the organism is not pathogenic for man or animals and does not produce pyrogens or toxins, (ii) the culture is demonstrated to be pure, (iii) transfer of test cultures to culture media shall be limited to the sterility test area or areas designated for work with spore-forming organisms, (iv) each culture be labeled with the name of the microorganism and the statement "Caution: microbial spores. See directions for storage, use and disposition.", and (v) the container of each culture is designed to withstand handling without breaking.

(3) *Work with spore-forming microorganisms.* (i) Manufacturing processes using spore-forming microorganisms conducted in a multiproduct manufacturing site must be performed under appropriate controls to prevent contamination of other products and areas within the site. Prevention of spore contamination can be achieved by using a separate dedicated building or by using process containment if manufacturing is conducted in a multiproduct manufacturing building. All product and personnel movement between the area where the spore-forming microorganisms are manufactured and other manufacturing areas must be conducted under conditions that will prevent the introduction of spores into other areas of the facility.

(ii) If process containment is employed in a multiproduct manufacturing area, procedures must be in place to demonstrate adequate removal of the spore-forming microorganism(s) from the manufacturing area for subsequent manufacture of other products. These procedures must provide for adequate removal or decontamination of the spore-forming microorganisms on and within manufacturing equipment, facilities, and ancillary room items as well as the removal of disposable or product dedicated items from the manufacturing area. Environmental monitoring specific for the spore-forming microorganism(s) must be conducted in adjacent areas during manufacturing operations and in the manufacturing area after completion of cleaning and decontamination.

(4) *Live vaccine processing.* Live vaccine processing must be performed under appropriate controls to prevent cross contamination of other products and other manufacturing areas within the building. Appropriate controls must include, at a minimum:

(i)(A) Using a dedicated manufacturing area that is either in a separate building, in a separate wing of a building, or in quarters at the blind end of a corridor and includes adequate space and equipment for all processing steps up to, but not including, filling into final containers; and

(B) Not conducting test procedures that potentially involve the presence of microorganisms other than the vaccine strains or the use of tissue culture cell lines other than primary cultures in space used for processing live vaccine; or

(ii) If manufacturing is conducted in a multiproduct manufacturing building or area, using procedural controls, and where necessary, process containment. Process containment is deemed to be necessary unless procedural controls are sufficient to prevent cross contamination of other products and other manufacturing areas within the building. Process containment is a system designed to mechanically isolate equipment or an area that involves manufacturing using live vaccine organisms. All product, equipment, and personnel movement between distinct live vaccine processing areas and between live vaccine processing areas and other manufacturing areas, up to, but not including, filling in final containers, must be conducted under conditions that will prevent cross contamination of other products and manufacturing areas within the building, including the introduction of live vaccine organisms into other areas. In addition, written procedures and effective processes must be in place to adequately remove or decontaminate live vaccine organisms from the manufacturing area and equipment for subsequent manufacture of other products. Written procedures must be in place for verification that processes to remove or decontaminate live vaccine organisms have been followed.

(5) *Equipment and supplies—contamination.* Equipment and supplies used in work on or otherwise exposed to any pathogenic or potentially pathogenic agent shall be kept separated from

equipment and supplies used in the manufacture of products to the extent necessary to prevent cross-contamination.

(f) *Animals used in manufacture*—(1) *Care of animals used in manufacturing.* Caretakers and attendants for animals used for the manufacture of products shall be sufficient in number and have adequate experience to insure adequate care. Animal quarters and cages shall be kept in sanitary condition. Animals on production shall be inspected daily to observe response to production procedures. Animals that become ill for reasons not related to production shall be isolated from other animals and shall not be used for production until recovery is complete. Competent veterinary care shall be provided as needed.

(2) *Quarantine of animals*—(i) *General.* No animal shall be used in processing unless kept under competent daily inspection and preliminary quarantine for a period of at least 7 days before use, or as otherwise provided in this subchapter. Only healthy animals free from detectable communicable diseases shall be used. Animals must remain in overt good health throughout the quarantine periods and particular care shall be taken during the quarantine periods to reject animals of the equine genus which may be infected with glanders and animals which may be infected with tuberculosis.

(ii) *Quarantine of monkeys.* In addition to observing the pertinent general quarantine requirements, monkeys used as a source of tissue in the manufacture of vaccine shall be maintained in quarantine for at least 6 weeks prior to use, except when otherwise provided in this part. Only monkeys that have reacted negatively to tuberculin at the start of the quarantine period and again within 2 weeks prior to use shall be used in the manufacture of vaccine. Due precaution shall be taken to prevent cross-infection from any infected or potentially infected monkeys on the premises. Monkeys to be used in the manufacture of a live vaccine shall be maintained throughout the quarantine period in cages closed on all sides with solid materials except the front which shall be screened, with no more than two monkeys housed in one cage. Cage mates shall not be interchanged.

(3) *Immunization against tetanus.* Horses and other animals susceptible to tetanus, that are used in the processing steps of the manufacture of biological products, shall be treated adequately to maintain immunity to tetanus.

(4) *Immunization and bleeding of animals used as a source of products.* Toxins or other nonviable antigens administered in the immunization of animals used in the manufacture of products shall be sterile. Viable antigens, when so used, shall be free of contaminants, as determined by appropriate tests prior to use. Injections shall not be made into horses within 6 inches of bleeding site. Horses shall not be bled for manufacturing purposes while showing persistent general reaction or local reaction near the site of bleeding. Blood shall not be used if it was drawn within 5 days of injecting the animals with viable microorganisms. Animals shall not be bled for manufacturing purposes when they have an intercurrent disease. Blood intended for use as a source of a biological product shall be collected in clean, sterile vessels. When the product is intended for use by injection, such vessels shall also be pyrogen-free.

(5) [Reserved]

(6) *Reporting of certain diseases.* In cases of actual or suspected infection with foot and mouth disease, glanders, tetanus, anthrax, gas gangrene, equine infectious anemia; equine encephalomyelitis, or any of the pock diseases among animals intended for use or used in the manufacture of products, the manufacturer shall immediately notify the Director, Center for Biologics Evaluation and Research or the Director, Center for Drug Evaluation and Research (see mailing addresses in § 600.2(a) or (b)).

(7) *Monkeys used previously for experimental or test purposes.* Monkeys that have been used previously for experimental or test purposes with live microbiological agents shall not be used as a source of kidney tissue for the manufacture of vaccine. Except as provided otherwise in this subchapter, monkeys that have been used previously for other experimental or test purposes may be used as

a source of kidney tissue upon their return to a normal condition, provided all quarantine requirements have been met.

(8) *Necropsy examination of monkeys.* Each monkey used in the manufacture of vaccine shall be examined at necropsy under the direction of a qualified pathologist, physician, or veterinarian having experience with diseases of monkeys, for evidence of ill health, particularly for (i) evidence of tuberculosis, (ii) presence of herpes-like lesions, including eruptions or plaques on or around the lips, in the buccal cavity or on the gums, and (iii) signs of conjunctivitis. If there are any such signs or other significant gross pathological lesions, the tissue shall not be used in the manufacture of vaccine.

(g) *Filling procedures.* Filling procedures shall be such as will not affect adversely the safety, purity or potency of the product.

(h) *Containers and closures.* All final containers and closures shall be made of material that will not hasten the deterioration of the product or otherwise render it less suitable for the intended use. All final containers and closures shall be clean and free of surface solids, leachable contaminants and other materials that will hasten the deterioration of the product or otherwise render it less suitable for the intended use. After filling, sealing shall be performed in a manner that will maintain the integrity of the product during the dating period. In addition, final containers and closures for products intended for use by injection shall be sterile and free from pyrogens. Except as otherwise provided in the regulations of this subchapter, final containers for products intended for use by injection shall be colorless and sufficiently transparent to permit visual examination of the contents under normal light. As soon as possible after filling final containers shall be labeled as prescribed in §610.60 et seq. of this chapter, except that final containers may be stored without such prescribed labeling provided they are stored in a sealed receptacle labeled both inside and outside with at least the name of the product, the lot number, and the filling identification.

[38 FR 32048, Nov. 20, 1973, as amended at 41 FR 10428, Mar. 11, 1976; 49 FR 23833, June 8, 1984; 55 FR 11013, Mar. 26, 1990; 68 FR 75119, Dec. 30, 2003; 70 FR 14982, Mar. 24, 2005; 72 FR 59003, Oct. 18, 2007; 80 FR 18092, Apr. 3, 2015]

§600.12 Records.

(a) *Maintenance of records.* Records shall be made, concurrently with the performance, of each step in the manufacture and distribution of products, in such a manner that at any time successive steps in the manufacture and distribution of any lot may be traced by an inspector. Such records shall be legible and indelible, shall identify the person immediately responsible, shall include dates of the various steps, and be as detailed as necessary for clear understanding of each step by one experienced in the manufacture of products.

(b) *Records retention*—(1) *General.* Records shall be retained for such interval beyond the expiration date as is necessary for the individual product, to permit the return of any clinical report of unfavorable reactions. The retention period shall be no less than five years after the records of manufacture have been completed or six months after the latest expiration date for the individual product, whichever represents a later date.

(2) *Records of recall.* Complete records shall be maintained pertaining to the recall from distribution of any product upon notification by the Director, Center for Biologics Evaluation and Research or the Director, Center for Drug Evaluation and Research, to recall for failure to conform with the standards prescribed in the regulations of this subchapter, because of deterioration of the product or for any other factor by reason of which the distribution of the product would constitute a danger to health.

(3) *Suspension of requirement for retention.* The Director, Center for Biologics Evaluation and Research or the Director, Center for Drug Evaluation and Research, may authorize the suspension of the requirement to retain records of a specific manufacturing step upon a showing that such records

no longer have significance for the purposes for which they were made: Provided, That a summary of such records shall be retained.

(c) *Records of sterilization of equipment and supplies.* Records relating to the mode of sterilization, date, duration, temperature and other conditions relating to each sterilization of equipment and supplies used in the processing of products shall be made by means of automatic recording devices or by means of a system of recording which gives equivalent assurance of the accuracy and reliability of the record. Such records shall be maintained in a manner that permits an identification of the product with the particular manufacturing process to which the sterilization relates.

(d) *Animal necropsy records.* A necropsy record shall be kept on each animal from which a biological product has been obtained and which dies or is sacrificed while being so used.

(e) *Records in case of divided manufacturing responsibility.* If two or more establishments participate in the manufacture of a product, the records of each such establishment must show plainly the degree of its responsibility. In addition, each participating manufacturer shall furnish to the manufacturer who prepares the product in final form for sale, barter or exchange, a copy of all records relating to the manufacturing operations performed by such participating manufacturer insofar as they concern the safety, purity and potency of the lots of the product involved, and the manufacturer who prepares the product in final form shall retain a complete record of all the manufacturing operations relating to the product.

[38 FR 32048, Nov. 20, 1973, as amended at 49 FR 23833, June 8, 1984; 55 FR 11013, Mar. 26, 1990; 70 FR 14982, Mar. 24, 2005]

§ 600.13 Retention samples.

Manufacturers shall retain for a period of at least 6 months after the expiration date, unless a different time period is specified in additional standards, a quantity of representative material of each lot of each product, sufficient for examination and testing for safety and potency, except Whole Blood, Cryoprecipitated AHF, Platelets, Red Blood Cells, Plasma, and Source Plasma and Allergenic Products prepared to a physician's prescription. Samples so retained shall be selected at random from either final container material, or from bulk and final containers, provided they include at least one final container as a final package, or package-equivalent of such filling of each lot of the product as intended for distribution. Such sample material shall be stored at temperatures and under conditions which will maintain the identity and integrity of the product. Samples retained as required in this section shall be in addition to samples of specific products required to be submitted to the Center for Biologics Evaluation and Research or the Center for Drug Evaluation and Research (see mailing addresses in § 600.2). Exceptions may be authorized by the Director, Center for Biologics Evaluation and Research or the Director, Center for Drug Evaluation and Research, when the lot yields relatively few final containers and when such lots are prepared by the same method in large number and in close succession.

[41 FR 10428, Mar. 11, 1976, as amended at 49 FR 23833, June 8, 1984; 50 FR 4133, Jan. 29, 1985; 55 FR 11013, Mar. 26, 1990; 70 FR 14982, Mar. 24, 2005]

§ 600.14 Reporting of biological product deviations by licensed manufacturers.

(a) *Who must report under this section?* (1) You, the manufacturer who holds the biological product license and who had control over the product when the deviation occurred, must report under this section. If you arrange for another person to perform a manufacturing, holding, or distribution step, while the product is in your control, that step is performed under your control. You must establish, maintain, and follow a procedure for receiving information from that person on all deviations, complaints, and adverse events concerning the affected product.

(2) Exceptions:

(i) Persons who manufacture only in vitro diagnostic products that are not subject to licensing under section 351 of the Public Health Service Act do not report biological product deviations for those products under this section but must report in accordance with part 803 of this chapter;

(ii) Persons who manufacture blood and blood components, including licensed manufacturers, unlicensed registered blood establishments, and transfusion services, do not report biological product deviations for those products under this section but must report under § 606.171 of this chapter;

(iii) Persons who manufacture Source Plasma or any other blood component and use that Source Plasma or any other blood component in the further manufacture of another licensed biological product must report:

(A) Under § 606.171 of this chapter, if a biological product deviation occurs during the manufacture of that Source Plasma or any other blood component; or

(B) Under this section, if a biological product deviation occurs after the manufacture of that Source Plasma or any other blood component, and during manufacture of the licensed biological product.

(b) *What do I report under this section?* You must report any event, and information relevant to the event, associated with the manufacturing, to include testing, processing, packing, labeling, or storage, or with the holding or distribution, of a licensed biological product, if that event meets all the following criteria:

(1) Either:

(i) Represents a deviation from current good manufacturing practice, applicable regulations, applicable standards, or established specifications that may affect the safety, purity, or potency of that product; or

(ii) Represents an unexpected or unforeseeable event that may affect the safety, purity, or potency of that product; and

(2) Occurs in your facility or another facility under contract with you; and

(3) Involves a distributed biological product.

(c) *When do I report under this section?* You should report a biological product deviation as soon as possible but you must report at a date not to exceed 45-calendar days from the date you, your agent, or another person who performs a manufacturing, holding, or distribution step under your control, acquire information reasonably suggesting that a reportable event has occurred.

(d) *How do I report under this section?* You must report on Form FDA-3486.

(e) *Where do I report under this section?* (1) For biological products regulated by the Center for Biologics Evaluation and Research (CBER), send the completed Form FDA 3486 to the CBER Document Control Center (see mailing address in § 600.2(a)), or submit electronically using CBER's electronic Web-based application.

(2) For biological products regulated by the Center for Drug Evaluation and Research (CDER), send the completed Form FDA-3486 to the Division of Compliance Risk Management and Surveillance (HFD-330) (see mailing addresses in § 600.2). CDER does not currently accept electronic filings.

(3) If you make a paper filing, you should identify on the envelope that a biological product deviation report (BPDR) is enclosed.

(f) *How does this regulation affect other FDA regulations?* This part supplements and does not supersede other provisions of the regulations in this chapter. All biological product deviations, whether or not they are required to be reported under this section, should be investigated in accordance with the applicable provisions of parts 211 and 820 of this chapter.

[65 FR 66634, Nov. 7, 2000, as amended at 70 FR 14982, Mar. 24, 2005; 80 FR 18092, Apr. 3, 2015]

§ 600.15 Temperatures during shipment.

The following products shall be maintained during shipment at the specified temperatures:

(a) *Products.*

Product	Temperature
Cryoprecipitated AHF	−18 °C or colder.
Measles and Rubella Virus Vaccine Live	10 °C or colder.
Measles Live and Smallpox Vaccine	Do.
Measles, Mumps, and Rubella Virus Vaccine Live	Do.
Measles and Mumps Virus Vaccine Live	Do.
Measles Virus Vaccine Live	Do.
Mumps Virus Vaccine Live	Do.
Fresh Frozen Plasma	−18 °C or colder.
Liquid Plasma	1 to 10 °C.
Plasma	−18 °C or colder.
Platelet Rich Plasma	Between 1 and 10 °C if the label indicates storage between 1 and 6 °C, or all reasonable methods to maintain the temperature as close as possible to a range between 20 and 24 °C, if the label indicates storage between 20 and 24 °C.
Platelets	Between 1 and 10 °C if the label indicates storage between 1 and 6 °C, or all reasonable methods to maintain the temperature as close as possible to a range between 20 to 24 °C, if the label indicates storage between 20 and 24 °C.
Poliovirus Vaccine Live Oral Trivalent	0 °C or colder.
Poliovirus Vaccine Live Oral Type I	Do.
Poliovirus Vaccine Live Oral Type II	Do.
Poliovirus Vaccine Live Oral Type III	Do.
Red Blood Cells (liquid product)	Between 1 and 10 °C.
Red Blood Cells Frozen	−65 °C or colder.
Rubella and Mumps Virus Vaccine Live	10 °C or colder.
Rubella Virus Vaccine Live	Do.
Smallpox Vaccine (Liquid Product)	0 °C or colder.
Source Plasma	−5 °C or colder.
Source Plasma Liquid	10 °C or colder.

Product	Temperature
Whole Blood	Blood that is transported from the collecting facility to the processing facility shall be transported in an environment capable of continuously cooling the blood toward a temperature range of 1 to 10 °C, or at a temperature as close as possible to 20 to 24 °C for a period not to exceed 6 hours. Blood transported from the storage facility shall be placed in an appropriate environment to maintain a temperature range between 1 to 10 °C during shipment.
Yellow Fever Vaccine	0 °C or colder.

(b) *Exemptions.* Exemptions or modifications shall be made only upon written approval, in the form of a supplement to the biologics license application, approved by the Director, Center for Biologics Evaluation and Research.

[39 FR 39872, Nov. 12, 1974, as amended at 49 FR 23833, June 8, 1984; 50 FR 4133, Jan. 29, 1985; 50 FR 9000, Mar. 6, 1985; 55 FR 11013, Mar. 26, 1990; 59 FR 49351, Sept. 28, 1994; 64 FR 56449, Oct. 20, 1999]

Subpart C—Establishment Inspection

§ 600.20 Inspectors.

Inspections shall be made by an officer of the Food and Drug Administration having special knowledge of the methods used in the manufacture and control of products and designated for such purposes by the Commissioner of Food and Drugs, or by any officer, agent, or employee of the Department of Health and Human Services specifically designated for such purpose by the Secretary.

[38 FR 32048, Nov. 20, 1973]

§ 600.21 Time of inspection.

The inspection of an establishment for which a biologics license application is pending need not be made until the establishment is in operation and is manufacturing the complete product for which a biologics license is desired. In case the license is denied following inspection for the original license, no reinspection need be made until assurance has been received that the faulty conditions which were the basis of the denial have been corrected. An inspection of each licensed establishment and its additional location(s) shall be made at least once every 2 years. Inspections may be made with or without notice, and shall be made during regular business hours unless otherwise directed.

[38 FR 32048, Nov. 20, 1973, as amended at 48 FR 26314, June 7, 1983; 64 FR 56449, Oct. 20, 1999]

Effective date note: At 83 FR 3589, Jan. 26, 2018, § 600.21 was amended by removing the last three sentences, effective June 11, 2018.

§ 600.22 Duties of inspector.

The inspector shall:

(a) Call upon the active head of the establishment, stating the object of his visit,

(b) Interrogate the proprietor or other personnel of the establishment as he may deem necessary,

(c) Examine the details of location, construction, equipment and maintenance, including stables, barns, warehouses, manufacturing laboratories, bleeding clinics maintained for the collection of human blood, shipping rooms, record rooms, and any other structure or appliance used in any part of the manufacture of a product,

(d) Investigate as fully as he deems necessary the methods of propagation, processing, testing, storing, dispensing, recording, or other details of manufacture and distribution of each licensed product, or product for which a license has been requested, including observation of these procedures in actual operation,

(e) Obtain and cause to be sent to the Director, Center for Biologics Evaluation and Research or the Director, Center for Drug Evaluation and Research (see mailing addresses in § 600.2(c)), adequate samples for the examination of any product or ingredient used in its manufacture,

(f) Bring to the attention of the manufacturer any fault observed in the course of inspection in location, construction, manufacturing methods, or administration of a licensed establishment which might lead to impairment of a product,

(g) Inspect and copy, as circumstances may require, any records required to be kept pursuant to § 600.12,

(h) Certify as to the condition of the establishment and of the manufacturing methods followed and make recommendations as to action deemed appropriate with respect to any application for license or any license previously issued.

[38 FR 32048, Nov. 20, 1973, as amended at 49 FR 23833, June 8, 1984; 55 FR 11013, Mar. 26, 1990; 70 FR 14982, Mar. 24, 2005; 80 FR 18092, Apr. 3, 2015]

Effective date note: At 83 FR 3589, Jan. 26, 2018, § 600.22 was removed, effective June 11, 2018.

Subpart D—Reporting of Adverse Experiences

Source: 59 FR 54042, Oct. 27, 1994, unless otherwise noted.

§ 600.80 Postmarketing reporting of adverse experiences.

(a) *Definitions.* The following definitions of terms apply to this section:

Adverse experience. Any adverse event associated with the use of a biological product in humans, whether or not considered product related, including the following: An adverse event occurring in the course of the use of a biological product in professional practice; an adverse event occurring from overdose of the product whether accidental or intentional; an adverse event occurring from abuse of the product; an adverse event occurring from withdrawal of the product; and any failure of expected pharmacological action.

Blood Component. As defined in § 606.3(c) of this chapter.

Disability. A substantial disruption of a person's ability to conduct normal life functions.

Individual case safety report (ICSR). A description of an adverse experience related to an individual patient or subject.

ICSR attachments. Documents related to the adverse experience described in an ICSR, such as medical records, hospital discharge summaries, or other documentation.

Life-threatening adverse experience. Any adverse experience that places the patient, in the view of the initial reporter, at immediate risk of death from the adverse experience as it occurred, i.e., it does not include an adverse experience that, had it occurred in a more severe form, might have caused death.

Serious adverse experience. Any adverse experience occurring at any dose that results in any of the following outcomes: Death, a life-threatening adverse experience, inpatient hospitalization or prolongation of existing hospitalization, a persistent or significant disability/incapacity, or a congenital anomaly/birth defect. Important medical events that may not result in death, be life-threatening, or require hospitalization may be considered a serious adverse experience when, based upon appropriate medical judgment, they may jeopardize the patient or subject and may require medical or surgical intervention to prevent one of the outcomes listed in this definition. Examples of such medical events include allergic bronchospasm requiring intensive treatment in an emergency room or at home, blood dyscrasias or convulsions that do not result in inpatient hospitalization, or the development of drug dependency or drug abuse.

Unexpected adverse experience: Any adverse experience that is not listed in the current labeling for the biological product. This includes events that may be symptomatically and pathophysiologically related to an event listed in the labeling, but differ from the event because of greater severity or specificity. For example, under this definition, hepatic necrosis would be unexpected (by virtue of greater severity) if the labeling only referred to elevated hepatic enzymes or hepatitis. Similarly, cerebral thromboembolism and cerebral vasculitis would be unexpected (by virtue of greater specificity) if the labeling only listed cerebral vascular accidents. "Unexpected," as used in this definition, refers to an adverse experience that has not been previously observed (i.e., included in the labeling) rather than from the perspective of such experience not being anticipated from the pharmacological properties of the pharmaceutical product.

(b) Review of adverse experiences. Any person having a biologics license under §601.20 of this chapter must promptly review all adverse experience information pertaining to its product obtained or otherwise received by the applicant from any source, foreign or domestic, including information derived from commercial marketing experience, postmarketing clinical investigations, postmarketing epidemiological/surveillance studies, reports in the scientific literature, and unpublished scientific papers. Applicants are not required to resubmit to FDA adverse product experience reports forwarded to the applicant by FDA; applicants, however, must submit all followup information on such reports to FDA. Any person subject to the reporting requirements under paragraph (c) of this section must also develop written procedures for the surveillance, receipt, evaluation, and reporting of postmarketing adverse experiences to FDA.

(c) Reporting requirements. The applicant must submit to FDA postmarketing 15-day Alert reports and periodic safety reports pertaining to its biological product as described in this section. These reports must be submitted to the Agency in electronic format as described in paragraph (h)(1) of this section, except as provided in paragraph (h)(2) of this section.

(1)(i) Postmarketing 15-day "Alert reports". The applicant must report each adverse experience that is both serious and unexpected, whether foreign or domestic, as soon as possible but no later than 15 calendar days from initial receipt of the information by the applicant.

(ii) Postmarketing 15-day "Alert reports"—followup. The applicant must promptly investigate all adverse experiences that are the subject of these postmarketing 15-day Alert reports and must submit followup reports within 15 calendar days of receipt of new information or as requested by FDA. If additional information is not obtainable, records should be maintained of the unsuccessful steps taken to seek additional information.

(iii) Submission of reports. The requirements of paragraphs (c)(1)(i) and (c)(1)(ii) of this section, concerning the submission of postmarketing 15-day Alert reports, also apply to any person whose name appears on the label of a licensed biological product as a manufacturer, packer, distributor, shared manufacturer, joint manufacturer, or any other participant involved in divided manufactur-

ing. To avoid unnecessary duplication in the submission to FDA of reports required by paragraphs (c)(1)(i) and (c)(1)(ii) of this section, obligations of persons other than the applicant of the final biological product may be met by submission of all reports of serious adverse experiences to the applicant of the final product. If a person elects to submit adverse experience reports to the applicant rather than to FDA, the person must submit, by any appropriate means, each report to the applicant within 5 calendar days of initial receipt of the information by the person, and the applicant must then comply with the requirements of this section. Under this circumstance, a person who elects to submit reports to the applicant of the final product shall maintain a record of this action which must include:

(A) A copy of all adverse biological product experience reports submitted to the applicant of the final product;

(B) The date the report was received by the person;

(C) The date the report was submitted to the applicant of the final product; and—

(D) The name and address of the applicant of the final product.

(2) Periodic adverse experience reports. (i) The applicant must report each adverse experience not reported under paragraph (c)(1)(i) of this section at quarterly intervals, for 3 years from the date of issuance of the biologics license, and then at annual intervals. The applicant must submit each quarterly report within 30 days of the close of the quarter (the first quarter beginning on the date of issuance of the biologics license) and each annual report within 60 days of the anniversary date of the issuance of the biologics license. Upon written notice, FDA may extend or reestablish the requirement that an applicant submit quarterly reports, or require that the applicant submit reports under this section at different times than those stated. Followup information to adverse experiences submitted in a periodic report may be submitted in the next periodic report.

(ii) Each periodic report is required to contain:

(A) Descriptive information. (1) A narrative summary and analysis of the information in the report;

(2) An analysis of the 15-day Alert reports submitted during the reporting interval (all 15-day Alert reports being appropriately referenced by the applicant's patient identification code for nonvaccine biological product reports or by the unique case identification number for vaccine reports, adverse reaction term(s), and date of submission to FDA);

(3) A history of actions taken since the last report because of adverse experiences (for example, labeling changes or studies initiated);

(4) An index consisting of a line listing of the applicant's patient identification code for nonvaccine biological product reports or by the unique case identification number for vaccine reports and adverse reaction term(s) for ICSRs submitted under paragraph (c)(2)(ii)(B) of this section; and

(B) ICSRs for serious, expected and, nonserious adverse experiences. An ICSR for each adverse experience not reported under paragraph (c)(1)(i) of this section (all serious, expected and nonserious adverse experiences). All such ICSRs must be submitted to FDA (either individually or in one or more batches) within the timeframe specified in paragraph (c)(2)(i) of this section. ICSRs must only be submitted to FDA once.

(iii) Periodic reporting, except for information regarding 15-day Alert reports, does not apply to adverse experience information obtained from postmarketing studies (whether or not conducted under an investigational new drug application), from reports in the scientific literature, and from foreign marketing experience.

(d) Scientific literature. A 15-day Alert report based on information in the scientific literature must be accompanied by a copy of the published article. The 15-day Alert reporting requirements in paragraph (c)(1)(i) of this section (i.e., serious, unexpected adverse experiences) apply only to reports found in scientific and medical journals either as case reports or as the result of a formal clinical trial.

(e) Postmarketing studies. Applicants are not required to submit a 15-day Alert report under paragraph (c) of this section for an adverse experience obtained from a postmarketing clinical study (whether or not conducted under a biological investigational new drug application) unless the applicant concludes that there is a reasonable possibility that the product caused the adverse experience.

(f) Information reported on ICSRs for nonvaccine biological products. ICSRs for nonvaccine biological products include the following information:

(1) Patient information.

(i) Patient identification code;

(ii) Patient age at the time of adverse experience, or date of birth;

(iii) Patient gender; and

(iv) Patient weight.

(2) Adverse experience.

(i) Outcome attributed to adverse experience;

(ii) Date of adverse experience;

(iii) Date of report;

(iv) Description of adverse experience (including a concise medical narrative);

(v) Adverse experience term(s);

(vi) Description of relevant tests, including dates and laboratory data; and

(vii) Other relevant patient history, including preexisting medical conditions.

(3) Suspect medical product(s).

(i) Name;

(ii) Dose, frequency, and route of administration used;

(iii) Therapy dates;

(iv) Diagnosis for use (indication);

(v) Whether the product is a combination product as defined in § 3.2(e) of this chapter;

(vi) Whether the product is a prescription or nonprescription product;

(vii) Whether adverse experience abated after product use stopped or dose reduced;

(viii) Whether adverse experience reappeared after reintroduction of the product;

(ix) Lot number;

(x) Expiration date;

(xi) National Drug Code (NDC) number, or other unique identifier; and

(xii) Concomitant medical products and therapy dates.

(4) Initial reporter information.

(i) Name, address, and telephone number;

(ii) Whether the initial reporter is a health care professional; and

(iii) Occupation, if a health care professional.

(5) Applicant information.

(i) Applicant name and contact office address;

(ii) Telephone number;

(iii) Report source, such as spontaneous, literature, or study;

(iv) Date the report was received by applicant;

(v) Application number and type;

(vi) Whether the ICSR is a 15-day "Alert report";

(vii) Whether the ICSR is an initial report or followup report; and

(viii) Unique case identification number, which must be the same in the initial report and any subsequent followup report(s).

(g) Information reported on ICSRs for vaccine products. ICSRs for vaccine products include the following information:

(1) Patient information.

(i) Patient name, address, telephone number;

(ii) Patient age at the time of vaccination, or date of birth;

(iii) Patient gender; and

(iv) Patient birth weight for children under age 5.

(2) Adverse experience.

(i) Outcome attributed to adverse experience;

(ii) Date and time of adverse experience;

(iii) Date of report;

(iv) Description of adverse experience (including a concise medical narrative);

(v) Adverse experience term(s);

(vi) Illness at the time of vaccination;

(vii) Description of relevant tests, including dates and laboratory data; and

(viii) Other relevant patient history, including preexisting medical conditions.

(3) Suspect medical product(s), including vaccines administered on the same date.

(i) Name;

(ii) Dose, frequency, and route or site of administration used;

(iii) Number of previous vaccine doses;

(iv) Vaccination date(s) and time(s);

(v) Diagnosis for use (indication);

(vi) Whether the product is a combination product (as defined in § 3.2(e) of this chapter);

(vii) Whether the adverse experience abated after product use stopped or dose reduced;

(viii) Whether the adverse experience reappeared after reintroduction of the product;

(ix) Lot number;

(x) Expiration date;

(xi) National Drug Code (NDC) number, or other unique identifier; and

(xii) Concomitant medical products and therapy dates.

(4) Vaccine(s) administered in the 4 weeks prior to the vaccination date.

(i) Name of vaccine;

(ii) Manufacturer;

(iii) Lot number;

(iv) Route or site of administration;

(v) Date given; and

(vi) Number of previous doses.

(5) Initial reporter information.

(i) Name, address, and telephone number;

(ii) Whether the initial reporter is a health care professional; and

(iii) Occupation, if a health care professional.

(6) Facility and personnel where vaccine was administered.

(i) Name of person who administered vaccine;

(ii) Name of responsible physician at facility where vaccine was administered; and

(iii) Name, address (including city, county, and state), and telephone number of facility where vaccine was administered.

(7) Applicant information.

(i) Applicant name and contact office address;

(ii) Telephone number;

(iii) Report source, such as spontaneous, literature, or study;

(iv) Date received by applicant;

(v) Application number and type;

(vi) Whether the ICSR is a 15-day "Alert report";

(vii) Whether the ICSR is an initial report or followup report; and

(viii) Unique case identification number, which must be the same in the initial report and any subsequent followup report(s).

(h) Electronic format for submissions. (1) Safety report submissions, including ICSRs, ICSR attachments, and the descriptive information in periodic reports, must be in an electronic format that FDA can process, review, and archive. FDA will issue guidance on how to provide the electronic submission (e.g., method of transmission, media, file formats, preparation and organization of files).

(2) Persons subject to the requirements of paragraph (c) of this section may request, in writing, a temporary waiver of the requirements in paragraph (h)(1) of this section. These waivers will be granted on a limited basis for good cause shown. FDA will issue guidance on requesting a waiver of the requirements in paragraph (h)(1) of this section. Requests for waivers must be submitted in accordance with § 600.90.

(i) Multiple reports. An applicant should not include in reports under this section any adverse experience that occurred in clinical trials if they were previously submitted as part of the biologics license application. If a report refers to more than one biological product marketed by an applicant, the applicant should submit the report to the biologics license application for the product listed first in the report.

(j) Patient privacy. For nonvaccine biological products, an applicant should not include in reports under this section the names and addresses of individual patients; instead, the applicant should assign a unique code for identification of the patient. The applicant should include the name of the reporter from whom the information was received as part of the initial reporter information, even when the reporter is the patient. The names of patients, health care professionals, hospitals, and geographical identifiers in adverse experience reports are not releasable to the public under FDA's public information regulations in part 20 of this chapter. For vaccine adverse experience reports, these data will become part of the CDC Privacy Act System 09-20-0136, "Epidemiologic Studies and Surveillance of Disease Problems." Information identifying the person who received the vaccine or

that person's legal representative will not be made available to the public, but may be available to the vaccinee or legal representative.

(k) Recordkeeping. The applicant must maintain for a period of 10 years records of all adverse experiences known to the applicant, including raw data and any correspondence relating to the adverse experiences.

(l) Revocation of biologics license. If an applicant fails to establish and maintain records and make reports required under this section with respect to a licensed biological product, FDA may revoke the biologics license for such a product in accordance with the procedures of § 601.5 of this chapter.

(m) Exemptions. Manufacturers of the following listed products are not required to submit adverse experience reports under this section:

(1) Whole blood or components of whole blood.

(2) In vitro diagnostic products, including assay systems for the detection of antibodies or antigens to retroviruses. These products are subject to the reporting requirements for devices.

(n) Disclaimer. A report or information submitted by an applicant under this section (and any release by FDA of that report or information) does not necessarily reflect a conclusion by the applicant or FDA that the report or information constitutes an admission that the biological product caused or contributed to an adverse effect. An applicant need not admit, and may deny, that the report or information submitted under this section constitutes an admission that the biological product caused or contributed to an adverse effect. For purposes of this provision, this paragraph also includes any person reporting under paragraph (c)(1)(iii) of this section.

[59 FR 54042, Oct. 27, 1994, as amended at 62 FR 34168, June 25, 1997; 62 FR 52252, Oct. 7, 1997; 63 FR 14612, Mar. 26, 1998; 64 FR 56449, Oct. 20, 1999; 70 FR 14982, Mar. 24, 2005; 79 FR 33090, June 10, 2014]

§ 600.81 Distribution reports.

(a) *Reporting requirements.* The applicant must submit to the Center for Biologics Evaluation and Research or the Center for Drug Evaluation and Research, information about the quantity of the product distributed under the biologics license, including the quantity distributed to distributors. The interval between distribution reports must be 6 months. Upon written notice, FDA may require that the applicant submit distribution reports under this section at times other than every 6 months. The distribution report must consist of the bulk lot number (from which the final container was filled), the fill lot numbers for the total number of dosage units of each strength or potency distributed (e.g., fifty thousand per 10-milliliter vials), the label lot number (if different from fill lot number), labeled date of expiration, number of doses in fill lot/label lot, date of release of fill lot/label lot for distribution at that time. If any significant amount of a fill lot/label lot is returned, include this information. Disclosure of financial or pricing data is not required. As needed, FDA may require submission of more detailed product distribution information. Upon written notice, FDA may require that the applicant submit reports under this section at times other than those stated. Requests by an applicant to submit reports at times other than those stated should be made as a request for a waiver under § 600.90.

(b)(1) *Electronic format.* Except as provided for in paragraph (b)(2) of this section, the distribution reports required under paragraph (a) of this section must be submitted to the Agency in an electronic format that FDA can process, review, and archive. FDA will issue guidance on how to provide the electronic submission (e.g., method of transmission, media, file formats, preparation and organization of files).

(2) *Waivers.* An applicant may request, in writing, a temporary waiver of the requirements in paragraph (b)(1) of this section. These waivers will be granted on a limited basis for good cause shown. FDA will issue guidance on requesting a waiver of the requirements in paragraph (b)(1) of this section. Requests for waivers must be submitted in accordance with § 600.90.

[59 FR 54042, Oct. 27, 1994, as amended at 64 FR 56449, Oct. 20, 1999; 70 FR 14983, Mar. 24, 2005; 79 FR 33091, June 10, 2014]

§ 600.82 Notification of a permanent discontinuance or an interruption in manufacturing.

(a) *Notification of a permanent discontinuance or an interruption in manufacturing.* (1) An applicant of a biological product, other than blood or blood components for transfusion, which is licensed under section 351 of the Public Health Service Act, and which may be dispensed only under prescription under section 503(b)(1) of the Federal Food, Drug, and Cosmetic Act (21 U.S.C. 353(b)(1)), must notify FDA in writing of a permanent discontinuance of manufacture of the biological product or an interruption in manufacturing of the biological product that is likely to lead to a meaningful disruption in supply of that biological product in the United States if:

(i) The biological product is life supporting, life sustaining, or intended for use in the prevention or treatment of a debilitating disease or condition, including any such biological product used in emergency medical care or during surgery; and

(ii) The biological product is not a radiopharmaceutical biological product.

(2) An applicant of blood or blood components for transfusion, which is licensed under section 351 of the Public Health Service Act, and which may be dispensed only under prescription under section 503(b) of the Federal Food, Drug, and Cosmetic Act, must notify FDA in writing of a permanent discontinuance of manufacture of any product listed in its license or an interruption in manufacturing of any such product that is likely to lead to a significant disruption in supply of that product in the United States if:

(i) The product is life supporting, life sustaining, or intended for use in the prevention or treatment of a debilitating disease or condition, including any such product used in emergency medical care or during surgery; and

(ii) The applicant is a manufacturer of a significant percentage of the U.S. blood supply.

(b) *Submission and timing of notification.* Notifications required by paragraph (a) of this section must be submitted to FDA electronically in a format that FDA can process, review, and archive:

(1) At least 6 months prior to the date of the permanent discontinuance or interruption in manufacturing; or

(2) If 6 months' advance notice is not possible because the permanent discontinuance or interruption in manufacturing was not reasonably anticipated 6 months in advance, as soon as practicable thereafter, but in no case later than 5 business days after such a permanent discontinuance or interruption in manufacturing occurs.

(c) Information included in notification. Notifications required by paragraph (a) of this section must include the following information:

(1) The name of the biological product subject to the notification, including the National Drug Code for such biological product, or an alternative standard for identification and labeling that has been recognized as acceptable by the Center Director;

(2) The name of the applicant of the biological product;

(3) Whether the notification relates to a permanent discontinuance of the biological product or an interruption in manufacturing of the biological product;

(4) A description of the reason for the permanent discontinuance or interruption in manufacturing; and

(5) The estimated duration of the interruption in manufacturing.

(d)(1) *Public list of biological product shortages.* FDA will maintain a publicly available list of biological products that are determined by FDA to be in shortage. This biological product shortages list will include the following information:

(i) The names and National Drug Codes for such biological products, or the alternative standards for identification and labeling that have been recognized as acceptable by the Center Director;

(ii) The name of each applicant for such biological products;

(iii) The reason for the shortage, as determined by FDA, selecting from the following categories: Requirements related to complying with good manufacturing practices; regulatory delay; shortage of an active ingredient; shortage of an inactive ingredient component; discontinuation of the manufacture of the biological product; delay in shipping of the biological product; demand increase for the biological product; or other reason; and

(iv) The estimated duration of the shortage.

(2) *Confidentiality.* FDA may choose not to make information collected to implement this paragraph available on the biological product shortages list or available under section 506C(c) of the Federal Food, Drug, and Cosmetic Act (21 U.S.C. 356c(c)) if FDA determines that disclosure of such information would adversely affect the public health (such as by increasing the possibility of hoarding or other disruption of the availability of the biological product to patients). FDA will also not provide information on the public shortages list or under section 506C(c) of the Federal Food, Drug, and Cosmetic Act that is protected by 18 U.S.C. 1905 or 5 U.S.C. 552(b)(4), including trade secrets and commercial or financial information that is considered confidential or privileged under § 20.61 of this chapter.

(e) *Noncompliance letters.* If an applicant fails to submit a notification as required under paragraph (a) of this section and in accordance with paragraph (b) of this section, FDA will issue a letter to the applicant informing it of such failure.

(1) Not later than 30 calendar days after the issuance of such a letter, the applicant must submit to FDA a written response setting forth the basis for noncompliance and providing the required notification under paragraph (a) of this section and including the information required under paragraph (c) of this section; and

(2) Not later than 45 calendar days after the issuance of a letter under this paragraph, FDA will make the letter and the applicant's response to the letter public, unless, after review of the applicant's response, FDA determines that the applicant had a reasonable basis for not notifying FDA as required under paragraph (a) of this section.

(f) *Definitions.* The following definitions of terms apply to this section:

Biological product shortage or *shortage* means a period of time when the demand or projected demand for the biological product within the United States exceeds the supply of the biological product.

Intended for use in the prevention or treatment of a debilitating disease or condition means a biological product intended for use in the prevention or treatment of a disease or condition associated with mortality or morbidity that has a substantial impact on day-to-day functioning.

Life supporting or *life sustaining* means a biological product that is essential to, or that yields information that is essential to, the restoration or continuation of a bodily function important to the continuation of human life.

Meaningful disruption means a change in production that is reasonably likely to lead to a reduction in the supply of a biological product by a manufacturer that is more than negligible and affects the ability of the manufacturer to fill orders or meet expected demand for its product, and does not include interruptions in manufacturing due to matters such as routine maintenance or insignificant changes in manufacturing so long as the manufacturer expects to resume operations in a short period of time.

Significant disruption means a change in production that is reasonably likely to lead to a reduction in the supply of blood or blood components by a manufacturer that substantially affects the ability of the manufacturer to fill orders or meet expected demand for its product, and does not include interruptions in manufacturing due to matters such as routine maintenance or insignificant changes in manufacturing so long as the manufacturer expects to resume operations in a short period of time.

[80 FR 38939, July 8, 2015]

§ 600.90 Waivers.

(a) An applicant may ask the Food and Drug Administration to waive under this section any requirement that applies to the applicant under §§ 600.80 and 600.81. A waiver request under this section is required to be submitted with supporting documentation. The waiver request is required to contain one of the following:

(1) An explanation why the applicant's compliance with the requirement is unnecessary or cannot be achieved,

(2) A description of an alternative submission that satisfies the purpose of the requirement, or

(3) Other information justifying a waiver.

(b) FDA may grant a waiver if it finds one of the following:

(1) The applicant's compliance with the requirement is unnecessary or cannot be achieved,

(2) The applicant's alternative submission satisfies the requirement, or

(3) The applicant's submission otherwise justifies a waiver.

[59 FR 54042, Oct. 27, 1994, as amended at 79 FR 33092, June 10, 2014]

• • •

PART 601—LICENSING

Subpart A—General Provisions

Authority: 15 U.S.C. 1451-1561; 21 U.S.C. 321, 351, 352, 353, 355, 356b, 360, 360c-360f, 360h-360j, 371, 374, 379e, 381; 42 U.S.C. 216, 241, 262, 263, 264; sec 122, Pub. L. 105-115, 111 Stat. 2322 (21 U.S.C. 355 note).

Source: 38 FR 32052, Nov. 20, 1973, unless otherwise noted.

Cross references: For U.S. Customs Service regulations relating to viruses, serums, and toxins, see 19 CFR 12.21-12.23. For U.S. Postal Service regulations relating to the admissibility to the United States mails see parts 124 and 125 of the Domestic Mail Manual, that is incorporated by reference in 39 CFR part 111.

Subpart A—General Provisions

§ 601.2 Applications for biologics licenses; procedures for filing.

(a) *General.* To obtain a biologics license under section 351 of the Public Health Service Act for any biological product, the manufacturer shall submit an application to the Director, Center for Biologics Evaluation and Research or the Director, Center for Drug Evaluation and Research (see mailing addresses in § 600.2(a) or (b) of this chapter), on forms prescribed for such purposes, and shall submit data derived from nonclinical laboratory and clinical studies which demonstrate that the manufactured product meets prescribed requirements of safety, purity, and potency; with respect to each nonclinical laboratory study, either a statement that the study was conducted in compliance with the requirements set forth in part 58 of this chapter, or, if the study was not conducted in compliance with such regulations, a brief statement of the reason for the noncompliance; statements regarding each clinical investigation involving human subjects contained in the application, that it either was conducted in compliance with the requirements for institutional review set forth in part 56 of this chapter; or was not subject to such requirements in accordance with § 56.104 or § 56.105, and was conducted in compliance with requirements for informed consent set forth in part 50 of this chapter. A full description of manufacturing methods; data establishing stability of the product through the dating period; sample(s) representative of the product for introduction or delivery for introduction into interstate commerce; summaries of results of tests performed on the lot(s) represented by the submitted sample(s); specimens of the labels, enclosures, and containers, and if applicable, any Medication Guide required under part 208 of this chapter proposed to be used for the product; and the address of each location involved in the manufacture of the biological product shall be listed in the biologics license application. The applicant shall also include a financial certification or disclosure statement(s) or both for clinical investigators as required by part 54 of this chapter. An application for a biologics license shall not be considered as filed until all pertinent information and data have been received by the Food and Drug Administration. The applicant shall also include either a claim for categorical exclusion under § 25.30 or § 25.31 of this chapter or an environmental assessment under § 25.40 of this chapter. The applicant, or the applicant's attorney, agent, or other authorized official shall sign the application. An application for any of the following specified categories of biological products subject to licensure shall be handled as set forth in paragraph (c) of this section:

(1) Therapeutic DNA plasmid products;

(2) Therapeutic synthetic peptide products of 40 or fewer amino acids;

(3) Monoclonal antibody products for in vivo use; and

(4) Therapeutic recombinant DNA-derived products.

(b) [Reserved]

(c)(1) To obtain marketing approval for a biological product subject to licensure which is a therapeutic DNA plasmid product, therapeutic synthetic peptide product of 40 or fewer amino acids, monoclonal antibody product for in vivo use, or therapeutic recombinant DNA-derived product, an applicant shall submit a biologics license application in accordance with paragraph (a) of this section except that the following sections in parts 600 through 680 of this chapter shall not be applicable to such products: §§ 600.10(b) and (c), 600.11, 600.12, 600.13, 610.53, and 610.62 of this chapter.

(2) To the extent that the requirements in this paragraph (c) conflict with other requirements in this subchapter, this paragraph (c) shall supersede other requirements.

(d) Approval of a biologics license application or issuance of a biologics license shall constitute a determination that the establishment(s) and the product meet applicable requirements to ensure the continued safety, purity, and potency of such products. Applicable requirements for the maintenance of establishments for the manufacture of a product subject to this section shall include but not be limited to the good manufacturing practice requirements set forth in parts 210, 211, 600, 606, and 820 of this chapter.

(e) Any establishment and product license for a biological product issued under section 351 of the Public Health Service Act (42 U.S.C. 201 et seq.) that has not been revoked or suspended as of December 20, 1999, shall constitute an approved biologics license application in effect under the same terms and conditions set forth in such product license and such portions of the establishment license relating to such product.

(f) *Withdrawal from sale of approved biological products.* A holder of a biologics license application (BLA) must report to FDA, in accordance with the requirements of §§ 207.61 and 207.65, the withdrawal from sale of an approved biological product. The information must be submitted to FDA within 30 working days of the biological product's withdrawal from sale. The following information must be submitted: The holder's name; product name; BLA number; the National Drug Code; and the date on which the product is expected to be no longer in commercial distribution. The reason for the withdrawal of the biological product is requested but not required to be submitted.

[64 FR 56450, Oct. 20, 1999, as amended at 70 FR 14983, Mar. 24, 2005; 80 FR 18092, Apr. 3, 2015; 80 FR 37974, July 2, 2015; 81 FR 60221, Aug. 31, 2016]

§ 601.3 Complete response letter to the applicant.

(a) *Complete response letter.* The Food and Drug Administration will send the biologics license applicant or supplement applicant a complete response letter if the agency determines that it will not approve the biologics license application or supplement in its present form.

(1) *Description of specific deficiencies.* A complete response letter will describe all of the deficiencies that the agency has identified in a biologics license application or supplement, except as stated in paragraph (a)(2) of this section.

(2) *Inadequate data.* If FDA determines, after a biologics license application or supplement is filed, that the data submitted are inadequate to support approval, the agency might issue a complete response letter without first conducting required inspections, testing submitted product lots, and/or reviewing proposed product labeling.

(3) *Recommendation of actions for approval.* When possible, a complete response letter will recommend actions that the applicant might take to place its biologics license application or supplement in condition for approval.

(b) *Applicant actions.* After receiving a complete response letter, the biologics license applicant or supplement applicant must take either of the following actions:

(1) *Resubmission.* Resubmit the application or supplement, addressing all deficiencies identified in the complete response letter.

(2) *Withdrawal.* Withdraw the application or supplement. A decision to withdraw the application or supplement is without prejudice to a subsequent submission.

(c) *Failure to take action.* (1) FDA may consider a biologics license applicant or supplement applicant's failure to either resubmit or withdraw the application or supplement within 1 year after issuance of a complete response letter to be a request by the applicant to withdraw the application or supplement, unless the applicant has requested an extension of time in which to resubmit the application or supplement. FDA will grant any reasonable request for such an extension. FDA may consider an applicant's failure to resubmit the application or supplement within the extended time period or request an additional extension to be a request by the applicant to withdraw the application.

(2) If FDA considers an applicant's failure to take action in accordance with paragraph (c)(1) of this section to be a request to withdraw the application, the agency will notify the applicant in writing. The applicant will have 30 days from the date of the notification to explain why the application or supplement should not be withdrawn and to request an extension of time in which to resubmit the application or supplement. FDA will grant any reasonable request for an extension. If the applicant does not respond to the notification within 30 days, the application or supplement will be deemed to be withdrawn.

[73 FR 39611, July 10, 2008]

§ 601.4 Issuance and denial of license.

(a) A biologics license shall be issued upon a determination by the Director, Center for Biologics Evaluation and Research or the Director, Center for Drug Evaluation and Research that the establishment(s) and the product meet the applicable requirements established in this chapter. A biologics license shall be valid until suspended or revoked.

(b) If the Commissioner determines that the establishment or product does not meet the requirements established in this chapter, the biologics license application shall be denied and the applicant shall be informed of the grounds for, and of an opportunity for a hearing on, the decision. If the applicant so requests, the Commissioner shall issue a notice of opportunity for hearing on the matter pursuant to § 12.21(b) of this chapter.

[42 FR 4718, Jan. 25, 1977, as amended at 42 FR 15676, Mar. 22, 1977; 42 FR 19142, Apr. 12, 1977; 64 FR 56450, Oct. 20, 1999; 70 FR 14983, Mar. 24, 2005]

§ 601.5 Revocation of license.

(a) A biologics license shall be revoked upon application of the manufacturer giving notice of intention to discontinue the manufacture of all products manufactured under such license or to discontinue the manufacture of a particular product for which a license is held and waiving an opportunity for a hearing on the matter.

(b)(1) The Commissioner shall notify the licensed manufacturer of the intention to revoke the biologics license, setting forth the grounds for, and offering an opportunity for a hearing on the proposed revocation if the Commissioner finds any of the following:

(i) Authorized Food and Drug Administration employees after reasonable efforts have been unable to gain access to an establishment or a location for the purpose of carrying out the inspection required under § 600.21 of this chapter,

(ii) Manufacturing of products or of a product has been discontinued to an extent that a meaningful inspection or evaluation cannot be made,

(iii) The manufacturer has failed to report a change as required by § 601.12 of this chapter,

(iv) The establishment or any location thereof, or the product for which the license has been issued, fails to conform to the applicable standards established in the license and in this chapter designed to ensure the continued safety, purity, and potency of the manufactured product,

(v) The establishment or the manufacturing methods have been so changed as to require a new showing that the establishment or product meets the requirements established in this chapter in order to protect the public health, or

(vi) The licensed product is not safe and effective for all of its intended uses or is misbranded with respect to any such use.

(2) Except as provided in § 601.6 of this chapter, or in cases involving willfulness, the notification required in this paragraph shall provide a reasonable period for the licensed manufacturer to demonstrate or achieve compliance with the requirements of this chapter, before proceedings will be instituted for the revocation of the license. If compliance is not demonstrated or achieved and the licensed manufacturer does not waive the opportunity for a hearing, the Commissioner shall issue a notice of opportunity for hearing on the matter under § 12.21(b) of this chapter.

[64 FR 56451, Oct. 20, 1999]

§ 601.6 Suspension of license.

(a) Whenever the Commissioner has reasonable grounds to believe that any of the grounds for revocation of a license exist and that by reason thereof there is a danger to health, the Commissioner may notify the licensed manufacturer that the biologics license is suspended and require that the licensed manufacturer do the following:

(1) Notify the selling agents and distributors to whom such product or products have been delivered of such suspension, and

(2) Furnish to the Center for Biologics Evaluation and Research or the Center for Drug Evaluation and Research, complete records of such deliveries and notice of suspension.

(b) Upon suspension of a license, the Commissioner shall either:

(1) Proceed under the provisions of § 601.5(b) of this chapter to revoke the license, or

(2) If the licensed manufacturer agrees, hold revocation in abeyance pending resolution of the matters involved.

[64 FR 56451, Oct. 20, 1999, as amended at 70 FR 14983, Mar. 24, 2005]

§ 601.7 Procedure for hearings.

(a) A notice of opportunity for hearing, notice of appearance and request for hearing, and grant or denial of hearing for a biological drug pursuant to this part, for which the exemption from the Federal Food, Drug, and Cosmetic Act in § 310.4 of this chapter has been revoked, shall be subject to the provisions of § 314.200 of this chapter except to the extent that the notice of opportunity for hearing on the matter issued pursuant to § 12.21(b) of this chapter specifically provides otherwise.

(b) Hearings pursuant to §§ 601.4 through 601.6 shall be governed by part 12 of this chapter.

(c) When a license has been suspended pursuant to § 601.6 and a hearing request has been granted, the hearing shall proceed on an expedited basis.

[42 FR 4718, Jan. 25, 1977, as amended at 42 FR 15676, Mar. 22, 1977; 42 FR 19143, Apr. 12, 1977]

§ 601.8 Publication of revocation.

The Commissioner, following revocation of a biologics license under 21 CFR 601.5(b), will publish a notice in the Federal Register with a statement of the specific grounds for the revocation.

[74 FR 20585, May 5, 2009]

§ 601.9 Licenses; reissuance.

(a) *Compliance with requirements.* A biologics license, previously suspended or revoked, may be reissued or reinstated upon a showing of compliance with requirements and upon such inspection and examination as may be considered necessary by the Director, Center for Biologics Evaluation and Research or the Director, Center for Drug Evaluation and Research.

(b) *Exclusion of noncomplying location.* A biologics license, excluding a location or locations that fail to comply with the requirements in this chapter, may be issued without further application and concurrently with the suspension or revocation of the license for noncompliance at the excluded location or locations.

(c) *Exclusion of noncomplying product(s).* In the case of multiple products included under a single biologics license application, a biologics license may be issued, excluding the noncompliant product(s), without further application and concurrently with the suspension or revocation of the biologics license for a noncompliant product(s).

[64 FR 56451, Oct. 20, 1999, as amended at 70 FR 14983, Mar. 24, 2005]

Subpart B—[Reserved]

Subpart C—Biologics Licensing

§ 601.12 Changes to an approved application.

(a) *General.* (1) As provided by this section, an applicant must inform the Food and Drug Administration (FDA) (see mailing addresses in § 600.2 of this chapter) about each change in the product, production process, quality controls, equipment, facilities, responsible personnel, or labeling established in the approved license application(s).

(2) Before distributing a product made using a change, an applicant must assess the effects of the change and demonstrate through appropriate validation and/or other clinical and/or nonclinical laboratory studies the lack of adverse effect of the change on the identity, strength, quality, purity, or potency of the product as they may relate to the safety or effectiveness of the product.

(3) Notwithstanding the requirements of paragraphs (b), (c), and (f) of this section, an applicant must make a change provided for in those paragraphs in accordance with a regulation or guidance that provides for a less burdensome notification of the change (for example, by submission of a supplement that does not require approval prior to distribution of the product or in an annual report).

(4) The applicant must promptly revise all promotional labeling and advertising to make it consistent with any labeling change implemented in accordance with paragraphs (f)(1) and (f)(2) of this section.

(5) A supplement or annual report must include a list of all changes contained in the supplement or annual report. For supplements, this list must be provided in the cover letter.

(b) *Changes requiring supplement submission and approval prior to distribution of the product made using the change (major changes).* (1) A supplement shall be submitted for any change in the product, production process, quality controls, equipment, facilities, or responsible personnel that has a substantial potential to have an adverse effect on the identity, strength, quality, purity, or potency of the product as they may relate to the safety or effectiveness of the product.

(2) These changes include, but are not limited to:

(i) Except as provided in paragraphs (c) and (d) of this section, changes in the qualitative or quantitative formulation, including inactive ingredients, or in the specifications provided in the approved application;

(ii) Changes requiring completion of an appropriate human study to demonstrate the equivalence of the identity, strength, quality, purity, or potency of the product as they may relate to the safety or effectiveness of the product;

(iii) Changes in the virus or adventitious agent removal or inactivation method(s);

(iv) Changes in the source material or cell line;

(v) Establishment of a new master cell bank or seed; and

(vi) Changes which may affect product sterility assurance, such as changes in product or component sterilization method(s), or an addition, deletion, or substitution of steps in an aseptic processing operation.

(3) The applicant must obtain approval of the supplement from FDA prior to distribution of the product made using the change. Except for submissions under paragraph (e) of this section, the following shall be contained in the supplement:

(i) A detailed description of the proposed change;

(ii) The product(s) involved;

(iii) The manufacturing site(s) or area(s) affected;

(iv) A description of the methods used and studies performed to evaluate the effect of the change on the identity, strength, quality, purity, or potency of the product as they may relate to the safety or effectiveness of the product;

(v) The data derived from such studies;

(vi) Relevant validation protocols and data; and

(vii) A reference list of relevant standard operating procedures (SOP's).

(4) An applicant may ask FDA to expedite its review of a supplement for public health reasons or if a delay in making the change described in it would impose an extraordinary hardship on the applicant. Such a supplement and its mailing cover should be plainly marked: "Prior Approval Supplement-Expedited Review Requested.

(c) *Changes requiring supplement submission at least 30 days prior to distribution of the product made using the change.* (1) A supplement shall be submitted for any change in the product, production process, quality controls, equipment, facilities, or responsible personnel that has a moderate potential to have an adverse effect on the identity, strength, quality, purity, or potency of the product as they may relate to the safety or effectiveness of the product. The supplement shall be labeled "Supplement—Changes Being Effected in 30 Days" or, if applicable under paragraph (c)(5) of this section, "Supplement—Changes Being Effected."

(2) These changes include, but are not limited to:

(i) [Reserved]

(ii) An increase or decrease in production scale during finishing steps that involves different equipment; and

(iii) Replacement of equipment with that of similar, but not identical, design and operating principle that does not affect the process methodology or process operating parameters.

(iv) Relaxation of an acceptance criterion or deletion of a test to comply with an official compendium that is consistent with FDA statutory and regulatory requirements.

(3) Pending approval of the supplement by FDA, and except as provided in paragraph (c)(5) of this section, distribution of the product made using the change may begin not less than 30 days after receipt of the supplement by FDA. The information listed in paragraph (b)(3)(i) through (b)(3)(vii) of this section shall be contained in the supplement.

(4) If within 30 days following FDA's receipt of the supplement, FDA informs the applicant that either:

(i) The change requires approval prior to distribution of the product in accordance with paragraph (b) of this section; or

(ii) Any of the information required under paragraph (c)(3) of this section is missing; the applicant shall not distribute the product made using the change until FDA determines that compliance with this section is achieved.

(5) In certain circumstances, FDA may determine that, based on experience with a particular type of change, the supplement for such change is usually complete and provides the proper information, and on particular assurances that the proposed change has been appropriately submitted, the product made using the change may be distributed immediately upon receipt of the supplement by FDA. These circumstances may include substantial similarity with a type of change regularly involving a "Supplement—Changes Being Effected" supplement or a situation in which the applicant presents evidence that the proposed change has been validated in accordance with an approved protocol for such change under paragraph (e) of this section.

(6) If the agency disapproves the supplemental application, it may order the manufacturer to cease distribution of the products made with the manufacturing change.

(d) *Changes to be described in an annual report (minor changes).* (1) Changes in the product, production process, quality controls, equipment, facilities, or responsible personnel that have a minimal potential to have an adverse effect on the identity, strength, quality, purity, or potency of the product as they may relate to the safety or effectiveness of the product shall be documented by the applicant in an annual report submitted each year within 60 days of the anniversary date of approval of the application. The Director, Center for Biologics Evaluation and Research or the Director, Center for Drug Evaluation and Research, may approve a written request for an alternative date to combine annual reports for multiple approved applications into a single annual report submission.

(2) These changes include, but are not limited to:

(i) Any change made to comply with a change to an official compendium, except a change described in paragraph (c)(2)(iv) of this section, that is consistent with FDA statutory and regulatory requirements.

(ii) The deletion or reduction of an ingredient intended only to affect the color of the product, except that a change intended only to affect Blood Grouping Reagents requires supplement submission and approval prior to distribution of the product made using the change in accordance with the requirements set forth in paragraph (b) of this section;

(iii) An extension of an expiration dating period based upon full shelf life data on production batches obtained from a protocol approved in the application;

(iv) A change within the container closure system for a nonsterile product, based upon a showing of equivalency to the approved system under a protocol approved in the application or published in an official compendium;

(v) A change in the size and/or shape of a container containing the same number of dosage units for a nonsterile solid dosage form product, without a change from one container closure system to another;

(vi) The addition by embossing, debossing, or engraving of a code imprint to a solid dosage form biological product other than a modified release dosage form, or a minor change in an existing code imprint; and

(vii) The addition or revision of an alternative analytical procedure that provides the same or increased assurance of the identity, strength, quality, purity, or potency of the material being tested as the analytical procedure described in the approved application, or deletion of an alternative analytical procedure.

(3) The following information for each change shall be contained in the annual report:

(i) A list of all products involved; and

(ii) A full description of the manufacturing and controls changes including: the manufacturing site(s) or area(s) involved; the date the change was made; a cross-reference to relevant validation protocols and/or SOP's; and relevant data from studies and tests performed to evaluate the effect of the change on the identity, strength, quality, purity, or potency of the product as they may relate to the safety or effectiveness of the product.

(iii) A statement by the holder of the approved application or license that the effects of the change have been assessed.

(4) The applicant shall submit the report to the FDA office responsible for reviewing the application. The report shall include all the information required under this paragraph for each change made during the annual reporting interval which ends on the anniversary date in the order in which they were implemented.

(e) An applicant may submit one or more protocols describing the specific tests and validation studies and acceptable limits to be achieved to demonstrate the lack of adverse effect for specified types of manufacturing changes on the identity, strength, quality, purity, or potency of the product as they may relate to the safety or effectiveness of the product. Any such protocols, or change to a protocol, shall be submitted as a supplement requiring approval from FDA prior to distribution of the product which, if approved, may justify a reduced reporting category for the particular change because the use of the protocol for that type of change reduces the potential risk of an adverse effect.

(f) *Labeling changes.* (1) Labeling changes requiring supplement submission—FDA approval must be obtained before distribution of the product with the labeling change. Except as described in paragraphs (f)(2) and (f)(3) of this section, an applicant shall submit a supplement describing a proposed change in the package insert, package label, container label, or, if applicable, a Medication Guide required under part 208 of this chapter, and include the information necessary to support the proposed change. An applicant cannot use paragraph (f)(2) of this section to make any change to the information required in § 201.57(a) of this chapter. An applicant may report the minor changes to the information specified in paragraph (f)(3)(i)(D) of this section in an annual report. The supplement shall clearly highlight the proposed change in the labeling. The applicant shall obtain approval from FDA prior to distribution of the product with the labeling change.

(2) *Labeling changes requiring supplement submission—product with a labeling change that may be distributed before FDA approval.* (i) An applicant shall submit, at the time such change is made, a supplement for any change in the package insert, package label, or container label to reflect newly acquired information, except for changes to the package insert required in § 201.57(a) of this chapter (which must be made under paragraph (f)(1) of this section), to accomplish any of the following:

(A) To add or strengthen a contraindication, warning, precaution, or adverse reaction for which the evidence of a causal association satisfies the standard for inclusion in the labeling under § 201.57(c) of this chapter;

(B) To add or strengthen a statement about abuse, dependence, psychological effect, or overdosage;

(C) To add or strengthen an instruction about dosage and administration that is intended to increase the safety of the use of the product; and

(D) To delete false, misleading, or unsupported indications for use or claims for effectiveness.

(E) Any labeling change normally requiring a supplement submission and approval prior to distribution of the product that FDA specifically requests be submitted under this provision.

(ii) Pending approval of the supplement by FDA, the applicant may distribute a product with a package insert, package label, or container label bearing such change at the time the supplement is submitted. The supplement shall clearly identify the change being made and include necessary supporting data. The supplement and its mailing cover shall be plainly marked: "Special Labeling Supplement—Changes Being Effected."

(3) *Labeling changes requiring submission in an annual report.* (i) An applicant shall submit any final printed package insert, package label, container label, or Medication Guide required under part 208 of this chapter incorporating the following changes in an annual report submitted to FDA each year as provided in paragraph (d)(1) of this section:

(A) Editorial or similar minor changes;

(B) A change in the information on how the product is supplied that does not involve a change in the dosage strength or dosage form;

(C) A change in the information specified in § 208.20(b)(8)(iii) and (b)(8)(iv) of this chapter for a Medication Guide; and

(D) A change to the information required in § 201.57(a) of this chapter as follows:

(1) Removal of a listed section(s) specified in § 201.57(a)(5) of this chapter; and

(2) Changes to the most recent revision date of the labeling as specified in § 201.57(a)(15) of this chapter.

(E) A change made pursuant to an exception or alternative granted under § 201.26 or § 610.68 of this chapter.

(ii) The applicant may distribute a product with a package insert, package label, or container label bearing such change at the time the change is made.

(4) *Advertisements and promotional labeling.* Advertisements and promotional labeling shall be submitted to the Center for Biologics Evaluation and Research or Center for Drug Evaluation and Research in accordance with the requirements set forth in § 314.81(b)(3)(i) of this chapter.

(5) The submission and grant of a written request for an exception or alternative under § 201.26 or § 610.68 of this chapter satisfies the requirements in paragraphs (f)(1) through (f)(2) of this section.

(6) For purposes of paragraph (f)(2) of this section, information will be considered newly acquired if it consists of data, analyses, or other information not previously submitted to the agency, which may include (but are not limited to) data derived from new clinical studies, reports of adverse events, or new analyses of previously submitted data (e.g., meta-analyses) if the studies, events or analyses reveal risks of a different type or greater severity or frequency than previously included in submissions to FDA.

(g) *Failure to comply.* In addition to other remedies available in law and regulations, in the event of repeated failure of the applicant to comply with this section, FDA may require that the applicant submit a supplement for any proposed change and obtain approval of the supplement by FDA prior to distribution of the product made using the change.

(h) *Administrative review.* Under § 10.75 of this chapter, an applicant may request internal FDA review of FDA employee decisions under this section.

[62 FR 39901, July 24, 1997, as amended at 63 FR 66399, Dec. 1, 1998. Redesignated at 65 FR 59718, Oct. 6, 2000, and amended at 69 FR 18766, Apr. 8, 2004; 70 FR 14983, Mar. 24, 2005; 71 FR 3997, Jan. 24, 2006; 72 FR 73600, Dec. 28, 2007; 73 FR 49609, Aug. 22, 2008; 73 FR 68333, Nov. 18, 2008; 80 FR 18092, Apr. 3, 2015]

§ 601.14 Regulatory submissions in electronic format.

(a) *General.* Electronic format submissions must be in a form that FDA can process, review, and archive. FDA will periodically issue guidance on how to provide the electronic submission (e.g., method of transmission, media, file formats, preparation and organization of files.)

(b) *Labeling.* The content of labeling required under § 201.100(d)(3) of this chapter (commonly referred to as the package insert or professional labeling), including all text, tables, and figures, must be submitted to the agency in electronic format as described in paragraph (a) of this section. This requirement is in addition to the provisions of §§ 601.2(a) and 601.12(f) that require applicants to submit specimens of the labels, enclosures, and containers, or to submit other final printed labeling. Submissions under this paragraph must be made in accordance with part 11 of this chapter except for the requirements of § 11.10(a), (c) through (h), and (k), and the corresponding requirements of § 11.30.

[68 FR 69020, Dec. 11, 2003]

§ 601.15 Foreign establishments and products: samples for each importation.

Random samples of each importation, obtained by the District Director of Customs and forwarded to the Director, Center for Biologics Evaluation and Research or the Director, Center for Drug Evaluation and Research (see mailing addresses in § 600.2(c) of this chapter) must be at least two final containers of each lot of product. A copy of the associated documents which describe and identify the shipment must accompany the shipment for forwarding with the samples to the Director, Center for Biologics Evaluation and Research or the Director, Center for Drug Evaluation and Research (see mailing addresses in §600.2(c)). For shipments of 20 or less final containers, samples need not be forwarded, provided a copy of an official release from the Center for Biologics Evaluation and Research or Center for Drug Evaluation and Research accompanies each shipment.

[70 FR 14983, Mar. 24, 2005, as amended at 80 FR 18092, Apr. 3, 2015]

§601.20 Biologics licenses; issuance and conditions.

(a) Examination—compliance with requirements. A biologics license application shall be approved only upon examination of the product and upon a determination that the product complies with the standards established in the biologics license application and the requirements prescribed in the regulations in this chapter including but not limited to the good manufacturing practice requirements set forth in parts 210, 211, 600, 606, and 820 of this chapter.

(b) *Availability of product.* No biologics license shall be issued unless:

(1) The product intended for introduction into interstate commerce is available for examination, and

(2) Such product is available for inspection during all phases of manufacture.

(c) *Manufacturing process—impairment of assurances.* No product shall be licensed if any part of the process of or relating to the manufacture of such product, in the judgment of the Director, Center for Biologics Evaluation and Research or the Director, Center for Drug Evaluation and Research, would impair the assurances of continued safety, purity, and potency as provided by the regulations contained in this chapter.

(d) *Inspection—compliance with requirements.* A biologics license shall be issued or a biologics license application approved only after inspection of the establishment(s) listed in the biologics license application and upon a determination that the establishment(s) complies with the standards established in the biologics license application and the requirements prescribed in applicable regulations.

(e) *One biologics license to cover all locations.* One biologics license shall be issued to cover all locations meeting the establishment standards identified in the approved biologics license application and each location shall be subject to inspection by FDA officials.

[64 FR 56451, Oct. 20, 1999, as amended at 70 FR 14983, Mar. 24, 2005]

§601.21 Products under development.

A biological product undergoing development, but not yet ready for a biologics license, may be shipped or otherwise delivered from one State or possession into another State or possession provided such shipment or delivery is not for introduction or delivery for introduction into interstate commerce, except as provided in sections 505(i) and 520(g) of the Federal Food, Drug, and Cosmetic Act, as amended, and the regulations thereunder (21 CFR parts 312 and 812).

[64 FR 56451, Oct. 20, 1999]

§601.22 Products in short supply; initial manufacturing at other than licensed location.

A biologics license issued to a manufacturer and covering all locations of manufacture shall authorize persons other than such manufacturer to conduct at places other than such locations the initial, and partial manufacturing of a product for shipment solely to such manufacturer only to the extent that the names of such persons and places are registered with the Commissioner of Food and Drugs and it is found upon application of such manufacturer, that the product is in short supply due either to the peculiar growth requirements of the organism involved or to the scarcity of the animal required for manufacturing purposes, and such manufacturer has established with respect to such persons and places such procedures, inspections, tests or other arrangements as will ensure full compliance with the applicable regulations of this subchapter related to continued safety, purity, and potency. Such persons and places shall be subject to all regulations of this subchapter except §§601.2 to 601.6, 601.9, 601.10, 601.20, 601.21 to 601.33, and 610.60 to 610.65 of this chapter. For persons and places authorized under this section to conduct the initial and partial manufacturing of a product for shipment solely to a manufacturer of a product subject to licensure under §601.2(c), the following additional regulations shall not be applicable: §§600.10(b) and (c), 600.11, 600.12, 600.13, and 610.53 of this chapter. Failure of such manufacturer to maintain such procedures, inspections, tests, or other arrangements, or failure of any person conducting such partial manufacturing to comply with applicable regulations shall constitute a ground for suspension or revocation of the authority conferred pursuant to this section on the same basis as provided in §§601.6 to 601.8 with respect to the suspension and the revocation of licenses.

[42 FR 4718, Jan. 25, 1977, as amended at 61 FR 24233, May 14, 1996; 64 FR 56452, Oct. 20, 1999; 80 FR 37974, July 2, 2015]

§601.27 Pediatric studies.

(a) *Required assessment.* Except as provided in paragraphs (b), (c), and (d) of this section, each application for a new active ingredient, new indication, new dosage form, new dosing regimen, or new route of administration shall contain data that are adequate to assess the safety and effectiveness of the product for the claimed indications in all relevant pediatric subpopulations, and to support dosing and administration for each pediatric subpopulation for which the product is safe and effective. Where the course of the disease and the effects of the product are similar in adults and pediatric patients, FDA may conclude that pediatric effectiveness can be extrapolated from adequate and well-controlled effectiveness studies in adults, usually supplemented with other information in pediatric patients, such as pharmacokinetic studies. In addition, studies may not be needed in each pediatric age group, if data from one age group can be extrapolated to another. Assessments required under this section for a product that represents a meaningful therapeutic benefit over existing treatments must be carried out using appropriate formulations for the age group(s) for which the assessment is required.

(b) *Deferred submission.* (1) FDA may, on its own initiative or at the request of an applicant, defer submission of some or all assessments of safety and effectiveness described in paragraph (a) of this section until after licensing of the product for use in adults. Deferral may be granted if, among other reasons, the product is ready for approval in adults before studies in pediatric patients are complete, pediatric studies should be delayed until additional safety or effectiveness data have been collected. If an applicant requests deferred submission, the request must provide an adequate justification for delaying pediatric studies, a description of the planned or ongoing studies, and evidence that the studies are being or will be conducted with due diligence and at the earliest possible time.

(2) If FDA determines that there is an adequate justification for temporarily delaying the submission of assessments of pediatric safety and effectiveness, the product may be licensed for use in adults subject to the requirement that the applicant submit the required assessments within a specified time.

(c) *Waivers*—(1) *General.* FDA may grant a full or partial waiver of the requirements of paragraph (a) of this section on its own initiative or at the request of an applicant. A request for a waiver must provide an adequate justification.

(2) *Full waiver.* An applicant may request a waiver of the requirements of paragraph (a) of this section if the applicant certifies that:

(i) The product does not represent a meaningful therapeutic benefit over existing therapies for pediatric patients and is not likely to be used in a substantial number of pediatric patients;

(ii) Necessary studies are impossible or highly impractical because, e.g., the number of such patients is so small or geographically dispersed; or

(iii) There is evidence strongly suggesting that the product would be ineffective or unsafe in all pediatric age groups.

(3) Partial waiver. An applicant may request a waiver of the requirements of paragraph (a) of this section with respect to a specified pediatric age group, if the applicant certifies that:

(i) The product does not represent a meaningful therapeutic benefit over existing therapies for pediatric patients in that age group, and is not likely to be used in a substantial number of patients in that age group;

(ii) Necessary studies are impossible or highly impractical because, e.g., the number of patients in that age group is so small or geographically dispersed;

(iii) There is evidence strongly suggesting that the product would be ineffective or unsafe in that age group; or

(iv) The applicant can demonstrate that reasonable attempts to produce a pediatric formulation necessary for that age group have failed.

(4) *FDA action on waiver.* FDA shall grant a full or partial waiver, as appropriate, if the agency finds that there is a reasonable basis on which to conclude that one or more of the grounds for waiver specified in paragraphs (c)(2) or (c)(3) of this section have been met. If a waiver is granted on the ground that it is not possible to develop a pediatric formulation, the waiver will cover only those pediatric age groups requiring that formulation. If a waiver is granted because there is evidence that the product would be ineffective or unsafe in pediatric populations, this information will be included in the product's labeling.

(5) *Definition of "meaningful therapeutic benefit".* For purposes of this section, a product will be considered to offer a meaningful therapeutic benefit over existing therapies if FDA estimates that:

(i) If approved, the product would represent a significant improvement in the treatment, diagnosis, or prevention of a disease, compared to marketed products adequately labeled for that use in the relevant pediatric population. Examples of how improvement might be demonstrated include, e.g., evidence of increased effectiveness in treatment, prevention, or diagnosis of disease; elimination or substantial reduction of a treatment-limiting drug reaction; documented enhancement of compliance; or evidence of safety and effectiveness in a new subpopulation; or

(ii) The product is in a class of products or for an indication for which there is a need for additional therapeutic options.

(d) *Exemption for orphan drugs.* This section does not apply to any product for an indication or indications for which orphan designation has been granted under part 316, subpart C, of this chapter.

[63 FR 66671, Dec. 2, 1998]

§ 601.28 Annual reports of postmarketing pediatric studies.

Sponsors of licensed biological products shall submit the following information each year within 60 days of the anniversary date of approval of each product under the license to the Director, Center for Biologics Evaluation and Research or the Director, Center for Drug Evaluation and Research (see mailing addresses in § 600.2(a) or (b) of this chapter):

(a) *Summary.* A brief summary stating whether labeling supplements for pediatric use have been submitted and whether new studies in the pediatric population to support appropriate labeling for the pediatric population have been initiated. Where possible, an estimate of patient exposure to the drug product, with special reference to the pediatric population (neonates, infants, children, and adolescents) shall be provided, including dosage form.

(b) *Clinical data.* Analysis of available safety and efficacy data in the pediatric population and changes proposed in the labeling based on this information. An assessment of data needed to ensure appropriate labeling for the pediatric population shall be included.

(c) *Status reports.* A statement on the current status of any postmarketing studies in the pediatric population performed by, or on behalf of, the applicant. The statement shall include whether postmarketing clinical studies in pediatric populations were required or agreed to, and, if so, the status of these studies shall be reported to FDA in annual progress reports of postmarketing studies under § 601.70 rather than under this section.

[65 FR 59718, Oct. 6, 2000, as amended at 65 FR 64618, Oct. 30, 2000; 70 FR 14984, Mar. 24, 2005; 80 FR 18092, Apr. 3, 2015]

§ 601.29 Guidance documents.

(a) FDA has made available guidance documents under § 10.115 of this chapter to help you comply with certain requirements of this part.

(b) The Center for Biologics Evaluation and Research (CBER) maintains a list of guidance documents that apply to the center's regulations. The lists are maintained on the Internet and are published annually in the Federal Register. You may request a copy of the CBER list from the Food and Drug Administration, Center for Biologics Evaluation and Research, Office of Communication, Outreach and Development, 10903 New Hampshire Ave., Bldg. 71, Rm. 3103, Silver Spring, MD 20993-0002.

[65 FR 56480, Sept. 19, 2000, as amended at 70 FR 14984, Mar. 24, 2005; 80 FR 18092, Apr. 3, 2015]

Subpart D—Diagnostic Radiopharmaceuticals

Source: 64 FR 26668, May 17, 1999, unless otherwise noted.

§ 601.30 Scope.

This subpart applies to radiopharmaceuticals intended for in vivo administration for diagnostic and monitoring use. It does not apply to radiopharmaceuticals intended for therapeutic purposes. In situations where a particular radiopharmaceutical is proposed for both diagnostic and therapeutic uses, the radiopharmaceutical must be evaluated taking into account each intended use.

§ 601.31 Definition.

For purposes of this part, *diagnostic radiopharmaceutical means:*

(a) An article that is intended for use in the diagnosis or monitoring of a disease or a manifestation of a disease in humans and that exhibits spontaneous disintegration of unstable nuclei with the emission of nuclear particles or photons; or

(b) Any nonradioactive reagent kit or nuclide generator that is intended to be used in the preparation of such article as defined in paragraph (a) of this section.

§ 601.32 General factors relevant to safety and effectiveness.

FDA's determination of the safety and effectiveness of a diagnostic radiopharmaceutical includes consideration of the following:

(a) The proposed use of the diagnostic radiopharmaceutical in the practice of medicine;

(b) The pharmacological and toxicological activity of the diagnostic radiopharmaceutical (including any carrier or ligand component of the diagnostic radiopharmaceutical); and

(c) The estimated absorbed radiation dose of the diagnostic radiopharmaceutical.

§ 601.33 Indications.

(a) For diagnostic radiopharmaceuticals, the categories of proposed indications for use include, but are not limited to, the following:

(1) Structure delineation;

(2) Functional, physiological, or biochemical assessment;

(3) Disease or pathology detection or assessment; and

(4) Diagnostic or therapeutic patient management.

(b) Where a diagnostic radiopharmaceutical is not intended to provide disease-specific information, the proposed indications for use may refer to a biochemical, physiological, anatomical, or pathological process or to more than one disease or condition.

§ 601.34 Evaluation of effectiveness.

(a) The effectiveness of a diagnostic radiopharmaceutical is assessed by evaluating its ability to provide useful clinical information related to its proposed indications for use. The method of this evaluation varies depending upon the proposed indication(s) and may use one or more of the following criteria:

(1) The claim of structure delineation is established by demonstrating in a defined clinical setting the ability to locate anatomical structures and to characterize their anatomy.

(2) The claim of functional, physiological, or biochemical assessment is established by demonstrating in a defined clinical setting reliable measurement of function(s) or physiological, biochemical, or molecular process(es).

(3) The claim of disease or pathology detection or assessment is established by demonstrating in a defined clinical setting that the diagnostic radiopharmaceutical has sufficient accuracy in identifying or characterizing the disease or pathology.

(4) The claim of diagnostic or therapeutic patient management is established by demonstrating in a defined clinical setting that the test is useful in diagnostic or therapeutic patient management.

(5) For a claim that does not fall within the indication categories identified in § 601.33, the applicant or sponsor should consult FDA on how to establish the effectiveness of the diagnostic radiopharmaceutical for the claim.

(b) The accuracy and usefulness of the diagnostic information is determined by comparison with a reliable assessment of actual clinical status. A reliable assessment of actual clinical status may be provided by a diagnostic standard or standards of demonstrated accuracy. In the absence of such diagnostic standard(s), the actual clinical status must be established in another manner, e.g., patient followup.

§ 601.35 Evaluation of safety.

(a) Factors considered in the safety assessment of a diagnostic radiopharmaceutical include, among others, the following:

(1) The radiation dose;

(2) The pharmacology and toxicology of the radiopharmaceutical, including any radionuclide, carrier, or ligand;

(3) The risks of an incorrect diagnostic determination;

(4) The adverse reaction profile of the drug;

(5) Results of human experience with the radiopharmaceutical for other uses; and

(6) Results of any previous human experience with the carrier or ligand of the radiopharmaceutical when the same chemical entity as the carrier or ligand has been used in a previously studied product.

(b) The assessment of the adverse reaction profile includes, but is not limited to, an evaluation of the potential of the diagnostic radiopharmaceutical, including the carrier or ligand, to elicit the following:

(1) Allergic or hypersensitivity responses,

(2) Immunologic responses,

(3) Changes in the physiologic or biochemical function of the target and nontarget tissues, and

(4) Clinically detectable signs or symptoms.

(c)(1) To establish the safety of a diagnostic radiopharmaceutical, FDA may require, among other information, the following types of data:

(A) Pharmacology data,

(B) Toxicology data,

(C) Clinical adverse event data, and

(D) Radiation safety assessment.

(2) The amount of new safety data required will depend on the characteristics of the product and available information regarding the safety of the diagnostic radiopharmaceutical, and its carrier or ligand, obtained from other studies and uses. Such information may include, but is not limited to, the dose, route of administration, frequency of use, half-life of the ligand or carrier, half-life of the radionuclide, and results of clinical and preclinical studies. FDA will establish categories of diagnostic radiopharmaceuticals based on defined characteristics relevant to risk and will specify the amount and type of safety data that are appropriate for each category (e.g., required safety data may be limited for diagnostic radiopharmaceuticals with a well established, low-risk profile). Upon reviewing the relevant product characteristics and safety information, FDA will place each diagnostic radiopharmaceutical into the appropriate safety risk category.

(d) *Radiation safety assessment.* The radiation safety assessment must establish the radiation dose of a diagnostic radiopharmaceutical by radiation dosimetry evaluations in humans and appropriate animal models. The maximum tolerated dose need not be established.

Subpart E—Accelerated Approval of Biological Products for Serious or Life-Threatening Illnesses

Source: 57 FR 58959, Dec. 11, 1992, unless otherwise noted.

§ 601.40 Scope.

This subpart applies to certain biological products that have been studied for their safety and effectiveness in treating serious or life-threatening illnesses and that provide meaningful therapeutic benefit to patients over existing treatments (e.g., ability to treat patients unresponsive to, or intolerant of, available therapy, or improved patient response over available therapy).

§ 601.41 Approval based on a surrogate endpoint or on an effect on a clinical endpoint other than survival or irreversible morbidity.

FDA may grant marketing approval for a biological product on the basis of adequate and well-controlled clinical trials establishing that the biological product has an effect on a surrogate endpoint that is reasonably likely, based on epidemiologic, therapeutic, pathophysiologic, or other evidence, to predict clinical benefit or on the basis of an effect on a clinical endpoint other than survival or irreversible morbidity. Approval under this section will be subject to the requirement that the applicant study the biological product further, to verify and describe its clinical benefit, where there is uncertainty as to the relation of the surrogate endpoint to clinical benefit, or of the observed clinical benefit to ultimate outcome. Postmarketing studies would usually be studies already underway. When required to be conducted, such studies must also be adequate and well-controlled. The applicant shall carry out any such studies with due diligence.

§ 601.42 Approval with restrictions to assure safe use.

(a) If FDA concludes that a biological product shown to be effective can be safely used only if distribution or use is restricted, FDA will require such postmarketing restrictions as are needed to assure safe use of the biological product, such as:

(1) Distribution restricted to certain facilities or physicians with special training or experience; or

(2) Distribution conditioned on the performance of specified medical procedures.

(b) The limitations imposed will be commensurate with the specific safety concerns presented by the biological product.

§ 601.43 Withdrawal procedures.

(a) For biological products approved under § 601.41 or § 601.42, FDA may withdraw approval, following a hearing as provided in part 15 of this chapter, as modified by this section, if:

(1) A postmarketing clinical study fails to verify clinical benefit;

(2) The applicant fails to perform the required postmarketing study with due diligence;

(3) Use after marketing demonstrates that postmarketing restrictions are inadequate to ensure safe use of the biological product;

(4) The applicant fails to adhere to the postmarketing restrictions agreed upon;

(5) The promotional materials are false or misleading; or

(6) Other evidence demonstrates that the biological product is not shown to be safe or effective under its conditions of use.

(b) *Notice of opportunity for a hearing.* The Director of the Center for Biologics Evaluation and Research or the Director of the Center for Drug Evaluation and Research will give the applicant notice of an opportunity for a hearing on the Center's proposal to withdraw the approval of an application approved under § 601.41 or § 601.42. The notice, which will ordinarily be a letter, will state generally the reasons for the action and the proposed grounds for the order.

(c) *Submission of data and information.* (1) If the applicant fails to file a written request for a hearing within 15 days of receipt of the notice, the applicant waives the opportunity for a hearing.

(2) If the applicant files a timely request for a hearing, the agency will publish a notice of hearing in the Federal Register in accordance with §§ 12.32(e) and 15.20 of this chapter.

(3) An applicant who requests a hearing under this section must, within 30 days of receipt of the notice of opportunity for a hearing, submit the data and information upon which the applicant intends to rely at the hearing.

(d) *Separation of functions.* Separation of functions (as specified in § 10.55 of this chapter) will not apply at any point in withdrawal proceedings under this section.

(e) *Procedures for hearings.* Hearings held under this section will be conducted in accordance with the provisions of part 15 of this chapter, with the following modifications:

(1) An advisory committee duly constituted under part 14 of this chapter will be present at the hearing. The committee will be asked to review the issues involved and to provide advice and recommendations to the Commissioner of Food and Drugs.

(2) The presiding officer, the advisory committee members, up to three representatives of the applicant, and up to three representatives of the Center may question any person during or at the

conclusion of the person's presentation. No other person attending the hearing may question a person making a presentation. The presiding officer may, as a matter of discretion, permit questions to be submitted to the presiding officer for response by a person making a presentation.

(f) *Judicial review.* The Commissioner's decision constitutes final agency action from which the applicant may petition for judicial review. Before requesting an order from a court for a stay of action pending review, an applicant must first submit a petition for a stay of action under § 10.35 of this chapter.

[57 FR 58959, Dec. 11, 1992, as amended at 68 FR 34797, June 11, 2003; 70 FR 14984, Mar. 24, 2005]

§ 601.44 Postmarketing safety reporting.

Biological products approved under this program are subject to the postmarketing recordkeeping and safety reporting applicable to all approved biological products.

§ 601.45 Promotional materials.

For biological products being considered for approval under this subpart, unless otherwise informed by the agency, applicants must submit to the agency for consideration during the preapproval review period copies of all promotional materials, including promotional labeling as well as advertisements, intended for dissemination or publication within 120 days following marketing approval. After 120 days following marketing approval, unless otherwise informed by the agency, the applicant must submit promotional materials at least 30 days prior to the intended time of initial dissemination of the labeling or initial publication of the advertisement.

§ 601.46 Termination of requirements.

If FDA determines after approval that the requirements established in § 601.42, § 601.43, or § 601.45 are no longer necessary for the safe and effective use of a biological product, it will so notify the applicant. Ordinarily, for biological products approved under § 601.41, these requirements will no longer apply when FDA determines that the required postmarketing study verifies and describes the biological product's clinical benefit and the biological product would be appropriate for approval under traditional procedures. For biological products approved under § 601.42, the restrictions would no longer apply when FDA determines that safe use of the biological product can be assured through appropriate labeling. FDA also retains the discretion to remove specific postapproval requirements upon review of a petition submitted by the sponsor in accordance with § 10.30.

Subpart F—Confidentiality of Information

§ 601.50 Confidentiality of data and information in an investigational new drug notice for a biological product.

(a) The existence of an IND notice for a biological product will not be disclosed by the Food and Drug Administration unless it has previously been publicly disclosed or acknowledged.

(b) The availability for public disclosure of all data and information in an IND file for a biological product shall be handled in accordance with the provisions established in § 601.51.

(c) Notwithstanding the provisions of § 601.51, the Food and Drug Administration shall disclose upon request to an individual on whom an investigational biological product has been used a copy of any adverse reaction report relating to such use.

[39 FR 44656, Dec. 24, 1974]

§ 601.51 Confidentiality of data and information in applications for biologics licenses.

(a) For purposes of this section the biological product file includes all data and information submitted with or incorporated by reference in any application for a biologics license, IND's incorporated into any such application, master files, and other related submissions. The availability for public disclosure of any record in the biological product file shall be handled in accordance with the provisions of this section.

(b) The existence of a biological product file will not be disclosed by the Food and Drug Administration before a biologics license application has been approved unless it has previously been publicly disclosed or acknowledged. The Food and Drug Administration will maintain a list available for public disclosure of biological products for which a license application has been approved.

(c) If the existence of a biological product file has not been publicly disclosed or acknowledged, no data or information in the biological product file is available for public disclosure.

(d)(1) If the existence of a biological product file has been publicly disclosed or acknowledged before a license has been issued, no data or information contained in the file is available for public disclosure before such license is issued, but the Commissioner may, in his discretion, disclose a summary of such selected portions of the safety and effectiveness data as are appropriate for public consideration of a specific pending issue, e.g., at an open session of a Food and Drug Administration advisory committee or pursuant to an exchange of important regulatory information with a foreign government.

(2) Notwithstanding paragraph (d)(1) of this section, FDA will make available to the public upon request the information in the IND that was required to be filed in Docket Number 95S-0158 in the Division of Dockets Management (HFA-305), Food and Drug Administration, 5630 Fishers Lane, rm. 1061, Rockville, MD 20852, for investigations involving an exception from informed consent under § 50.24 of this chapter. Persons wishing to request this information shall submit a request under the Freedom of Information Act.

(e) After a license has been issued, the following data and information in the biological product file are immediately available for public disclosure unless extraordinary circumstances are shown:

(1) All safety and effectiveness data and information.

(2) A protocol for a test or study, unless it is shown to fall within the exemption established for trade secrets and confidential commercial or financial information in § 20.61 of this chapter.

(3) Adverse reaction reports, product experience reports, consumer complaints, and other similar data and information, after deletion of:

(i) Names and any information that would identify the person using the product.

(ii) Names and any information that would identify any third party involved with the report, such as a physician or hospital or other institution.

(4) A list of all active ingredients and any inactive ingredients previously disclosed to the public, as defined in § 20.81 of this chapter.

(5) An assay method or other analytical method, unless it serves no regulatory or compliance purpose and it is shown to fall within the exemption established in § 20.61 of this chapter.

(6) All correspondence and written summaries of oral discussions relating to the biological product file, in accordance with the provisions of part 20 of this chapter.

(7) All records showing the manufacturer's testing of a particular lot, after deletion of data or information that would show the volume of the drug produced, manufacturing procedures and controls, yield from raw materials, costs, or other material falling within § 20.61 of this chapter.

(8) All records showing the testing of and action on a particular lot by the Food and Drug Administration.

(f) The following data and information in a biological product file are not available for public disclosure unless they have been previously disclosed to the public as defined in § 20.81 of this chapter or they relate to a product or ingredient that has been abandoned and they no longer represent a trade secret or confidential commercial or financial information as defined in § 20.61 of this chapter:

(1) Manufacturing methods or processes, including quality control procedures.

(2) Production, sales, distribution, and similar data and information, except that any compilation of such data and information aggregated and prepared in a way that does not reveal data or information which is not available for public disclosure under this provision is available for public disclosure.

(3) Quantitative or semiquantitative formulas.

(g) For purposes of this regulation, safety and effectiveness data include all studies and tests of a biological product on animals and humans and all studies and tests on the drug for identity, stability, purity, potency, and bioavailability.

[39 FR 44656, Dec. 24, 1974, as amended at 42 FR 15676, Mar. 22, 1977; 49 FR 23833, June 8, 1984; 55 FR 11013, Mar. 26, 1990; 61 FR 51530, Oct. 2, 1996; 64 FR 56452, Oct. 20, 1999; 68 FR 24879, May 9, 2003; 69 FR 13717, Mar. 24, 2004; 70 FR 14984, Mar. 24, 2005]

Subpart G—Postmarketing Studies

Source: 65 FR 64618, Oct. 30, 2000, unless otherwise noted.

§ 601.70 Annual progress reports of postmarketing studies.

(a) *General requirements.* This section applies to all required postmarketing studies (e.g., accelerated approval clinical benefit studies, pediatric studies) and postmarketing studies that an applicant has committed, in writing, to conduct either at the time of approval of an application or a supplement to an application, or after approval of an application or a supplement. Postmarketing studies within the meaning of this section are those that concern:

(1) Clinical safety;

(2) Clinical efficacy;

(3) Clinical pharmacology; and

(4) Nonclinical toxicology.

(b) *What to report.* Each applicant of a licensed biological product shall submit a report to FDA on the status of postmarketing studies for each approved product application. The status of these postmarketing studies shall be reported annually until FDA notifies the applicant, in writing, that the agency concurs with the applicant's determination that the study commitment has been fulfilled, or that the study is either no longer feasible or would no longer provide useful information. Each annual progress report shall be accompanied by a completed transmittal Form FDA-2252, and shall include all the information required under this section that the applicant received or otherwise obtained during the annual reporting interval which ends on the U.S. anniversary date. The report must provide the following information for each postmarketing study:

(1) *Applicant's name.*

(2) *Product name.* Include the approved product's proper name and the proprietary name, if any.

(3) *Biologics license application (BLA) and supplement number.*

(4) *Date of U.S. approval of BLA.*

(5) *Date of postmarketing study commitment.*

(6) *Description of postmarketing study commitment.* The description must include sufficient information to uniquely describe the study. This information may include the purpose of the study, the type of study, the patient population addressed by the study and the indication(s) and dosage(s) that are to be studied.

(7) *Schedule for completion and reporting of the postmarketing study commitment.* The schedule should include the actual or projected dates for submission of the study protocol to FDA, comple-

tion of patient accrual or initiation of an animal study, completion of the study, submission of the final study report to FDA, and any additional milestones or submissions for which projected dates were specified as part of the commitment. In addition, it should include a revised schedule, as appropriate. If the schedule has been previously revised, provide both the original schedule and the most recent, previously submitted revision.

(8) Current status of the postmarketing study commitment. The status of each postmarketing study should be categorized using one of the following terms that describes the study's status on the anniversary date of U.S. approval of the application or other agreed upon date:

(i) *Pending*. The study has not been initiated, but does not meet the criterion for delayed.

(ii) *Ongoing*. The study is proceeding according to or ahead of the original schedule described under paragraph (b)(7) of this section.

(iii) *Delayed*. The study is behind the original schedule described under paragraph (b)(7) of this section.

(iv) *Terminated*. The study was ended before completion but a final study report has not been submitted to FDA.

(v) *Submitted*. The study has been completed or terminated and a final study report has been submitted to FDA.

(9) *Explanation of the study's status*. Provide a brief description of the status of the study, including the patient accrual rate (expressed by providing the number of patients or subjects enrolled to date, and the total planned enrollment), and an explanation of the study's status identified under paragraph (b)(8) of this section. If the study has been completed, include the date the study was completed and the date the final study report was submitted to FDA, as applicable. Provide a revised schedule, as well as the reason(s) for the revision, if the schedule under paragraph (b)(7) of this section has changed since the previous report.

(c) *When to report*. Annual progress reports for postmarketing study commitments entered into by applicants shall be reported to FDA within 60 days of the anniversary date of the U.S. approval of the application for the product.

(d) *Where to report*. Submit two copies of the annual progress report of postmarketing studies to the Center for Biologics Evaluation and Research or Center for Drug Evaluation and Research (see mailing addresses in § 600.2(a) or (b) of this chapter).

(e) *Public disclosure of information*. Except for the information described in this paragraph, FDA may publicly disclose any information concerning a postmarketing study, within the meaning of this section, if the agency determines that the information is necessary to identify an applicant or to establish the status of the study including the reasons, if any, for failure to conduct, complete, and report the study. Under this section, FDA will not publicly disclose trade secrets, as defined in § 20.61 of this chapter, or information, described in § 20.63 of this chapter, the disclosure of which would constitute an unwarranted invasion of personal privacy.

[65 FR 64618, Oct. 30, 2000, as amended at 70 FR 14984, Mar. 24, 2005; 80 FR 18092, Apr. 3, 2015]

Subpart H—Approval of Biological Products When Human Efficacy Studies Are Not Ethical or Feasible

Source: 67 FR 37996, May 31, 2002, unless otherwise noted.

§ 601.90 Scope.

This subpart applies to certain biological products that have been studied for their safety and efficacy in ameliorating or preventing serious or life-threatening conditions caused by exposure to lethal or permanently disabling toxic biological, chemical, radiological, or nuclear substances. This subpart applies only to those biological products for which: Definitive human efficacy studies cannot be conducted because it would be unethical to deliberately expose healthy human volunteers to a lethal or permanently disabling toxic biological, chemical, radiological, or nuclear substance; and field trials to study the product's efficacy after an accidental or hostile exposure have not been feasible. This subpart does not apply to products that can be approved based on efficacy standards described elsewhere in FDA's regulations (e.g., accelerated approval based on surrogate markers or clinical endpoints other than survival or irreversible morbidity), nor does it address the safety evaluation for the products to which it does apply.

§ 601.91 Approval based on evidence of effectiveness from studies in animals.

(a) FDA may grant marketing approval for a biological product for which safety has been established and for which the requirements of § 601.90 are met based on adequate and well-controlled animal studies when the results of those animal studies establish that the biological product is reasonably likely to produce clinical benefit in humans. In assessing the sufficiency of animal data, the agency may take into account other data, including human data, available to the agency. FDA will rely on the evidence from studies in animals to provide substantial evidence of the effectiveness of these products only when:

(1) There is a reasonably well-understood pathophysiological mechanism of the toxicity of the substance and its prevention or substantial reduction by the product;

(2) The effect is demonstrated in more than one animal species expected to react with a response predictive for humans, unless the effect is demonstrated in a single animal species that represents a sufficiently well-characterized animal model for predicting the response in humans;

(3) The animal study endpoint is clearly related to the desired benefit in humans, generally the enhancement of survival or prevention of major morbidity; and

(4) The data or information on the kinetics and pharmacodynamics of the product or other relevant data or information, in animals and humans, allows selection of an effective dose in humans.

(b) Approval under this subpart will be subject to three requirements:

(1) *Postmarketing studies.* The applicant must conduct postmarketing studies, such as field studies, to verify and describe the biological product's clinical benefit and to assess its safety when used as indicated when such studies are feasible and ethical. Such postmarketing studies would not be feasible until an exigency arises. When such studies are feasible, the applicant must conduct such studies with due diligence. Applicants must include as part of their application a plan or approach to postmarketing study commitments in the event such studies become ethical and feasible.

(2) *Approval with restrictions to ensure safe use.* If FDA concludes that a biological product shown to be effective under this subpart can be safely used only if distribution or use is restricted, FDA will require such postmarketing restrictions as are needed to ensure safe use of the biological product, commensurate with the specific safety concerns presented by the biological product, such as:

(i) Distribution restricted to certain facilities or health care practitioners with special training or experience;

(ii) Distribution conditioned on the performance of specified medical procedures, including medical followup; and

(iii) Distribution conditioned on specified recordkeeping requirements.

(3) *Information to be provided to patient recipients.* For biological products or specific indications approved under this subpart, applicants must prepare, as part of their proposed labeling, labeling to be provided to patient recipients. The patient labeling must explain that, for ethical or feasibility reasons, the biological product's approval was based on efficacy studies conducted in animals alone and must give the biological product's indication(s), directions for use (dosage and administration), contraindications, a description of any reasonably foreseeable risks, adverse reactions, anticipated

benefits, drug interactions, and any other relevant information required by FDA at the time of approval. The patient labeling must be available with the product to be provided to patients prior to administration or dispensing of the biological product for the use approved under this subpart, if possible.

§601.92 Withdrawal procedures.

(a) *Reasons to withdraw approval.* For biological products approved under this subpart, FDA may withdraw approval, following a hearing as provided in part 15 of this chapter, as modified by this section, if:

(1) A postmarketing clinical study fails to verify clinical benefit;

(2) The applicant fails to perform the postmarketing study with due diligence;

(3) Use after marketing demonstrates that postmarketing restrictions are inadequate to ensure safe use of the biological product;

(4) The applicant fails to adhere to the postmarketing restrictions applied at the time of approval under this subpart;

(5) The promotional materials are false or misleading; or

(6) Other evidence demonstrates that the biological product is not shown to be safe or effective under its conditions of use.

(b) *Notice of opportunity for a hearing.* The Director of the Center for Biologics Evaluation and Research or the Director of the Center for Drug Evaluation and Research will give the applicant notice of an opportunity for a hearing on the proposal to withdraw the approval of an application approved under this subpart. The notice, which will ordinarily be a letter, will state generally the reasons for the action and the proposed grounds for the order.

(c) *Submission of data and information.* (1) If the applicant fails to file a written request for a hearing within 15 days of receipt of the notice, the applicant waives the opportunity for a hearing.

(2) If the applicant files a timely request for a hearing, the agency will publish a notice of hearing in the Federal Register in accordance with §§ 12.32(e) and 15.20 of this chapter.

(3) An applicant who requests a hearing under this section must, within 30 days of receipt of the notice of opportunity for a hearing, submit the data and information upon which the applicant intends to rely at the hearing.

(d) *Separation of functions.* Separation of functions (as specified in § 10.55 of this chapter) will not apply at any point in withdrawal proceedings under this section.

(e) *Procedures for hearings.* Hearings held under this section will be conducted in accordance with the provisions of part 15 of this chapter, with the following modifications:

(1) An advisory committee duly constituted under part 14 of this chapter will be present at the hearing. The committee will be asked to review the issues involved and to provide advice and recommendations to the Commissioner of Food and Drugs.

(2) The presiding officer, the advisory committee members, up to three representatives of the applicant, and up to three representatives of CBER may question any person during or at the conclusion of the person's presentation. No other person attending the hearing may question a person making a presentation. The presiding officer may, as a matter of discretion, permit questions to be submitted to the presiding officer for response by a person making a presentation.

(f) *Judicial review.* The Commissioner of Food and Drugs' decision constitutes final agency action from which the applicant may petition for judicial review. Before requesting an order from a court for a stay of action pending review, an applicant must first submit a petition for a stay of action under § 10.35 of this chapter.

[67 FR 37996, May 31, 2002, as amended at 70 FR 14984, Mar. 24, 2005]

§ 601.93 Postmarketing safety reporting.

Biological products approved under this subpart are subject to the postmarketing recordkeeping and safety reporting applicable to all approved biological products.

§ 601.94 Promotional materials.

For biological products being considered for approval under this subpart, unless otherwise informed by the agency, applicants must submit to the agency for consideration during the preapproval review period copies of all promotional materials, including promotional labeling as well as advertisements, intended for dissemination or publication within 120 days following marketing approval. After 120 days following marketing approval, unless otherwise informed by the agency, the applicant must submit promotional materials at least 30 days prior to the intended time of initial dissemination of the labeling or initial publication of the advertisement.

§ 601.95 Termination of requirements.

If FDA determines after approval under this subpart that the requirements established in §§ 601.91(b)(2), 601.92, and 601.93 are no longer necessary for the safe and effective use of a biological product, FDA will so notify the applicant. Ordinarily, for biological products approved under § 601.91, these requirements will no longer apply when FDA determines that the postmarketing study verifies and describes the biological product's clinical benefit. For biological products approved under § 601.91, the restrictions would no longer apply when FDA determines that safe use of the biological product can be ensured through appropriate labeling. FDA also retains the discretion to remove specific postapproval requirements upon review of a petition submitted by the sponsor in accordance with § 10.30 of this chapter.

• • •

PART 610—GENERAL BIOLOGICAL PRODUCTS STANDARDS

Authority: 21 U.S.C. 321, 331, 351, 352, 353, 355, 360, 360c, 360d, 360h, 360i, 371, 372, 374, 381; 42 U.S.C. 216, 262, 263, 263a, 264.

Source: 38 FR 32056, Nov. 20, 1973, unless otherwise noted.

Cross references: For U.S. Customs Service regulations relating to viruses, serums, and toxins, see 19 CFR 12.21-12.23. For U.S. Postal Service regulations relating to the admissibility to the United States mails see parts 124 and 125 of the Domestic Mail Manual, that is incorporated by reference in 39 CFR part 111.

Subpart A—Release Requirements

§ 610.1 Tests prior to release required for each lot.

No lot of any licensed product shall be released by the manufacturer prior to the completion of tests for conformity with standards applicable to such product. Each applicable test shall be made on each lot after completion of all processes of manufacture which may affect compliance with the standard to which the test applies. The results of all tests performed shall be considered in determining whether or not the test results meet the test objective, except that a test result may be disregarded when it is established that the test is invalid due to causes unrelated to the product.

§610.2 Requests for samples and protocols; official release.

(a) *Licensed biological products regulated by CBER.* Samples of any lot of any licensed product together with the protocols showing results of applicable tests, may at any time be required to be sent to the Director, Center for Biologics Evaluation and Research (see mailing addresses in §600.2(c) of this chapter). Upon notification by the Director, Center for Biologics Evaluation and Research, a manufacturer shall not distribute a lot of a product until the lot is released by the Director, Center for Biologics Evaluation and Research: Provided, That the Director, Center for Biologics Evaluation and Research, shall not issue such notification except when deemed necessary for the safety, purity, or potency of the product.

(b) *Licensed biological products regulated by CDER.* Samples of any lot of any licensed product together with the protocols showing results of applicable tests, may at any time be required to be sent to the Director, Center for Drug Evaluation and Research (see mailing addresses in §600.2(c) of this chapter) for official release. Upon notification by the Director, Center for Drug Evaluation and Research, a manufacturer shall not distribute a lot of a biological product until the lot is released by the Director, Center for Drug Evaluation and Research: Provided, That the Director, Center for Drug Evaluation and Research shall not issue such notification except when deemed necessary for the safety, purity, or potency of the product.

[40 FR 31313, July 25, 1975, as amended at 49 FR 23834, June 8, 1984; 50 FR 10941, Mar. 19, 1985; 55 FR 11013, 11014, Mar. 26, 1990; 67 FR 9587, Mar. 4, 2002; 70 FR 14984, Mar. 24, 2005; 80 FR 18093, Apr. 3, 2015]

Subpart B—General Provisions

§610.9 Equivalent methods and processes.

Modification of any particular test method or manufacturing process or the conditions under which it is conducted as required in this part or in the additional standards for specific biological products in parts 620 through 680 of this chapter shall be permitted only under the following conditions:

(a) The applicant presents evidence, in the form of a license application, or a supplement to the application submitted in accordance with §601.12(b) or (c), demonstrating that the modification will provide assurances of the safety, purity, potency, and effectiveness of the biological product equal to or greater than the assurances provided by the method or process specified in the general standards or additional standards for the biological product; and

(b) Approval of the modification is received in writing from the Director, Center for Biologics Evaluation and Research or the Director, Center for Drug Evaluation and Research.

[62 FR 39903, July 24, 1997, as amended at 70 FR 14984, Mar. 24, 2005]

§610.10 Potency.

Tests for potency shall consist of either in vitro or in vivo tests, or both, which have been specifically designed for each product so as to indicate its potency in a manner adequate to satisfy the interpretation of potency given by the definition in §600.3(s) of this chapter.

§610.11-610.11a [Reserved]

§610.12 Sterility.

(a) *The test.* Except as provided in paragraph (h) of this section, manufacturers of biological products must perform sterility testing of each lot of each biological product's final container material or other material, as appropriate and as approved in the biologics license application or supplement for that product.

(b) *Test requirements.* (1) The sterility test must be appropriate to the material being tested such that the material does not interfere with or otherwise hinder the test.

(2) The sterility test must be validated to demonstrate that the test is capable of reliably and consistently detecting the presence of viable contaminating microorganisms.

(3) The sterility test and test components must be verified to demonstrate that the test method can consistently detect the presence of viable contaminating microorganisms.

(c) *Written procedures.* Manufacturers must establish, implement, and follow written procedures for sterility testing that describe, at a minimum, the following:

(1) The sterility test method to be used;

(i) If culture-based test methods are used, include, at a minimum:

(A) Composition of the culture media;

(B) Growth-promotion test requirements; and

(C) Incubation conditions (time and temperature).

(ii) If non-culture-based test methods are used, include, at a minimum:

(A) Composition of test components;

(B) Test parameters, including acceptance criteria; and

(C) Controls used to verify the method's ability to detect the presence of viable contaminating microorganisms.

(2) The method of sampling, including the number, volume, and size of articles to be tested;

(3) Written specifications for the acceptance or rejection of each lot; and

(4) A statement of any other function critical to the particular sterility test method to ensure consistent and accurate results.

(d) *The sample.* The sample must be appropriate to the material being tested, considering, at a minimum:

(1) The size and volume of the final product lot;

(2) The duration of manufacturing of the drug product;

(3) The final container configuration and size;

(4) The quantity or concentration of inhibitors, neutralizers, and preservatives, if present, in the tested material;

(5) For a culture-based test method, the volume of test material that results in a dilution of the product that is not bacteriostatic or fungistatic; and

(6) For a non-culture-based test method, the volume of test material that results in a dilution of the product that does not inhibit or otherwise hinder the detection of viable contaminating microorganisms.

(e) *Verification.* (1) For culture-based test methods, studies must be conducted to demonstrate that the performance of the test organisms and culture media are suitable to consistently detect the presence of viable contaminating microorganisms, including tests for each lot of culture media to verify its growth-promoting properties over the shelf-life of the media.

(2) For non-culture-based test methods, within the test itself, appropriate controls must be used to demonstrate the ability of the test method to continue to consistently detect the presence of viable contaminating microorganisms.

(f) *Repeat test procedures.* (1) If the initial test indicates the presence of microorganisms, the product does not comply with the sterility test requirements unless a thorough investigation by the quality control unit can ascribe definitively the microbial presence to a laboratory error or faulty materials used in conducting the sterility testing.

(2) If the investigation described in paragraph (f)(1) of this section finds that the initial test indicated the presence of microorganisms due to laboratory error or the use of faulty materials, a sterility test may be repeated one time. If no evidence of microorganisms is found in the repeat test, the product examined complies with the sterility test requirements. If evidence of microorganisms is found in the repeat test, the product examined does not comply with the sterility test requirements.

(3) If a repeat test is conducted, the same test method must be used for both the initial and repeat tests, and the repeat test must be conducted with comparable product that is reflective of the initial sample in terms of sample location and the stage in the manufacturing process from which it was obtained.

(g) *Records*. The records related to the test requirements of this section must be prepared and maintained as required by §§ 211.167 and 211.194 of this chapter.

(h) *Exceptions*. Sterility testing must be performed on final container material or other appropriate material as defined in the approved biologics license application or supplement and as described in this section, except as follows:

(1) This section does not require sterility testing for Whole Blood, Cryoprecipitated Antihemophilic Factor, Platelets, Red Blood Cells, Plasma, Source Plasma, Smallpox Vaccine, Reagent Red Blood Cells, Anti-Human Globulin, and Blood Grouping Reagents.

(2) A manufacturer is not required to comply with the sterility test requirements if the Director of the Center for Biologics Evaluation and Research or the Director of the Center for Drug Evaluation and Research, as appropriate, determines that data submitted in the biologics license application or supplement adequately establish that the route of administration, the method of preparation, or any other aspect of the product precludes or does not necessitate a sterility test to assure the safety, purity, and potency of the product.

[77 FR 26174, May 3, 2012]

§ 610.13 Purity.

Products shall be free of extraneous material except that which is unavoidable in the manufacturing process described in the approved biologics license application. In addition, products shall be tested as provided in paragraphs (a) and (b) of this section.

(a)(1) *Test for residual moisture.* Each lot of dried product shall be tested for residual moisture and shall meet and not exceed established limits as specified by an approved method on file in the biologics license application. The test for residual moisture may be exempted by the Director, Center for Biologics Evaluation and Research or the Director, Center for Drug Evaluation and Research, when deemed not necessary for the continued safety, purity, and potency of the product.

(2) *Records*. Appropriate records for residual moisture under paragraph (a)(1) of this section shall be prepared and maintained as required by the applicable provisions of §§ 211.188 and 211.194 of this chapter.

(b) *Test for pyrogenic substances.* Each lot of final containers of any product intended for use by injection shall be tested for pyrogenic substances by intravenous injection into rabbits as provided in paragraphs (b) (1) and (2) of this section: Provided, That notwithstanding any other provision of Subchapter F of this chapter, the test for pyrogenic substances is not required for the following products: Products containing formed blood elements; Cryoprecipitate; Plasma; Source Plasma; Normal Horse Serum; bacterial, viral, and rickettsial vaccines and antigens; toxoids; toxins; allergenic extracts; venoms; diagnostic substances and trivalent organic arsenicals.

(1) *Test dose.* The test dose for each rabbit shall be at least 3 milliliters per kilogram of body weight of the rabbit and also shall be at least equivalent proportionately, on a body weight basis, to the maximum single human dose recommended, but need not exceed 10 milliliters per kilogram of body weight of the rabbit, except that: (i) Regardless of the human dose recommended, the test dose per kilogram of body weight of each rabbit shall be at least 1 milliliter for immune globulins derived from human blood; (ii) for Streptokinase, the test dose shall be at least equivalent proportionately, on a body weight basis, to the maximum single human dose recommended.

(2) *Test procedure, results, and interpretation; standards to be met.* The test for pyrogenic substances shall be performed according to the requirements specified in United States Pharmacopeia XX.

(3) *Retest.* If the lot fails to meet the test requirements prescribed in paragraph (b)(2) of this section, the test may be repeated once using five other rabbits. The temperature rises recorded for all eight rabbits used in testing shall be included in determining whether the requirements are met. The lot meets the requirements for absence of pyrogens if not more than three of the eight rabbits show individual rises in temperature of 0.6 °C or more, and if the sum of the eight individual maximum temperature rises does not exceed 3.7 °C.

[38 FR 32056, Nov. 20, 1973, as amended at 40 FR 29710, July 15, 1975; 41 FR 10429, Mar. 11, 1976; 41 FR 41424, Sept. 22, 1976; 44 FR 40289, July 10, 1979; 46 FR 62845, Dec. 29, 1981; 49 FR 15187, Apr. 18, 1984; 50 FR 4134, Jan. 29, 1985; 55 FR 28381, July 11, 1990; 64 FR 56453, Oct. 20, 1999; 67 FR 9587, Mar. 4, 2002; 70 FR 14985, Mar. 24, 2005]

§610.14 Identity.

The contents of a final container of each filling of each lot shall be tested for identity after all labeling operations shall have been completed. The identity test shall be specific for each product in a manner that will adequately identify it as the product designated on final container and package labels and circulars, and distinguish it from any other product being processed in the same laboratory. Identity may be established either through the physical or chemical characteristics of the product, inspection by macroscopic or microscopic methods, specific cultural tests, or in vitro or in vivo immunological tests.

§610.15 Constituent materials.

(a) *Ingredients, preservatives, diluents, adjuvants.* All ingredients used in a licensed product, and any diluent provided as an aid in the administration of the product, shall meet generally accepted standards of purity and quality. Any preservative used shall be sufficiently nontoxic so that the amount present in the recommended dose of the product will not be toxic to the recipient, and in the combination used it shall not denature the specific substances in the product to result in a decrease below the minimum acceptable potency within the dating period when stored at the recommended temperature. Products in multiple-dose containers shall contain a preservative, except that a preservative need not be added to Yellow Fever Vaccine; Poliovirus Vaccine Live Oral; viral vaccines labeled for use with the jet injector; dried vaccines when the accompanying diluent contains a preservative; or to an Allergenic Product in 50 percent or more volume in volume (v/v) glycerin. An adjuvant shall not be introduced into a product unless there is satisfactory evidence that it does not affect adversely the safety or potency of the product. The amount of aluminum in the recommended individual dose of a biological product shall not exceed:

(1) 0.85 milligrams if determined by assay;

(2) 1.14 milligrams if determined by calculation on the basis of the amount of aluminum compound added; or

(3) 1.25 milligrams determined by assay provided that data demonstrating that the amount of aluminum used is safe and necessary to produce the intended effect are submitted to and approved

by the Director, Center for Biologics Evaluation and Research or the Director, Center for Drug Evaluation and Research (see mailing addresses in § 600.2(a) or (b) of this chapter).

(b) *Extraneous protein; cell culture produced vaccines.* Extraneous protein known to be capable of producing allergenic effects in human subjects shall not be added to a final virus medium of cell culture produced vaccines intended for injection. If serum is used at any stage, its calculated concentration in the final medium shall not exceed 1:1,000,000.

(c) *Antibiotics.* A minimum concentration of antibiotics, other than penicillin, may be added to the production substrate of viral vaccines.

(d) The Director of the Center for Biologics Evaluation and Research or the Director of the Center for Drug Evaluation and Research may approve an exception or alternative to any requirement in this section. Requests for such exceptions or alternatives must be in writing.

[38 FR 32056, Nov. 20, 1973, as amended at 46 FR 51903, Oct. 23, 1981; 48 FR 13025, Mar. 29, 1983; 48 FR 37023, Aug. 16, 1983; 49 FR 23834, June 8, 1984; 50 FR 4134, Jan. 29, 1985; 51 FR 15607, Apr. 25, 1986; 55 FR 11013, Mar. 26, 1990; 70 FR 14985, Mar. 24, 2005; 76 FR 20518, Apr. 13, 2011; 80 FR 18093, Apr. 3, 2015]

§ 610.16 Total solids in serums.

Except as otherwise provided by regulation, no liquid serum or antitoxin shall contain more than 20 percent total solids.

§ 610.17 Permissible combinations.

Licensed products may not be combined with other licensed products either therapeutic, prophylactic or diagnostic, except as a license is obtained for the combined product. Licensed products may not be combined with nonlicensable therapeutic, prophylactic, or diagnostic substances except as a license is obtained for such combination.

§ 610.18 Cultures.

(a) *Storage and maintenance.* Cultures used in the manufacture of products shall be stored in a secure and orderly manner, at a temperature and by a method that will retain the initial characteristics of the organisms and insure freedom from contamination and deterioration.

(b) *Identity and verification.* Each culture shall be clearly identified as to source strain. A complete identification of the strain shall be made for each new stock culture preparation. Primary and subsequent seed lots shall be identified by lot number and date of preparation. Periodic tests shall be performed as often as necessary to verify the integrity of the strain characteristics and freedom from extraneous organisms. Results of all periodic tests for verification of cultures and determination of freedom from extraneous organisms shall be recorded and retained.

(c) *Cell lines used for manufacturing biological products*—(1) *General requirements.* Cell lines used for manufacturing biological products shall be:

(i) Identified by history;

(ii) Described with respect to cytogenetic characteristics and tumorigenicity;

(iii) Characterized with respect to in vitro growth characteristics and life potential; and

(iv) Tested for the presence of detectable microbial agents.

(2) *Tests.* Tests that are necessary to assure the safety, purity, and potency of a product may be required by the Director, Center for Biologics Evaluation and Research or the Director, Center for Drug Evaluation and Research.

(3) *Applicability.* This paragraph applies to diploid and nondiploid cell lines. Primary cell cultures that are not subcultivated and primary cell cultures that are subsequently subcultivated for only a very limited number of population doublings are not subject to the provisions of this paragraph (c).

(d) *Records*. The records appropriate for cultures under this section shall be prepared and maintained as required by the applicable provisions of §§ 211.188 and 211.194 of this chapter.

[38 FR 32056, Nov. 20, 1973, as amended at 51 FR 44453, Dec. 10, 1986; 55 FR 11013, Mar. 26, 1990; 67 FR 9587, Mar. 4, 2002; 70 FR 14985, Mar. 24, 2005]

Subpart D—[Reserved]

§§ 610.20-610.21 [Reserved]

Subpart D—Mycoplasma

§ 610.30 Test for Mycoplasma.

Except as provided otherwise in this subchapter, prior to clarification or filtration in the case of live virus vaccines produced from in vitro living cell cultures, and prior to inactivation in the case of inactivated virus vaccines produced from such living cell cultures, each virus harvest pool and control fluid pool shall be tested for the presence of *Mycoplasma*, as follows:

> Samples of the virus for this test shall be stored either (1) between 2 and 8 °C for no longer than 24 hours, or (2) at −20 °C or lower if stored for longer than 24 hours. The test shall be performed on samples of the viral harvest pool and on control fluid pool obtained at the time of viral harvest, as follows: No less than 2.0 ml. of each sample shall be inoculated in evenly distributed amounts over the surface of no less than 10 plates of at least two agar media. No less than 1.0 ml. of sample shall be inoculated into each of four tubes containing 10 ml. of a semisolid broth medium. The media shall be such as have been shown to be capable of detecting known Mycoplasma and each test shall include control cultures of at least two known strains of Mycoplasma, one of which must be M. pneumoniae. One half of the plates and two tubes of broth shall be incubated aerobically at 36 °C ±1 °C and the remaining plates and tubes shall be incubated anaerobically at 36 °C ±1 °C in an environment of 5-10 percent CO2 in N2. Aerobic incubation shall be for a period of no less than 14 days and the broth in the two tubes shall be tested after 3 days and 14 days, at which times 0.5 ml. of broth from each of the two tubes shall be combined and subinoculated on to no less than 4 additional plates and incubated aerobically. Anaerobic incubation shall be for no less than 14 days and the broth in the two tubes shall be tested after 3 days and 14 days, at which times 0.5 ml. of broth from each of the two tubes shall be combined and subinoculated onto no less than four additional plates and incubated anaerobically. All inoculated plates shall be incubated for no less than 14 days, at which time observation for growth of Mycoplasma shall be made at a magnification of no less than 300 ×. If the Dienes Methylene Blue-Azure dye or an equivalent staining procedure is used, no less than a one square cm. plug of the agar shall be excised from the inoculated area and examined for the presence of Mycoplasma. The presence of the Mycoplasma shall be determined by comparison of the growth obtained from the test samples with that of the control cultures, with respect to typical colonial and microscopic morphology. The virus pool is satisfactory for vaccine manufacture if none of the tests on the samples show evidence of the presence of Mycoplasma.

[38 FR 32056, Nov. 20, 1973, as amended at 63 FR 16685, Apr. 6, 1998]

Subpart E—Testing Requirements for Relevant Transfusion-Transmitted Infections

§ 610.39 Definitions.

The definitions set out in § 630.3 of this chapter apply to this subpart.

[80 FR 29896, May 22, 2015]

§610.40 Test requirements.

(a) *Human blood and blood components.* Except as specified in paragraphs (c) and (d) of this section, you, an establishment that collects blood and blood components for transfusion or for use in manufacturing a product, including donations intended as a component of, or used to manufacture, a medical device, must comply with the following requirements:

(1) Test each donation for evidence of infection due to the relevant transfusion-transmitted infections described in §630.3(h)(1)(i) through (iii) of this chapter (HIV, HBV, and HCV).

(2) Test each donation for evidence of infection due to the relevant transfusion-transmitted infections described in §630.3(h)(1)(iv) through (vii) of this chapter (HTLV, syphilis, West Nile virus, and Chagas disease). The following exceptions apply:

(i) To identify evidence of infection with syphilis in donors of Source Plasma, you must test donors for evidence of such infection in accordance with §640.65(b) of this chapter, and not under this section.

(ii) You are not required to test donations of Source Plasma for evidence of infection due to the relevant transfusion-transmitted infections described in §630.3(h)(1)(iv), (vi), and (vii) of this chapter (HTLV, West Nile virus, and Chagas disease).

(iii) For each of the relevant transfusion-transmitted infections described in §630.3(h)(1)(iv) through (vii) of this chapter (HTLV, syphilis, West Nile virus, and Chagas disease):

(A) If, based on evidence related to the risk of transmission of that relevant transfusion-transmitted infection, testing each donation is not necessary to reduce adequately and appropriately the risk of transmission of such infection by blood or a blood component, you may adopt an adequate and appropriate alternative testing procedure that has been found acceptable for this purpose by FDA.

(B) If, based on evidence related to the risk of transmission of that relevant transfusion-transmitted infection, testing previously required for that infection is no longer necessary to reduce adequately and appropriately the risk of transmission of such infection by blood or a blood component, you may stop such testing in accordance with procedures found acceptable for this purpose by FDA.

(3) For each of the relevant transfusion-transmitted infections described in §630.3(h)(1)(viii) through (x) of this chapter (CJD, vCJD, malaria) and §630.3(h)(2) of this chapter (other transfusion-transmitted infections):

(i) You must test for evidence of infection when the following conditions are met:

(A) A test(s) for the relevant transfusion-transmitted infection is licensed, approved or cleared by FDA for use as a donor screening test and is available for such use; and

(B) Testing for the relevant transfusion-transmitted infection is necessary to reduce adequately and appropriately the risk of transmission of the relevant transfusion-transmitted infection by blood, or blood component, or blood derivative product manufactured from the collected blood or blood component.

(ii) You must perform this testing on each donation, unless one of the following exceptions applies:

(A) Testing of each donation is not necessary to reduce adequately and appropriately the risk of transmission of such infection by blood, blood component, or blood derivative product manufactured from the collected blood or blood component. When evidence related to the risk of transmission of such infection supports this determination, you may adopt an adequate and appropriate alternative testing procedure that has been found acceptable for this purpose by FDA.

(B) Testing of each donation is not necessary to reduce adequately and appropriately the risk of transmission of such infection by blood, blood component, or blood derivative product manufactured from the collected blood or blood component. When evidence related to the risk of transmission of such infection supports this determination, you may stop such testing in accordance with procedures found acceptable for this purpose by FDA.

(4) Evidence related to the risk of transmission of a relevant transfusion-transmitted infection that would support a determination that testing is not necessary, or that testing of each donation is not necessary, to reduce adequately and appropriately the risk of transmission of such infection by blood or blood component, as described in paragraphs (a)(2)(iii)(A) and (B) of this section, or by blood, blood component, or blood derivative, as described in paragraphs (a)(3)(ii)(A) and (B) of this section, includes epidemiological or other scientific evidence. It may include evidence related to the seasonality or geographic limitation of risk of transmission of such infection by blood or blood component, or other information related to when and how a donation is at risk of transmitting a relevant transfusion-transmitted infection. It may also include evidence related to the effectiveness of manufacturing steps (for example, the use of pathogen reduction technology) that reduce the risk of transmission of the relevant transfusion-transmitted infection by blood, blood components, or blood derivatives, as applicable.

(b) *Testing using one or more licensed, approved, or cleared screening tests.* To perform testing for evidence of infection due to relevant transfusion-transmitted infections as required in paragraph (a) of this section, you must use screening tests that FDA has licensed, approved, or cleared for such use, in accordance with the manufacturer's instructions. You must perform one or more such tests as necessary to reduce adequately and appropriately the risk of transmission of relevant transfusion-transmitted infections.

(c) *Exceptions to testing for dedicated donations, medical devices, and samples.*—(1) *Dedicated donations.* (i) You must test donations of human blood and blood components from a donor whose donations are dedicated to and used solely by a single identified recipient under paragraphs (a), (b), and (e) of this section; except that, if the donor makes multiple donations for a single identified recipient, you may perform such testing only on the first donation in each 30-day period. If an untested dedicated donation is made available for any use other than transfusion to the single, identified recipient, then this exemption from the testing required under this section no longer applies.

(ii) Each donation must be labeled as required under §606.121 of this chapter and with a label entitled "INTENDED RECIPIENT INFORMATION LABEL" containing the name and identifying information of the recipient. Each donation must also have the following label, as appropriate:

Donor Testing Status	**Label**
Tests negative	Label as required under §606.121
Tested negative within the last 30 days	"DONOR TESTED WITHIN THE LAST 30 DAYS"

(2) *Medical device.* (i) You are not required to test donations of human blood or blood components intended solely as a component of, or used to prepare, a medical device for evidence of infection due to the relevant transfusion-transmitted infections listed in §630.3(h)(iv) of this chapter unless the final device contains viable leukocytes.

(ii) Donations of human blood and blood components intended solely as a component of, or used to prepare, a medical device must be labeled "Caution: For Further Manufacturing Use as a Component of, or to Prepare, a Medical Device."

(3) *Samples.* You are not required to test samples of blood, blood components, plasma, or sera if used or distributed for clinical laboratory testing or research purposes and not intended for administration to humans or in the manufacture of a product.

(d) Autologous donations. You, an establishment that collects human blood or blood components from autologous donors, or you, an establishment that is a consignee of a collecting establishment, are not required to test donations of human blood or blood components from autologous donors for evidence of infection due to relevant transfusion-transmitted infections listed in paragraph (a) of this section, except:

(1) If you allow any autologous donation to be used for allogeneic transfusion, you must assure that all autologous donations are tested under this section.

(2) If you ship autologous donations to another establishment that allows autologous donations to be used for allogeneic transfusion, you must assure that all autologous donations shipped to that establishment are tested under this section.

(3) If you ship autologous donations to another establishment that does not allow autologous donations to be used for allogeneic transfusion, you must assure that, at a minimum, the first donation in each 30-day period is tested under this section.

(4) Each autologous donation must be labeled as required under § 606.121 of this chapter and with the following label, as appropriate:

Donor Testing Status	**Label**
Untested	"DONOR UNTESTED"
Tests negative	Label as required under § 606.121
Reactive on current collection/reactive in the last 30 days	"BIOHAZARD" legend in § 610.40(h)(2)(ii)(B)
Tested negative within the last 30 days	"DONOR TESTED WITHIN THE LAST 30 DAYS"

(e) *Further testing.* You must further test each donation, including autologous donations, found to be reactive by a donor screening test performed under paragraphs (a) and (b) of this section using a licensed, approved, or cleared supplemental test, when available. If no such supplemental test is available, you must perform one or more licensed, approved, or cleared tests as adequate and appropriate to provide additional information concerning the reactive donor's infection status. Except:

(1) For autologous donations:

(i) You must further test under this section, at a minimum, the first reactive donation in each 30 calendar day period; or

(ii) If you have a record for that donor of a positive result on further testing performed under this section, you do not have to further test an autologous donation.

(2) You are not required to perform further testing of a donation found to be reactive by a treponemal donor screening test for syphilis.

(f) *Testing responsibility.* Required testing under this section, must be performed by a laboratory registered in accordance with part 607 of this chapter and either certified to perform such testing on human specimens under the Clinical Laboratory Improvement Amendments of 1988 (42 U.S.C. 263a) under 42 CFR part 493 or has met equivalent requirements as determined by the Centers for Medicare and Medicaid Services in accordance with those provisions.

(g) *Release or shipment prior to testing.* Human blood or blood components that are required to be tested for evidence of infection due to relevant transfusion-transmitted infections designated in paragraph (a) of this section may be released or shipped prior to completion of testing in the following circumstances provided that you label the blood or blood components under § 606.121(h) of this chapter, you complete the tests for evidence of infection due to relevant transfusion-transmitted infections as soon as possible after release or shipment, and that you provide the results promptly to the consignee:

(1) Only in appropriately documented medical emergency situations; or

(2) For further manufacturing use as approved in writing by FDA.

(h) *Restrictions on shipment or use*—(1) *Reactive screening test.* You must not ship or use human blood or blood components that have a reactive screening test for evidence of infection due to relevant transfusion-transmitted infection(s) designated in paragraph (a) of this section or that are collected from a donor with a previous record of a reactive screening test for evidence of infection due to relevant transfusion-transmitted infection(s) designated in paragraph (a) of this section, except as provided in paragraphs (h)(2)(i) through (h)(2)(vii) of this section.

(2) *Exceptions.* (i) You may ship or use blood or blood components intended for autologous use, including reactive donations, as described in paragraph (d) of this section.

(ii) You must not ship or use human blood or blood components that have a reactive screening test for evidence of infection due to a relevant transfusion-transmitted infection(s) designated in paragraph (a) of this section or that are collected from a donor deferred under §610.41(a) unless you meet the following conditions:

(A) Except for autologous donations, you must obtain from FDA written approval for the shipment or use;

(B) You must appropriately label such blood or blood components as required under §606.121 of this chapter, and with the "BIOHAZARD" legend;

(C) Except for autologous donations, you must label such human blood and blood components as reactive for the appropriate screening test for evidence of infection due to the identified relevant transfusion-transmitted infection(s);

(D) If the blood or blood components are intended for further manufacturing use into injectable products, you must include a statement on the container label indicating the exempted use specifically approved by FDA.

(E) Each blood or blood component with a reactive screening test and intended solely as a component of, or used to prepare a medical device, must be labeled with the following label, as appropriate:

Type of Medical Device	**Label**
A medical device other than an in vitro diagnostic reagent	"Caution: For Further Manufacturing Use as a Component of a Medical Device For Which There Are No Alternative Sources"
An in vitro diagnostic reagent	"Caution: For Further Manufacturing Into In Vitro Diagnostic Reagents For Which There Are No Alternative Sources"

(iii) The restrictions on shipment or use do not apply to samples of blood, blood components, plasma, or sera if used or distributed for clinical laboratory testing or research purposes, and not intended for administration in humans or in the manufacture of a product.

(iv) You may use human blood or blood components from a donor with a previous record of a reactive screening test(s) for evidence of infection due to a relevant transfusion-transmitted infection(s) designated in paragraph (a) of this section, if:

(A) At the time of donation, the donor is shown or was previously shown to be eligible by a requalification method or process found acceptable for such purposes by FDA under §610.41(b); and

(B) tests performed under paragraphs (a) and (b) of this section are nonreactive.

(v) Anti-HBc reactive donations, otherwise nonreactive when tested as required under this section, may be used for further manufacturing into plasma derivatives without prior FDA approval or a "BIOHAZARD" legend as required under paragraphs (h)(2)(ii)(A) and (h)(2)(ii)(B) of this section.

(vi) You may use human blood or blood components, excluding Source Plasma, that test reactive by a screening test for syphilis as required under paragraph (a) of this section if, the donation is further tested by an adequate and appropriate test which demonstrates that the reactive screening test is a biological false positive. You must label the blood or blood components with both test results.

(vii) You may use Source Plasma from a donor who tests reactive by a screening test for syphilis as required under § 640.65(a)(2)(ii) and (b)(1)(i) of this chapter, if the donor meets the requirements of § 640.65(b)(2)(i) through (b)(2)(iv) of this chapter.

[66 FR 31162, June 11, 2001, as amended at 77 FR 18, Jan. 3, 2012; 80 FR 29896, May 22, 2015]

§ 610.41 Donor deferral.

(a) You, an establishment that collects human blood or blood components, must defer donors testing reactive by a screening test for evidence of infection due to a relevant transfusion-transmitted infection(s) under § 610.40(a), from future donations of human blood and blood components, except:

(1) You are not required to defer a donor who tests reactive for anti-HBc or anti-HTLV, types I and II, on only one occasion. However, you must defer the donor if further testing for HBV or HTLV has been performed under § 610.40(e) and the donor is found to be positive, or if a second, licensed, cleared, or approved screening test for HBV or HTLV has been performed on the same donation under § 610.40(a) and is reactive, or if the donor tests reactive for anti-HBc or anti-HTLV, types I and II, on more than one occasion;

(2) A deferred donor who tests reactive for evidence of infection due to a relevant transfusion-transmitted infection(s) under § 610.40(a) may serve as a donor for blood or blood components shipped or used under § 610.40(h)(2)(ii);

(3) A deferred donor who showed evidence of infection due to hepatitis B surface antigen (HBsAg) when previously tested under § 610.40(a), (b), and (e) subsequently may donate Source Plasma for use in the preparation of Hepatitis B Immune Globulin (Human) provided the current donation tests nonreactive for HBsAg and the donor is otherwise determined to be eligible;

(4) A deferred donor, who otherwise is determined to be eligible for donation and tests reactive for anti-HBc or for evidence of infection due to HTLV, types I and II, may serve as a donor of Source Plasma;

(5) A deferred donor who tests reactive for a relevant transfusion-transmitted infections(s) under § 610.40(a), may serve as an autologous donor under § 610.40(d).

(b) A deferred donor subsequently may be found to be eligible as a donor of blood or blood components by a requalification method or process found acceptable for such purposes by FDA. Such a donor is considered no longer deferred.

(c) You must comply with the requirements under §§ 610.46 and 610.47 when a donor tests reactive by a screening test for HIV or HCV required under § 610.40(a) and (b), or when you are aware of other reliable test results or information indicating evidence of HIV or HCV infection.

[66 FR 31164, June 11, 2001, as amended at 72 FR 48798, Aug. 24, 2007; 80 FR 29897, May 22, 2015]

§ 610.42 Restrictions on use for further manufacture of medical devices.

(a) In addition to labeling requirements in subchapter H of this chapter, when a medical device contains human blood or a blood component as a component of the final device, and the human blood or blood component was found to be reactive by a screening test performed under §610.40(a) and (b), then you must include in the device labeling a statement of warning indicating that the product was manufactured from a donation found to be reactive by a screening test for evidence of infection due to the identified relevant transfusion-transmitted infection(s).

(b) FDA may approve an exception or alternative to the statement of warning required in paragraph (a) of this section based on evidence that the reactivity of the human blood or blood component in the medical device presents no significant health risk through use of the medical device.

[66 FR 31164, June 11, 2001, as amended at 80 FR 29897, May 22, 2015]

§610.44 Use of reference panels by manufacturers of test kits.

(a) When available and appropriate to verify acceptable sensitivity and specificity, you, a manufacturer of test kits, must use a reference panel you obtain from FDA or from an FDA designated source to test lots of the following products. You must test each lot of the following products, unless FDA informs you that less frequent testing is appropriate, based on your consistent prior production of products of acceptable sensitivity and specificity:

(1) A test kit approved for use in testing donations of human blood and blood components for evidence of infection due to relevant transfusion-transmitted infections under §610.40(a); and

(2) Human immunodeficiency virus (HIV) test kit approved for use in the diagnosis, prognosis, or monitoring of this relevant transfusion-transmitted infection.

(b) You must not distribute a lot that is found to be not acceptable for sensitivity and specificity under §610.44(a). FDA may approve an exception or alternative to this requirement. Applicants must submit such requests in writing. However, in limited circumstances, such requests may be made orally and permission may be given orally by FDA. Oral requests and approvals must be promptly followed by written requests and written approvals.

[66 FR 31164, June 11, 2001, as amended at 80 FR 29897, May 22, 2015]

§610.46 Human immunodeficiency virus (HIV) "lookback" requirements.

(a) If you are an establishment that collects Whole Blood or blood components, including Source Plasma and Source Leukocytes, you must establish, maintain, and follow an appropriate system for the following actions:

(1) Within 3 calendar days after a donor tests reactive for evidence of human immunodeficiency virus (HIV) infection when tested under §610.40(a) and (b) or when you are made aware of other reliable test results or information indicating evidence of HIV infection, you must review all records required under §606.160(d) of this chapter, to identify blood and blood components previously donated by such a donor. For those identified blood and blood components collected:

(i) Twelve months and less before the donor's most recent nonreactive screening tests, or

(ii) Twelve months and less before the donor's reactive direct viral detection test, e.g., nucleic acid test or HIV p24 antigen test, and nonreactive antibody screening test, whichever is the lesser period, you must:

(A) Quarantine all previously collected in-date blood and blood components identified under paragraph (a)(1) of this section if intended for use in another person or for further manufacture into injectable products, except pooled blood components intended solely for further manufacturing into products that are manufactured using validated viral clearance procedures; and

(B) Notify consignees to quarantine all previously collected in-date blood and blood components identified under paragraph (a)(1) of this section if intended for use in another person or for further manufacture into injectable products, except pooled blood components intended solely for further manufacturing into products that are manufactured using validated viral clearance procedures;

(2) You must perform further testing for HIV as required under §610.40(e) of this chapter on the reactive donation.

(3) You must notify consignees of the results of further testing for HIV, or the results of the reactive screening test if further testing under paragraph (a)(2) of this section is not available, or if under an investigational new drug application (IND) or investigational device exemption (IDE), is exempted for such use by FDA, within 45 calendar days after the donor tests reactive for evidence of HIV infection under §610.40(a) and (b) of this chapter. Notification of consignees must include the test results for blood and blood components identified under paragraph (a)(1) of this section that were previously collected from donors who later test reactive for evidence of HIV infection.

(4) You must release from quarantine, destroy, or relabel quarantined in-date blood and blood components, consistent with the results of the further testing performed under paragraph (a)(2) of this section or the results of the reactive screening test if further testing is not available, or if under an IND or IDE, exempted for such use by FDA.

(b) If you are a consignee of Whole Blood or blood components, including Source Plasma and Source Leukocytes, you must establish, maintain, and follow an appropriate system for the following actions:

(1) You must quarantine all previously collected in-date blood and blood components identified under paragraph (a)(1) of this section, except pooled blood components intended solely for further manufacturing into products that are manufactured using validated viral clearance procedures, when notified by the collecting establishment.

(2) You must release from quarantine, destroy, or relabel quarantined in-date blood and blood components consistent with the results of the further testing performed under paragraph (a)(2) of this section, or the results of the reactive screening test if further testing is not available, or if under an IND or IDE, is exempted for such use by FDA.

(3) When further testing for HIV is positive or when the screening test is reactive and further testing is not available, or if under an IND or IDE is exempted for such use by FDA, you must notify transfusion recipients of previous collections of blood and blood components at increased risk of transmitting HIV infection, or the recipient's physician of record, of the need for recipient HIV testing and counseling. You must notify the recipient's physician of record or a legal representative or relative if the recipient is a minor, deceased, adjudged incompetent by a State court, or, if the recipient is competent but State law permits a legal representative or relative to receive information on behalf of the recipient. You must make reasonable attempts to perform the notification within 12 weeks after receiving the results of further testing for evidence of HIV infection from the collecting establishment, or after receiving the donor's reactive screening test result for HIV if further testing is not available, or if under an IND or IDE is exempted for such use by FDA.

(c) Actions under this section do not constitute a recall as defined in §7.3 of this chapter.

[72 FR 48799, Aug. 24, 2007, as amended at 80 FR 29897, May 22, 2015]

§610.47 Hepatitis C virus (HCV) "lookback" requirements.

(a) If you are an establishment that collects Whole Blood or blood components, including Source Plasma and Source Leukocytes, you must establish, maintain, and follow an appropriate system for the following actions:

(1) Within 3 calendar days after a donor tests reactive for evidence of hepatitis C virus (HCV) infection when tested under §610.40(a) and (b) of this chapter or when you are made aware of other reliable test results or information indicating evidence of HCV infection, you must review all records required under §606.160(d) of this chapter, to identify blood and blood components previously donated by such a donor. For those identified blood and blood components collected:

(i) Twelve months and less before the donor's most recent nonreactive screening tests, or

(ii) Twelve months and less before the donor's reactive direct viral detection test, e.g., nucleic acid test and nonreactive antibody screening test, whichever is the lesser period, you must:

(A) Quarantine all previously collected in-date blood and blood components identified under paragraph (a)(1) of this section if intended for use in another person or for further manufacture into injectable products, except pooled blood components intended solely for further manufacturing into products that are manufactured using validated viral clearance procedures; and

(B) Notify consignees to quarantine all previously collected in-date blood and blood components identified under paragraph (a)(1) of this section if intended for use in another person or for further manufacture into injectable products, except pooled blood components intended solely for further manufacturing into products that are manufactured using validated viral clearance procedures;

(2) You must perform further testing for HCV as required under §610.40(e) on the reactive donation.

(3) You must notify consignees of the results of further testing for HCV, or the results of the reactive screening test if further testing is not available, or if under an investigational new drug application (IND) or investigational device exemption (IDE), is exempted for such use by FDA, within 45 calendar days after the donor tests reactive for evidence of HCV infection under §610.40(a) and (b). Notification of consignees must include the test results for blood and blood components identified under paragraph (a)(1) of this section that were previously collected from donors who later test reactive for evidence of HCV infection.

(4) You must release from quarantine, destroy, or relabel quarantined in-date blood and blood components consistent with the results of the further testing performed under paragraph (a)(2) of this section, or the results of the reactive screening test if further testing is not available, or if under an IND or IDE, exempted for such use by FDA.

(b) If you are a consignee of Whole Blood or blood components, including Source Plasma or Source Leukocytes, you must establish, maintain, and follow an appropriate system for the following actions:

(1) You must quarantine all previously collected in-date blood and blood components identified under paragraph (a)(1) of this section, except pooled blood components intended solely for further manufacturing into products that are manufactured using validated viral clearance procedures, when notified by the collecting establishment.

(2) You must release from quarantine, destroy, or relabel quarantined in-date blood and blood components, consistent with the results of the further testing performed under paragraph (a)(2) of this section, or the results of the reactive screening test if further testing is not available, or if under an IND or IDE, is exempted for such use by FDA.

(3) When the further testing for HCV is positive or when the screening test is reactive and further testing is not available, or if under an IND or IDE, is exempted for such use by FDA, you must notify transfusion recipients of previous collections of blood and blood components at increased risk of transmitting HCV infection, or the recipient's physician of record, of the need for recipient HCV testing and counseling. You must notify the recipient's physician of record or a legal representative or relative if the recipient is a minor, adjudged incompetent by a State court, or if the recipient is competent but State law permits a legal representative or relative to receive information on behalf of the recipient. You must make reasonable attempts to perform the notification within 12 weeks after receiving the results of further testing for evidence of HCV infection from the collecting establishment, or after receiving the donor's reactive screening test result for HCV if further testing is not available, or if under an IND or IDE, is exempted for such use by FDA.

(c) Actions under this section do not constitute a recall as defined in §7.3 of this chapter.

[72 FR 48799, Aug. 24, 2007, as amended at 80 FR 29897, May 22, 2015]

§610.48 [Reserved]

Subpart F—Dating Period Limitations

§610.50 Date of manufacture for biological products.

(a) *When the dating period begins.* The dating period for a product must begin on the date of manufacture as described in paragraphs (b) and (c) of this section. The dating period for a combination of two or more products must be no longer than the dating period of the component with the shortest dating period.

(b) *Determining the date of manufacture for biological products other than Whole Blood and blood components.* The date of manufacture for biological products, other than Whole Blood and blood components, must be identified in the approved biologics license application as one of the following, whichever is applicable: The date of:

(1) Potency test or other specific test as described in a biologics license application or supplement to the application;

(2) Removal from animals or humans;

(3) Extraction;

(4) Solution;

(5) Cessation of growth;

(6) Final sterile filtration of a bulk solution;

(7) Manufacture as described in part 660 of this chapter; or

(8) Other specific manufacturing activity described in a biologics license application or supplement to the biologics license application.

(c) *Determining the date of manufacture for Whole Blood and blood components.* (1) The date of manufacture for Whole Blood and blood components must be one of the following, whichever is applicable:

(i) Collection date and/or time;

(ii) Irradiation date;

(iii) The time the red blood cell product was removed from frozen storage for deglycerolization;

(iv) The time the additive or rejuvenation solution was added;

(v) The time the product was entered for washing or removing plasma (if prepared in an open system);

(vi) As specified in the instructions for use by the blood collection, processing, and storage system approved or cleared for such use by FDA; or

(vii) As approved by the Director, Center for Biologics Evaluation and Research, in a biologics license application or supplement to the application.

(2) For licensed Whole Blood and blood components, the date of manufacture must be identified in the approved biologics license application or supplement to the application.

[81 FR 26691, May 4, 2016]

§610.53 Dating periods for Whole Blood and blood components.

(a) *General.* Dating periods for Whole Blood and blood components are specified in the table in paragraph (b) of this section.

(b) *Table of dating periods.* In using the table in this paragraph, when a product in column A is stored at the storage temperature prescribed in column B, storage of a product must not exceed the dating period specified in column C, unless a different dating period is specified in the instructions for use by the blood collection, processing and storage system approved or cleared for such use by FDA. Container labels for each product must include the recommended storage temperatures.

Whole Blood and Blood Components Storage Temperatures and Dating Periods

A	B	C
Product	**Storage temperature**	**Dating period**
	Whole Blood	
ACD, CPD, CP2D	Between 1 and 6 °C	21 days from date of collection.
CPDA-1	do[1]	35 days from date of collection.
	Red Blood Cells	
ACD, CPD, CP2D	Between 1 and 6 °C	21 days from date of collection.
CPDA-1	do	35 days from date of collection.
Additive solutions	do	42 days from date of collection.
Open system(e.g., deglycerolized, washed)	do	24 hours after entering bag.
Deglycerolized in closed system with additive solution added	do	14 days after entering bag.
Irradiated	do	28 days from date of irradiation or original dating, whichever is shorter.
Frozen	−65 °C or colder	10 years from date of collection.
	Platelets	
Platelets	Between 20 and 24 °C	5 days from date of collection.
Platelets	Other temperatures according to storage bag instructions	As specified in the instructions for use by the blood collection, processing and storage system approved or cleared for such use by FDA.
	Plasma	
Fresh Frozen Plasma	−18 °C or colder	1 year from date of collection.
Plasma Frozen Within 24 Hours After Phlebotomy	do	1 year from date of collection.

Plasma		
Plasma Frozen Within 24 Hours After Phlebotomy Held at Room Temperature Up To 24 Hours After Phlebotomy	do	1 year from date of collection.
Plasma Cryoprecipitate Reduced	do	1 year from date of collection.
Plasma	do	5 years from date of collection.
Liquid Plasma	Between 1 and 6 °C	5 days from end of Whole Blood dating period.
Source Plasma (frozen injectable)	−20 °C or colder	10 years from date of collection.
Source Plasma Liquid (injectable)	10 °C or colder	According to approved biologics license application.
Source Plasma (noninjectable)	Temperature appropriate for final product	10 years from date of collection.
Therapeutic Exchange Plasma	−20 °C or colder	10 years from date of collection.
Cryoprecipitated AHF		
Cryoprecipitated AHF	−18 °C or colder	1 year from date of collection of source blood or from date of collection of oldest source blood in pre-storage pool.
Source Leukocytes		
Source Leukocytes	Temperature appropriate for final product	In lieu of expiration date, the collection date must appear on the label.

1.The abbreviation "do." for ditto is used in the table to indicate that the previous line is being repeated.

[81 FR 26691, May 4, 2016]

Subpart G—Labeling Standards

§610.60 Container label.

(a) *Full label.* The following items shall appear on the label affixed to each container of a product capable of bearing a full label:

(1) The proper name of the product;

(2) The name, address, and license number of manufacturer;

(3) The lot number or other lot identification;

(4) The expiration date;

(5) The recommended individual dose, for multiple dose containers.

(6) The statement: "'Rx only'" for prescription biologicals.

(7) If a Medication Guide is required under part 208 of this chapter, the statement required under § 208.24(d) of this chapter instructing the authorized dispenser to provide a Medication Guide to each patient to whom the drug is dispensed and stating how the Medication Guide is provided, except where the container label is too small, the required statement may be placed on the package label.

(b) *Package label information.* If the container is not enclosed in a package, all the items required for a package label shall appear on the container label.

(c) *Partial label.* If the container is capable of bearing only a partial label, the container shall show as a minimum the name (expressed either as the proper or common name), the lot number or other lot identification and the name of the manufacturer; in addition, for multiple dose containers, the recommended individual dose. Containers bearing partial labels shall be placed in a package which bears all the items required for a package label.

(d) No container label. If the container is incapable of bearing any label, the items required for a container label may be omitted, provided the container is placed in a package which bears all the items required for a package label.

(e) *Visual inspection.* When the label has been affixed to the container a sufficient area of the container shall remain uncovered for its full length or circumference to permit inspection of the contents.

[38 FR 32056, Nov. 20, 1973, as amended at 47 FR 22518, May 25, 1982; 63 FR 66400, Dec. 1, 1998; 67 FR 4907, Feb. 1, 2002]

§ 610.61 Package label.

The following items shall appear on the label affixed to each package containing a product:

(a) The proper name of the product;

(b) The name, address, and license number of manufacturer;

(c) The lot number or other lot identification;

(d) The expiration date;

(e) The preservative used and its concentration, or if no preservative is used and the absence of a preservative is a safety factor, the words "no preservative";

(f) The number of containers, if more than one;

(g) The amount of product in the container expressed as (1) the number of doses, (2) volume, (3) units of potency, (4) weight, (5) equivalent volume (for dried product to be reconstituted), or (6) such combination of the foregoing as needed for an accurate description of the contents, whichever is applicable;

(h) The recommended storage temperature;

(i) The words "Shake Well", "Do not Freeze" or the equivalent, as well as other instructions, when indicated by the character of the product;

(j) The recommended individual dose if the enclosed container(s) is a multiple-dose container;

(k) The route of administration recommended, or reference to such directions in an enclosed circular;

(l) Known sensitizing substances, or reference to an enclosed circular containing appropriate information;

(m) The type and calculated amount of antibiotics added during manufacture;

(n) The inactive ingredients when a safety factor, or reference to an enclosed circular containing appropriate information;

(o) The adjuvant, if present;

(p) The source of the product when a factor in safe administration;

(q) The identity of each microorganism used in manufacture, and, where applicable, the production medium and the method of inactivation, or reference to an enclosed circular containing appropriate information;

(r) Minimum potency of product expressed in terms of official standard of potency or, if potency is a factor and no U.S. standard of potency has been prescribed, the words "No U.S. standard of potency."

(s) The statement: "'Rx only'" for prescription biologicals.

[38 FR 32056, Nov. 20, 1973, as amended at 47 FR 22518, May 25, 1982; 55 FR 10423, Mar. 21, 1990; 67 FR 4907, Feb. 1, 2002]

§ 610.62 Proper name; package label; legible type.

(a) *Position*. The proper name of the product on the package label shall be placed above any trademark or trade name identifying the product and symmetrically arranged with respect to other printing on the label.

(b) *Prominence*. The point size and typeface of the proper name shall be at least as prominent as the point size and typeface used in designating the trademark and trade name. The contrast in color value between the proper name and the background shall be at least as great as the color value between the trademark and trade name and the background. Typography, layout, contrast, and other printing features shall not be used in a manner that will affect adversely the prominence of the proper name.

(c) *Legible type*. All items required to be on the container label and package label shall be in legible type. "Legible type" is type of a size and character which can be read with ease when held in a good light and with normal vision.

§ 610.63 Divided manufacturing responsibility to be shown.

If two or more licensed manufacturers participate in the manufacture of a biological product, the name, address, and license number of each must appear on the package label, and on the label of the container if capable of bearing a full label.

[64 FR 56453, Oct. 20, 1999]

§ 610.64 Name and address of distributor.

The name and address of the distributor of a product may appear on the label provided that the name, address, and license number of the manufacturer also appears on the label and the name of the distributor is qualified by one of the following phrases: "Manufactured for ______", "Distributed by ______", "Manufactured by ______ for ______", "Manufactured for ______ by ______", "Distributor: ______", or "Marketed by ______". The qualifying phrases may be abbreviated.

[61 FR 57330, Nov. 6, 1996]

§ 610.65 Products for export.

Labels on packages or containers of products for export may be adapted to meet specific requirements of the regulations of the country to which the product is to be exported provided that in all such cases the minimum label requirements prescribed in § 610.60 are observed.

§ 610.67 Bar code label requirements.

Biological products must comply with the bar code requirements at § 201.25 of this chapter. However, the bar code requirements do not apply to devices regulated by the Center for Biologics Evaluation and Research or to blood and blood components intended for transfusion. For blood and blood components intended for transfusion, the requirements at §606.121(c)(13) of this chapter apply instead.

[69 FR 9171, Feb. 26, 2004]

§610.68 Exceptions or alternatives to labeling requirements for biological products held by the Strategic National Stockpile.

(a) The appropriate FDA Center Director may grant an exception or alternative to any provision listed in paragraph (f) of this section and not explicitly required by statute, for specified lots, batches, or other units of a biological product, if the Center Director determines that compliance with such labeling requirement could adversely affect the safety, effectiveness, or availability of such product that is or will be included in the Strategic National Stockpile.

(b)(1)(i) A Strategic National Stockpile official or any entity that manufactures (including labeling, packing, relabeling, or repackaging), distributes, or stores a biological product that is or will be included in the Strategic National Stockpile may submit, with written concurrence from a Strategic National Stockpile official, a written request for an exception or alternative described in paragraph (a) of this section to the Center Director.

(ii) The Center Director may grant an exception or alternative described in paragraph (a) of this section on his or her own initiative.

(2) A written request for an exception or alternative described in paragraph (a) of this section must:

(i) Identify the specified lots, batches, or other units of the biological product that would be subject to the exception or alternative;

(ii) Identify the labeling provision(s) listed in paragraph (f) of this section that are the subject of the exception or alternative request;

(iii) Explain why compliance with such labeling provision(s) could adversely affect the safety, effectiveness, or availability of the specified lots, batches, or other units of the biological product that are or will be included in the Strategic National Stockpile;

(iv) Describe any proposed safeguards or conditions that will be implemented so that the labeling of the product includes appropriate information necessary for the safe and effective use of the product, given the anticipated circumstances of use of the product;

(v) Provide a draft of the proposed labeling of the specified lots, batches, or other units of the biological product subject to the exception or alternative; and

(vi) Provide any other information requested by the Center Director in support of the request.

(c) The Center Director must respond in writing to all requests under this section.

(d) A grant of an exception or alternative under this section will include any safeguards or conditions deemed appropriate by the Center Director so that the labeling of product subject to the exception or alternative includes the information necessary for the safe and effective use of the product, given the anticipated circumstances of use.

(e) If you are a sponsor receiving a grant of a request for an exception or alternative to the labeling requirements under this section:

(1) You need not submit a supplement under §601.12(f)(1) through (f)(2) of this chapter; however,

(2) You must report any grant of a request for an exception or alternative under this section as part of your annual report under §601.12(f)(3) of this chapter.

(f) The Center Director may grant an exception or alternative under this section to the following provisions of this chapter, to the extent that the requirements in these provisions are not explicitly required by statute:

(1) § 610.60;

(2) § 610.61(c) and (e) through (r);

(3) § 610.62;

(4) § 610.63;

(5) § 610.64;

(6) § 610.65; and

(7) § 312.6.

[72 FR 73600, Dec. 28, 2007]

• • •

SUBCHAPTER H—MEDICAL DEVICES

PART 812—INVESTIGATIONAL DEVICE EXEMPTIONS

Authority: 21 U.S.C. 331, 351, 352, 353, 355, 360, 360c-360f, 360h-360j, 360bbb-8b, 371, 372, 374, 379e, 381, 382, 383; 42 U.S.C. 216, 241, 262, 263b-263n.

Source: 45 FR 3751, Jan. 18, 1980, unless otherwise noted.

Subpart A—General Provisions

§ 812.1 Scope.

(a) The purpose of this part is to encourage, to the extent consistent with the protection of public health and safety and with ethical standards, the discovery and development of useful devices intended for human use, and to that end to maintain optimum freedom for scientific investigators in their pursuit of this purpose. This part provides procedures for the conduct of clinical investigations of devices. An approved investigational device exemption (IDE) permits a device that otherwise would be required to comply with a performance standard or to have premarket approval to be shipped lawfully for the purpose of conducting investigations of that device. An IDE approved under § 812.30 or considered approved under § 812.2(b) exempts a device from the requirements of the following sections of the Federal Food, Drug, and Cosmetic Act (the act) and regulations issued thereunder: Misbranding under section 502 of the act, registration, listing, and premarket notification under section 510, performance standards under section 514, premarket approval under section 515, a banned device regulation under section 516, records and reports under section 519, restricted device requirements under section 520(e), good manufacturing practice requirements under section 520(f) except for the requirements found in § 820.30, if applicable (unless the sponsor states an intention to comply with these requirements under § 812.20(b)(3) or § 812.140(b)(4)(v)) and color additive requirements under section 721.

(b) References in this part to regulatory sections of the Code of Federal Regulations are to chapter I of title 21, unless otherwise noted.

[45 FR 3751, Jan. 18, 1980, as amended at 59 FR 14366, Mar. 28, 1994; 61 FR 52654, Oct. 7, 1996]

§812.2 Applicability.

(a) *General.* This part applies to all clinical investigations of devices to determine safety and effectiveness, except as provided in paragraph (c) of this section.

(b) *Abbreviated requirements.* The following categories of investigations are considered to have approved applications for IDE's, unless FDA has notified a sponsor under §812.20(a) that approval of an application is required:

(1) An investigation of a device other than a significant risk device, if the device is not a banned device and the sponsor:

(i) Labels the device in accordance with §812.5;

(ii) Obtains IRB approval of the investigation after presenting the reviewing IRB with a brief explanation of why the device is not a significant risk device, and maintains such approval;

(iii) Ensures that each investigator participating in an investigation of the device obtains from each subject under the investigator's care, informed consent under part 50 and documents it, unless documentation is waived by an IRB under §56.109(c).

(iv) Complies with the requirements of §812.46 with respect to monitoring investigations;

(v) Maintains the records required under §812.140(b) (4) and (5) and makes the reports required under §812.150(b) (1) through (3) and (5) through (10);

(vi) Ensures that participating investigators maintain the records required by §812.140(a)(3)(i) and make the reports required under §812.150(a) (1), (2), (5), and (7); and

(vii) Complies with the prohibitions in §812.7 against promotion and other practices.

(2) An investigation of a device other than one subject to paragraph (e) of this section, if the investigation was begun on or before July 16, 1980, and to be completed, and is completed, on or before January 19, 1981.

(c) *Exempted investigations.* This part, with the exception of §812.119, does not apply to investigations of the following categories of devices:

(1) A device, other than a transitional device, in commercial distribution immediately before May 28, 1976, when used or investigated in accordance with the indications in labeling in effect at that time.

(2) A device, other than a transitional device, introduced into commercial distribution on or after May 28, 1976, that FDA has determined to be substantially equivalent to a device in commercial distribution immediately before May 28, 1976, and that is used or investigated in accordance with the indications in the labeling FDA reviewed under subpart E of part 807 in determining substantial equivalence.

(3) A diagnostic device, if the sponsor complies with applicable requirements in §809.10(c) and if the testing:

(i) Is noninvasive,

(ii) Does not require an invasive sampling procedure that presents significant risk,

(iii) Does not by design or intention introduce energy into a subject, and

(iv) Is not used as a diagnostic procedure without confirmation of the diagnosis by another, medically established diagnostic product or procedure.

(4) A device undergoing consumer preference testing, testing of a modification, or testing of a combination of two or more devices in commercial distribution, if the testing is not for the purpose of determining safety or effectiveness and does not put subjects at risk.

(5) A device intended solely for veterinary use.

(6) A device shipped solely for research on or with laboratory animals and labeled in accordance with §812.5(c).

(7) A custom device as defined in §812.3(b), unless the device is being used to determine safety or effectiveness for commercial distribution.

(d) *Limit on certain exemptions.* In the case of class II or class III device described in paragraph (c)(1) or (2) of this section, this part applies beginning on the date stipulated in an FDA regulation or order that calls for the submission of premarket approval applications for an unapproved class III device, or establishes a performance standard for a class II device.

(e) *Investigations subject to IND's.* A sponsor that, on July 16, 1980, has an effective investigational new drug application (IND) for an investigation of a device shall continue to comply with the requirements of part 312 until 90 days after that date. To continue the investigation after that date, a sponsor shall comply with paragraph (b)(1) of this section, if the device is not a significant risk device, or shall have obtained FDA approval under §812.30 of an IDE application for the investigation of the device.

[45 FR 3751, Jan. 18, 1980, as amended at 46 FR 8956, Jan. 27, 1981; 46 FR 14340, Feb. 27, 1981; 53 FR 11252, Apr. 6, 1988; 62 FR 4165, Jan. 29, 1997; 62 FR 12096, Mar. 14, 1997]

§812.3 Definitions.

(a) *Act* means the Federal Food, Drug, and Cosmetic Act (sections 201-901, 52 Stat. 1040 et seq., as amended (21 U.S.C. 301-392)).

(b) A custom device means a device within the meaning of section 520(b) of the Federal Food, Drug, and Cosmetic Act.

(c) *FDA* means the Food and Drug Administration.

(d) *Implant* means a device that is placed into a surgically or naturally formed cavity of the human body if it is intended to remain there for a period of 30 days or more. FDA may, in order to protect public health, determine that devices placed in subjects for shorter periods are also "implants" for purposes of this part.

(e) *Institution* means a person, other than an individual, who engages in the conduct of research on subjects or in the delivery of medical services to individuals as a primary activity or as an adjunct to providing residential or custodial care to humans. The term includes, for example, a hospital, retirement home, confinement facility, academic establishment, and device manufacturer. The term has the same meaning as "facility" in section 520(g) of the act.

(f) *Institutional review board* (IRB) means any board, committee, or other group formally designated by an institution to review biomedical research involving subjects and established, operated, and functioning in conformance with part 56. The term has the same meaning as "institutional review committee" in section 520(g) of the act.

(g) *Investigational device* means a device, including a transitional device, that is the object of an investigation.

(h) *Investigation* means a clinical investigation or research involving one or more subjects to determine the safety or effectiveness of a device.

(i) *Investigator* means an individual who actually conducts a clinical investigation, i.e., under whose immediate direction the test article is administered or dispensed to, or used involving, a subject, or, in the event of an investigation conducted by a team of individuals, is the responsible leader of that team.

(j) *Monitor,* when used as a noun, means an individual designated by a sponsor or contract research organization to oversee the progress of an investigation. The monitor may be an employee of a sponsor or a consultant to the sponsor, or an employee of or consultant to a contract research organization. Monitor, when used as a verb, means to oversee an investigation.

(k) *Noninvasive*, when applied to a diagnostic device or procedure, means one that does not by design or intention: (1) Penetrate or pierce the skin or mucous membranes of the body, the ocular cavity, or the urethra, or (2) enter the ear beyond the external auditory canal, the nose beyond the nares, the mouth beyond the pharynx, the anal canal beyond the rectum, or the vagina beyond the cervical os. For purposes of this part, blood sampling that involves simple venipuncture is considered noninvasive, and the use of surplus samples of body fluids or tissues that are left over from samples taken for noninvestigational purposes is also considered noninvasive.

(l) *Person* includes any individual, partnership, corporation, association, scientific or academic establishment, Government agency or organizational unit of a Government agency, and any other legal entity.

(m) *Significant risk device* means an investigational device that:

(1) Is intended as an implant and presents a potential for serious risk to the health, safety, or welfare of a subject;

(2) Is purported or represented to be for a use in supporting or sustaining human life and presents a potential for serious risk to the health, safety, or welfare of a subject;

(3) Is for a use of substantial importance in diagnosing, curing, mitigating, or treating disease, or otherwise preventing impairment of human health and presents a potential for serious risk to the health, safety, or welfare of a subject; or

(4) Otherwise presents a potential for serious risk to the health, safety, or welfare of a subject.

(n) *Sponsor* means a person who initiates, but who does not actually conduct, the investigation, that is, the investigational device is administered, dispensed, or used under the immediate direction of another individual. A person other than an individual that uses one or more of its own employees to conduct an investigation that it has initiated is a sponsor, not a sponsor-investigator, and the employees are investigators.

(o) *Sponsor-investigator* means an individual who both initiates and actually conducts, alone or with others, an investigation, that is, under whose immediate direction the investigational device is administered, dispensed, or used. The term does not include any person other than an individual. The obligations of a sponsor-investigator under this part include those of an investigator and those of a sponsor.

(p) *Subject* means a human who participates in an investigation, either as an individual on whom or on whose specimen an investigational device is used or as a control. A subject may be in normal health or may have a medical condition or disease.

(q) *Termination* means a discontinuance, by sponsor or by withdrawal of IRB or FDA approval, of an investigation before completion.

(r) *Transitional device* means a device subject to section 520(l) of the act, that is, a device that FDA considered to be a new drug or an antibiotic drug before May 28, 1976.

(s) *Unanticipated adverse device effect* means any serious adverse effect on health or safety or any life-threatening problem or death caused by, or associated with, a device, if that effect, problem, or death was not previously identified in nature, severity, or degree of incidence in the investigational plan or application (including a supplementary plan or application), or any other unanticipated serious problem associated with a device that relates to the rights, safety, or welfare of subjects.

(t) *Independent ethics committee (IEC)* means an independent review panel that is responsible for ensuring the protection of the rights, safety, and well-being of subjects involved in a clinical investigation and is adequately constituted to ensure that protection. An institutional review board (IRB), as defined in paragraph (f) of this section and subject to the requirements of part 56 of this chapter, is one type of IEC.

[45 FR 3751, Jan. 18, 1980, as amended at 46 FR 8956, Jan. 27, 1981; 48 FR 15622, Apr. 12, 1983; 81 FR 70340, Oct. 12, 2016; 83 FR 7385, Feb. 21, 2018]

§ 812.5 Labeling of investigational devices.

(a) *Contents*. An investigational device or its immediate package shall bear a label with the following information: the name and place of business of the manufacturer, packer, or distributor (in accordance with § 801.1), the quantity of contents, if appropriate, and the following statement: "CAUTION—Investigational device. Limited by Federal (or United States) law to investigational use." The label or other labeling shall describe all relevant contraindications, hazards, adverse effects, interfering substances or devices, warnings, and precautions.

(b) *Prohibitions*. The labeling of an investigational device shall not bear any statement that is false or misleading in any particular and shall not represent that the device is safe or effective for the purposes for which it is being investigated.

(c) *Animal research*. An investigational device shipped solely for research on or with laboratory animals shall bear on its label the following statement: "CAUTION—Device for investigational use in laboratory animals or other tests that do not involve human subjects."

(d) The appropriate FDA Center Director, according to the procedures set forth in § 801.128 or § 809.11 of this chapter, may grant an exception or alternative to the provisions in paragraphs (a) and (c) of this section, to the extent that these provisions are not explicitly required by statute, for specified lots, batches, or other units of a device that are or will be included in the Strategic National Stockpile.

[45 FR 3751, Jan. 18, 1980, as amended at 45 FR 58842, Sept. 5, 1980; 72 FR 73602, Dec. 28, 2007]

§ 812.7 Prohibition of promotion and other practices.

A sponsor, investigator, or any person acting for or on behalf of a sponsor or investigator shall not:

(a) Promote or test market an investigational device, until after FDA has approved the device for commercial distribution.

(b) Commercialize an investigational device by charging the subjects or investigators for a device a price larger than that necessary to recover costs of manufacture, research, development, and handling.

(c) Unduly prolong an investigation. If data developed by the investigation indicate in the case of a class III device that premarket approval cannot be justified or in the case of a class II device that it will not comply with an applicable performance standard or an amendment to that standard, the sponsor shall promptly terminate the investigation.

(d) Represent that an investigational device is safe or effective for the purposes for which it is being investigated.

§ 812.10 Waivers.

(a) *Request*. A sponsor may request FDA to waive any requirement of this part. A waiver request, with supporting documentation, may be submitted separately or as part of an application to the address in § 812.19.

(b) FDA action. FDA may by letter grant a waiver of any requirement that FDA finds is not required by the act and is unnecessary to protect the rights, safety, or welfare of human subjects.

(c) *Effect of request*. Any requirement shall continue to apply unless and until FDA waives it.

§812.18 Import and export requirements.

(a) *Imports.* In addition to complying with other requirements of this part, a person who imports or offers for importation an investigational device subject to this part shall be the agent of the foreign exporter with respect to investigations of the device and shall act as the sponsor of the clinical investigation, or ensure that another person acts as the agent of the foreign exporter and the sponsor of the investigation.

(b) *Exports.* A person exporting an investigational device subject to this part shall obtain FDA's prior approval, as required by section 801(e) of the act or comply with section 802 of the act.

[45 FR 3751, Jan. 18, 1980, as amended at 62 FR 26229, May 13, 1997]

§812.19 Address for IDE correspondence.

(a) If you are sending an application, supplemental application, report, request for waiver, request for import or export approval, or other correspondence relating to matters covered by this part, you must send the submission to the appropriate address as follows:

(1) For devices regulated by the Center for Devices and Radiological Health, send it to Food and Drug Administration, Center for Devices and Radiological Health, Document Mail Center, 10903 New Hampshire Ave., Bldg. 66, rm. G609, Silver Spring, MD 20993-0002.

(2) For devices regulated by the Center for Biologics Evaluation and Research, send it to the Food and Drug Administration, Center for Biologics Evaluation and Research, Document Control Center, 10903 New Hampshire Ave., Bldg. 71, Rm. G112, Silver Spring, MD 20993-0002.

(3) For devices regulated by the Center for Drug Evaluation and Research, send it to Central Document Control Room, Center for Drug Evaluation and Research, Food and Drug Administration, 5901-B Ammendale Rd., Beltsville, MD 20705-1266.

(b) You must state on the outside wrapper of each submission what the submission is, for example, an "IDE application," a "supplemental IDE application," or a "correspondence concerning an IDE (or an IDE application)."

[71 FR 42048, July 25, 2006, as amended at 75 FR 20915, Apr. 22, 2010; 80 FR 18094, Apr. 3, 2015]

Subpart B—Application and Administrative Action

§812.20 Application.

(a) *Submission.* (1) A sponsor shall submit an application to FDA if the sponsor intends to use a significant risk device in an investigation, intends to conduct an investigation that involves an exception from informed consent under §50.24 of this chapter, or if FDA notifies the sponsor that an application is required for an investigation.

(2) A sponsor shall not begin an investigation for which FDA's approval of an application is required until FDA has approved the application.

(3) A sponsor shall submit three copies of a signed "Application for an Investigational Device Exemption" (IDE application), together with accompanying materials, by registered mail or by hand to the address in §812.19. Subsequent correspondence concerning an application or a supplemental application shall be submitted by registered mail or by hand.

(4)(i) A sponsor shall submit a separate IDE for any clinical investigation involving an exception from informed consent under §50.24 of this chapter. Such a clinical investigation is not permitted to proceed without the prior written authorization of FDA. FDA shall provide a written determination 30 days after FDA receives the IDE or earlier.

(ii) If the investigation involves an exception from informed consent under §50.24 of this chapter, the sponsor shall prominently identify on the cover sheet that the investigation is subject to the requirements in §50.24 of this chapter.

(b) *Contents.* An IDE application shall include, in the following order:

(1) The name and address of the sponsor.

(2) A complete report of prior investigations of the device and an accurate summary of those sections of the investigational plan described in §812.25(a) through (e) or, in lieu of the summary, the complete plan. The sponsor shall submit to FDA a complete investigational plan and a complete report of prior investigations of the device if no IRB has reviewed them, if FDA has found an IRB's review inadequate, or if FDA requests them.

(3) A description of the methods, facilities, and controls used for the manufacture, processing, packing, storage, and, where appropriate, installation of the device, in sufficient detail so that a person generally familiar with good manufacturing practices can make a knowledgeable judgment about the quality control used in the manufacture of the device.

(4) An example of the agreements to be entered into by all investigators to comply with investigator obligations under this part, and a list of the names and addresses of all investigators who have signed the agreement.

(5) A certification that all investigators who will participate in the investigation have signed the agreement, that the list of investigators includes all the investigators participating in the investigation, and that no investigators will be added to the investigation until they have signed the agreement.

(6) A list of the name, address, and chairperson of each IRB that has been or will be asked to review the investigation and a certification of the action concerning the investigation taken by each such IRB.

(7) The name and address of any institution at which a part of the investigation may be conducted that has not been identified in accordance with paragraph (b)(6) of this section.

(8) If the device is to be sold, the amount to be charged and an explanation of why sale does not constitute commercialization of the device.

(9) A claim for categorical exclusion under §25.30 or §25.34 or an environmental assessment under §25.40.

(10) Copies of all labeling for the device.

(11) Copies of all forms and informational materials to be provided to subjects to obtain informed consent.

(12) Any other relevant information FDA requests for review of the application.

(c) *Additional information.* FDA may request additional information concerning an investigation or revision in the investigational plan. The sponsor may treat such a request as a disapproval of the application for purposes of requesting a hearing under part 16.

(d) *Information previously submitted.* Information previously submitted to the Center for Devices and Radiological Health, the Center for Biologics Evaluation and Research, or the Center for Drug Evaluation and Research, as applicable, in accordance with this chapter ordinarily need not be resubmitted, but may be incorporated by reference.

[45 FR 3751, Jan. 18, 1980, as amended at 46 FR 8956, Jan. 27, 1981; 50 FR 16669, Apr. 26, 1985; 53 FR 11252, Apr. 6, 1988; 61 FR 51530, Oct. 2, 1996; 62 FR 40600, July 29, 1997; 64 FR 10942, Mar. 8, 1999; 73 FR 49942, Aug. 25, 2008]

§812.25 Investigational plan.

The investigational plan shall include, in the following order:

(a) *Purpose.* The name and intended use of the device and the objectives and duration of the investigation.

(b) *Protocol.* A written protocol describing the methodology to be used and an analysis of the protocol demonstrating that the investigation is scientifically sound.

(c) *Risk analysis.* A description and analysis of all increased risks to which subjects will be exposed by the investigation; the manner in which these risks will be minimized; a justification for the investigation; and a description of the patient population, including the number, age, sex, and condition.

(d) *Description of device.* A description of each important component, ingredient, property, and principle of operation of the device and of each anticipated change in the device during the course of the investigation.

(e) *Monitoring procedures.* The sponsor's written procedures for monitoring the investigation and the name and address of any monitor.

(f) *Labeling.* Copies of all labeling for the device.

(g) *Consent materials.* Copies of all forms and informational materials to be provided to subjects to obtain informed consent.

(h) *IRB information.* A list of the names, locations, and chairpersons of all IRB's that have been or will be asked to review the investigation, and a certification of any action taken by any of those IRB's with respect to the investigation.

(i) *Other institutions.* The name and address of each institution at which a part of the investigation may be conducted that has not been identified in paragraph (h) of this section.

(j) *Additional records and reports.* A description of records and reports that will be maintained on the investigation in addition to those prescribed in subpart G.

§ 812.27 Report of prior investigations.

(a) *General.* The report of prior investigations shall include reports of all prior clinical, animal, and laboratory testing of the device and shall be comprehensive and adequate to justify the proposed investigation.

(b) *Specific contents.* The report also shall include:

(1) A bibliography of all publications, whether adverse or supportive, that are relevant to an evaluation of the safety or effectiveness of the device, copies of all published and unpublished adverse information, and, if requested by an IRB or FDA, copies of other significant publications.

(2) A summary of all other unpublished information (whether adverse or supportive) in the possession of, or reasonably obtainable by, the sponsor that is relevant to an evaluation of the safety or effectiveness of the device.

(3) If information on nonclinical laboratory studies is provided, a statement that all such studies have been conducted in compliance with applicable requirements in the good laboratory practice regulations in part 58, or if any such study was not conducted in compliance with such regulations, a brief statement of the reason for the noncompliance. Failure or inability to comply with this requirement does not justify failure to provide information on a relevant nonclinical test study.

(4)(i) If data from clinical investigations conducted in the United States are provided, a statement that each investigation was conducted in compliance with applicable requirements in the protection of human subjects regulations in part 50 of this chapter, the institutional review boards regulations in part 56 of this chapter, or was not subject to the regulations under § 56.104 or § 56.105, and the investigational device exemptions regulations in this part, or if any such investigation was not conducted in compliance with those regulations, a brief statement of the reason for the noncompliance. Failure or inability to comply with these requirements does not justify failure to provide information on a relevant clinical investigation.

(ii) If data from clinical investigations conducted outside the United States are provided to support the IDE, the requirements under § 812.28 apply. If any such investigation was not conducted in accordance with good clinical practice (GCP) as described in § 812.28(a), the report of prior investigations shall include either a waiver request in accordance with § 812.28(c) or a brief statement of the reason for not conducting the investigation in accordance with GCP and a description of steps taken to ensure that the data and results are credible and accurate and that the rights, safety, and well-being of subjects have been adequately protected. Failure or inability to comply with these requirements does not justify failure to provide information on a relevant clinical investigation.

[45 FR 3751, Jan. 18, 1980, as amended at 50 FR 7518, Feb. 22, 1985; 83 FR 7385, Feb. 21, 2018]

§ 812.28 Acceptance of data from clinical investigations conducted outside the United States.

(a) *Acceptance of data from clinical investigations conducted outside the United States to support an IDE or a device marketing application or submission (an application under section 515 or 520(m) of the Federal Food, Drug, and Cosmetic Act, a premarket notification submission under section 510(k) of the Federal Food, Drug, and Cosmetic Act, or a request for De Novo classification under section 513(f)(2) of the Federal Food, Drug, and Cosmetic Act).* FDA will accept information on a clinical investigation conducted outside the United States to support an IDE or a device marketing application or submission if the investigation is well-designed and well-conducted and the following conditions are met:

(1) A statement is provided that the investigation was conducted in accordance with good clinical practice (GCP). For the purposes of this section, GCP is defined as a standard for the design, conduct, performance, monitoring, auditing, recording, analysis, and reporting of clinical investigations in a way that provides assurance that the data and results are credible and accurate and that the rights, safety, and well-being of subjects are protected. GCP includes review and approval (or provision of a favorable opinion) by an independent ethics committee (IEC) before initiating an investigation, continuing review of an ongoing investigation by an IEC, and obtaining and documenting the freely given informed consent of the subject (or a subject's legally authorized representative, if the subject is unable to provide informed consent) before initiating an investigation. GCP does not require informed consent in life-threatening situations when the IEC reviewing the investigation finds, before initiation of the investigation, that informed consent is not feasible and either that the conditions present are consistent with those described in § 50.23 or § 50.24(a) of this chapter, or that the measures described in the protocol or elsewhere will protect the rights, safety, and well-being of subjects.

(2) In addition to the information required elsewhere in parts 807, 812, and 814 of this chapter, as applicable, the information in paragraph (b) of this section is submitted, as follows:

(i) For an investigation of a significant risk device, as defined in § 812.3(m), the supporting information as described in paragraph (b) of this section is submitted.

(ii) For an investigation of a device, other than a significant risk device, the supporting information as described in paragraphs (b)(1), (4), (5), (7) through (9), and (11) of this section is submitted, and the supporting information as described in paragraph (b)(10) of this section and the rationale for determining the investigation is of a device other than a significant risk device are made available for agency review upon request by FDA.

(iii) For a device investigation that meets the exemption criteria in § 812.2(c), the supporting information as described in paragraphs (b)(1), (4), (5), (7) through (11) of this section and the rationale for determining the investigation meets the exemption criteria in § 812.2(c) are made available for agency review upon request by FDA.

(3) FDA is able to validate the data from the investigation through an onsite inspection, or through other appropriate means, if the agency deems it necessary.

(b) *Supporting information.* A sponsor or applicant who submits data from a clinical investigation conducted outside the United States to support an IDE or a device marketing application or submission, in addition to information required elsewhere in parts 807, 812, and 814 of this chapter, as applicable, shall provide a description of the actions the sponsor or applicant took to ensure that the research conformed to GCP as described in paragraph (a)(1) of this section. The description is not required to duplicate information already submitted in the application or submission. Instead, the description must provide either the following information, as specified in paragraph (a)(2) of this section, or a cross-reference to another section of the application or submission where the information is located:

(1) The names of the investigators and the names and addresses of the research facilities and sites where records relating to the investigation are maintained;

(2) The investigator's qualifications;

(3) A description of the research facility(ies);

(4) A detailed summary of the protocol and results of the investigation and, should FDA request, case records maintained by the investigator or additional background data such as hospital or other institutional records;

(5) Either a statement that the device used in the investigation conducted outside the United States is identical to the device that is the subject of the submission or application, or a detailed description of the device and each important component (including all materials and specifications), ingredient, property, and principle of operation of the device used in the investigation conducted outside the United States and a comparison to the device that is the subject of the submission or application that indicates how the device used in the investigation is similar to and/or different from the device that is the subject of the submission or application;

(6) If the investigation is intended to support the safety and effectiveness of a device, a discussion demonstrating that the data and information constitute valid scientific evidence within the meaning of § 860.7 of this chapter;

(7) The name and address of the IEC that reviewed the investigation and a statement that the IEC meets the definition in § 812.3(t). The sponsor or applicant must maintain records supporting such statement, including records describing the qualifications of IEC members, and make these records available for agency review upon request;

(8) A summary of the IEC's decision to approve or modify and approve the investigation, or to provide a favorable opinion;

(9) A description of how informed consent was obtained;

(10) A description of what incentives, if any, were provided to subjects to participate in the investigation; (11) A description of how the sponsor(s) monitored the investigation and ensured that the investigation was carried out consistently with the protocol; and

(12) A description of how investigators were trained to comply with GCP (as described in paragraph (a)(1) of this section) and to conduct the investigation in accordance with the protocol, and a statement on whether written commitments by investigators to comply with GCP and the protocol were obtained. Any signed written commitments by investigators must be maintained by the sponsor or applicant and made available for agency review upon request.

(c) *Waivers.* (1) A sponsor or applicant may ask FDA to waive any applicable requirements under paragraphs (a)(1) and (b) of this section. A waiver request may be submitted in an IDE or in an amendment or supplement to an IDE, in a device marketing application or submission (an application under section 515 or 520(m) of the Federal Food, Drug, and Cosmetic Act, a premarket notification submission under section 510(k) of the Federal Food, Drug, and Cosmetic Act, or a request for De Novo classification under section 513(f)(2) of the Federal Food, Drug, and Cosmetic Act) or in an amendment or supplement to a device marketing application or submission, or in a pre-submission. A waiver request is required to contain at least one of the following:

(i) An explanation why the sponsor's or applicant's compliance with the requirement is unnecessary or cannot be achieved;

(ii) A description of an alternative submission or course of action that satisfies the purpose of the requirement; or

(iii) Other information justifying a waiver.

(2) FDA may grant a waiver if it finds that doing so would be in the interest of the public health.

(d) *Records.* A sponsor or applicant must retain the records required by this section for a clinical investigation conducted outside the United States as follows:

(1) If the investigation is submitted in support of an IDE, for 2 years after the termination or completion of the IDE; and

(2) If the investigation is submitted in support of a premarket approval application, a notice of completion of a product development protocol, a humanitarian device exemption application, a premarket notification submission, or a request for De Novo classification, for 2 years after an agency decision on that submission or application.

(e) *Clinical investigations conducted outside of the United States that do not meet conditions.* For clinical investigations conducted outside the United States that do not meet the conditions under paragraph (a) of this section, FDA may accept the information from such clinical investigations to support an IDE or a device marketing application or submission if FDA believes that the data and results from such clinical investigation are credible and accurate and that the rights, safety, and well-being of subjects have been adequately protected.

[83 FR 7386, Feb. 21, 2018]

§ 812.30 FDA action on applications.

(a) *Approval or disapproval.* FDA will notify the sponsor in writing of the date it receives an application. FDA may approve an investigation as proposed, approve it with modifications, or disapprove it. An investigation may not begin until:

(1) Thirty days after FDA receives the application at the address in § 812.19 for the investigation of a device other than a banned device, unless FDA notifies the sponsor that the investigation may not begin; or

(2) FDA approves, by order, an IDE for the investigation.

(b) *Grounds for disapproval or withdrawal.* FDA may disapprove or withdraw approval of an application if FDA finds that:

(1) There has been a failure to comply with any requirement of this part or the act, any other applicable regulation or statute, or any condition of approval imposed by an IRB or FDA.

(2) The application or a report contains an untrue statement of a material fact, or omits material information required by this part.

(3) The sponsor fails to respond to a request for additional information within the time prescribed by FDA.

(4) There is reason to believe that the risks to the subjects are not outweighed by the anticipated benefits to the subjects and the importance of the knowledge to be gained, or informed consent is inadequate, or the investigation is scientifically unsound, or there is reason to believe that the device as used is ineffective.

(5) It is otherwise unreasonable to begin or to continue the investigation owing to the way in which the device is used or the inadequacy of:

(i) The report of prior investigations or the investigational plan;

(ii) The methods, facilities, and controls used for the manufacturing, processing, packaging, storage, and, where appropriate, installation of the device; or

(iii) Monitoring and review of the investigation.

(c) *Notice of disapproval or withdrawal.* If FDA disapproves an application or proposes to withdraw approval of an application, FDA will notify the sponsor in writing.

(1) A disapproval order will contain a complete statement of the reasons for disapproval and a statement that the sponsor has an opportunity to request a hearing under part 16.

(2) A notice of a proposed withdrawal of approval will contain a complete statement of the reasons for withdrawal and a statement that the sponsor has an opportunity to request a hearing under part 16. FDA will provide the opportunity for hearing before withdrawal of approval, unless FDA determines in the notice that continuation of testing under the exemption will result in an unreasonble risk to the public health and orders withdrawal of approval before any hearing.

[45 FR 3751, Jan. 18, 1980, as amended at 45 FR 58842, Sept. 5, 1980]

§ 812.35 Supplemental applications.

(a) *Changes in investigational plan*—(1) *Changes requiring prior approval.* Except as described in paragraphs (a)(2) through (a)(4) of this section, a sponsor must obtain approval of a supplemental application under § 812.30(a), and IRB approval when appropriate (see §§ 56.110 and 56.111 of this chapter), prior to implementing a change to an investigational plan. If a sponsor intends to conduct an investigation that involves an exception to informed consent under § 50.24 of this chapter, the sponsor shall submit a separate investigational device exemption (IDE) application in accordance with § 812.20(a).

(2) *Changes effected for emergency use.* The requirements of paragraph (a)(1) of this section regarding FDA approval of a supplement do not apply in the case of a deviation from the investigational plan to protect the life or physical well-being of a subject in an emergency. Such deviation shall be reported to FDA within 5-working days after the sponsor learns of it (see § 812.150(a)(4)).

(3) *Changes effected with notice to FDA within 5 days.* A sponsor may make certain changes without prior approval of a supplemental application under paragraph (a)(1) of this section if the sponsor determines that these changes meet the criteria described in paragraphs (a)(3)(i) and (a)(3)(ii) of this section, on the basis of credible information defined in paragraph (a)(3)(iii) of this section, and the sponsor provides notice to FDA within 5-working days of making these changes.

(i) *Developmental changes.* The requirements in paragraph (a)(1) of this section regarding FDA approval of a supplement do not apply to developmental changes in the device (including manufacturing changes) that do not constitute a significant change in design or basic principles of operation and that are made in response to information gathered during the course of an investigation.

(ii) *Changes to clinical protocol.* The requirements in paragraph (a)(1) of this section regarding FDA approval of a supplement do not apply to changes to clinical protocols that do not affect:

(A) The validity of the data or information resulting from the completion of the approved protocol, or the relationship of likely patient risk to benefit relied upon to approve the protocol;

(B) The scientific soundness of the investigational plan; or

(C) The rights, safety, or welfare of the human subjects involved in the investigation.

(iii) *Definition of credible information.* (A) Credible information to support developmental changes in the device (including manufacturing changes) includes data generated under the design control procedures of § 820.30, preclinical/animal testing, peer reviewed published literature, or other reliable information such as clinical information gathered during a trial or marketing.

(B) Credible information to support changes to clinical protocols is defined as the sponsor's documentation supporting the conclusion that a change does not have a significant impact on the study design or planned statistical analysis, and that the change does not affect the rights, safety, or welfare of the subjects. Documentation shall include information such as peer reviewed published literature, the recommendation of the clinical investigator(s), and/or the data gathered during the clinical trial or marketing.

(iv) *Notice of IDE change.* Changes meeting the criteria in paragraphs (a)(3)(i) and (a)(3)(ii) of this section that are supported by credible information as defined in paragraph (a)(3)(iii) of this section may be made without prior FDA approval if the sponsor submits a notice of the change to the IDE not later than 5-working days after making the change. Changes to devices are deemed to occur on the date the device, manufactured incorporating the design or manufacturing change, is distributed to the investigator(s). Changes to a clinical protocol are deemed to occur when a clinical investigator is notified by the sponsor that the change should be implemented in the protocol or, for sponsor-investigator studies, when a sponsor-investigator incorporates the change in the protocol. Such notices shall be identified as a "notice of IDE change."

(A) For a developmental or manufacturing change to the device, the notice shall include a summary of the relevant information gathered during the course of the investigation upon which the change was based; a description of the change to the device or manufacturing process (cross-referenced to the appropriate sections of the original device description or manufacturing process); and, if design controls were used to assess the change, a statement that no new risks were identified by appropriate risk analysis and that the verification and validation testing, as appropriate, demonstrated that the design outputs met the design input requirements. If another method of assessment was used, the notice shall include a summary of the information which served as the credible information supporting the change.

(B) For a protocol change, the notice shall include a description of the change (cross-referenced to the appropriate sections of the original protocol); an assessment supporting the conclusion that the change does not have a significant impact on the study design or planned statistical analysis; and a summary of the information that served as the credible information supporting the sponsor's determination that the change does not affect the rights, safety, or welfare of the subjects.

(4) *Changes submitted in annual report.* The requirements of paragraph (a)(1) of this section do not apply to minor changes to the purpose of the study, risk analysis, monitoring procedures, labeling, informed consent materials, and IRB information that do not affect:

(i) The validity of the data or information resulting from the completion of the approved protocol, or the relationship of likely patient risk to benefit relied upon to approve the protocol;

(ii) The scientific soundness of the investigational plan; or

(iii) The rights, safety, or welfare of the human subjects involved in the investigation. Such changes shall be reported in the annual progress report for the IDE, under § 812.150(b)(5).

(b) *IRB approval for new facilities.* A sponsor shall submit to FDA a certification of any IRB approval of an investigation or a part of an investigation not included in the IDE application. If the investigation is otherwise unchanged, the supplemental application shall consist of an updating of the information required by § 812.20(b) and (c) and a description of any modifications in the investigational plan required by the IRB as a condition of approval. A certification of IRB approval need not be included in the initial submission of the supplemental application, and such certification is not a precondition for agency consideration of the application. Nevertheless, a sponsor may not begin a part of an investigation at a facility until the IRB has approved the investigation, FDA has received the certification of IRB approval, and FDA, under § 812.30(a), has approved the supplemental application relating to that part of the investigation (see § 56.103(a)).

[50 FR 25909, June 24, 1985; 50 FR 28932, July 17, 1985, as amended at 61 FR 51531, Oct. 2, 1996; 63 FR 64625, Nov. 23, 1998]

§ 812.36 Treatment use of an investigational device.

(a) *General.* A device that is not approved for marketing may be under clinical investigation for a serious or immediately life-threatening disease or condition in patients for whom no comparable or satisfactory alternative device or other therapy is available. During the clinical trial or prior to final action on the marketing application, it may be appropriate to use the device in the treatment of patients not in the trial under the provisions of a treatment investigational device exemption (IDE). The purpose of this section is to facilitate the availability of promising new devices to desperately ill patients as early in the device development process as possible, before general marketing begins, and to obtain additional data on the device's safety and effectiveness. In the case of a serious disease, a device ordinarily may be made available for treatment use under this section after all clinical trials have been completed. In the case of an immediately life-threatening disease, a device may be made available for treatment use under this section prior to the completion of all clinical trials. For the purpose of this section, an "immediately life-threatening" disease means a stage of a disease in which there is a reasonable likelihood that death will occur within a matter of months or in which premature death is likely without early treatment. For purposes of this section, "treatment use"of a device includes the use of a device for diagnostic purposes.

(b) *Criteria.* FDA shall consider the use of an investigational device under a treatment IDE if:

(1) The device is intended to treat or diagnose a serious or immediately life-threatening disease or condition;

(2) There is no comparable or satisfactory alternative device or other therapy available to treat or diagnose that stage of the disease or condition in the intended patient population;

(3) The device is under investigation in a controlled clinical trial for the same use under an approved IDE, or such clinical trials have been completed; and

(4) The sponsor of the investigation is actively pursuing marketing approval/clearance of the investigational device with due diligence.

(c) *Applications for treatment use.* (1) A treatment IDE application shall include, in the following order:

(i) The name, address, and telephone number of the sponsor of the treatment IDE;

(ii) The intended use of the device, the criteria for patient selection, and a written protocol describing the treatment use;

(iii) An explanation of the rationale for use of the device, including, as appropriate, either a list of the available regimens that ordinarily should be tried before using the investigational device or an explanation of why the use of the investigational device is preferable to the use of available marketed treatments;

(iv) A description of clinical procedures, laboratory tests, or other measures that will be used to evaluate the effects of the device and to minimize risk;

(v) Written procedures for monitoring the treatment use and the name and address of the monitor;

(vi) Instructions for use for the device and all other labeling as required under § 812.5(a) and (b);

(vii) Information that is relevant to the safety and effectiveness of the device for the intended treatment use. Information from other IDE's may be incorporated by reference to support the treatment use;

(viii) A statement of the sponsor's commitment to meet all applicable responsibilities under this part and part 56 of this chapter and to ensure compliance of all participating investigators with the informed consent requirements of part 50 of this chapter;

(ix) An example of the agreement to be signed by all investigators participating in the treatment IDE and certification that no investigator will be added to the treatment IDE before the agreement is signed; and

(x) If the device is to be sold, the price to be charged and a statement indicating that the price is based on manufacturing and handling costs only.

(2) A licensed practitioner who receives an investigational device for treatment use under a treatment IDE is an "investigator" under the IDE and is responsible for meeting all applicable investigator responsibilities under this part and parts 50 and 56 of this chapter.

(d) *FDA action on treatment IDE applications*—(1) *Approval of treatment IDE's.* Treatment use may begin 30 days after FDA receives the treatment IDE submission at the address specified in §812.19, unless FDA notifies the sponsor in writing earlier than the 30 days that the treatment use may or may not begin. FDA may approve the treatment use as proposed or approve it with modifications.

(2) *Disapproval or withdrawal of approval of treatment IDE's.* FDA may disapprove or withdraw approval of a treatment IDE if:

(i) The criteria specified in §812.36(b) are not met or the treatment IDE does not contain the information required in §812.36(c);

(ii) FDA determines that any of the grounds for disapproval or withdrawal of approval listed in §812.30(b)(1) through (b)(5) apply;

(iii) The device is intended for a serious disease or condition and there is insufficient evidence of safety and effectiveness to support such use;

(iv) The device is intended for an immediately life-threatening disease or condition and the available scientific evidence, taken as a whole, fails to provide a reasonable basis for concluding that the device:

(A) May be effective for its intended use in its intended population; or

(B) Would not expose the patients to whom the device is to be administered to an unreasonable and significant additional risk of illness or injury;

(v) There is reasonable evidence that the treatment use is impeding enrollment in, or otherwise interfering with the conduct or completion of, a controlled investigation of the same or another investigational device;

(vi) The device has received marketing approval/clearance or a comparable device or therapy becomes available to treat or diagnose the same indication in the same patient population for which the investigational device is being used;

(vii) The sponsor of the controlled clinical trial is not pursuing marketing approval/clearance with due diligence;

(viii) Approval of the IDE for the controlled clinical investigation of the device has been withdrawn; or

(ix) The clinical investigator(s) named in the treatment IDE are not qualified by reason of their scientific training and/or experience to use the investigational device for the intended treatment use.

(3) *Notice of disapproval or withdrawal.* If FDA disapproves or proposes to withdraw approval of a treatment IDE, FDA will follow the procedures set forth in §812.30(c).

(e) *Safeguards.* Treatment use of an investigational device is conditioned upon the sponsor and investigators complying with the safeguards of the IDE process and the regulations governing informed consent (part 50 of this chapter) and institutional review boards (part 56 of this chapter).

(f) *Reporting requirements.* The sponsor of a treatment IDE shall submit progress reports on a semi-annual basis to all reviewing IRB's and FDA until the filing of a marketing application. These reports shall be based on the period of time since initial approval of the treatment IDE and shall include the number of patients treated with the device under the treatment IDE, the names of the investigators participating in the treatment IDE, and a brief description of the sponsor's efforts to pursue marketing approval/clearance of the device. Upon filing of a marketing application, progress reports shall be submitted annually in accordance with § 812.150(b)(5). The sponsor of a treatment IDE is responsible for submitting all other reports required under § 812.150.

[62 FR 48947, Sept. 18, 1997]

§ 812.38 Confidentiality of data and information.

(a) *Existence of IDE.* FDA will not disclose the existence of an IDE unless its existence has previously been publicly disclosed or acknowledged, until FDA approves an application for premarket approval of the device subject to the IDE; or a notice of completion of a product development protocol for the device has become effective.

(b) *Availability of summaries or data.* (1) FDA will make publicly available, upon request, a detailed summary of information concerning the safety and effectiveness of the device that was the basis for an order approving, disapproving, or withdrawing approval of an application for an IDE for a banned device. The summary shall include information on any adverse effect on health caused by the device.

(2) If a device is a banned device or if the existence of an IDE has been publicly disclosed or acknowledged, data or information contained in the file is not available for public disclosure before approval of an application for premarket approval or the effective date of a notice of completion of a product development protocol except as provided in this section. FDA may, in its discretion, disclose a summary of selected portions of the safety and effectiveness data, that is, clinical, animal, or laboratory studies and tests of the device, for public consideration of a specific pending issue.

(3) If the existence of an IDE file has not been publicly disclosed or acknowledged, no data or information in the file are available for public disclosure except as provided in paragraphs (b)(1) and (c) of this section.

(4) Notwithstanding paragraph (b)(2) of this section, FDA will make available to the public, upon request, the information in the IDE that was required to be filed in Docket Number 95S-0158 in the Division of Dockets Management (HFA-305), Food and Drug Administration, 5630 Fishers Lane, rm. 1061, Rockville, MD 20852, for investigations involving an exception from informed consent under § 50.24 of this chapter. Persons wishing to request this information shall submit a request under the Freedom of Information Act.

(c) *Reports of adverse effects.* Upon request or on its own initiative, FDA shall disclose to an individual on whom an investigational device has been used a copy of a report of adverse device effects relating to that use.

(d) *Other rules.* Except as otherwise provided in this section, the availability for public disclosure of data and information in an IDE file shall be handled in accordance with § 814.9.

[45 FR 3751, Jan. 18, 1980, as amended at 53 FR 11253, Apr. 6, 1988; 61 FR 51531, Oct. 2, 1996]

Subpart C—Responsibilities of Sponsors

§812.40 General responsibilities of sponsors.

Sponsors are responsible for selecting qualified investigators and providing them with the information they need to conduct the investigation properly, ensuring proper monitoring of the investigation, ensuring that IRB review and approval are obtained, submitting an IDE application to FDA, and ensuring that any reviewing IRB and FDA are promptly informed of significant new information about an investigation. Additional responsibilities of sponsors are described in subparts B and G.

§812.42 FDA and IRB approval.

A sponsor shall not begin an investigation or part of an investigation until an IRB and FDA have both approved the application or supplemental application relating to the investigation or part of an investigation.

[46 FR 8957, Jan. 27, 1981]

§812.43 Selecting investigators and monitors.

(a) *Selecting investigators.* A sponsor shall select investigators qualified by training and experience to investigate the device.

(b) *Control of device.* A sponsor shall ship investigational devices only to qualified investigators participating in the investigation.

(c) *Obtaining agreements.* A sponsor shall obtain from each participating investigator a signed agreement that includes:

(1) The investigator's curriculum vitae.

(2) Where applicable, a statement of the investigator's relevant experience, including the dates, location, extent, and type of experience.

(3) If the investigator was involved in an investigation or other research that was terminated, an explanation of the circumstances that led to termination.

(4) A statement of the investigator's commitment to:

(i) Conduct the investigation in accordance with the agreement, the investigational plan, this part and other applicable FDA regulations, and conditions of approval imposed by the reviewing IRB or FDA;

(ii) Supervise all testing of the device involving human subjects; and

(iii) Ensure that the requirements for obtaining informed consent are met.

(5) Sufficient accurate financial disclosure information to allow the sponsor to submit a complete and accurate certification or disclosure statement as required under part 54 of this chapter. The sponsor shall obtain a commitment from the clinical investigator to promptly update this information if any relevant changes occur during the course of the investigation and for 1 year following completion of the study. This information shall not be submitted in an investigational device exemption application, but shall be submitted in any marketing application involving the device.

(d) *Selecting monitors.* A sponsor shall select monitors qualified by training and experience to monitor the investigational study in accordance with this part and other applicable FDA regulations.

[45 FR 3751, Jan. 18, 1980, as amended at 63 FR 5253, Feb. 2, 1998]

§812.45 Informing investigators.

A sponsor shall supply all investigators participating in the investigation with copies of the investigational plan and the report of prior investigations of the device.

§812.46 Monitoring investigations.

(a) *Securing compliance.* A sponsor who discovers that an investigator is not complying with the signed agreement, the investigational plan, the requirements of this part or other applicable FDA regulations, or any conditions of approval imposed by the reviewing IRB or FDA shall promptly either secure compliance, or discontinue shipments of the device to the investigator and terminate the investigator's participation in the investigation. A sponsor shall also require such an investigator to dispose of or return the device, unless this action would jeopardize the rights, safety, or welfare of a subject.

(b) *Unanticipated adverse device effects.* (1) A sponsor shall immediately conduct an evaluation of any unanticipated adverse device effect.

(2) A sponsor who determines that an unanticipated adverse device effect presents an unreasonable risk to subjects shall terminate all investigations or parts of investigations presenting that risk as soon as possible. Termination shall occur not later than 5 working days after the sponsor makes this determination and not later than 15 working days after the sponsor first received notice of the effect.

(c) *Resumption of terminated studies.* If the device is a significant risk device, a sponsor may not resume a terminated investigation without IRB and FDA approval. If the device is not a significant risk device, a sponsor may not resume a terminated investigation without IRB approval and, if the investigation was terminated under paragraph (b)(2) of this section, FDA approval.

§812.47 Emergency research under §50.24 of this chapter.

(a) The sponsor shall monitor the progress of all investigations involving an exception from informed consent under §50.24 of this chapter. When the sponsor receives from the IRB information concerning the public disclosures under §50.24(a)(7)(ii) and (a)(7)(iii) of this chapter, the sponsor shall promptly submit to the IDE file and to Docket Number 95S-0158 in the Division of Dockets Management (HFA-305), Food and Drug Administration, 5630 Fishers Lane, rm. 1061, Rockville, MD 20852, copies of the information that was disclosed, identified by the IDE number.

(b) The sponsor also shall monitor such investigations to determine when an IRB determines that it cannot approve the research because it does not meet the criteria in the exception in §50.24(a) of this chapter or because of other relevant ethical concerns. The sponsor promptly shall provide this information in writing to FDA, investigators who are asked to participate in this or a substantially equivalent clinical investigation, and other IRB's that are asked to review this or a substantially equivalent investigation.

[61 FR 51531, Oct. 2, 1996, as amended at 64 FR 10943, Mar. 8, 1999]

Subpart D—IRB Review and Approval

§812.60 IRB composition, duties, and functions.

An IRB reviewing and approving investigations under this part shall comply with the requirements of part 56 in all respects, including its composition, duties, and functions.

[46 FR 8957, Jan. 27, 1981]

§812.62 IRB approval.

(a) An IRB shall review and have authority to approve, require modifications in (to secure approval), or disapprove all investigations covered by this part.

(b) If no IRB exists or if FDA finds that an IRB's review is inadequate, a sponsor may submit an application to FDA.

[46 FR 8957, Jan. 27, 1981]

§ 812.64 IRB's continuing review.

The IRB shall conduct its continuing review of an investigation in accordance with part 56.

[46 FR 8957, Jan. 27, 1981]

§ 812.65 [Reserved]

§ 812.66 Significant risk device determinations.

If an IRB determines that an investigation, presented for approval under § 812.2(b)(1)(ii), involves a significant risk device, it shall so notify the investigator and, where appropriate, the sponsor. A sponsor may not begin the investigation except as provided in § 812.30(a).

[46 FR 8957, Jan. 27, 1981]

Subpart E—Responsibilities of Investigators

§ 812.100 General responsibilities of investigators.

An investigator is responsible for ensuring that an investigation is conducted according to the signed agreement, the investigational plan and applicable FDA regulations, for protecting the rights, safety, and welfare of subjects under the investigator's care, and for the control of devices under investigation. An investigator also is responsible for ensuring that informed consent is obtained in accordance with part 50 of this chapter. Additional responsibilities of investigators are described in subpart G.

[45 FR 3751, Jan. 18, 1980, as amended at 46 FR 8957, Jan. 27, 1981]

§ 812.110 Specific responsibilities of investigators.

(a) *Awaiting approval.* An investigator may determine whether potential subjects would be interested in participating in an investigation, but shall not request the written informed consent of any subject to participate, and shall not allow any subject to participate before obtaining IRB and FDA approval.

(b) *Compliance.* An investigator shall conduct an investigation in accordance with the signed agreement with the sponsor, the investigational plan, this part and other applicable FDA regulations, and any conditions of approval imposed by an IRB or FDA.

(c) *Supervising device use.* An investigator shall permit an investigational device to be used only with subjects under the investigator's supervision. An investigator shall not supply an investigational device to any person not authorized under this part to receive it.

(d) *Financial disclosure.* A clinical investigator shall disclose to the sponsor sufficient accurate financial information to allow the applicant to submit complete and accurate certification or disclosure statements required under part 54 of this chapter. The investigator shall promptly update this information if any relevant changes occur during the course of the investigation and for 1 year following completion of the study.

(e) *Disposing of device.* Upon completion or termination of a clinical investigation or the investigator's part of an investigation, or at the sponsor's request, an investigator shall return to the sponsor any remaining supply of the device or otherwise dispose of the device as the sponsor directs.

[45 FR 3751, Jan. 18, 1980, as amended at 63 FR 5253, Feb. 2, 1998]

§ 812.119 Disqualification of a clinical investigator.

(a) If FDA has information indicating that an investigator (including a sponsor-investigator) has repeatedly or deliberately failed to comply with the requirements of this part, part 50, or part 56 of this chapter, or has repeatedly or deliberately submitted to FDA or to the sponsor false information in any required report, the Center for Devices and Radiological Health, the Center for Biologics

Evaluation and Research, or the Center for Drug Evaluation and Research will furnish the investigator written notice of the matter complained of and offer the investigator an opportunity to explain the matter in writing, or, at the option of the investigator, in an informal conference. If an explanation is offered and accepted by the applicable Center, the Center will discontinue the disqualification proceeding. If an explanation is offered but not accepted by the applicable Center, the investigator will be given an opportunity for a regulatory hearing under part 16 of this chapter on the question of whether the investigator is eligible to receive test articles under this part and eligible to conduct any clinical investigation that supports an application for a research or marketing permit for products regulated by FDA.

(b) After evaluating all available information, including any explanation presented by the investigator, if the Commissioner determines that the investigator has repeatedly or deliberately failed to comply with the requirements of this part, part 50, or part 56 of this chapter, or has repeatedly or deliberately submitted to FDA or to the sponsor false information in any required report, the Commissioner will notify the investigator, the sponsor of any investigation in which the investigator has been named as a participant, and the reviewing investigational review boards (IRBs) that the investigator is not eligible to receive test articles under this part. The notification to the investigator, sponsor and IRBs will provide a statement of the basis for such determination. The notification also will explain that an investigator determined to be ineligible to receive test articles under this part will be ineligible to conduct any clinical investigation that supports an application for a research or marketing permit for products regulated by FDA, including drugs, biologics, devices, new animal drugs, foods, including dietary supplements, that bear a nutrient content claim or a health claim, infant formulas, food and color additives, and tobacco products.

(c) Each application or submission to FDA under the provisions of this chapter containing data reported by an investigator who has been determined to be ineligible to receive FDA-regulated test articles is subject to examination to determine whether the investigator has submitted unreliable data that are essential to the continuation of an investigation or essential to the clearance or approval of a marketing application, or essential to the continued marketing of an FDA-regulated product.

(d) If the Commissioner determines, after the unreliable data submitted by the investigator are eliminated from consideration, that the data remaining are inadequate to support a conclusion that it is reasonably safe to continue the investigation, the Commissioner will notify the sponsor, who shall have an opportunity for a regulatory hearing under part 16 of this chapter. If a danger to the public health exists, however, the Commissioner shall terminate the investigational device exemption (IDE) immediately and notify the sponsor and the reviewing IRBs of the termination. In such case, the sponsor shall have an opportunity for a regulatory hearing before FDA under part 16 of this chapter on the question of whether the IDE should be reinstated. The determination that an investigation may not be considered in support of a research or marketing application or a notification or petition submission does not, however, relieve the sponsor of any obligation under any other applicable regulation to submit to FDA the results of the investigation.

(e) If the Commissioner determines, after the unreliable data submitted by the investigator are eliminated from consideration, that the continued clearance or approval of the product for which the data were submitted cannot be justified, the Commissioner will proceed to rescind clearance or withdraw approval of the product in accordance with the applicable provisions of the relevant statutes.

(f) An investigator who has been determined to be ineligible under paragraph (b) of this section may be reinstated as eligible when the Commissioner determines that the investigator has presented adequate assurances that the investigator will employ all test articles, and will conduct any clinical investigation that supports an application for a research or marketing permit for products regulated by FDA, solely in compliance with the applicable provisions of this chapter.

[77 FR 25360, Apr. 30, 2012]

Subpart F—[Reserved]

Subpart G—Records and Reports

§ 812.140 Records.

(a) *Investigator records.* A participating investigator shall maintain the following accurate, complete, and current records relating to the investigator's participation in an investigation:

(1) All correspondence with another investigator, an IRB, the sponsor, a monitor, or FDA, including required reports.

(2) Records of receipt, use or disposition of a device that relate to:

(i) The type and quantity of the device, the dates of its receipt, and the batch number or code mark.

(ii) The names of all persons who received, used, or disposed of each device.

(iii) Why and how many units of the device have been returned to the sponsor, repaired, or otherwise disposed of.

(3) Records of each subject's case history and exposure to the device. Case histories include the case report forms and supporting data including, for example, signed and dated consent forms and medical records including, for example, progress notes of the physician, the individual's hospital chart(s), and the nurses' notes. Such records shall include:

(i) Documents evidencing informed consent and, for any use of a device by the investigator without informed consent, any written concurrence of a licensed physician and a brief description of the circumstances justifying the failure to obtain informed consent. The case history for each individual shall document that informed consent was obtained prior to participation in the study.

(ii) All relevant observations, including records concerning adverse device effects (whether anticipated or unanticipated), information and data on the condition of each subject upon entering, and during the course of, the investigation, including information about relevant previous medical history and the results of all diagnostic tests.

(iii) A record of the exposure of each subject to the investigational device, including the date and time of each use, and any other therapy.

(4) The protocol, with documents showing the dates of and reasons for each deviation from the protocol.

(5) Any other records that FDA requires to be maintained by regulation or by specific requirement for a category of investigations or a particular investigation.

(b) *Sponsor records.* A sponsor shall maintain the following accurate, complete, and current records relating to an investigation:

(1) All correspondence with another sponsor, a monitor, an investigator, an IRB, or FDA, including required reports.

(2) Records of shipment and disposition. Records of shipment shall include the name and address of the consignee, type and quantity of device, date of shipment, and batch number or code mark. Records of disposition shall describe the batch number or code marks of any devices returned to the sponsor, repaired, or disposed of in other ways by the investigator or another person, and the reasons for and method of disposal.

(3) Signed investigator agreements including the financial disclosure information required to be collected under § 812.43(c)(5) in accordance with part 54 of this chapter.

(4) For each investigation subject to § 812.2(b)(1) of a device other than a significant risk device, the records described in paragraph (b)(5) of this section and the following records, consolidated in one location and available for FDA inspection and copying:

(i) The name and intended use of the device and the objectives of the investigation;

(ii) A brief explanation of why the device is not a significant risk device:

(iii) The name and address of each investigator:

(iv) The name and address of each IRB that has reviewed the investigation:

(v) A statement of the extent to which the good manufacturing practice regulation in part 820 will be followed in manufacturing the device; and

(vi) Any other information required by FDA.

(5) Records concerning adverse device effects (whether anticipated or unanticipated) and complaints and

(6) Any other records that FDA requires to be maintained by regulation or by specific requirement for a category of investigation or a particular investigation.

(c) *IRB records.* An IRB shall maintain records in accordance with part 56 of this chapter.

(d) *Retention period.* An investigator or sponsor shall maintain the records required by this subpart during the investigation and for a period of 2 years after the latter of the following two dates: The date on which the investigation is terminated or completed, or the date that the records are no longer required for purposes of supporting a premarket approval application, a notice of completion of a product development protocol, a humanitarian device exemption application, a premarket notification submission, or a request for De Novo classification.

(e) *Records custody.* An investigator or sponsor may withdraw from the responsibility to maintain records for the period required in paragraph (d) of this section and transfer custody of the records to any other person who will accept responsibility for them under this part, including the requirements of § 812.145. Notice of a transfer shall be given to FDA not later than 10 working days after transfer occurs.

[45 FR 3751, Jan. 18, 1980, as amended at 45 FR 58843, Sept. 5, 1980; 46 FR 8957, Jan. 27, 1981; 61 FR 57280, Nov. 5, 1996; 63 FR 5253, Feb. 2, 1998; 83 FR 7387, Feb. 21, 2018]

§ 812.145 Inspections.

(a) Entry and inspection. A sponsor or an investigator who has authority to grant access shall permit authorized FDA employees, at reasonable times and in a reasonable manner, to enter and inspect any establishment where devices are held (including any establishment where devices are manufactured, processed, packed, installed, used, or implanted or where records of results from use of devices are kept).

(b) *Records inspection.* A sponsor, IRB, or investigator, or any other person acting on behalf of such a person with respect to an investigation, shall permit authorized FDA employees, at reasonable times and in a reasonable manner, to inspect and copy all records relating to an investigation.

(c) *Records identifying subjects.* An investigator shall permit authorized FDA employees to inspect and copy records that identify subjects, upon notice that FDA has reason to suspect that adequate informed consent was not obtained, or that reports required to be submitted by the investigator to the sponsor or IRB have not been submitted or are incomplete, inaccurate, false, or misleading.

§ 812.150 Reports.

(a) *Investigator reports.* An investigator shall prepare and submit the following complete, accurate, and timely reports:

(1) *Unanticipated adverse device effects.* An investigator shall submit to the sponsor and to the reviewing IRB a report of any unanticipated adverse device effect occurring during an investigation as soon as possible, but in no event later than 10 working days after the investigator first learns of the effect.

(2) *Withdrawal of IRB approval.* An investigator shall report to the sponsor, within 5 working days, a withdrawal of approval by the reviewing IRB of the investigator's part of an investigation.

(3) *Progress.* An investigator shall submit progress reports on the investigation to the sponsor, the monitor, and the reviewing IRB at regular intervals, but in no event less often than yearly.

(4) *Deviations from the investigational plan.* An investigator shall notify the sponsor and the reviewing IRB (see § 56.108(a) (3) and (4)) of any deviation from the investigational plan to protect the life or physical well-being of a subject in an emergency. Such notice shall be given as soon as possible, but in no event later than 5 working days after the emergency occurred. Except in such an emergency, prior approval by the sponsor is required for changes in or deviations from a plan, and if these changes or deviations may affect the scientific soundness of the plan or the rights, safety, or welfare of human subjects, FDA and IRB in accordance with § 812.35(a) also is required.

(5) *Informed consent.* If an investigator uses a device without obtaining informed consent, the investigator shall report such use to the sponsor and the reviewing IRB within 5 working days after the use occurs.

(6) *Final report.* An investigator shall, within 3 months after termination or completion of the investigation or the investigator's part of the investigation, submit a final report to the sponsor and the reviewing IRB.

(7) *Other.* An investigator shall, upon request by a reviewing IRB or FDA, provide accurate, complete, and current information about any aspect of the investigation.

(b) *Sponsor reports.* A sponsor shall prepare and submit the following complete, accurate, and timely reports:

(1) *Unanticipated adverse device effects.* A sponsor who conducts an evaluation of an unanticipated adverse device effect under § 812.46(b) shall report the results of such evaluation to FDA and to all reviewing IRB's and participating investigators within 10 working days after the sponsor first receives notice of the effect. Thereafter the sponsor shall submit such additional reports concerning the effect as FDA requests.

(2) *Withdrawal of IRB approval.* A sponsor shall notify FDA and all reviewing IRB's and participating investigators of any withdrawal of approval of an investigation or a part of an investigation by a reviewing IRB within 5 working days after receipt of the withdrawal of approval.

(3) *Withdrawal of FDA approval.* A sponsor shall notify all reviewing IRB's and participating investigators of any withdrawal of FDA approval of the investigation, and shall do so within 5 working days after receipt of notice of the withdrawal of approval.

(4) *Current investigator list.* A sponsor shall submit to FDA, at 6-month intervals, a current list of the names and addresses of all investigators participating in the investigation. The sponsor shall submit the first such list 6 months after FDA approval.

(5) *Progress reports.* At regular intervals, and at least yearly, a sponsor shall submit progress reports to all reviewing IRB's. In the case of a significant risk device, a sponsor shall also submit progress reports to FDA. A sponsor of a treatment IDE shall submit semi-annual progress reports to all reviewing IRB's and FDA in accordance with § 812.36(f) and annual reports in accordance with this section.

(6) *Recall and device disposition.* A sponsor shall notify FDA and all reviewing IRB's of any request that an investigator return, repair, or otherwise dispose of any units of a device. Such notice shall occur within 30 working days after the request is made and shall state why the request was made.

(7) *Final report.* In the case of a significant risk device, the sponsor shall notify FDA within 30 working days of the completion or termination of the investigation and shall submit a final report to FDA and all reviewing the IRB's and participating investigators within 6 months after completion or termination. In the case of a device that is not a significant risk device, the sponsor shall submit a final report to all reviewing IRB's within 6 months after termination or completion.

(8) *Informed consent.* A sponsor shall submit to FDA a copy of any report by an investigator under paragraph (a)(5) of this section of use of a device without obtaining informed consent, within 5 working days of receipt of notice of such use.

(9) *Significant risk device determinations.* If an IRB determines that a device is a significant risk device, and the sponsor had proposed that the IRB consider the device not to be a significant risk device, the sponsor shall submit to FDA a report of the IRB's determination within 5 working days after the sponsor first learns of the IRB's determination.

(10) *Other.* A sponsor shall, upon request by a reviewing IRB or FDA, provide accurate, complete, and current information about any aspect of the investigation.

[45 FR 3751, Jan. 18, 1980, as amended at 45 FR 58843, Sept. 5, 1980; 48 FR 15622, Apr. 12, 1983; 62 FR 48948, Sept. 18, 1997]

• • •

PART 814—PREMARKET APPROVAL OF MEDICAL DEVICES

Authority: 21 U.S.C. 351, 352, 353, 360, 360c-360j, 360bbb-8b, 371, 372, 373, 374, 375, 379, 379e, 381.

Source: 51 FR 26364, July 22, 1986, unless otherwise noted.

Subpart A—General

§ 814.1 Scope.

(a) This section implements sections 515 and 515A of the act by providing procedures for the premarket approval of medical devices intended for human use.

(b) References in this part to regulatory sections of the Code of Federal Regulations are to chapter I of title 21, unless otherwise noted.

(c) This part applies to any class III medical device, unless exempt under section 520(g) of the act, that:

(1) Was not on the market (introduced or delivered for introduction into commerce for commercial distribution) before May 28, 1976, and is not substantially equivalent to a device on the market before May 28, 1976, or to a device first marketed on, or after that date, which has been classified into class I or class II; or

(2) Is required to have an approved premarket approval application (PMA) or a declared completed product development protocol under a regulation issued under section 515(b) of the act; or

(3) Was regulated by FDA as a new drug or antibiotic drug before May 28, 1976, and therefore is governed by section 520(1) of the act.

(d) This part amends the conditions to approval for any PMA approved before the effective date of this part. Any condition to approval for an approved PMA that is inconsistent with this part is revoked. Any condition to approval for an approved PMA that is consistent with this part remains in effect.

[51 FR 26364, July 22, 1986, as amended at 79 FR 1740, Jan. 10, 2014]

§814.2 Purpose.

The purpose of this part is to establish an efficient and thorough device review process—

(a) To facilitate the approval of PMA's for devices that have been shown to be safe and effective and that otherwise meet the statutory criteria for approval; and

(b) To ensure the disapproval of PMA's for devices that have not been shown to be safe and effective or that do not otherwise meet the statutory criteria for approval. This part shall be construed in light of these objectives.

§814.3 Definitions.

For the purposes of this part:

(a) *Act* means the Federal Food, Drug, and Cosmetic Act (sections 201-902, 52 Stat. 1040 et seq., as amended (21 U.S.C. 321-392)).

(b) *FDA* means the Food and Drug Administration.

(c) *IDE* means an approved or considered approved investigational device exemption under section 520(g) of the act and parts 812 and 813.

(d) *Master file* means a reference source that a person submits to FDA. A master file may contain detailed information on a specific manufacturing facility, process, methodology, or component used in the manufacture, processing, or packaging of a medical device.

(e) *PMA* means any premarket approval application for a class III medical device, including all information submitted with or incorporated by reference therein. "PMA" includes a new drug application for a device under section 520(1) of the act.

(f) *PMA amendment* means information an applicant submits to FDA to modify a pending PMA or a pending PMA supplement.

(g) *PMA supplement* means a supplemental application to an approved PMA for approval of a change or modification in a class III medical device, including all information submitted with or incorporated by reference therein.

(h) *Person* includes any individual, partnership, corporation, association, scientific or academic establishment, Government agency, or organizational unit thereof, or any other legal entity.

(i) *Statement of material fact* means a representation that tends to show that the safety or effectiveness of a device is more probable than it would be in the absence of such a representation. A false affirmation or silence or an omission that would lead a reasonable person to draw a particular conclusion as to the safety or effectiveness of a device also may be a false statement of material fact, even if the statement was not intended by the person making it to be misleading or to have any probative effect.

(j) *30-day PMA supplement* means a supplemental application to an approved PMA in accordance with §814.39(e).

(k) *Reasonable probability* means that it is more likely than not that an event will occur.

(l) *Serious, adverse health consequences* means any significant adverse experience, including those which may be either life-threatening or involve permanent or long term injuries, but excluding injuries that are nonlife-threatening and that are temporary and reasonably reversible.

(m) *HDE* means a premarket approval application submitted pursuant to this subpart seeking a humanitarian device exemption from the effectiveness requirements of sections 514 and 515 of the act as authorized by section 520(m)(2) of the act.

(n) *HUD (humanitarian use device)* means a medical device intended to benefit patients in the treatment or diagnosis of a disease or condition that affects or is manifested in not more than 8,000 individuals in the United States per year.

(o) *Newly acquired information* means data, analyses, or other information not previously submitted to the agency, which may include (but are not limited to) data derived from new clinical studies, reports of adverse events, or new analyses of previously submitted data (e.g., meta-analyses) if the studies, events or analyses reveal risks of a different type or greater severity or frequency than previously included in submissions to FDA.

(p) *Human cell, tissue, or cellular or tissue-based product (HCT/P) regulated as a device* means an HCT/P as defined in § 1271.3(d) of this chapter that does not meet the criteria in § 1271.10(a) and that is also regulated as a device.

(q) *Unique device identifier (UDI)* means an identifier that adequately identifies a device through its distribution and use by meeting the requirements of § 830.20 of this chapter. A unique device identifier is composed of:

(1) *A device identifier*—a mandatory, fixed portion of a UDI that identifies the specific version or model of a device and the labeler of that device; and

(2) *A production identifier*—a conditional, variable portion of a UDI that identifies one or more of the following when included on the label of the device:

(i) The lot or batch within which a device was manufactured;

(ii) The serial number of a specific device;

(iii) The expiration date of a specific device;

(iv) The date a specific device was manufactured.

(v) For an HCT/P regulated as a device, the distinct identification code required by § 1271.290(c) of this chapter.

(r) *Universal product code (UPC)* means the product identifier used to identify an item sold at retail in the United States.

(s) *Pediatric patients* means patients who are 21 years of age or younger (that is, from birth through the twenty-first year of life, up to but not including the twenty-second birthday) at the time of the diagnosis or treatment.

(t) *Readily available* means available in the public domain through commonly used public resources for conducting biomedical, regulatory, and medical product research.

[51 FR 26364, July 22, 1986, as amended at 61 FR 15190, Apr. 5, 1996; 61 FR 33244, June 26, 1996; 73 FR 49610, Aug. 22, 2008; 78 FR 55821, Sept. 24, 2013; 79 FR 1740, Jan. 10, 2014; 82 FR 26349, June 7, 2017]

§ 814.9 Confidentiality of data and information in a premarket approval application (PMA) file.

(a) A "PMA file" includes all data and information submitted with or incorporated by reference in the PMA, any IDE incorporated into the PMA, any PMA supplement, any report under § 814.82, any master file, or any other related submission. Any record in the PMA file will be available for public disclosure in accordance with the provisions of this section and part 20. The confidentiality of information in a color additive petition submitted as part of a PMA is governed by § 71.15.

(b) The existence of a PMA file may not be disclosed by FDA before an approval order is issued to the applicant unless it previously has been publicly disclosed or acknowledged.

(c) If the existence of a PMA file has not been publicly disclosed or acknowledged, data or information in the PMA file are not available for public disclosure.

(d)(1) If the existence of a PMA file has been publicly disclosed or acknowledged before an order approving, or an order denying approval of the PMA is issued, data or information contained in the file are not available for public disclosure before such order issues. FDA may, however, disclose a summary of portions of the safety and effectiveness data before an approval order or an order denying approval of the PMA issues if disclosure is relevant to public consideration of a specific pending issue.

(2) Notwithstanding paragraph (d)(1) of this section, FDA will make available to the public upon request the information in the IDE that was required to be filed in Docket Number 95S-0158 in the Division of Dockets Management (HFA-305), Food and Drug Administration, 12420 Parklawn Dr., rm. 1-23, Rockville, MD 20857, for investigations involving an exception from informed consent under § 50.24 of this chapter. Persons wishing to request this information shall submit a request under the Freedom of Information Act.

(e) Upon issuance of an order approving, or an order denying approval of any PMA, FDA will make available to the public the fact of the existence of the PMA and a detailed summary of information submitted to FDA respecting the safety and effectiveness of the device that is the subject of the PMA and that is the basis for the order.

(f) After FDA issues an order approving, or an order denying approval of any PMA, the following data and information in the PMA file are immediately available for public disclosure:

(1) All safety and effectiveness data and information previously disclosed to the public, as such disclosure is defined in § 20.81.

(2) Any protocol for a test or study unless the protocol is shown to constitute trade secret or confidential commercial or financial information under § 20.61.

(3) Any adverse reaction report, product experience report, consumer complaint, and other similar data and information, after deletion of:

(i) Any information that constitutes trade secret or confidential commercial or financial information under § 20.61; and

(ii) Any personnel, medical, and similar information disclosure of which would constitute a clearly unwarranted invasion of personal privacy under § 20.63; provided, however, that except for the information that constitutes trade secret or confidential commercial or financial information under § 20.61, FDA will disclose to a patient who requests a report all the information in the report concerning that patient.

(4) A list of components previously disclosed to the public, as such disclosure is defined in § 20.81.

(5) An assay method or other analytical method, unless it does not serve any regulatory purpose and is shown to fall within the exemption in § 20.61 for trade secret or confidential commercial or financial information.

(6) All correspondence and written summaries of oral discussions relating to the PMA file, in accordance with the provisions of §§ 20.103 and 20.104.

(g) All safety and effectiveness data and other information not previously disclosed to the public are available for public disclosure if any one of the following events occurs and the data and information do not constitute trade secret or confidential commercial or financial information under § 20.61:

(1) The PMA has been abandoned. FDA will consider a PMA abandoned if:

(i)(A) The applicant fails to respond to a request for additional information within 180 days after the date FDA issues the request or

(B) Other circumstances indicate that further work is not being undertaken with respect to it, and

(ii) The applicant fails to communicate with FDA within 7 days after the date on which FDA notifies the applicant that the PMA appears to have been abandoned.

(2) An order denying approval of the PMA has issued, and all legal appeals have been exhausted.

(3) An order withdrawing approval of the PMA has issued, and all legal appeals have been exhausted.

(4) The device has been reclassified.

(5) The device has been found to be substantially equivalent to a class I or class II device.

(6) The PMA is considered voluntarily withdrawn under § 814.44(g).

(h) The following data and information in a PMA file are not available for public disclosure unless they have been previously disclosed to the public, as such disclosure is defined in § 20.81, or they relate to a device for which a PMA has been abandoned and they no longer represent a trade secret or confidential commercial or financial information as defined in § 20.61:

(1) Manufacturing methods or processes, including quality control procedures.

(2) Production, sales, distribution, and similar data and information, except that any compilation of such data and information aggregated and prepared in a way that does not reveal data or information which are not available for public disclosure under this provision is available for public disclosure.

(3) Quantitative or semiquantitative formulas.

[51 FR 26364, July 22, 1986, as amended at 61 FR 51531, Oct. 2, 1996]

§ 814.15 Research conducted outside the United States.

(a) *Data to support PMA.* If data from clinical investigations conducted outside the United States are submitted to support a PMA, the applicant shall comply with the provisions in § 812.28 of this chapter, as applicable.

(b) *As sole basis for marketing approval.* A PMA based solely on foreign clinical data and otherwise meeting the criteria for approval under this part may be approved if:

(1) The foreign data are applicable to the U.S. population and U.S. medical practice;

(2) The studies have been performed by clinical investigators of recognized competence; and

(3) The data may be considered valid without the need for an on-site inspection by FDA or, if FDA considers such an inspection to be necessary, FDA can validate the data through an on-site inspection or other appropriate means.

(c) *Consultation between FDA and applicants.* Applicants are encouraged to meet with FDA officials in a "presubmission" meeting when approval based solely on foreign data will be sought.

[51 FR 26364, July 22, 1986; 51 FR 40415, Nov. 7, 1986, as amended at 51 FR 43344, Dec. 2, 1986; 83 FR 7387, Feb. 21, 2018]

§ 814.17 Service of orders.

Orders issued under this part will be served in person by a designated officer or employee of FDA on, or by registered mail to, the applicant or the designated agent at the applicant's or designated agent's last known address in FDA's records.

§ 814.19 Product development protocol (PDP).

A class III device for which a product development protocol has been declared completed by FDA under this chapter will be considered to have an approved PMA.

Subpart B—Premarket Approval Application (PMA)

§814.20 Application.

(a) The applicant or an authorized representative shall sign the PMA. If the applicant does not reside or have a place of business within the United States, the PMA shall be countersigned by an authorized representative residing or maintaining a place of business in the United States and shall identify the representative's name and address.

(b) Unless the applicant justifies an omission in accordance with paragraph (d) of this section, a PMA shall include:

(1) The name and address of the applicant.

(2) A table of contents that specifies the volume and page number for each item referred to in the table. A PMA shall include separate sections on nonclinical laboratory studies and on clinical investigations involving human subjects. A PMA shall be submitted in six copies each bound in one or more numbered volumes of reasonable size. The applicant shall include information that it believes to be trade secret or confidential commercial or financial information in all copies of the PMA and identify in at least one copy the information that it believes to be trade secret or confidential commercial or financial information.

(3) A summary in sufficient detail that the reader may gain a general understanding of the data and information in the application. The summary shall contain the following information:

(i) *Indications for use.* A general description of the disease or condition the device will diagnose, treat, prevent, cure, or mitigate, including a description of the patient population for which the device is intended.

(ii) *Device description.* An explanation of how the device functions, the basic scientific concepts that form the basis for the device, and the significant physical and performance characteristics of the device. A brief description of the manufacturing process should be included if it will significantly enhance the reader's understanding of the device. The generic name of the device as well as any proprietary name or trade name should be included.

(iii) *Alternative practices and procedures.* A description of existing alternative practices or procedures for diagnosing, treating, preventing, curing, or mitigating the disease or condition for which the device is intended.

(iv) *Marketing history.* A brief description of the foreign and U.S. marketing history, if any, of the device, including a list of all countries in which the device has been marketed and a list of all countries in which the device has been withdrawn from marketing for any reason related to the safety or effectiveness of the device. The description shall include the history of the marketing of the device by the applicant and, if known, the history of the marketing of the device by any other person.

(v) *Summary of studies.* An abstract of any information or report described in the PMA under paragraph (b)(8)(ii) of this section and a summary of the results of technical data submitted under paragraph (b)(6) of this section. Such summary shall include a description of the objective of the study, a description of the experimental design of the study, a brief description of how the data were collected and analyzed, and a brief description of the results, whether positive, negative, or inconclusive. This section shall include the following:

(A) A summary of the nonclinical laboratory studies submitted in the application;

(B) A summary of the clinical investigations involving human subjects submitted in the application including a discussion of subject selection and exclusion criteria, study population, study period, safety and effectiveness data, adverse reactions and complications, patient discontinuation, patient complaints, device failures and replacements, results of statistical analyses of the clinical investigations, contraindications and precautions for use of the device, and other information from the clinical investigations as appropriate (any investigation conducted under an IDE shall be identified as such).

(vi) *Conclusions drawn from the studies.* A discussion demonstrating that the data and information in the application constitute valid scientific evidence within the meaning of §860.7 and provide reasonable assurance that the device is safe and effective for its intended use. A concluding discussion shall present benefit and risk considerations related to the device including a discussion of any adverse effects of the device on health and any proposed additional studies or surveillance the applicant intends to conduct following approval of the PMA.

(4) A complete description of:

(i) The device, including pictorial representations;

(ii) Each of the functional components or ingredients of the device if the device consists of more than one physical component or ingredient;

(iii) The properties of the device relevant to the diagnosis, treatment, prevention, cure, or mitigation of a disease or condition;

(iv) The principles of operation of the device; and

(v) The methods used in, and the facilities and controls used for, the manufacture, processing, packing, storage, and, where appropriate, installation of the device, in sufficient detail so that a person generally familiar with current good manufacturing practice can make a knowledgeable judgment about the quality control used in the manufacture of the device.

(5) Reference to any performance standard under section 514 of the act or under section 534 of Subchapter C—Electronic Product Radiation Control of the Federal Food, Drug, and Cosmetic Act (formerly the Radiation Control for Health and Safety Act of 1968) in effect or proposed at the time of the submission and to any voluntary standard that is relevant to any aspect of the safety or effectiveness of the device and that is known to or that should reasonably be known to the applicant. The applicant shall—

(i) Provide adequate information to demonstrate how the device meets, or justify any deviation from, any performance standard established under section 514 of the act or under section 534 of Subchapter C—Electronic Product Radiation Control of the Federal Food, Drug, and Cosmetic Act (formerly the Radiation Control for Health and Safety Act of 1968), and

(ii) Explain any deviation from a voluntary standard.

(6) The following technical sections which shall contain data and information in sufficient detail to permit FDA to determine whether to approve or deny approval of the application:

(i) A section containing results of the nonclinical laboratory studies with the device including microbiological, toxicological, immunological, biocompatibility, stress, wear, shelf life, and other laboratory or animal tests as appropriate. Information on nonclinical laboratory studies shall include a statement that each such study was conducted in compliance with part 58, or, if the study was not conducted in compliance with such regulations, a brief statement of the reason for the noncompliance.

(ii) A section containing results of the clinical investigations involving human subjects with the device including clinical protocols, number of investigators and subjects per investigator, subject selection and exclusion criteria, study population, study period, safety and effectiveness data, adverse reactions and complications, patient discontinuation, patient complaints, device failures and replacements, tabulations of data from all individual subject report forms and copies of such forms for each subject who died during a clinical investigation or who did not complete the investigation, results of statistical analyses of the clinical investigations, device failures and replacements, contraindications and precautions for use of the device, and any other appropriate information from the clinical investigations. Any investigation conducted under an IDE shall be identified as such. Information on clinical investigations involving human subjects shall include the following:

(A) For clinical investigations conducted in the United States, a statement with respect to each investigation that it either was conducted in compliance with the institutional review board regulations in part 56 of this chapter, or was not subject to the regulations under § 56.104 or § 56.105, and that it was conducted in compliance with the informed consent regulations in part 50 of this chapter; or if the investigation was not conducted in compliance with those regulations, a brief statement of the reason for the noncompliance. Failure or inability to comply with these requirements does not justify failure to provide information on a relevant clinical investigation.

(B) For clinical investigations conducted in the United States, a statement that each investigation was conducted in compliance with part 812 of this chapter concerning sponsors of clinical investigations and clinical investigators, or if the investigation was not conducted in compliance with those regulations, a brief statement of the reason for the noncompliance. Failure or inability to comply with these requirements does not justify failure to provide information on a relevant clinical investigation.

(C) For clinical investigations conducted outside the United States that are intended to support the PMA, the requirements under § 812.28 of this chapter apply. If any such investigation was not conducted in accordance with good clinical practice (GCP) as described in § 812.28(a), include either a waiver request in accordance with § 812.28(c) or a brief statement of the reason for not conducting the investigation in accordance with GCP and a description of steps taken to ensure that the data and results are credible and accurate and that the rights, safety, and well-being of subjects have been adequately protected. Failure or inability to comply with these requirements does not justify failure to provide information on a relevant clinical investigation.

(7) For a PMA supported solely by data from one investigation, a justification showing that data and other information from a single investigator are sufficient to demonstrate the safety and effectiveness of the device and to ensure reproducibility of test results.

(8)(i) A bibliography of all published reports not submitted under paragraph (b)(6) of this section, whether adverse or supportive, known to or that should reasonably be known to the applicant and that concern the safety or effectiveness of the device.

(ii) An identification, discussion, and analysis of any other data, information, or report relevant to an evaluation of the safety and effectiveness of the device known to or that should reasonably be known to the applicant from any source, foreign or domestic, including information derived from investigations other than those proposed in the application and from commercial marketing experience.

(iii) Copies of such published reports or unpublished information in the possession of or reasonably obtainable by the applicant if an FDA advisory committee or FDA requests.

(9) One or more samples of the device and its components, if requested by FDA. If it is impractical to submit a requested sample of the device, the applicant shall name the location at which FDA may examine and test one or more devices.

(10) Copies of all proposed labeling for the device. Such labeling may include, e.g., instructions for installation and any information, literature, or advertising that constitutes labeling under section 201(m) of the act.

(11) An environmental assessment under § 25.20(n) prepared in the applicable format in § 25.40, unless the action qualifies for exclusion under § 25.30 or § 25.34. If the applicant believes that the action qualifies for exclusion, the PMA shall under § 25.15(a) and (d) provide information that establishes to FDA's satisfaction that the action requested is included within the excluded category and meets the criteria for the applicable exclusion.

(12) A financial certification or disclosure statement or both as required by part 54 of this chapter.

(13) *Information concerning uses in pediatric patients.* The application must include the following information, if readily available:

(i) A description of any pediatric subpopulations (neonates, infants, children, adolescents) that suffer from the disease or condition that the device is intended to treat, diagnose, or cure; and

(ii) The number of affected pediatric patients.

(14) Such other information as FDA may request. If necessary, FDA will obtain the concurrence of the appropriate FDA advisory committee before requesting additional information.

(c) Pertinent information in FDA files specifically referred to by an applicant may be incorporated into a PMA by reference. Information in a master file or other information submitted to FDA by a person other than the applicant will not be considered part of a PMA unless such reference is authorized in writing by the person who submitted the information or the master file. If a master file is not referenced within 5 years after the date that it is submitted to FDA, FDA will return the master file to the person who submitted it.

(d) If the applicant believes that certain information required under paragraph (b) of this section to be in a PMA is not applicable to the device that is the subject of the PMA, and omits any such information from its PMA, the applicant shall submit a statement that identifies the omitted information and justifies the omission. The statement shall be submitted as a separate section in the PMA and identified in the table of contents. If the justification for the omission is not accepted by the agency, FDA will so notify the applicant.

(e) The applicant shall periodically update its pending application with new safety and effectiveness information learned about the device from ongoing or completed studies that may reasonably affect an evaluation of the safety or effectiveness of the device or that may reasonably affect the statement of contraindications, warnings, precautions, and adverse reactions in the draft labeling. The update report shall be consistent with the data reporting provisions of the protocol. The applicant shall submit three copies of any update report and shall include in the report the number assigned by FDA to the PMA. These updates are considered to be amendments to the PMA. The time frame for review of a PMA will not be extended due to the submission of an update report unless the update is a major amendment under § 814.37(c)(1). The applicant shall submit these reports—

(1) 3 months after the filing date,

(2) Following receipt of an approvable letter, and

(3) At any other time as requested by FDA.

(f) If a color additive subject to section 721 of the act is used in or on the device and has not previously been listed for such use, then, in lieu of submitting a color additive petition under part 71, at the option of the applicant, the information required to be submitted under part 71 may be submitted as part of the PMA. When submitted as part of the PMA, the information shall be submitted in three copies each bound in one or more numbered volumes of reasonable size. A PMA for a device that contains a color additive that is subject to section 721 of the act will not be approved until the color additive is listed for use in or on the device.

(g) Additional information on FDA policies and procedures, as well as links to PMA guidance documents, is available on the Internet at *http://www.fda.gov/MedicalDevices/DeviceRegulationandGuidance/HowtoMarketYourDevice/PremarketSubmissions/PremarketApprovalPMA/default.htm.*

(h) If you are sending a PMA, PMA amendment, PMA supplement, or correspondence with respect to a PMA, you must send the submission to the appropriate address as follows:

(1) For devices regulated by the Center for Devices and Radiological Health, Food and Drug Administration, Center for Devices and Radiological Health, Document Mail Center, 10903 New Hampshire Ave., Bldg. 66, rm. G609, Silver Spring, MD 20993-0002.

(2) For devices regulated by the Center for Biologics Evaluation and Research, send it to: Food and Drug Administration, Center for Biologics Evaluation and Research, Document Control Center, 10903 New Hampshire Ave., Bldg. 71, Rm. G112, Silver Spring, MD 20993-0002.

(3) For devices regulated by the Center for Drug Evaluation and Research, send it to: Central Document Control Room, Center for Drug Evaluation and Research, Food and Drug Administration, 5901-B Ammendale Rd., Beltsville, MD 20705-1266.

[51 FR 26364, July 22, 1986; 51 FR 40415, Nov. 7, 1986, as amended at 51 FR 43344, Dec. 2, 1986; 55 FR 11169, Mar. 27, 1990; 62 FR 40600, July 29, 1997; 63 FR 5253, Feb. 2, 1998; 65 FR 17137, Mar. 31, 2000; 65 FR 56480, Sept. 19, 2000; 67 FR 9587, Mar. 4, 2002; 71 FR 42048, July 25, 2006; 72 FR 17399, Apr. 9, 2007; 73 FR 34859, June 19, 2008; 74 FR 14478, Mar. 31, 2009; 75 FR 20915, Apr. 22, 2010; 78 FR 18233, Mar. 26, 2013; 79 FR 1740, Jan. 10, 2014; 80 FR 18094, Apr. 3, 2015; 83 FR 7387, Feb. 21, 2018]

§ 814.37 PMA amendments and resubmitted PMAs.

(a) An applicant may amend a pending PMA or PMA supplement to revise existing information or provide additional information.

(b)(1) FDA may request the applicant to amend a PMA or PMA supplement with any information regarding the device that is necessary for FDA or the appropriate advisory committee to complete the review of the PMA or PMA supplement.

(2) FDA may request the applicant to amend a PMA or PMA supplement with information concerning pediatric uses as required under §§ 814.20(b)(13) and 814.39(c)(2).

(c) A PMA amendment submitted to FDA shall include the PMA or PMA supplement number assigned to the original submission and, if submitted on the applicant's own initiative, the reason for submitting the amendment. FDA may extend the time required for its review of the PMA, or PMA supplement, as follows:

(1) If the applicant on its own initiative or at FDA's request submits a major PMA amendment (e.g., an amendment that contains significant new data from a previously unreported study, significant updated data from a previously reported study, detailed new analyses of previously submitted data, or significant required information previously omitted), the review period may be extended up to 180 days.

(2) If an applicant declines to submit a major amendment requested by FDA, the review period may be extended for the number of days that elapse between the date of such request and the date that FDA receives the written response declining to submit the requested amendment.

(d) An applicant may on its own initiative withdraw a PMA or PMA supplement. If FDA requests an applicant to submit a PMA amendment and a written response to FDA's request is not received within 180 days of the date of the request, FDA will consider the pending PMA or PMA supplement to be withdrawn voluntarily by the applicant.

(e) An applicant may resubmit a PMA or PMA supplement after withdrawing it or after it is considered withdrawn under paragraph (d) of this section, or after FDA has refused to accept it for filing, or has denied approval of the PMA or PMA supplement. A resubmitted PMA or PMA supplement shall comply with the requirements of § 814.20 or § 814.39, respectively, and shall include the PMA number assigned to the original submission and the applicant's reasons for resubmission of the PMA or PMA supplement.

[51 FR 26364, July 22, 1986, as amended at 79 FR 1740, Jan. 10, 2014]

§814.39 PMA supplements.

(a) After FDA's approval of a PMA, an applicant shall submit a PMA supplement for review and approval by FDA before making a change affecting the safety or effectiveness of the device for which the applicant has an approved PMA, unless the change is of a type for which FDA, under paragraph (e) of this section, has advised that an alternate submission is permitted or is of a type which, under section 515(d)(6)(A) of the act and paragraph (f) of this section, does not require a PMA supplement under this paragraph. While the burden for determining whether a supplement is required is primarily on the PMA holder, changes for which an applicant shall submit a PMA supplement include, but are not limited to, the following types of changes if they affect the safety or effectiveness of the device:

(1) New indications for use of the device.

(2) Labeling changes.

(3) The use of a different facility or establishment to manufacture, process, or package the device.

(4) Changes in sterilization procedures.

(5) Changes in packaging.

(6) Changes in the performance or design specifications, circuits, components, ingredients, principle of operation, or physical layout of the device.

(7) Extension of the expiration date of the device based on data obtained under a new or revised stability or sterility testing protocol that has not been approved by FDA. If the protocol has been approved, the change shall be reported to FDA under paragraph (b) of this section.

(b) An applicant may make a change in a device after FDA's approval of a PMA for the device without submitting a PMA supplement if the change does not affect the device's safety or effectiveness and the change is reported to FDA in postapproval periodic reports required as a condition to approval of the device, e.g., an editorial change in labeling which does not affect the safety or effectiveness of the device.

(c)(1) All procedures and actions that apply to an application under §814.20 also apply to PMA supplements except that the information required in a supplement is limited to that needed to support the change. A summary under §814.20(b)(3) is required for only a supplement submitted for new indications for use of the device, significant changes in the performance or design specifications, circuits, components, ingredients, principles of operation, or physical layout of the device, or when otherwise required by FDA. The applicant shall submit three copies of a PMA supplement and shall include information relevant to the proposed changes in the device. A PMA supplement shall include a separate section that identifies each change for which approval is being requested and explains the reason for each such change. The applicant shall submit additional copies and additional information if requested by FDA. The time frames for review of, and FDA action on, a PMA supplement are the same as those provided in §814.40 for a PMA.

(2) The supplement must include the following information:

(i) Information concerning pediatric uses as required under §814.20(b)(13).

(ii) If information concerning the device that is the subject of the supplement was previously submitted under §814.20(b)(13) or under this section in a previous supplement, that information may be included by referencing a previous application or submission that contains the information. However, if additional information required under §814.20(b)(13) has become readily available to the applicant since the previous submission, the applicant must submit that information as part of the supplement.

(d)(1) After FDA approves a PMA, any change described in paragraph (d)(2) of this section to reflect newly acquired information that enhances the safety of the device or the safety in the use of the device may be placed into effect by the applicant prior to the receipt under § 814.17 of a written FDA order approving the PMA supplement provided that:

(i) The PMA supplement and its mailing cover are plainly marked "Special PMA Supplement—Changes Being Effected";

(ii) The PMA supplement provides a full explanation of the basis for the changes;

(iii) The applicant has received acknowledgement from FDA of receipt of the supplement; and

(iv) The PMA supplement specifically identifies the date that such changes are being effected.

(2) The following changes are permitted by paragraph (d)(1) of this section:

(i) Labeling changes that add or strengthen a contraindication, warning, precaution, or information about an adverse reaction for which there is reasonable evidence of a causal association.

(ii) Labeling changes that add or strengthen an instruction that is intended to enhance the safe use of the device.

(iii) Labeling changes that delete misleading, false, or unsupported indications.

(iv) Changes in quality controls or manufacturing process that add a new specification or test method, or otherwise provide additional assurance of purity, identity, strength, or reliability of the device.

(e)(1) FDA will identify a change to a device for which an applicant has an approved PMA and for which a PMA supplement under paragraph (a) is not required. FDA will identify such a change in an advisory opinion under § 10.85, if the change applies to a generic type of device, or in correspondence to the applicant, if the change applies only to the applicant's device. FDA will require that a change for which a PMA supplement under paragraph (a) is not required be reported to FDA in:

(i) A periodic report under § 814.84 or

(ii) A 30-day PMA supplement under this paragraph.

(2) FDA will identify, in the advisory opinion or correspondence, the type of information that is to be included in the report or 30-day PMA supplement. If the change is required to be reported to FDA in a periodic report, the change may be made before it is reported to FDA. If the change is required to be reported in a 30-day PMA supplement, the change may be made 30 days after FDA files the 30-day PMA supplement unless FDA requires the PMA holder to provide additional information, informs the PMA holder that the supplement is not approvable, or disapproves the supplement. The 30-day PMA supplement shall follow the instructions in the correspondence or advisory opinion. Any 30-day PMA supplement that does not meet the requirements of the correspondence or advisory opinion will not be filed and, therefore, will not be deemed approved 30 days after receipt.

(f) Under section 515(d) of the act, modifications to manufacturing procedures or methods of manufacture that affect the safety and effectiveness of a device subject to an approved PMA do not require submission of a PMA supplement under paragraph (a) of this section and are eligible to be the subject of a 30-day notice. A 30-day notice shall describe in detail the change, summarize the data or information supporting the change, and state that the change has been made in accordance with the requirements of part 820 of this chapter. The manufacturer may distribute the device 30 days after the date on which FDA receives the 30-day notice, unless FDA notifies the applicant within 30 days from receipt of the notice that the notice is not adequate. If the notice is not adequate, FDA shall inform the applicant in writing that a 135-day PMA supplement is needed and shall describe what further information or action is required for acceptance of such change. The number of days under review as a 30-day notice shall be deducted from the 135-day PMA supplement review period if the notice meets appropriate content requirements for a PMA supplement.

(g) The submission and grant of a written request for an exception or alternative under § 801.128 or § 809.11 of this chapter satisfies the requirement in paragraph (a) of this section.

[51 FR 26364, July 22, 1986, as amended at 51 FR 43344, Dec. 2, 1986; 63 FR 54044, Oct. 8, 1998; 67 FR 9587, Mar. 4, 2002; 69 FR 11313, Mar. 10, 2004; 72 FR 73602, Dec. 28, 2007; 73 FR 49610, Aug. 22, 2008; 79 FR 1740, Jan. 10, 2014]

Subpart C—FDA Action on a PMA

§ 814.40 Time frames for reviewing a PMA.

Within 180 days after receipt of an application that is accepted for filing and to which the applicant does not submit a major amendment, FDA will review the PMA and, after receiving the report and recommendation of the appropriate FDA advisory committee, send the applicant an approval order under § 814.44(d), an approvable letter under § 814.44(e), a not approvable letter under § 814.44(f), or an order denying approval under § 814.45. The approvable letter and the not approvable letter will provide an opportunity for the applicant to amend or withdraw the application, or to consider the letter to be a denial of approval of the PMA under § 814.45 and to request administrative review under section 515 (d)(3) and (g) of the act.

§ 814.42 Filing a PMA.

(a) The filing of an application means that FDA has made a threshold determination that the application is sufficiently complete to permit a substantive review. Within 45 days after a PMA is received by FDA, the agency will notify the applicant whether the application has been filed.

(b) If FDA does not find that any of the reasons in paragraph (e) of this section for refusing to file the PMA applies, the agency will file the PMA and will notify the applicant in writing of the filing. The notice will include the PMA reference number and the date FDA filed the PMA. The date of filing is the date that a PMA accepted for filing was received by the agency. The 180-day period for review of a PMA starts on the date of filing.

(c) If FDA refuses to file a PMA, the agency will notify the applicant of the reasons for the refusal. This notice will identify the deficiencies in the application that prevent filing and will include the PMA reference number.

(d) If FDA refuses to file the PMA, the applicant may:

(1) Resubmit the PMA with additional information necessary to comply with the requirements of section 515(c)(1) (A)-(G) of the act and § 814.20. A resubmitted PMA shall include the PMA reference number of the original submission. If the resubmitted PMA is accepted for filing, the date of filing is the date FDA receives the resubmission;

(2) Request in writing within 10 working days of the date of receipt of the notice refusing to file the PMA, an informal conference with the Director of the Office of Device Evaluation to review FDA's decision not to file the PMA. FDA will hold the informal conference within 10 working days of its receipt of the request and will render its decision on filing within 5 working days after the informal conference. If, after the informal conference, FDA accepts the PMA for filing, the date of filing will be the date of the decision to accept the PMA for filing. If FDA does not reverse its decision not to file the PMA, the applicant may request reconsideration of the decision from the Director of the Center for Devices and Radiological Health, the Director of the Center for Biologics Evaluation and Research, or the Director of the Center for Drug Evaluation and Research, as applicable. The Director's decision will constitute final administrative action for the purpose of judicial review.

(e) FDA may refuse to file a PMA if any of the following applies:

(1) The application is incomplete because it does not on its face contain all the information required under section 515(c)(1) (A)-(G) of the act;

(2) The PMA does not contain each of the items required under § 814.20 and justification for omission of any item is inadequate;

(3) The applicant has a pending premarket notification under section 510(k) of the act with respect to the same device, and FDA has not determined whether the device falls within the scope of § 814.1(c).

(4) The PMA contains a false statement of material fact.

(5) The PMA is not accompanied by a statement of either certification or disclosure as required by part 54 of this chapter.

[51 FR 26364, July 22, 1986, as amended at 63 FR 5254, Feb. 2, 1998; 73 FR 49942, Aug. 25, 2008]

§ 814.44 Procedures for review of a PMA.

(a) FDA will begin substantive review of a PMA after the PMA is accepted for filing under § 814.42. FDA may refer the PMA to a panel on its own initiative, and will do so upon request of an applicant, unless FDA determines that the application substantially duplicates information previously reviewed by a panel. If FDA refers an application to a panel, FDA will forward the PMA, or relevant portions thereof, to each member of the appropriate FDA panel for review. During the review process, FDA may communicate with the applicant as set forth under § 814.37(b), or with a panel to respond to questions that may be posed by panel members or to provide additional information to the panel. FDA will maintain a record of all communications with the applicant and with the panel.

(b) The advisory committee shall submit a report to FDA which includes the committee's recommendation and the basis for such recommendation on the PMA. Before submission of this report, the committee shall hold a public meeting to review the PMA in accordance with part 14. This meeting may be held by a telephone conference under § 14.22(g). The advisory committee report and recommendation may be in the form of a meeting transcript signed by the chairperson of the committee.

(c) FDA will complete its review of the PMA and the advisory committee report and recommendation and, within the later of 180 days from the date of filing of the PMA under § 814.42 or the number of days after the date of filing as determined under § 814.37(c), issue an approval order under paragraph (d) of this section, an approvable letter under paragraph (e) of this section, a not approvable letter under paragraph (f) of this section, or an order denying approval of the application under § 814.45(a).

(d)(1) FDA will issue to the applicant an order approving a PMA if none of the reasons in § 814.45 for denying approval of the application applies. FDA will approve an application on the basis of draft final labeling if the only deficiencies in the application concern editorial or similar minor deficiencies in the draft final labeling. Such approval will be conditioned upon the applicant incorporating the specified labeling changes exactly as directed and upon the applicant submitting to FDA a copy of the final printed labeling before marketing. FDA will also give the public notice of the order, including notice of and opportunity for any interested persons to request review under section 515(d)(3) of the act. The notice of approval will be placed on FDA's home page on the Internet (*http://www.fda.gov*), and it will state that a detailed summary of information respecting the safety and effectiveness of the device, which was the basis for the order approving the PMA, including information about any adverse effects of the device on health, is available on the Internet and has been placed on public display, and that copies are available upon request. FDA will publish in the Federal Register after each quarter a list of the approvals announced in that quarter. When a notice of approval is published, data and information in the PMA file will be available for public disclosure in accordance with § 814.9.

(2) A request for copies of the current PMA approvals and denials document and for copies of summaries of safety and effectiveness shall be sent in writing to the Division of Dockets Management (HFA-305), Food and Drug Administration, 5630 Fishers Lane, rm. 1061, Rockville, MD 20852.

(e) FDA will send the applicant an approvable letter if the application substantially meets the requirements of this part and the agency believes it can approve the application if specific additional information is submitted or specific conditions are agreed to by the applicant.

(1) The approvable letter will describe the information FDA requires to be provided by the applicant or the conditions the applicant is required to meet to obtain approval. For example, FDA may require, as a condition to approval:

(i) The submission of certain information identified in the approvable letter, e.g., final labeling;

(ii) The submission of additional information concerning pediatric uses required by § 814.20(b)(13);

(iii) An FDA inspection that finds the manufacturing facilities, methods, and controls in compliance with part 820 and, if applicable, that verifies records pertinent to the PMA;

(iv) Restrictions imposed on the device under section 515(d)(1)(B)(ii) or 520(e) of the act;

(v) Postapproval requirements as described in subpart E of this part.

(2) In response to an approvable letter the applicant may:

(i) Amend the PMA as requested in the approvable letter; or

(ii) Consider the approvable letter to be a denial of approval of the PMA under § 814.45 and request administrative review under section 515(d)(3) of the act by filing a petition in the form of a petition for reconsideration under § 10.33; or

(iii) Withdraw the PMA.

(f) FDA will send the applicant a not approvable letter if the agency believes that the application may not be approved for one or more of the reasons given in § 814.45(a). The not approvable letter will describe the deficiencies in the application, including each applicable ground for denial under section 515(d)(2) (A)-(E) of the act, and, where practical, will identify measures required to place the PMA in approvable form. In response to a not approvable letter, the applicant may:

(1) Amend the PMA as requested in the not approvable letter (such an amendment will be considered a major amendment under § 814.37(c)(1)); or

(2) Consider the not approvable letter to be a denial of approval of the PMA under § 814.45 and request administrative review under section 515(d)(3) of the act by filing a petition in the form of a petition for reconsideration under § 10.33; or

(3) Withdraw the PMA.

(g) FDA will consider a PMA to have been withdrawn voluntarily if:

(1) The applicant fails to respond in writing to a written request for an amendment within 180 days after the date FDA issues such request;

(2) The applicant fails to respond in writing to an approvable or not approvable letter within 180 days after the date FDA issues such letter; or

(3) The applicant submits a written notice to FDA that the PMA has been withdrawn.

[51 FR 26364, July 22, 1986, as amended at 57 FR 58403, Dec. 10, 1992; 63 FR 4572, Jan. 30, 1998; 79 FR 1740, Jan. 10, 2014]

§ 814.45 Denial of approval of a PMA.

(a) FDA may issue an order denying approval of a PMA if the applicant fails to follow the requirements of this part or if, upon the basis of the information submitted in the PMA or any other information before the agency, FDA determines that any of the grounds for denying approval of a PMA specified in section 515(d)(2) (A)-(E) of the act applies. In addition, FDA may deny approval of a PMA for any of the following reasons:

(1) The PMA contains a false statement of material fact;

(2) The device's proposed labeling does not comply with the requirements in part 801 or part 809;

(3) The applicant does not permit an authorized FDA employee an opportunity to inspect at a reasonable time and in a reasonable manner the facilities, controls, and to have access to and to copy and verify all records pertinent to the application;

(4) A nonclinical laboratory study that is described in the PMA and that is essential to show that the device is safe for use under the conditions prescribed, recommended, or suggested in its proposed labeling, was not conducted in compliance with the good laboratory practice regulations in part 58 and no reason for the noncompliance is provided or, if it is, the differences between the practices used in conducting the study and the good laboratory practice regulations do not support the validity of the study; or

(5) Any clinical investigation involving human subjects described in the PMA, subject to the institutional review board regulations in part 56 of this chapter or informed consent regulations in part 50 of this chapter or GCP referenced in § 814.15(a) and described in § 812.28(a) of this chapter, was not conducted in compliance with those regulations such that the rights or safety of human subjects were not adequately protected or the supporting data were determined to be otherwise unreliable.

(b) FDA will issue any order denying approval of the PMA in accordance with § 814.17. The order will inform the applicant of the deficiencies in the PMA, including each applicable ground for denial under section 515(d)(2) of the act and the regulations under this part, and, where practical, will identify measures required to place the PMA in approvable form. The order will include a notice of an opportunity to request review under section 515(d)(4) of the act.

(c) FDA will use the criteria specified in § 860.7 to determine the safety and effectiveness of a device in deciding whether to approve or deny approval of a PMA. FDA may use information other than that submitted by the applicant in making such determination.

(d)(1) FDA will give the public notice of an order denying approval of the PMA. The notice will be placed on the FDA's home page on the Internet (*http://www.fda.gov*), and it will state that a detailed summary of information respecting the safety and effectiveness of the device, including information about any adverse effects of the device on health, is available on the Internet and has been placed on public display and that copies are available upon request. FDA will publish in the Federal Register after each quarter a list of the denials announced in that quarter. When a notice of denial of approval is made publicly available, data and information in the PMA file will be available for public disclosure in accordance with § 814.9.

(2) A request for copies of the current PMA approvals and denials document and copies of summaries of safety and effectiveness shall be sent in writing to the Freedom of Information Staff's address listed on the Agency's Web site at *http://www.fda.gov.*

(e) FDA will issue an order denying approval of a PMA after an approvable or not approvable letter has been sent and the applicant:

(1) Submits a requested amendment but any ground for denying approval of the application under section 515(d)(2) of the act still applies; or

(2) Notifies FDA in writing that the requested amendment will not be submitted; or

(3) Petitions for review under section 515(d)(3) of the act by filing a petition in the form of a petition for reconsideration under § 10.33.

[51 FR 26364, July 22, 1986, as amended at 63 FR 4572, Jan. 30, 1998; 73 FR 34859, June 19, 2008; 76 FR 31470, June 1, 2011; 79 FR 68115, Nov. 14, 2014; 83 FR 7387, Feb. 21, 2018]

§814.46 Withdrawal of approval of a PMA.

(a) FDA may issue an order withdrawing approval of a PMA if, from any information available to the agency, FDA determines that:

(1) Any of the grounds under section 515(e)(1) (A)-(G) of the act applies.

(2) Any postapproval requirement imposed by the PMA approval order or by regulation has not been met.

(3) A nonclinical laboratory study that is described in the PMA and that is essential to show that the device is safe for use under the conditions prescribed, recommended, or suggested in its proposed labeling, was not conducted in compliance with the good laboratory practice regulations in part 58 and no reason for the noncompliance is provided or, if it is, the differences between the practices used in conducting the study and the good laboratory practice regulations do not support the validity of the study.

(4) Any clinical investigation involving human subjects described in the PMA, subject to the institutional review board regulations in part 56 of this chapter or informed consent regulations in part 50 of this chapter or GCP referenced in §814.15(a) and described in §812.28(a) of this chapter, was not conducted in compliance with those regulations such that the rights or safety of human subjects were not adequately protected or the supporting data were determined to be otherwise unreliable.

(b)(1) FDA may seek advice on scientific matters from any appropriate FDA advisory committee in deciding whether to withdraw approval of a PMA.

(2) FDA may use information other than that submitted by the applicant in deciding whether to withdraw approval of a PMA.

(c) Before issuing an order withdrawing approval of a PMA, FDA will issue the holder of the approved application a notice of opportunity for an informal hearing under part 16.

(d) If the applicant does not request a hearing or if after the part 16 hearing is held the agency decides to proceed with the withdrawal, FDA will issue to the holder of the approved application an order withdrawing approval of the application. The order will be issued under §814.17, will state each ground for withdrawing approval, and will include a notice of an opportunity for administrative review under section 515(e)(2) of the act.

(e) FDA will give the public notice of an order withdrawing approval of a PMA. The notice will be published in the Federal Register and will state that a detailed summary of information respecting the safety and effectiveness of the device, including information about any adverse effects of the device on health, has been placed on public display and that copies are available upon request. When a notice of withdrawal of approval is published, data and information in the PMA file will be available for public disclosure in accordance with §814.9.

[51 FR 26364, July 22, 1986, as amended at 83 FR 7387, Feb. 21, 2018]

§814.47 Temporary suspension of approval of a PMA.

(a) *Scope.* (1) This section describes the procedures that FDA will follow in exercising its authority under section 515(e)(3) of the act (21 U.S.C. 360e(e)(3)). This authority applies to the original PMA, as well as any PMA supplement(s), for a medical device.

(2) FDA will issue an order temporarily suspending approval of a PMA if FDA determines that there is a reasonable probability that continued distribution of the device would cause serious, adverse health consequences or death.

(b) *Regulatory hearing.* (1) If FDA believes that there is a reasonable probability that the continued distribution of a device subject to an approved PMA would cause serious, adverse health consequences or death, FDA may initiate and conduct a regulatory hearing to determine whether to issue an order temporarily suspending approval of the PMA.

(2) Any regulatory hearing to determine whether to issue an order temporarily suspending approval of a PMA shall be initiated and conducted by FDA pursuant to part 16 of this chapter. If FDA believes that immediate action to remove a dangerous device from the market is necessary to protect the public health, the agency may, in accordance with § 16.60(h) of this chapter, waive, suspend, or modify any part 16 procedure pursuant to § 10.19 of this chapter.

(3) FDA shall deem the PMA holder's failure to request a hearing within the timeframe specified by FDA in the notice of opportunity for hearing to be a waiver.

(c) *Temporary suspension order.* If the PMA holder does not request a regulatory hearing or if, after the hearing, and after consideration of the administrative record of the hearing, FDA determines that there is a reasonable probability that the continued distribution of a device under an approved PMA would cause serious, adverse health consequences or death, the agency shall, under the authority of section 515(e)(3) of the act, issue an order to the PMA holder temporarily suspending approval of the PMA.

(d) *Permanent withdrawal of approval of the PMA.* If FDA issues an order temporarily suspending approval of a PMA, the agency shall proceed expeditiously, but within 60 days, to hold a hearing on whether to permanently withdraw approval of the PMA in accordance with section 515(e)(1) of the act and the procedures set out in § 814.46.

[61 FR 15190, Apr. 5, 1996]

Subpart D—Administrative Review [Reserved]

Subpart E—Postapproval Requirements

§ 814.80 General.

A device may not be manufactured, packaged, stored, labeled, distributed, or advertised in a manner that is inconsistent with any conditions to approval specified in the PMA approval order for the device.

§ 814.82 Postapproval requirements.

(a) FDA may impose postapproval requirements in a PMA approval order or by regulation at the time of approval of the PMA or by regulation subsequent to approval. Postapproval requirements may include as a condition to approval of the device:

(1) Restriction of the sale, distribution, or use of the device as provided by section 515(d)(1)(B)(ii) or 520(e) of the act.

(2) Continuing evaluation and periodic reporting on the safety, effectiveness, and reliability of the device for its intended use. FDA will state in the PMA approval order the reason or purpose for such requirement and the number of patients to be evaluated and the reports required to be submitted.

(3) Prominent display in the labeling of a device and in the advertising of any restricted device of warnings, hazards, or precautions important for the device's safe and effective use, including patient information, e.g., information provided to the patient on alternative modes of therapy and on risks and benefits associated with the use of the device.

(4) Inclusion of identification codes on the device or its labeling, or in the case of an implant, on cards given to patients if necessary to protect the public health.

(5) Maintenance of records that will enable the applicant to submit to FDA information needed to trace patients if such information is necessary to protect the public health. Under section 519(a)(4) of the act, FDA will require that the identity of any patient be disclosed in records maintained under this paragraph only to the extent required for the medical welfare of the individual, to determine

the safety or effectiveness of the device, or to verify a record, report, or information submitted to the agency.

(6) Maintenance of records for specified periods of time and organization and indexing of records into identifiable files to enable FDA to determine whether there is reasonable assurance of the continued safety and effectiveness of the device.

(7) Submission to FDA at intervals specified in the approval order of periodic reports containing the information required by §814.84(b).

(8) Batch testing of the device.

(9) Such other requirements as FDA determines are necessary to provide reasonable assurance, or continued reasonable assurance, of the safety and effectiveness of the device.

(b) An applicant shall grant to FDA access to any records and reports required under the provisions of this part, and shall permit authorized FDA employees to copy and verify such records and reports and to inspect at a reasonable time and in a reasonable manner all manufacturing facilities to verify that the device is being manufactured, stored, labeled, and shipped under approved conditions.

(c) Failure to comply with any postapproval requirement constitutes a ground for withdrawal of approval of a PMA.

(Approved by the Office of Management and Budget under control number 0910-0231)

[51 FR 26364, July 22, 1986, as amended at 51 FR 43344, Dec. 2, 1986]

§814.84 Reports.

(a) The holder of an approved PMA shall comply with the requirements of part 803 and with any other requirements applicable to the device by other regulations in this subchapter or by order approving the device.

(b) Unless FDA specifies otherwise, any periodic report shall:

(1) Identify changes described in §814.39(a) and changes required to be reported to FDA under §814.39(b).

(2) Contain a summary and bibliography of the following information not previously submitted as part of the PMA:

(i) Unpublished reports of data from any clinical investigations or nonclinical laboratory studies involving the device or related devices and known to or that reasonably should be known to the applicant.

(ii) Reports in the scientific literature concerning the device and known to or that reasonably should be known to the applicant. If, after reviewing the summary and bibliography, FDA concludes that the agency needs a copy of the unpublished or published reports, FDA will notify the applicant that copies of such reports shall be submitted.

(3) Identify changes made pursuant to an exception or alternative granted under §801.128 or §809.11 of this chapter.

(4) Identify each device identifier currently in use for the device, and each device identifier for the device that has been discontinued since the previous periodic report. It is not necessary to identify any device identifier discontinued prior to December 23, 2013.

[51 FR 26364, July 22, 1986, as amended at 51 FR 43344, Dec. 2, 1986; 67 FR 9587, Mar. 4, 2002; 72 FR 73602, Dec. 28, 2007; 78 FR 58822, Sept. 24, 2013]

Subparts F-G [Reserved]

Subpart H—Humanitarian Use Devices

Source: 61 FR 33244, June 26, 1996, unless otherwise noted.

§ 814.100 Purpose and scope.

(a) This subpart H implements sections 515A and 520(m) of the act.

(b) The purpose of section 520(m) is, to the extent consistent with the protection of the public health and safety and with ethical standards, to encourage the discovery and use of devices intended to benefit patients in the treatment or diagnosis of diseases or conditions that affect or are manifested in not more than 8,000 individuals in the United States per year. This subpart provides procedures for obtaining:

(1) HUD designation of a medical device; and

(2) Marketing approval for the HUD notwithstanding the absence of reasonable assurance of effectiveness that would otherwise be required under sections 514 and 515 of the act.

(c) Section 515A of the act is intended to ensure the submission of readily available information concerning:

(1) Any pediatric subpopulations (neonates, infants, children, adolescents) that suffer from the disease or condition that the device is intended to treat, diagnose, or cure; and

(2) The number of affected pediatric patients.

(d) Although a HUD may also have uses that differ from the humanitarian use, applicants seeking approval of any non-HUD use shall submit a PMA as required under § 814.20, or a premarket notification as required under part 807 of this chapter.

(e) Obtaining marketing approval for a HUD involves two steps:

(1) Obtaining designation of the device as a HUD from FDA's Office of Orphan Products Development, and

(2) Submitting an HDE to the Office of Device Evaluation (ODE), Center for Devices and Radiological Health (CDRH), the Center for Biologics Evaluation and Research (CBER), or the Center for Drug Evaluation and Research (CDER), as applicable.

(f) A person granted an exemption under section 520(m) of the act shall submit periodic reports as described in § 814.126(b).

(g) FDA may suspend or withdraw approval of an HDE after providing notice and an opportunity for an informal hearing.

[61 FR 33244, June 26, 1996, as amended at 63 FR 59220, Nov. 3, 1998; 73 FR 49942, Aug. 25, 2008; 79 FR 1740, Jan. 10, 2014; 82 FR 26349, June 7, 2017]

§ 814.102 Designation of HUD status.

(a) *Request for designation.* Prior to submitting an HDE application, the applicant shall submit a request for HUD designation to FDA's Office of Orphan Products Development. The request shall contain the following:

(1) A statement that the applicant requests HUD designation for a rare disease or condition or a valid subset of a disease or condition which shall be identified with specificity;

(2) The name and address of the applicant, the name of the applicant's primary contact person and/or resident agent, including title, address, and telephone number;

(3) A description of the rare disease or condition for which the device is to be used, the proposed indication or indications for use of the device, and the reasons why such therapy is needed. If the

device is proposed for an indication that represents a subset of a common disease or condition, a demonstration that the subset is medically plausible should be included;

(4) A description of the device and a discussion of the scientific rationale for the use of the device for the rare disease or condition; and

(5) Documentation, with appended authoritative references, to demonstrate that the device is designed to treat or diagnose a disease or condition that affects or is manifested in not more than 8,000 people in the United States per year. If the device is for diagnostic purposes, the documentation must demonstrate that not more than 8,000 patients per year would be subjected to diagnosis by the device in the United States. Authoritative references include literature citations in specialized medical journals, textbooks, specialized medical society proceedings, or governmental statistics publications. When no such studies or literature citations exist, the applicant may be able to demonstrate the prevalence of the disease or condition in the United States by providing credible conclusions from appropriate research or surveys.

(b) *FDA action.* Within 45 days of receipt of a request for HUD designation, FDA will take one of the following actions:

(1) Approve the request and notify the applicant that the device has been designated as a HUD based on the information submitted;

(2) Return the request to the applicant pending further review upon submission of additional information. This action will ensue if the request is incomplete because it does not on its face contain all of the information required under § 814.102(a). Upon receipt of this additional information, the review period may be extended up to 45 days; or

(3) Disapprove the request for HUD designation based on a substantive review of the information submitted. FDA may disapprove a request for HUD designation if:

(i) There is insufficient evidence to support the estimate that the disease or condition for which the device is designed to treat or diagnose affects or is manifested in not more than 8,000 people in the United States per year;

(ii) FDA determines that, for a diagnostic device, more than 8,000 patients in the United States would be subjected to diagnosis using the device per year; or

(iii) FDA determines that the patient population defined in the request is not a medically plausible subset of a larger population.

(c) *Revocation of designation.* FDA may revoke a HUD designation if the agency finds that:

(1) The request for designation contained an untrue statement of material fact or omitted material information; or

(2) Based on the evidence available, the device is not eligible for HUD designation.

(d) *Submission.* The applicant shall submit two copies of a completed, dated, and signed request for HUD designation to: Office of Orphan Products Development (HF-35), Food and Drug Administration, 5600 Fishers Lane, Rockville, MD 20857.

[61 FR 33244, June 26, 1996, as amended at 82 FR 26349, June 7, 2017]

§ 814.104 Original applications.

(a) *United States applicant or representative.* The applicant or an authorized representative shall sign the HDE. If the applicant does not reside or have a place of business within the United States, the HDE shall be countersigned by an authorized representative residing or maintaining a place of business in the United States and shall identify the representative's name and address.

(b) *Contents.* Unless the applicant justifies an omission in accordance with paragraph (d) of this section, an HDE shall include:

(1) A copy of or reference to the determination made by FDA's Office of Orphan Products Development (in accordance with § 814.102) that the device qualifies as a HUD;

(2) An explanation of why the device would not be available unless an HDE were granted and a statement that no comparable device (other than another HUD approved under this subpart or a device under an approved IDE) is available to treat or diagnose the disease or condition. The application also shall contain a discussion of the risks and benefits of currently available devices or alternative forms of treatment in the United States;

(3) An explanation of why the probable benefit to health from the use of the device outweighs the risk of injury or illness from its use, taking into account the probable risks and benefits of currently available devices or alternative forms of treatment. Such explanation shall include a description, explanation, or theory of the underlying disease process or condition, and known or postulated mechanism(s) of action of the device in relation to the disease process or condition;

(4) All of the information required to be submitted under § 814.20(b), except that:

(i) In lieu of the summaries, conclusions, and results from clinical investigations required under § 814.20(b)(3)(v)(B), (b)(3)(vi), and the introductory text of (b)(6)(ii), the applicant shall include the summaries, conclusions, and results of all clinical experience or investigations (whether adverse or supportive) reasonably obtainable by the applicant that are relevant to an assessment of the risks and probable benefits of the device and to the extent the applicant includes data from clinical investigations, the applicant shall include the statements described in § 814.20(b)(6)(ii)(A) and (B) with respect to clinical investigations conducted in the United States and the information described in § 814.20(b)(6)(ii)(C) with respect to clinical investigations conducted outside the United States; and

(ii) In addition to the proposed labeling requirement set forth in § 814.20(b)(10), the labeling shall bear the following statement: Humanitarian Device. Authorized by Federal law for use in the [treatment or diagnosis] of [specify disease or condition]. The effectiveness of this device for this use has not been demonstrated;

(5) The amount to be charged for the device and, if the amount is more than $250, a report by an independent certified public accountant, made in accordance with the Statement on Standards for Attestation established by the American Institute of Certified Public Accountants, or in lieu of such a report, an attestation by a responsible individual of the organization, verifying that the amount charged does not exceed the costs of the device's research, development, fabrication, and distribution. If the amount charged is $250 or less, the requirement for a report by an independent certified public accountant or an attestation by a responsible individual of the organization is waived; and

(6) Information concerning pediatric uses of the device, as required by § 814.20(b)(13).

(c) *Omission of information.* If the applicant believes that certain information required under paragraph (b) of this section is not applicable to the device that is the subject of the HDE, and omits any such information from its HDE, the applicant shall submit a statement that identifies and justifies the omission. The statement shall be submitted as a separate section in the HDE and identified in the table of contents. If the justification for the omission is not accepted by the agency, FDA will so notify the applicant.

(d) *Address for submissions and correspondence.* Copies of all original HDEs amendments and supplements, as well as any correspondence relating to an HDE, must be sent or delivered to the following:

(1) For devices regulated by the Center for Devices and Radiological Health, send to Document Mail Center, 10903 New Hampshire Ave., Bldg. 66, rm. G609, Silver Spring, MD 20993-0002.

(2) For devices regulated by the Center for Biologics Evaluation and Research, send this information to the Food and Drug Administration, Center for Biologics Evaluation and Research, Document Control Center, 10903 New Hampshire Ave., Bldg. 71, Rm. G112, Silver Spring, MD 20993-0002.

(3) For devices regulated by the Center for Drug Evaluation and Research, send this information to the Central Document Control Room, Center for Drug Evaluation and Research, Food and Drug Administration, 5901-B Ammendale Rd., Beltsville, MD 20705-1266.

[61 FR 33244, June 26, 1996, as amended at 63 FR 59220, Nov. 3, 1998; 73 FR 49942, Aug. 25, 2008; 75 FR 20915, Apr. 22, 2010; 79 FR 1740, Jan. 10, 2014; 80 FR 18094, Apr. 3, 2015; 83 FR 7388, Feb. 21, 2018]

§ 814.106 HDE amendments and resubmitted HDE's.

An HDE or HDE supplement may be amended or resubmitted upon an applicant's own initiative, or at the request of FDA, for the same reasons and in the same manner as prescribed for PMA's in § 814.37, except that the timeframes set forth in § 814.37(c)(1) and (d) do not apply. If FDA requests an HDE applicant to submit an HDE amendment, and a written response to FDA's request is not received within 75 days of the date of the request, FDA will consider the pending HDE or HDE supplement to be withdrawn voluntarily by the applicant. Furthermore, if the HDE applicant, on its own initiative or at FDA's request, submits a major amendment as described in § 814.37(c)(1), the review period may be extended up to 75 days.

[63 FR 59220, Nov. 3, 1998]

§ 814.108 Supplemental applications.

After FDA approval of an original HDE, an applicant shall submit supplements in accordance with the requirements for PMA's under § 814.39, except that a request for a new indication for use of a HUD shall comply with requirements set forth in § 814.110. The timeframes for review of, and FDA action on, an HDE supplement are the same as those provided in § 814.114 for an HDE.

[63 FR 59220, Nov. 3, 1998]

§ 814.110 New indications for use.

(a) An applicant seeking a new indication for use of a HUD approved under this subpart H shall obtain a new designation of HUD status in accordance with § 814.102 and shall submit an original HDE in accordance with § 814.104.

(b) An application for a new indication for use made under § 814.104 may incorporate by reference any information or data previously submitted to the agency under an HDE.

§ 814.112 Filing an HDE.

(a) The filing of an HDE means that FDA has made a threshold determination that the application is sufficiently complete to permit substantive review. Within 30 days from the date an HDE is received by FDA, the agency will notify the applicant whether the application has been filed. FDA may refuse to file an HDE if any of the following applies:

(1) The application is incomplete because it does not on its face contain all the information required under § 814.104(b);

(2) FDA determines that there is a comparable device available (other than another HUD approved under this subpart or a device under an approved IDE) to treat or diagnose the disease or condition for which approval of the HUD is being sought; or

(3) The application contains an untrue statement of material fact or omits material information.

(4) The HDE is not accompanied by a statement of either certification or disclosure, or both, as required by part 54 of this chapter.

(b) The provisions contained in § 814.42(b), (c), and (d) regarding notification of filing decisions, filing dates, the start of the 75-day review period, and applicant's options in response to FDA refuse to file decisions shall apply to HDE's.

[61 FR 33244, June 26, 1996, as amended at 63 FR 5254, Feb. 2, 1998; 63 FR 59221, Nov. 3, 1998]

§814.114 Timeframes for reviewing an HDE.

Within 75 days after receipt of an HDE that is accepted for filing and to which the applicant does not submit a major amendment, FDA shall send the applicant an approval order, an approvable letter, a not approvable letter (under §814.116), or an order denying approval (under §814.118).

[63 FR 59221, Nov. 3, 1998]

§814.116 Procedures for review of an HDE.

(a) *Substantive review.* FDA will begin substantive review of an HDE after the HDE is accepted for filing under §814.112. FDA may refer an original HDE application to a panel on its own initiative, and shall do so upon the request of an applicant, unless FDA determines that the application substantially duplicates information previously reviewed by a panel. If the HDE is referred to a panel, the agency shall follow the procedures set forth under §814.44, with the exception that FDA will complete its review of the HDE and the advisory committee report and recommendations within 75 days from receipt of an HDE that is accepted for filing under §814.112 or the date of filing as determined under §814.106, whichever is later. Within the later of these two timeframes, FDA will issue an approval order under paragraph (b) of this section, an approvable letter under paragraph (c) of this section, a not approvable letter under paragraph (d) of this section, or an order denying approval of the application under §814.118(a).

(b) Approval order. FDA will issue to the applicant an order approving an HDE if none of the reasons in §814.118 for denying approval of the application applies. FDA will approve an application on the basis of draft final labeling if the only deficiencies in the application concern editorial or similar minor deficiencies in the draft final labeling. Such approval will be conditioned upon the applicant incorporating the specified labeling changes exactly as directed and upon the applicant submitting to FDA a copy of the final printed labeling before marketing. The notice of approval of an HDE will be published in the Federal Register in accordance with the rules and policies applicable to PMA's submitted under §814.20. Following the issuance of an approval order, data and information in the HDE file will be available for public disclosure in accordance with §814.9(b) through (h), as applicable.

(c) *Approvable letter.* FDA will send the applicant an approvable letter if the application substantially meets the requirements of this subpart and the agency believes it can approve the application if specific additional information is submitted or specific conditions are agreed to by the applicant. The approvable letter will describe the information FDA requires to be provided by the applicant or the conditions the applicant is required to meet to obtain approval. For example, FDA may require as a condition to approval:

(1) The submission of certain information identified in the approvable letter, e.g., final labeling;

(2) The submission of additional information concerning pediatric uses of the device, as required by §814.20(b)(13);

(3) Restrictions imposed on the device under section 520(e) of the act;

(4) Postapproval requirements as described in subpart E of this part; and

(5) An FDA inspection that finds the manufacturing facilities, methods, and controls in compliance with part 820 of this chapter and, if applicable, that verifies records pertinent to the HDE.

(d) *Not approvable letter.* FDA will send the applicant a not approvable letter if the agency believes that the application may not be approved for one or more of the reasons given in §814.118. The not approvable letter will describe the deficiencies in the application and, where practical, will identify measures required to place the HDE in approvable form. The applicant may respond to the not approvable letter in the same manner as permitted for not approvable letters for PMA's under §814.44(f), with the exception that if a major HDE amendment is submitted, the review period may be extended up to 75 days.

(e) FDA will consider an HDE to have been withdrawn voluntarily if:

(1) The applicant fails to respond in writing to a written request for an amendment within 75 days after the date FDA issues such request;

(2) The applicant fails to respond in writing to an approvable or not approvable letter within 75 days after the date FDA issues such letter; or

(3) The applicant submits a written notice to FDA that the HDE has been withdrawn.

[61 FR 33244, June 26, 1996, as amended at 63 FR 59221, Nov. 3, 1998; 79 FR 1741, Jan. 10, 2014]

§814.118 Denial of approval or withdrawal of approval of an HDE.

(a) FDA may deny approval or withdraw approval of an application if the applicant fails to meet the requirements of section 520(m) of the act or of this part, or of any condition of approval imposed by an IRB or by FDA, or any postapproval requirements imposed under §814.126. In addition, FDA may deny approval or withdraw approval of an application if, upon the basis of the information submitted in the HDE or any other information before the agency, FDA determines that:

(1) There is a lack of a showing of reasonable assurance that the device is safe under the conditions of use prescribed, recommended, or suggested in the labeling thereof;

(2) The device is ineffective under the conditions of use prescribed, recommended, or suggested in the labeling thereof;

(3) The applicant has not demonstrated that there is a reasonable basis from which to conclude that the probable benefit to health from the use of the device outweighs the risk of injury or illness, taking into account the probable risks and benefits of currently available devices or alternative forms of treatment;

(4) The application or a report submitted by or on behalf of the applicant contains an untrue statement of material fact, or omits material information;

(5) The device's labeling does not comply with the requirements in part 801 or part 809 of this chapter;

(6) A nonclinical laboratory study that is described in the HDE and that is essential to show that the device is safe for use under the conditions prescribed, recommended, or suggested in its proposed labeling, was not conducted in compliance with the good laboratory practice regulations in part 58 of this chapter and no reason for the noncompliance is provided or, if it is, the differences between the practices used in conducting the study and the good laboratory practice regulations do not support the validity of the study;

(7) Any clinical investigation involving human subjects described in the HDE, subject to the institutional review board regulations in part 56 of this chapter or the informed consent regulations in part 50 of this chapter, was not conducted in compliance with those regulations such that the rights or safety of human subjects were not adequately protected;

(8) The applicant does not permit an authorized FDA employee an opportunity to inspect at a reasonable time and in a reasonable manner the facilities and controls, and to have access to and to copy and verify all records pertinent to the application; or

(9) The device's HUD designation should be revoked in accordance with §814.102(c).

(b) If FDA issues an order denying approval of an application, the agency will comply with the same notice and disclosure provisions required for PMA's under §814.45(b) and (d), as applicable.

(c) FDA will issue an order denying approval of an HDE after an approvable or not approvable letter has been sent and the applicant:

(1) Submits a requested amendment but any ground for denying approval of the application under §814.118(a) still applies;

(2) Notifies FDA in writing that the requested amendment will not be submitted; or

(3) Petitions for review under section 515(d)(3) of the act by filing a petition in the form of a petition for reconsideration under § 10.33 of this chapter.

(d) Before issuing an order withdrawing approval of an HDE, FDA will provide the applicant with notice and an opportunity for a hearing as required for PMA's under § 814.46(c) and (d), and will provide the public with notice in accordance with § 814.46(e), as applicable.

[61 FR 33244, June 26, 1996, as amended at 63 FR 59221, Nov. 3, 1998]

§ 814.120 Temporary suspension of approval of an HDE.

An HDE or HDE supplement may be temporarily suspended for the same reasons and in the same manner as prescribed for PMA's in § 814.47.

[63 FR 59221, Nov. 3, 1998]

§ 814.122 Confidentiality of data and information.

(a) *Requirement for disclosure.* The "HDE file" includes all data and information submitted with or referenced in the HDE, any IDE incorporated into the HDE, any HDE amendment or supplement, any report submitted under § 814.126, any master file, or any other related submission. Any record in the HDE file will be available for public disclosure in accordance with the provisions of this section and part 20 of this chapter.

(b) Extent of disclosure. Disclosure by FDA of the existence and contents of an HDE file shall be subject to the same rules that pertain to PMA's under § 814.9(b) through (h), as applicable.

§ 814.124 Institutional Review Board requirements.

(a) *IRB approval.* The HDE holder is responsible for ensuring that a HUD approved under this subpart is administered only in facilities having oversight by an Institutional Review Board (IRB) constituted and acting pursuant to part 56 of this chapter, including continuing review of use of the device. In addition, a HUD may be administered only if such use has been approved by an IRB. If, however, a physician in an emergency situation determines that approval from an IRB cannot be obtained in time to prevent serious harm or death to a patient, a HUD may be administered without prior approval by an IRB. In such an emergency situation, the physician shall, within 5 days after the use of the device, provide written notification to the chairman of the IRB of such use. Such written notification shall include the identification of the patient involved, the date on which the device was used, and the reason for the use.

(b) *Withdrawal of IRB approval.* A holder of an approved HDE shall notify FDA of any withdrawal of approval for the use of a HUD by a reviewing IRB within 5 working days after being notified of the withdrawal of approval.

[61 FR 33244, June 26, 1996, as amended at 63 FR 59221, Nov. 3, 1998; 82 FR 26349, June 7, 2017]

§ 814.126 Postapproval requirements and reports.

(a) An HDE approved under this subpart H shall be subject to the postapproval requirements and reports set forth under subpart E of this part, as applicable, with the exception of § 814.82(a)(7). In addition, medical device reports submitted to FDA in compliance with the requirements of part 803 of this chapter shall also be submitted to the IRB of record.

(b) In addition to the reports identified in paragraph (a) of this section, the holder of an approved HDE shall prepare and submit the following complete, accurate, and timely reports:

(1) *Periodic reports.* An HDE applicant is required to submit reports in accordance with the approval order. Unless FDA specifies otherwise, any periodic report shall include:

(i) An update of the information required under § 814.102(a) in a separately bound volume;

(ii) An update of the information required under §814.104(b)(2), (b)(3), and (b)(5);

(iii) The number of devices that have been shipped or sold since initial marketing approval under this subpart H and, if the number shipped or sold exceeds 8,000, an explanation and estimate of the number of devices used per patient. If a single device is used on multiple patients, the applicant shall submit an estimate of the number of patients treated or diagnosed using the device together with an explanation of the basis for the estimate;

(iv) Information describing the applicant's clinical experience with the device since the HDE was initially approved. This information shall include safety information that is known or reasonably should be known to the applicant, medical device reports made under part 803 of this chapter, any data generated from the postmarketing studies, and information (whether published or unpublished) that is known or reasonably expected to be known by the applicant that may affect an evaluation of the safety of the device or that may affect the statement of contraindications, warnings, precautions, and adverse reactions in the device's labeling; and

(v) A summary of any changes made to the device in accordance with supplements submitted under §814.108. If information provided in the periodic reports, or any other information in the possession of FDA, gives the agency reason to believe that a device raises public health concerns or that the criteria for exemption are no longer met, the agency may require the HDE holder to submit additional information to demonstrate continued compliance with the HDE requirements.

(2) *Other*. An HDE holder shall maintain records of the names and addresses of the facilities to which the HUD has been shipped, correspondence with reviewing IRB's, as well as any other information requested by a reviewing IRB or FDA. Such records shall be maintained in accordance with the HDE approval order.

[61 FR 33244, June 26, 1996, as amended at 63 FR 59221, Nov. 3, 1998; 71 FR 16228, Mar. 31, 2006; 82 FR 26349, June 7, 2017]

APPENDIX F

Integrated Addendum to ICH E6(R1): Guideline for Good Clinical Practice E6(R2)

Current *Step 4* version dated 9 November 2016

Introduction

Good Clinical Practice (GCP) is an international ethical and scientific quality standard for designing, conducting, recording and reporting trials that involve the participation of human subjects. Compliance with this standard provides public assurance that the rights, safety and well-being of trial subjects are protected, consistent with the principles that have their origin in the Declaration of Helsinki, and that the clinical trial data are credible.

The objective of this ICH GCP Guideline is to provide a unified standard for the European Union (EU), Japan and the United States to facilitate the mutual acceptance of clinical data by the regulatory authorities in these jurisdictions.

The guideline was developed with consideration of the current good clinical practices of the European Union, Japan, and the United States, as well as those of Australia, Canada, the Nordic countries and the World Health Organization (WHO).

This guideline should be followed when generating clinical trial data that are intended to be submitted to regulatory authorities.

The principles established in this guideline may also be applied to other clinical investigations that may have an impact on the safety and well-being of human subjects.

Addendum

Since the development of the ICH GCP Guideline, the scale, complexity, and cost of clinical trials have increased. Evolutions in technology and risk management processes offer new opportunities to increase efficiency and focus on relevant activities. When the original ICH E6(R1) text was prepared, clinical trials were performed in a largely paper-based process. Advances in use of electronic data recording and reporting facilitate implementation of other approaches. For example, centralized monitoring can now offer a greater advantage, to a broader range of trials than is suggested in the original text. Therefore, this guideline has been amended to encourage implementation of improved and more efficient approaches to clinical trial design, conduct, oversight, recording and reporting while continuing to ensure human subject protection and reliability of trial results. Standards regarding electronic records and essential documents intended to increase clinical trial quality and efficiency have also been updated.

This guideline should be read in conjunction with other ICH guidelines relevant to the conduct of clinical trials (e.g., E2A (clinical safety data management), E3 (clinical study reporting), E7 (geriatric populations), E8 (general considerations for clinical trials), E9 (statistical principles), and E11 (pediatric populations)).

This ICH GCP Guideline Integrated Addendum provides a unified standard for the European Union, Japan, the United States, Canada, and Switzerland to facilitate the mutual acceptance of data from clinical trials by the regulatory authorities in these jurisdictions. In the event of any conflict between the E6(R1) text and the E6(R2) addendum text, the E6(R2) addendum text should take priority.

1. GLOSSARY

1.1 Adverse Drug Reaction (ADR)

In the pre-approval clinical experience with a new medicinal product or its new usages, particularly as the therapeutic dose(s) may not be established: all noxious and unintended responses to a medicinal product related to any dose should be considered adverse drug reactions. The phrase responses to a medicinal product means that a causal relationship between a medicinal product and an adverse event is at least a reasonable possibility, i.e., the relationship cannot be ruled out.

Regarding marketed medicinal products: a response to a drug which is noxious and unintended and which occurs at doses normally used in man for prophylaxis, diagnosis, or therapy of diseases or for modification of physiological function (see the ICH Guideline for Clinical Safety Data Management: Definitions and Standards for Expedited Reporting).

1.2 Adverse Event (AE)

Any untoward medical occurrence in a patient or clinical investigation subject administered a pharmaceutical product and which does not necessarily have a causal relationship with this treatment. An adverse event (AE) can therefore be any unfavourable and unintended sign (including an abnormal laboratory finding), symptom, or disease temporally associated with the use of a medicinal (investigational) product, whether or not related to the medicinal (investigational) product (see the ICH Guideline for Clinical Safety Data Management: Definitions and Standards for Expedited Reporting).

1.3 Amendment (to the protocol)

See Protocol Amendment.

1.4 Applicable Regulatory Requirement(s)

Any law(s) and regulation(s) addressing the conduct of clinical trials of investigational products.

1.5 Approval (in relation to Institutional Review Boards)

The affirmative decision of the IRB that the clinical trial has been reviewed and may be conducted at the institution site within the constraints set forth by the IRB, the institution, Good Clinical Practice (GCP), and the applicable regulatory requirements.

1.6 Audit

A systematic and independent examination of trial related activities and documents to determine whether the evaluated trial related activities were conducted, and the data were recorded, analyzed and accurately reported according to the protocol, sponsor's standard operating procedures (SOPs), Good Clinical Practice (GCP), and the applicable regulatory requirement(s).

1.7 Audit Certificate

A declaration of confirmation by the auditor that an audit has taken place.

1.8 Audit Report

A written evaluation by the sponsor's auditor of the results of the audit.

1.9 Audit Trail

Documentation that allows reconstruction of the course of events.

1.10 Blinding/Masking

A procedure in which one or more parties to the trial are kept unaware of the treatment assignment(s). Single-blinding usually refers to the subject(s) being unaware, and double-blinding usually refers to the subject(s), investigator(s), monitor, and, in some cases, data analyst(s) being unaware of the treatment assignment(s).

1.11 Case Report Form (CRF)

A printed, optical, or electronic document designed to record all of the protocol required information to be reported to the sponsor on each trial subject.

1.12 Clinical Trial/Study

Any investigation in human subjects intended to discover or verify the clinical, pharmacological and/or other pharmacodynamic effects of an investigational product(s), and/or to identify any adverse reactions to an investigational product(s), and/or to study absorption, distribution, metabolism, and excretion of an investigational product(s) with the object of ascertaining its safety and/or efficacy. The terms clinical trial and clinical study are synonymous.

1.13 Clinical Trial/Study Report

A written description of a trial/study of any therapeutic, prophylactic, or diagnostic agent conducted in human subjects, in which the clinical and statistical description, presentations, and analyses are fully integrated into a single report (see the ICH Guideline for Structure and Content of Clinical Study Reports).

1.14 Comparator (Product)

An investigational or marketed product (i.e., active control), or placebo, used as a reference in a clinical trial.

1.15 Compliance (in relation to trials)

Adherence to all the trial-related requirements, Good Clinical Practice (GCP) requirements, and the applicable regulatory requirements.

1.16 Confidentiality

Prevention of disclosure, to other than authorized individuals, of a sponsor's proprietary information or of a subject's identity.

1.17 Contract

A written, dated, and signed agreement between two or more involved parties that sets out any arrangements on delegation and distribution of tasks and obligations and, if appropriate, on financial matters. The protocol may serve as the basis of a contract.

1.18 Coordinating Committee

A committee that a sponsor may organize to coordinate the conduct of a multicentre trial.

1.19 Coordinating Investigator

An investigator assigned the responsibility for the coordination of investigators at different centres participating in a multicentre trial.

1.20 Contract Research Organization (CRO)

A person or an organization (commercial, academic, or other) contracted by the sponsor to perform one or more of a sponsor's trial-related duties and functions.

1.21 Direct Access

Permission to examine, analyze, verify, and reproduce any records and reports that are important to evaluation of a clinical trial. Any party (e.g., domestic and foreign regulatory authorities, sponsor's monitors and auditors) with direct access should take all reasonable precautions within the constraints of the applicable regulatory requirement(s) to maintain the confidentiality of subjects' identities and sponsor's proprietary information.

1.22 Documentation

All records, in any form (including, but not limited to, written, electronic, magnetic, and optical records, and scans, x-rays, and electrocardiograms) that describe or record the methods, conduct, and/or results of a trial, the factors affecting a trial, and the actions taken.

1.23 Essential Documents

Documents which individually and collectively permit evaluation of the conduct of a study and the quality of the data produced (see 8. Essential Documents for the Conduct of a Clinical Trial).

1.24 Good Clinical Practice (GCP)

A standard for the design, conduct, performance, monitoring, auditing, recording, analyses, and reporting of clinical trials that provides assurance that the data and reported results are credible and accurate, and that the rights, integrity, and confidentiality of trial subjects are protected.

1.25 Independent Data-Monitoring Committee (IDMC) (Data and Safety Monitoring Board, Monitoring Committee, Data Monitoring Committee)

An independent data-monitoring committee that may be established by the sponsor to assess at intervals the progress of a clinical trial, the safety data, and the critical efficacy endpoints, and to recommend to the sponsor whether to continue, modify, or stop a trial.

1.26 Impartial Witness

A person, who is independent of the trial, who cannot be unfairly influenced by people involved with the trial, who attends the informed consent process if the subject or the subject's legally acceptable representative cannot read, and who reads the informed consent form and any other written information supplied to the subject.

1.27 Independent Ethics Committee (IEC)

An independent body (a review board or a committee, institutional, regional, national, or supranational), constituted of medical professionals and non-medical members, whose responsibility it is to ensure the protection of the rights, safety and well-being of human subjects involved in a trial and to provide public assurance of that protection, by, among other things, reviewing and approving/ providing favourable opinion on, the trial protocol, the suitability of the investigator(s), facilities, and the methods and material to be used in obtaining and documenting informed consent of the trial subjects.

The legal status, composition, function, operations and regulatory requirements pertaining to Independent Ethics Committees may differ among countries, but should allow the Independent Ethics Committee to act in agreement with GCP as described in this guideline.

1.28 Informed Consent

A process by which a subject voluntarily confirms his or her willingness to participate in a particular trial, after having been informed of all aspects of the trial that are relevant to the subject's decision to participate. Informed consent is documented by means of a written, signed and dated informed consent form.

1.29 Inspection

The act by a regulatory authority(ies) of conducting an official review of documents, facilities, records, and any other resources that are deemed by the authority(ies) to be related to the clinical trial and that may be located at the site of the trial, at the sponsor's and/or contract research organization's (CRO's) facilities, or at other establishments deemed appropriate by the regulatory authority(ies).

1.30 Institution (medical)

Any public or private entity or agency or medical or dental facility where clinical trials are conducted.

1.31 Institutional Review Board (IRB)

An independent body constituted of medical, scientific, and non-scientific members, whose responsibility is to ensure the protection of the rights, safety and well-being of human subjects involved in a trial by, among other things, reviewing, approving, and providing continuing review of trial protocol and amendments and of the methods and material to be used in obtaining and documenting informed consent of the trial subjects.

1.32 Interim Clinical Trial/Study Report

A report of intermediate results and their evaluation based on analyses performed during the course of a trial.

1.33 Investigational Product

A pharmaceutical form of an active ingredient or placebo being tested or used as a reference in a clinical trial, including a product with a marketing authorization when used or assembled (formulated or packaged) in a way different from the approved form, or when used for an unapproved indication, or when used to gain further information about an approved use.

1.34 Investigator

A person responsible for the conduct of the clinical trial at a trial site. If a trial is conducted by a team of individuals at a trial site, the investigator is the responsible leader of the team and may be called the principal investigator. See also Subinvestigator.

1.35 Investigator/Institution

An expression meaning "the investigator and/or institution, where required by the applicable regulatory requirements".

1.36 Investigator's Brochure

A compilation of the clinical and nonclinical data on the investigational product(s) which is relevant to the study of the investigational product(s) in human subjects (see 7. Investigator's Brochure).

1.37 Legally Acceptable Representative

An individual or juridical or other body authorized under applicable law to consent, on behalf of a prospective subject, to the subject's participation in the clinical trial.

1.38 Monitoring

The act of overseeing the progress of a clinical trial, and of ensuring that it is conducted, recorded, and reported in accordance with the protocol, Standard Operating Procedures (SOPs), Good Clinical Practice (GCP), and the applicable regulatory requirement(s).

1.39 Monitoring Report

A written report from the monitor to the sponsor after each site visit and/or other trial-related communication according to the sponsor's SOPs.

1.40 Multicentre Trial

A clinical trial conducted according to a single protocol but at more than one site, and therefore, carried out by more than one investigator.

1.41 Nonclinical Study

Biomedical studies not performed on human subjects.

1.42 Opinion (in relation to Independent Ethics Committee)

The judgement and/or the advice provided by an Independent Ethics Committee (IEC).

1.43 Original Medical Record

See Source Documents.

1.44 Protocol

A document that describes the objective(s), design, methodology, statistical considerations, and organization of a trial. The protocol usually also gives the background and rationale for the trial, but these could be provided in other protocol referenced documents. Throughout the ICH GCP Guideline the term protocol refers to protocol and protocol amendments.

1.45 Protocol Amendment

A written description of a change(s) to or formal clarification of a protocol.

1.46 Quality Assurance (QA)

All those planned and systematic actions that are established to ensure that the trial is performed and the data are generated, documented (recorded), and reported in compliance with Good Clinical Practice (GCP) and the applicable regulatory requirement(s).

1.47 Quality Control (QC)

The operational techniques and activities undertaken within the quality assurance system to verify that the requirements for quality of the trial-related activities have been fulfilled.

1.48 Randomization

The process of assigning trial subjects to treatment or control groups using an element of chance to determine the assignments in order to reduce bias.

1.49 Regulatory Authorities

Bodies having the power to regulate. In the ICH GCP Guideline the expression Regulatory Authorities includes the authorities that review submitted clinical data and those that conduct inspections (see 1.29). These bodies are sometimes referred to as competent authorities.

1.50 Serious Adverse Event (SAE) or Serious Adverse Drug Reaction (Serious ADR)

Any untoward medical occurrence that at any dose:

- results in death,
- is life-threatening,
- requires inpatient hospitalization or prolongation of existing hospitalization,
- results in persistent or significant disability/incapacity,

or

- is a congenital anomaly/birth defect

(see the ICH Guideline for Clinical Safety Data Management: Definitions and Standards for Expedited Reporting).

1.51 Source Data

All information in original records and certified copies of original records of clinical findings, observations, or other activities in a clinical trial necessary for the reconstruction and evaluation of the trial. Source data are contained in source documents (original records or certified copies).

1.52 Source Documents

Original documents, data, and records (e.g., hospital records, clinical and office charts, laboratory notes, memoranda, subjects' diaries or evaluation checklists, pharmacy dispensing records, recorded data from automated instruments, copies or transcriptions certified after verification as being accurate copies, microfiches, photographic negatives, microfilm or magnetic media, x-rays, subject files, and records kept at the pharmacy, at the laboratories and at medico-technical departments involved in the clinical trial).

1.53 Sponsor

An individual, company, institution, or organization which takes responsibility for the initiation, management, and/or financing of a clinical trial.

1.54 Sponsor-Investigator

An individual who both initiates and conducts, alone or with others, a clinical trial, and under whose immediate direction the investigational product is administered to, dispensed to, or used by a subject. The term does not include any person other than an individual (e.g., it does not include a corporation or an agency). The obligations of a sponsor-investigator include both those of a sponsor and those of an investigator.

1.55 Standard Operating Procedures (SOPs)

Detailed, written instructions to achieve uniformity of the performance of a specific function.

1.56 Subinvestigator

Any individual member of the clinical trial team designated and supervised by the investigator at a trial site to perform critical trial-related procedures and/or to make important trial-related decisions (e.g., associates, residents, research fellows). See also Investigator.

1.57 Subject/Trial Subject

An individual who participates in a clinical trial, either as a recipient of the investigational product(s) or as a control.

1.58 Subject Identification Code

A unique identifier assigned by the investigator to each trial subject to protect the subject's identity and used in lieu of the subject's name when the investigator reports adverse events and/or other trial related data.

1.59 Trial Site

The location(s) where trial-related activities are actually conducted.

1.60 Unexpected Adverse Drug Reaction

An adverse reaction, the nature or severity of which is not consistent with the applicable product information (e.g., Investigator's Brochure for an unapproved investigational product or package insert/summary of product characteristics for an approved product) (see the ICH Guideline for Clinical Safety Data Management: Definitions and Standards for Expedited Reporting).

1.61 Vulnerable Subjects

Individuals whose willingness to volunteer in a clinical trial may be unduly influenced by the expectation, whether justified or not, of benefits associated with participation, or of a retaliatory response from senior members of a hierarchy in case of refusal to participate. Examples are members of a group with a hierarchical structure, such as medical, pharmacy, dental, and nursing students, subordinate hospital and laboratory personnel, employees of the pharmaceutical industry, members of the armed forces, and persons kept in detention. Other vulnerable subjects include patients with incurable diseases, persons in nursing homes, unemployed or impoverished persons, patients in emergency situations, ethnic minority groups, homeless persons, nomads, refugees, minors, and those incapable of giving consent.

1.62 Well-being (of the trial subjects)

The physical and mental integrity of the subjects participating in a clinical trial.

ADDENDUM

1.63 Certified Copy

A copy (irrespective of the type of media used) of the original record that has been verified (i.e., by a dated signature or by generation through a validated process) to have the same information, including data that describe the context, content, and structure, as the original.

1.64 Monitoring Plan

A document that describes the strategy, methods, responsibilities, and requirements for monitoring the trial.

1.65 Validation of Computerized Systems

A process of establishing and documenting that the specified requirements of a computerized system can be consistently fulfilled from design until decommissioning of the system or transition to a new system. The approach to validation should be based on a risk assessment that takes into consideration the intended use of the system and the potential of the system to affect human subject protection and reliability of trial results.

2. THE PRINCIPLES OF ICH GCP

2.1 Clinical trials should be conducted in accordance with the ethical principles that have their origin in the Declaration of Helsinki, and that are consistent with GCP and the applicable regulatory requirement(s).

2.2 Before a trial is initiated, foreseeable risks and inconveniences should be weighed against the anticipated benefit for the individual trial subject and society. A trial should be initiated and continued only if the anticipated benefits justify the risks.

2.3 The rights, safety, and well-being of the trial subjects are the most important considerations and should prevail over interests of science and society.

2.4 The available nonclinical and clinical information on an investigational product should be adequate to support the proposed clinical trial.

2.5 Clinical trials should be scientifically sound, and described in a clear, detailed protocol.

2.6 A trial should be conducted in compliance with the protocol that has received prior institutional review board (IRB)/independent ethics committee (IEC) approval/favourable opinion.

2.7 The medical care given to, and medical decisions made on behalf of, subjects should always be the responsibility of a qualified physician or, when appropriate, of a qualified dentist.

2.8 Each individual involved in conducting a trial should be qualified by education, training, and experience to perform his or her respective task(s).

2.9 Freely given informed consent should be obtained from every subject prior to clinical trial participation.

2.10 All clinical trial information should be recorded, handled, and stored in a way that allows its accurate reporting, interpretation and verification.

ADDENDUM

This principle applies to all records referenced in this guideline, irrespective of the type of media used.

2.11 The confidentiality of records that could identify subjects should be protected, respecting the privacy and confidentiality rules in accordance with the applicable regulatory requirement(s).

2.12 Investigational products should be manufactured, handled, and stored in accordance with applicable good manufacturing practice (GMP). They should be used in accordance with the approved protocol.

2.13 Systems with procedures that assure the quality of every aspect of the trial should be implemented.

ADDENDUM

Aspects of the trial that are essential to ensure human subject protection and reliability of trial results should be the focus of such systems.

3. INSTITUTIONAL REVIEW BOARD/INDEPENDENT ETHICS COMMITTEE (IRB/IEC)

3.1 Responsibilities

3.1.1 An IRB/IEC should safeguard the rights, safety, and well-being of all trial subjects. Special attention should be paid to trials that may include vulnerable subjects.

3.1.2 The IRB/IEC should obtain the following documents:
trial protocol(s)/amendment(s), written informed consent form(s) and consent form updates that the investigator proposes for use in the trial, subject recruitment procedures (e.g., advertisements), written information to be provided to subjects, Investigator's Brochure (IB), available safety information, information about payments and compensation available to subjects, the investigator's current curriculum vitae and/or other documentation evidencing qualifications, and any other documents that the IRB/IEC may need to fulfil its responsibilities.

The IRB/IEC should review a proposed clinical trial within a reasonable time and document its views in writing, clearly identifying the trial, the documents reviewed and the dates for the following:

- approval/favourable opinion;
- modifications required prior to its approval/favourable opinion;
- disapproval / negative opinion; and
- termination/suspension of any prior approval/favourable opinion.

3.1.3 The IRB/IEC should consider the qualifications of the investigator for the proposed trial, as documented by a current curriculum vitae and/or by any other relevant documentation the IRB/IEC requests.

3.1.4 The IRB/IEC should conduct continuing review of each ongoing trial at intervals appropriate to the degree of risk to human subjects, but at least once per year.

3.1.5 The IRB/IEC may request more information than is outlined in paragraph 4.8.10 be given to subjects when, in the judgement of the IRB/IEC, the additional information would add meaningfully to the protection of the rights, safety and/or well-being of the subjects.

3.1.6 When a non-therapeutic trial is to be carried out with the consent of the subject's legally acceptable representative (see 4.8.12, 4.8.14), the IRB/IEC should determine that the proposed protocol and/or other document(s) adequately addresses relevant ethical concerns and meets applicable regulatory requirements for such trials.

3.1.7 Where the protocol indicates that prior consent of the trial subject or the subject's legally acceptable representative is not possible (see 4.8.15), the IRB/IEC should determine that the proposed protocol and/or other document(s) adequately addresses relevant ethical concerns and meets applicable regulatory requirements for such trials (i.e., in emergency situations).

3.1.8 The IRB/IEC should review both the amount and method of payment to subjects to assure that neither presents problems of coercion or undue influence on the trial subjects. Payments to a subject should be prorated and not wholly contingent on completion of the trial by the subject.

3.1.9 The IRB/IEC should ensure that information regarding payment to subjects, including the methods, amounts, and schedule of payment to trial subjects, is set forth in the written informed consent form and any other written information to be provided to subjects. The way payment will be prorated should be specified.

3.2 Composition, Functions and Operations

3.2.1 The IRB/IEC should consist of a reasonable number of members, who collectively have the qualifications and experience to review and evaluate the science, medical aspects, and ethics of the proposed trial. It is recommended that the IRB/IEC should include:

A. At least five members.

B. At least one member whose primary area of interest is in a nonscientific area.

C. At least one member who is independent of the institution/trial site.

Only those IRB/IEC members who are independent of the investigator and the sponsor of the trial should vote/provide opinion on a trial-related matter.

A list of IRB/IEC members and their qualifications should be maintained.

3.2.2 The IRB/IEC should perform its functions according to written operating procedures, should maintain written records of its activities and minutes of its meetings, and should comply with GCP and with the applicable regulatory requirement(s).

3.2.3 An IRB/IEC should make its decisions at announced meetings at which at least a quorum, as stipulated in its written operating procedures, is present.

3.2.4 Only members who participate in the IRB/IEC review and discussion should vote/provide their opinion and/or advise.

3.2.5 The investigator may provide information on any aspect of the trial, but should not participate in the deliberations of the IRB/IEC or in the vote/opinion of the IRB/IEC.

3.2.6 An IRB/IEC may invite nonmembers with expertise in special areas for assistance.

3.3 Procedures

The IRB/IEC should establish, document in writing, and follow its procedures, which should include:

3.3.1 Determining its composition (names and qualifications of the members) and the authority under which it is established.

3.3.2 Scheduling, notifying its members of, and conducting its meetings.

3.3.3 Conducting initial and continuing review of trials.

3.3.4 Determining the frequency of continuing review, as appropriate.

3.3.5 Providing, according to the applicable regulatory requirements, expedited review and approval/favourable opinion of minor change(s) in ongoing trials that have the approval/favourable opinion of the IRB/IEC.

3.3.6 Specifying that no subject should be admitted to a trial before the IRB/IEC issues its written approval/favourable opinion of the trial.

3.3.7 Specifying that no deviations from, or changes of, the protocol should be initiated without prior written IRB/IEC approval/favourable opinion of an appropriate amendment, except when necessary to eliminate immediate hazards to the subjects or when the change(s) involves only logistical or administrative aspects of the trial (e.g., change of monitor(s), telephone number(s)) (see 4.5.2).

3.3.8 Specifying that the investigator should promptly report to the IRB/IEC:

A. Deviations from, or changes of, the protocol to eliminate immediate hazards to the trial subjects (see 3.3.7, 4.5.2, 4.5.4).

B. Changes increasing the risk to subjects and/or affecting significantly the conduct of the trial (see 4.10.2).

C. All adverse drug reactions (ADRs) that are both serious and unexpected.

D. New information that may affect adversely the safety of the subjects or the conduct of the trial.

3.3.9 Ensuring that the IRB/IEC promptly notify in writing the investigator/institution concerning:

A. Its trial-related decisions/opinions.

B. The reasons for its decisions/opinions.

C. Procedures for appeal of its decisions/opinions.

3.4 Records

The IRB/IEC should retain all relevant records (e.g., written procedures, membership lists, lists of occupations/affiliations of members, submitted documents, minutes of meetings, and correspondence) for a period of at least 3-years after completion of the trial and make them available upon request from the regulatory authority(ies).

The IRB/IEC may be asked by investigators, sponsors or regulatory authorities to provide its written procedures and membership lists.

4. INVESTIGATOR

4.1 Investigator's Qualifications and Agreements

4.1.1 The investigator(s) should be qualified by education, training, and experience to assume responsibility for the proper conduct of the trial, should meet all the qualifications specified by the applicable regulatory requirement(s), and should provide evidence of such qualifications through up-to-date curriculum vitae and/or other relevant documentation requested by the sponsor, the IRB/IEC, and/or the regulatory authority(ies).

4.1.2 The investigator should be thoroughly familiar with the appropriate use of the investigational product(s), as described in the protocol, in the current Investigator's Brochure, in the product information and in other information sources provided by the sponsor.

4.1.3 The investigator should be aware of, and should comply with, GCP and the applicable regulatory requirements.

4.1.4 The investigator/institution should permit monitoring and auditing by the sponsor, and inspection by the appropriate regulatory authority(ies).

4.1.5 The investigator should maintain a list of appropriately qualified persons to whom the investigator has delegated significant trial-related duties.

4.2 Adequate Resources

4.2.1 The investigator should be able to demonstrate (e.g., based on retrospective data) a potential for recruiting the required number of suitable subjects within the agreed recruitment period.

4.2.2 The investigator should have sufficient time to properly conduct and complete the trial within the agreed trial period.

4.2.3 The investigator should have available an adequate number of qualified staff and adequate facilities for the foreseen duration of the trial to conduct the trial properly and safely.

4.2.4 The investigator should ensure that all persons assisting with the trial are adequately informed about the protocol, the investigational product(s), and their trial-related duties and functions.

ADDENDUM

4.2.5 The investigator is responsible for supervising any individual or party to whom the investigator delegates trial-related duties and functions conducted at the trial site.

4.2.6 If the investigator/institution retains the services of any individual or party to perform trial-related duties and functions, the investigator/institution should ensure this individual or party is qualified to perform those trial-related duties and functions and should implement procedures to ensure the integrity of the trial-related duties and functions performed and any data generated.

4.3 Medical Care of Trial Subjects

4.3.1 A qualified physician (or dentist, when appropriate), who is an investigator or a subinvestigator for the trial, should be responsible for all trial-related medical (or dental) decisions.

4.3.2 During and following a subject's participation in a trial, the investigator/institution should ensure that adequate medical care is provided to a subject for any adverse events, including clinically significant laboratory values, related to the trial. The investigator/institution should inform a subject when medical care is needed for intercurrent illness(es) of which the investigator becomes aware.

4.3.3 It is recommended that the investigator inform the subject's primary physician about the subject's participation in the trial if the subject has a primary physician and if the subject agrees to the primary physician being informed.

4.3.4 Although a subject is not obliged to give his/her reason(s) for withdrawing prematurely from a trial, the investigator should make a reasonable effort to ascertain the reason(s), while fully respecting the subject's rights.

4.4 Communication with IRB/IEC

4.4.1 Before initiating a trial, the investigator/institution should have written and dated approval/favourable opinion from the IRB/IEC for the trial protocol, written informed consent form, consent form updates, subject recruitment procedures (e.g., advertisements), and any other written information to be provided to subjects.

4.4.2 As part of the investigator's/institution's written application to the IRB/IEC, the investigator/institution should provide the IRB/IEC with a current copy of the Investigator's Brochure. If the

Investigator's Brochure is updated during the trial, the investigator/institution should supply a copy of the updated Investigator's Brochure to the IRB/IEC.

4.4.3 During the trial the investigator/institution should provide to the IRB/IEC all documents subject to review.

4.5 Compliance with Protocol

4.5.1 The investigator/institution should conduct the trial in compliance with the protocol agreed to by the sponsor and, if required, by the regulatory authority(ies) and which was given approval/favourable opinion by the IRB/IEC. The investigator/institution and the sponsor should sign the protocol, or an alternative contract, to confirm agreement.

4.5.2 The investigator should not implement any deviation from, or changes of the protocol without agreement by the sponsor and prior review and documented approval/favourable opinion from the IRB/IEC of an amendment, except where necessary to eliminate an immediate hazard(s) to trial subjects, or when the change(s) involves only logistical or administrative aspects of the trial (e.g., change in monitor(s), change of telephone number(s)).

4.5.3 The investigator, or person designated by the investigator, should document and explain any deviation from the approved protocol.

4.5.4 The investigator may implement a deviation from, or a change of, the protocol to eliminate an immediate hazard(s) to trial subjects without prior IRB/IEC approval/favourable opinion. As soon as possible, the implemented deviation or change, the reasons for it, and, if appropriate, the proposed protocol amendment(s) should be submitted:

A. to the IRB/IEC for review and approval/favourable opinion,

B. to the sponsor for agreement and, if required,

C. to the regulatory authority(ies).

4.6 Investigational Product(s)

4.6.1 Responsibility for investigational product(s) accountability at the trial site(s) rests with the investigator/institution.

4.6.2 Where allowed/required, the investigator/institution may/should assign some or all of the investigator's/institution's duties for investigational product(s) accountability at the trial site(s) to an appropriate pharmacist or another appropriate individual who is under the supervision of the investigator/institution..

4.6.3 The investigator/institution and/or a pharmacist or other appropriate individual, who is designated by the investigator/institution, should maintain records of the product's delivery to the trial site, the inventory at the site, the use by each subject, and the return to the sponsor or alternative disposition of unused product(s). These records should include dates, quantities, batch/serial numbers, expiration dates (if applicable), and the unique code numbers assigned to the investigational product(s) and trial subjects. Investigators should maintain records that document adequately that the subjects were provided the doses specified by the protocol and reconcile all investigational product(s) received from the sponsor.

4.6.4 The investigational product(s) should be stored as specified by the sponsor (see 5.13.2 and 5.14.3) and in accordance with applicable regulatory requirement(s).

4.6.5 The investigator should ensure that the investigational product(s) are used only in accordance with the approved protocol.

4.6.6 The investigator, or a person designated by the investigator/institution, should explain the correct use of the investigational product(s) to each subject and should check, at intervals appropriate for the trial, that each subject is following the instructions properly.

4.7 Randomization Procedures and Unblinding

The investigator should follow the trial's randomization procedures, if any, and should ensure that the code is broken only in accordance with the protocol. If the trial is blinded, the investigator should promptly document and explain to the sponsor any premature unblinding (e.g., accidental unblinding, unblinding due to a serious adverse event) of the investigational product(s).

4.8 Informed Consent of Trial Subjects

4.8.1 In obtaining and documenting informed consent, the investigator should comply with the applicable regulatory requirement(s), and should adhere to GCP and to the ethical principles that have their origin in the Declaration of Helsinki. Prior to the beginning of the trial, the investigator should have the IRB/IEC's written approval/favourable opinion of the written informed consent form and any other written information to be provided to subjects.

4.8.2 The written informed consent form and any other written information to be provided to subjects should be revised whenever important new information becomes available that may be relevant to the subject's consent. Any revised written informed consent form, and written information should receive the IRB/IEC's approval/favourable opinion in advance of use. The subject or the subject's legally acceptable representative should be informed in a timely manner if new information becomes available that may be relevant to the subject's willingness to continue participation in the trial. The communication of this information should be documented.

4.8.3 Neither the investigator, nor the trial staff, should coerce or unduly influence a subject to participate or to continue to participate in a trial.

4.8.4 None of the oral and written information concerning the trial, including the written informed consent form, should contain any language that causes the subject or the subject's legally acceptable representative to waive or to appear to waive any legal rights, or that releases or appears to release the investigator, the institution, the sponsor, or their agents from liability for negligence.

4.8.5 The investigator, or a person designated by the investigator, should fully inform the subject or, if the subject is unable to provide informed consent, the subject's legally acceptable representative, of all pertinent aspects of the trial including the written information and the approval/favourable opinion by the IRB/IEC.

4.8.6 The language used in the oral and written information about the trial, including the written informed consent form, should be as non-technical as practical and should be understandable to the subject or the subject's legally acceptable representative and the impartial witness, where applicable.

4.8.7 Before informed consent may be obtained, the investigator, or a person designated by the investigator, should provide the subject or the subject's legally acceptable representative ample time and opportunity to inquire about details of the trial and to decide whether or not to participate in the trial. All questions about the trial should be answered to the satisfaction of the subject or the subject's legally acceptable representative.

4.8.8 Prior to a subject's participation in the trial, the written informed consent form should be signed and personally dated by the subject or by the subject's legally acceptable representative, and by the person who conducted the informed consent discussion.

4.8.9 If a subject is unable to read or if a legally acceptable representative is unable to read, an impartial witness should be present during the entire informed consent discussion. After the written informed consent form and any other written information to be provided to subjects, is read and explained to the subject or the subject's legally acceptable representative, and after the subject or the subject's legally acceptable representative has orally consented to the subject's participation in the trial and, if capable of doing so, has signed and personally dated the informed consent form, the witness should sign and personally date the consent form. By signing the consent form, the witness attests that the information in the consent form and any other written information was accurately explained to, and apparently understood by, the subject or the subject's legally acceptable representative, and that informed consent was freely given by the subject or the subject's legally acceptable representative.

4.8.10 Both the informed consent discussion and the written informed consent form and any other written information to be provided to subjects should include explanations of the following:

A. That the trial involves research.

B. The purpose of the trial.

C. The trial treatment(s) and the probability for random assignment to each treatment.

D. The trial procedures to be followed, including all invasive procedures.

E. The subject's responsibilities.

F. Those aspects of the trial that are experimental.

G. The reasonably foreseeable risks or inconveniences to the subject and, when applicable, to an embryo, fetus, or nursing infant.

H. The reasonably expected benefits. When there is no intended clinical benefit to the subject, the subject should be made aware of this.

I. The alternative procedure(s) or course(s) of treatment that may be available to the subject, and their important potential benefits and risks.

J. The compensation and/or treatment available to the subject in the event of trial-related injury.

K. The anticipated prorated payment, if any, to the subject for participating in the trial.

L. The anticipated expenses, if any, to the subject for participating in the trial.

M. That the subject's participation in the trial is voluntary and that the subject may refuse to participate or withdraw from the trial, at any time, without penalty or loss of benefits to which the subject is otherwise entitled.

N. That the monitor(s), the auditor(s), the IRB/IEC, and the regulatory authority(ies) will be granted direct access to the subject's original medical records for verification of clinical trial procedures and/or data, without violating the confidentiality of the subject, to the extent permitted by the applicable laws and regulations and that, by signing a written informed consent form, the subject or the subject's legally acceptable representative is authorizing such access.

O. That records identifying the subject will be kept confidential and, to the extent permitted by the applicable laws and/or regulations, will not be made publicly available. If the results of the trial are published, the subject's identity will remain confidential.

P. That the subject or the subject's legally acceptable representative will be informed in a timely manner if information becomes available that may be relevant to the subject's willingness to continue participation in the trial.

Q. The person(s) to contact for further information regarding the trial and the rights of trial subjects, and whom to contact in the event of trial-related injury.

R. The foreseeable circumstances and/or reasons under which the subject's participation in the trial may be terminated.

S. The expected duration of the subject's participation in the trial.

T. The approximate number of subjects involved in the trial.

4.8.11 Prior to participation in the trial, the subject or the subject's legally acceptable representative should receive a copy of the signed and dated written informed consent form and any other written information provided to the subjects. During a subject's participation in the trial, the subject or the subject's legally acceptable representative should receive a copy of the signed and dated consent form updates and a copy of any amendments to the written information provided to subjects.

4.8.12 When a clinical trial (therapeutic or non-therapeutic) includes subjects who can only be enrolled in the trial with the consent of the subject's legally acceptable representative (e.g., minors, or patients with severe dementia), the subject should be informed about the trial to the extent compatible with the subject's understanding and, if capable, the subject should sign and personally date the written informed consent.

4.8.13 Except as described in 4.8.14, a non-therapeutic trial (i.e., a trial in which there is no anticipated direct clinical benefit to the subject), should be conducted in subjects who personally give consent and who sign and date the written informed consent form.

4.8.14 Non-therapeutic trials may be conducted in subjects with consent of a legally acceptable representative provided the following conditions are fulfilled:

A. The objectives of the trial can not be met by means of a trial in subjects who can give informed consent personally.

B. The foreseeable risks to the subjects are low.

C. The negative impact on the subject's well-being is minimized and low.

D. The trial is not prohibited by law.

E. The approval/favourable opinion of the IRB/IEC is expressly sought on the inclusion of such subjects, and the written approval/ favourable opinion covers this aspect.

Such trials, unless an exception is justified, should be conducted in patients having a disease or condition for which the investigational product is intended. Subjects in these trials should be particularly closely monitored and should be withdrawn if they appear to be unduly distressed.

4.8.15 In emergency situations, when prior consent of the subject is not possible, the consent of the subject's legally acceptable representative, if present, should be requested. When prior consent of the subject is not possible, and the subject's legally acceptable representative is not available, enrolment of the subject should require measures described in the protocol and/or elsewhere, with documented approval/favourable opinion by the IRB/IEC, to protect the rights, safety and well-being of the subject and to ensure compliance with applicable regulatory requirements. The subject or the subject's legally acceptable representative should be informed about the trial as soon as possible and consent to continue and other consent as appropriate (see 4.8.10) should be requested.

4.9 Records and Reports

ADDENDUM

4.9.0 The investigator/institution should maintain adequate and accurate source documents and trial records that include all pertinent observations on each of the site's trial subjects. Source data should be attributable, legible, contemporaneous, original, accurate, and complete. Changes to source data should be traceable, should not obscure the original entry, and should be explained if necessary (e.g., via an audit trail).

4.9.1 The investigator should ensure the accuracy, completeness, legibility, and timeliness of the data reported to the sponsor in the CRFs and in all required reports.

4.9.2 Data reported on the CRF, that are derived from source documents, should be consistent with the source documents or the discrepancies should be explained.

4.9.3 Any change or correction to a CRF should be dated, initialed, and explained (if necessary) and should not obscure the original entry (i.e., an audit trail should be maintained); this applies to both written and electronic changes or corrections (see 5.18.4 (n)). Sponsors should provide guidance to investigators and/or the investigators' designated representatives on making such corrections. Sponsors should have written procedures to assure that changes or corrections in CRFs made by sponsor's designated representatives are documented, are necessary, and are endorsed by the investigator. The investigator should retain records of the changes and corrections.

4.9.4 The investigator/institution should maintain the trial documents as specified in Essential Documents for the Conduct of a Clinical Trial (see 8.) and as required by the applicable regulatory requirement(s). The investigator/institution should take measures to prevent accidental or premature destruction of these documents.

4.9.5 Essential documents should be retained until at least 2-years after the last approval of a marketing application in an ICH region and until there are no pending or contemplated marketing applications in an ICH region or at least 2-years have elapsed since the formal discontinuation of clinical development of the investigational product. These documents should be retained for a longer period however if required by the applicable regulatory requirements or by an agreement with the sponsor. It is the responsibility of the sponsor to inform the investigator/institution as to when these documents no longer need to be retained (see 5.5.12).

4.9.6 The financial aspects of the trial should be documented in an agreement between the sponsor and the investigator/institution.

4.9.7 Upon request of the monitor, auditor, IRB/IEC, or regulatory authority, the investigator/institution should make available for direct access all requested trial-related records.

4.10 Progress Reports

4.10.1 The investigator should submit written summaries of the trial status to the IRB/IEC annually, or more frequently, if requested by the IRB/IEC.

4.10.2 The investigator should promptly provide written reports to the sponsor, the IRB/IEC (see 3.3.8) and, where applicable, the institution on any changes significantly affecting the conduct of the trial, and/or increasing the risk to subjects.

4.11 Safety Reporting

4.11.1 All serious adverse events (SAEs) should be reported immediately to the sponsor except for those SAEs that the protocol or other document (e.g., Investigator's Brochure) identifies as not needing immediate reporting. The immediate reports should be followed promptly by detailed, written reports. The immediate and follow-up reports should identify subjects by unique code numbers assigned to the trial subjects rather than by the subjects' names, personal identification numbers, and/or addresses. The investigator should also comply with the applicable regulatory requirement(s) related to the reporting of unexpected serious adverse drug reactions to the regulatory authority(ies) and the IRB/IEC.

4.11.2 Adverse events and/or laboratory abnormalities identified in the protocol as critical to safety evaluations should be reported to the sponsor according to the reporting requirements and within the time periods specified by the sponsor in the protocol.

4.11.3 For reported deaths, the investigator should supply the sponsor and the IRB/IEC with any additional requested information (e.g., autopsy reports and terminal medical reports).

4.12 Premature Termination or Suspension of a Trial

If the trial is prematurely terminated or suspended for any reason, the investigator/institution should promptly inform the trial subjects, should assure appropriate therapy and follow-up for the subjects, and, where required by the applicable regulatory requirement(s), should inform the regulatory authority(ies). In addition:

4.12.1 If the investigator terminates or suspends a trial without prior agreement of the sponsor, the investigator should inform the institution where applicable, and the investigator/institution should promptly inform the sponsor and the IRB/IEC, and should provide the sponsor and the IRB/IEC a detailed written explanation of the termination or suspension.

4.12.2 If the sponsor terminates or suspends a trial (see 5.21), the investigator should promptly inform the institution where applicable and the investigator/institution should promptly inform the IRB/IEC and provide the IRB/IEC a detailed written explanation of the termination or suspension.

4.12.3 If the IRB/IEC terminates or suspends its approval/favourable opinion of a trial (see 3.1.2 and 3.3.9), the investigator should inform the institution where applicable and the investigator/institution should promptly notify the sponsor and provide the sponsor with a detailed written explanation of the termination or suspension.

4.13 Final Report(s) by Investigator

Upon completion of the trial, the investigator, where applicable, should inform the institution; the investigator/institution should provide the IRB/IEC with a summary of the trial's outcome, and the regulatory authority(ies) with any reports required.

5. SPONSOR

ADDENDUM

5.0 Quality Management

The sponsor should implement a system to manage quality throughout all stages of the trial process.

Sponsors should focus on trial activities essential to ensuring human subject protection and the reliability of trial results. Quality management includes the design of efficient clinical trial protocols and tools and procedures for data collection and processing, as well as the collection of information that is essential to decision making.

The methods used to assure and control the quality of the trial should be proportionate to the risks inherent in the trial and the importance of the information collected. The sponsor should ensure that all aspects of the trial are operationally feasible and should avoid unnecessary complexity, procedures, and data collection. Protocols, case report forms, and other operational documents should be clear, concise, and consistent.

The quality management system should use a risk-based approach as described below.

5.0.1 *Critical Process and Data Identification*

During protocol development, the sponsor should identify those processes and data that are critical to ensure human subject protection and the reliability of trial results.

5.0.2 *Risk Identification*

The sponsor should identify risks to critical trial processes and data. Risks should be considered at both the system level (e.g., standard operating procedures, computerized systems, personnel) and clinical trial level (e.g., trial design, data collection, informed consent process).

5.0.3 *Risk Evaluation*

The sponsor should evaluate the identified risks, against existing risk controls by considering:

A. The likelihood of errors occurring.

B. The extent to which such errors would be detectable.

C. The impact of such errors on human subject protection and reliability of trial results.

5.0.4 *Risk Control*

The sponsor should decide which risks to reduce and/or which risks to accept. The approach used to reduce risk to an acceptable level should be proportionate to the significance of the risk. Risk reduction activities may be incorporated in protocol design and implementation, monitoring plans,

agreements between parties defining roles and responsibilities, systematic safeguards to ensure adherence to standard operating procedures, and training in processes and procedures.
Predefined quality tolerance limits should be established, taking into consideration the medical and statistical characteristics of the variables as well as the statistical design of the trial, to identify systematic issues that can impact subject safety or reliability of trial results. Detection of deviations from the predefined quality tolerance limits should trigger an evaluation to determine if action is needed.

5.0.5 Risk Communication

The sponsor should document quality management activities. The sponsor should communicate quality management activities to those who are involved in or affected by such activities, to facilitate risk review and continual improvement during clinical trial execution.

5.0.6 Risk Review

The sponsor should periodically review risk control measures to ascertain whether the implemented quality management activities remain effective and relevant, taking into account emerging knowledge and experience.

5.0.7 Risk Reporting

The sponsor should describe the quality management approach implemented in the trial and summarize important deviations from the predefined quality tolerance limits and remedial actions taken in the clinical study report (ICH E3, Section 9.6 Data Quality Assurance).

5.1 Quality Assurance and Quality Control

5.1.1 The sponsor is responsible for implementing and maintaining quality assurance and quality control systems with written SOPs to ensure that trials are conducted and data are generated, documented (recorded), and reported in compliance with the protocol, GCP, and the applicable regulatory requirement(s).

5.1.2 The sponsor is responsible for securing agreement from all involved parties to ensure direct access (see 1.21) to all trial related sites, source data/documents , and reports for the purpose of monitoring and auditing by the sponsor, and inspection by domestic and foreign regulatory authorities.

5.1.3 Quality control should be applied to each stage of data handling to ensure that all data are reliable and have been processed correctly.

5.1.4 Agreements, made by the sponsor with the investigator/institution and any other parties involved with the clinical trial, should be in writing, as part of the protocol or in a separate agreement.

5.2 Contract Research Organization (CRO)

5.2.1 A sponsor may transfer any or all of the sponsor's trial-related duties and functions to a CRO, but the ultimate responsibility for the quality and integrity of the trial data always resides with the sponsor. The CRO should implement quality assurance and quality control.

5.2.2 Any trial-related duty and function that is transferred to and assumed by a CRO should be specified in writing.

ADDENDUM

The sponsor should ensure oversight of any trial-related duties and functions carried out on its behalf, including trial-related duties and functions that are subcontracted to another party by the sponsor's contracted CRO(s).

5.2.3 Any trial-related duties and functions not specifically transferred to and assumed by a CRO are retained by the sponsor.

5.2.4 All references to a sponsor in this guideline also apply to a CRO to the extent that a CRO has assumed the trial related duties and functions of a sponsor.

5.3 Medical Expertise

The sponsor should designate appropriately qualified medical personnel who will be readily available to advise on trial related medical questions or problems. If necessary, outside consultant(s) may be appointed for this purpose.

5.4 Trial Design

5.4.1 The sponsor should utilize qualified individuals (e.g., biostatisticians, clinical pharmacologists, and physicians) as appropriate, throughout all stages of the trial process, from designing the protocol and CRFs and planning the analyses to analyzing and preparing interim and final clinical trial reports.

5.4.2 For further guidance: Clinical Trial Protocol and Protocol Amendment(s) (see 6.), the ICH Guideline for Structure and Content of Clinical Study Reports, and other appropriate ICH guidance on trial design, protocol and conduct.

5.5 Trial Management, Data Handling, and Record Keeping

5.5.1 The sponsor should utilize appropriately qualified individuals to supervise the overall conduct of the trial, to handle the data, to verify the data, to conduct the statistical analyses, and to prepare the trial reports.

5.5.2 The sponsor may consider establishing an independent data-monitoring committee (IDMC) to assess the progress of a clinical trial, including the safety data and the critical efficacy endpoints at intervals, and to recommend to the sponsor whether to continue, modify, or stop a trial. The IDMC should have written operating procedures and maintain written records of all its meetings.

5.5.3 When using electronic trial data handling and/or remote electronic trial data systems, the sponsor should:

A. Ensure and document that the electronic data processing system(s) conforms to the sponsor's established requirements for completeness, accuracy, reliability, and consistent intended performance (i.e., validation).

ADDENDUM

The sponsor should base their approach to validation of such systems on a risk assessment that takes into consideration the intended use of the system and the potential of the system to affect human subject protection and reliability of trial results.

B. Maintains SOPs for using these systems.

ADDENDUM

The SOPs should cover system setup, installation, and use. The SOPs should describe system validation and functionality testing, data collection and handling, system maintenance, system security measures, change control, data backup, recovery, contingency planning, and decommissioning. The responsibilities of the sponsor, investigator, and other parties with respect to the use of these computerized systems should be clear, and the users should be provided with training in their use.

C. Ensure that the systems are designed to permit data changes in such a way that the data changes are documented and that there is no deletion of entered data (i.e., maintain an audit trail, data trail, edit trail).

D. Maintain a security system that prevents unauthorized access to the data.

E. Maintain a list of the individuals who are authorized to make data changes (see 4.1.5 and 4.9.3).

F. Maintain adequate backup of the data.

G. Safeguard the blinding, if any (e.g., maintain the blinding during data entry and processing).

ADDENDUM

H. Ensure the integrity of the data including any data that describe the context, content, and structure. This is particularly important when making changes to the computerized systems, such as software upgrades or migration of data.

5.5.4 If data are transformed during processing, it should always be possible to compare the original data and observations with the processed data.

5.5.5 The sponsor should use an unambiguous subject identification code (see 1.58) that allows identification of all the data reported for each subject.

5.5.6 The sponsor, or other owners of the data, should retain all of the sponsor-specific essential documents pertaining to the trial (see 8. Essential Documents for the Conduct of a Clinical Trial).

5.5.7 The sponsor should retain all sponsor-specific essential documents in conformance with the applicable regulatory requirement(s) of the country(ies) where the product is approved, and/or where the sponsor intends to apply for approval(s).

5.5.8 If the sponsor discontinues the clinical development of an investigational product (i.e., for any or all indications, routes of administration, or dosage forms), the sponsor should maintain all sponsor-specific essential documents for at least 2-years after formal discontinuation or in conformance with the applicable regulatory requirement(s).

5.5.9 If the sponsor discontinues the clinical development of an investigational product, the sponsor should notify all the trial investigators/institutions and all the regulatory authorities.

5.5.10 Any transfer of ownership of the data should be reported to the appropriate authority(ies), as required by the applicable regulatory requirement(s).

5.5.11 The sponsor specific essential documents should be retained until at least 2-years after the last approval of a marketing application in an ICH region and until there are no pending or contemplated marketing applications in an ICH region or at least 2-years have elapsed since the formal discontinuation of clinical development of the investigational product. These documents should be retained for a longer period however if required by the applicable regulatory requirement(s) or if needed by the sponsor.

5.5.12 The sponsor should inform the investigator(s)/institution(s) in writing of the need for record retention and should notify the investigator(s)/institution(s) in writing when the trial related records are no longer needed.

5.6 Investigator Selection

5.6.1 The sponsor is responsible for selecting the investigator(s)/institution(s). Each investigator should be qualified by training and experience and should have adequate resources (see 4.1, 4.2) to properly conduct the trial for which the investigator is selected. If organization of a coordinating committee and/or selection of coordinating investigator(s) are to be utilized in multicentre trials, their organization and/or selection are the sponsor's responsibility.

5.6.2 Before entering an agreement with an investigator/institution to conduct a trial, the sponsor should provide the investigator(s)/institution(s) with the protocol and an up-to-date Investigator's Brochure, and should provide sufficient time for the investigator/institution to review the protocol and the information provided.

5.6.3 The sponsor should obtain the investigator's/institution's agreement:

A. to conduct the trial in compliance with GCP, with the applicable regulatory requirement(s) (see 4.1.3), and with the protocol agreed to by the sponsor and given approval/favourable opinion by the IRB/IEC (see 4.5.1);

B. to comply with procedures for data recording/reporting;

C. to permit monitoring, auditing and inspection (see 4.1.4) and

D. to retain the trial related essential documents until the sponsor informs the investigator/institution these documents are no longer needed (see 4.9.4 and 5.5.12).

The sponsor and the investigator/institution should sign the protocol, or an alternative document, to confirm this agreement.

5.7 Allocation of Responsibilities

Prior to initiating a trial, the sponsor should define, establish, and allocate all trial-related duties and functions.

5.8 Compensation to Subjects and Investigators

5.8.1 If required by the applicable regulatory requirement(s), the sponsor should provide insurance or should indemnify (legal and financial coverage) the investigator/the institution against claims arising from the trial, except for claims that arise from malpractice and/or negligence.

5.8.2 The sponsor's policies and procedures should address the costs of treatment of trial subjects in the event of trial-related injuries in accordance with the applicable regulatory requirement(s).

5.8.3 When trial subjects receive compensation, the method and manner of compensation should comply with applicable regulatory requirement(s).

5.9 Financing

The financial aspects of the trial should be documented in an agreement between the sponsor and the investigator/institution.

5.10 Notification/Submission to Regulatory Authority(ies)

Before initiating the clinical trial(s), the sponsor (or the sponsor and the investigator, if required by the applicable regulatory requirement(s)) should submit any required application(s) to the appropriate authority(ies) for review, acceptance, and/or permission (as required by the applicable regulatory requirement(s)) to begin the trial(s). Any notification/submission should be dated and contain sufficient information to identify the protocol.

5.11 Confirmation of Review by IRB/IEC

5.11.1 The sponsor should obtain from the investigator/institution:

A. The name and address of the investigator's/institution's IRB/IEC.

B. A statement obtained from the IRB/IEC that it is organized and operates according to GCP and the applicable laws and regulations.

C. Documented IRB/IEC approval/favourable opinion and, if requested by the sponsor, a current copy of protocol, written informed consent form(s) and any other written information to be provided to subjects, subject recruiting procedures, and documents related to payments and compensation available to the subjects, and any other documents that the IRB/IEC may have requested.

5.11.2 If the IRB/IEC conditions its approval/favourable opinion upon change(s) in any aspect of the trial, such as modification(s) of the protocol, written informed consent form and any other written information to be provided to subjects, and/or other procedures, the sponsor should obtain from the investigator/institution a copy of the modification(s) made and the date approval/favourable opinion was given by the IRB/IEC.

5.11.3 The sponsor should obtain from the investigator/institution documentation and dates of any IRB/IEC reapprovals/re-evaluations with favourable opinion, and of any withdrawals or suspensions of approval/favourable opinion.

5.12 Information on Investigational Product(s)

5.12.1 When planning trials, the sponsor should ensure that sufficient safety and efficacy data from nonclinical studies and/or clinical trials are available to support human exposure by the route, at the dosages, for the duration, and in the trial population to be studied.

5.12.2 The sponsor should update the Investigator's Brochure as significant new information becomes available (see 7. Investigator's Brochure).

5.13 Manufacturing, Packaging, Labelling, and Coding Investigational Product(s)

5.13.1 The sponsor should ensure that the investigational product(s) (including active comparator(s) and placebo, if applicable) is characterized as appropriate to the stage of development of the product(s), is manufactured in accordance with any applicable GMP, and is coded and labelled in a manner that protects the blinding, if applicable. In addition, the labelling should comply with applicable regulatory requirement(s).

5.13.2 The sponsor should determine, for the investigational product(s), acceptable storage temperatures, storage conditions (e.g., protection from light), storage times, reconstitution fluids and procedures, and devices for product infusion, if any. The sponsor should inform all involved parties (e.g., monitors, investigators, pharmacists, storage managers) of these determinations.

5.13.3 The investigational product(s) should be packaged to prevent contamination and unacceptable deterioration during transport and storage.

5.13.4 In blinded trials, the coding system for the investigational product(s) should include a mechanism that permits rapid identification of the product(s) in case of a medical emergency, but does not permit undetectable breaks of the blinding.

5.13.5 If significant formulation changes are made in the investigational or comparator product(s) during the course of clinical development, the results of any additional studies of the formulated product(s) (e.g., stability, dissolution rate, bioavailability) needed to assess whether these changes would significantly alter the pharmacokinetic profile of the product should be available prior to the use of the new formulation in clinical trials.

5.14 Supplying and Handling Investigational Product(s)

5.14.1 The sponsor is responsible for supplying the investigator(s)/institution(s) with the investigational product(s).

5.14.2 The sponsor should not supply an investigator/institution with the investigational product(s) until the sponsor obtains all required documentation (e.g., approval/favourable opinion from IRB/IEC and regulatory authority(ies)).

5.14.3 The sponsor should ensure that written procedures include instructions that the investigator/institution should follow for the handling and storage of investigational product(s) for the trial and documentation thereof. The procedures should address adequate and safe receipt, handling, storage, dispensing, retrieval of unused product from subjects, and return of unused investigational product(s) to the sponsor (or alternative disposition if authorized by the sponsor and in compliance with the applicable regulatory requirement(s)).

5.14.4 The sponsor should:

A. Ensure timely delivery of investigational product(s) to the investigator(s).

B. Maintain records that document shipment, receipt, disposition, return, and destruction of the investigational product(s) (see 8. Essential Documents for the Conduct of a Clinical Trial).

C. Maintain a system for retrieving investigational products and documenting this retrieval (e.g., for deficient product recall, reclaim after trial completion, expired product reclaim).

D. Maintain a system for the disposition of unused investigational product(s) and for the documentation of this disposition.

5.14.5 The sponsor should:

A. Take steps to ensure that the investigational product(s) are stable over the period of use.

B. Maintain sufficient quantities of the investigational product(s) used in the trials to reconfirm specifications, should this become necessary, and maintain records of batch sample analyses and characteristics. To the extent stability permits, samples should be retained either until the analyses of the trial data are complete or as required by the applicable regulatory requirement(s), whichever represents the longer retention period.

5.15 Record Access

5.15.1 The sponsor should ensure that it is specified in the protocol or other written agreement that the investigator(s)/institution(s) provide direct access to source data/documents for trial-related monitoring, audits, IRB/IEC review, and regulatory inspection.

5.15.2 The sponsor should verify that each subject has consented, in writing, to direct access to his/her original medical records for trial-related monitoring, audit, IRB/IEC review, and regulatory inspection.

5.16 Safety Information

5.16.1 The sponsor is responsible for the ongoing safety evaluation of the investigational product(s).

5.16.2 The sponsor should promptly notify all concerned investigator(s)/institution(s) and the regulatory authority(ies) of findings that could affect adversely the safety of subjects, impact the conduct of the trial, or alter the IRB/IEC's approval/favourable opinion to continue the trial.

5.17 Adverse Drug Reaction Reporting

5.17.1 The sponsor should expedite the reporting to all concerned investigator(s)/institutions(s), to the IRB(s)/IEC(s), where required, and to the regulatory authority(ies) of all adverse drug reactions (ADRs) that are both serious and unexpected.

5.17.2 Such expedited reports should comply with the applicable regulatory requirement(s) and with the ICH Guideline for Clinical Safety Data Management: Definitions and Standards for Expedited Reporting.

5.17.3 The sponsor should submit to the regulatory authority(ies) all safety updates and periodic reports, as required by applicable regulatory requirement(s).

5.18 Monitoring

5.18.1 *Purpose*
The purposes of trial monitoring are to verify that:

A. The rights and well-being of human subjects are protected.

B. The reported trial data are accurate, complete, and verifiable from source documents.

C. The conduct of the trial is in compliance with the currently approved protocol/amendment(s), with GCP, and with the applicable regulatory requirement(s).

5.18.2 *Selection and Qualifications of Monitors*

A. Monitors should be appointed by the sponsor.

B. Monitors should be appropriately trained, and should have the scientific and/or clinical knowledge needed to monitor the trial adequately. A monitor's qualifications should be documented.

C. Monitors should be thoroughly familiar with the investigational product(s), the protocol, written informed consent form and any other written information to be provided to subjects, the sponsor's SOPs, GCP, and the applicable regulatory requirement(s).

5.18.3 Extent and Nature of Monitoring

The sponsor should ensure that the trials are adequately monitored. The sponsor should determine the appropriate extent and nature of monitoring. The determination of the extent and nature of monitoring should be based on considerations such as the objective, purpose, design, complexity, blinding, size, and endpoints of the trial. In general there is a need for on-site monitoring, before, during, and after the trial; however in exceptional circumstances the sponsor may determine that central monitoring in conjunction with procedures such as investigators' training and meetings, and extensive written guidance can assure appropriate conduct of the trial in accordance with GCP. Statistically controlled sampling may be an acceptable method for selecting the data to be verified.

ADDENDUM

The sponsor should develop a systematic, prioritized, risk-based approach to monitoring clinical trials. The flexibility in the extent and nature of monitoring described in this section is intended to permit varied approaches that improve the effectiveness and efficiency of monitoring. The sponsor may choose on-site monitoring, a combination of on-site and centralized monitoring, or, where justified, centralized monitoring. The sponsor should document the rationale for the chosen monitoring strategy (e.g., in the monitoring plan).

On-site monitoring is performed at the sites at which the clinical trial is being conducted. Centralized monitoring is a remote evaluation of accumulating data, performed in a timely manner, supported by appropriately qualified and trained persons (e.g., data managers, biostatisticians).

Centralized monitoring processes provide additional monitoring capabilities that can complement and reduce the extent and/or frequency of on-site monitoring and help distinguish between reliable data and potentially unreliable data.

Review, that may include statistical analyses, of accumulating data from centralized monitoring can be used to:

A. identify missing data, inconsistent data, data outliers, unexpected lack of variability and protocol deviations.

B. examine data trends such as the range, consistency, and variability of data within and across sites.

C. evaluate for systematic or significant errors in data collection and reporting at a site or across sites; or potential data manipulation or data integrity problems.

D. analyze site characteristics and performance metrics.

E. select sites and/or processes for targeted on-site monitoring.

5.18.4 Monitor's Responsibilities

The monitor(s) in accordance with the sponsor's requirements should ensure that the trial is conducted and documented properly by carrying out the following activities when relevant and necessary to the trial and the trial site:

A. Acting as the main line of communication between the sponsor and the investigator.

B. Verifying that the investigator has adequate qualifications and resources (see 4.1, 4.2, 5.6) and remain adequate throughout the trial period, that facilities, including laboratories, equipment, and staff, are adequate to safely and properly conduct the trial and remain adequate throughout the trial period.

C. Verifying, for the investigational product(s):

    I. That storage times and conditions are acceptable, and that supplies are sufficient throughout the trial.

    II. That the investigational product(s) are supplied only to subjects who are eligible to receive it and at the protocol specified dose(s).

    III. That subjects are provided with necessary instruction on properly using, handling, storing, and returning the investigational product(s).

    IV. That the receipt, use, and return of the investigational product(s) at the trial sites are controlled and documented adequately.

    V. That the disposition of unused investigational product(s) at the trial sites complies with applicable regulatory requirement(s) and is in accordance with the sponsor.

D. Verifying that the investigator follows the approved protocol and all approved amendment(s), if any.

E. Verifying that written informed consent was obtained before each subject's participation in the trial.

F. Ensuring that the investigator receives the current Investigator's Brochure, all documents, and all trial supplies needed to conduct the trial properly and to comply with the applicable regulatory requirement(s).

G. Ensuring that the investigator and the investigator's trial staff are adequately informed about the trial.

H. Verifying that the investigator and the investigator's trial staff are performing the specified trial functions, in accordance with the protocol and any other written agreement between the sponsor and the investigator/institution, and have not delegated these functions to unauthorized individuals.

I. Verifying that the investigator is enroling only eligible subjects.

J. Reporting the subject recruitment rate.

K. Verifying that source documents and other trial records are accurate, complete, kept up-to-date and maintained.

L. Verifying that the investigator provides all the required reports, notifications, applications, and submissions, and that these documents are accurate, complete, timely, legible, dated, and identify the trial.

M. Checking the accuracy and completeness of the CRF entries, source documents and other trial-related records against each other. The monitor specifically should verify that:

   I. (i) The data required by the protocol are reported accurately on the CRFs and are consistent with the source documents.

   II. (ii) Any dose and/or therapy modifications are well documented for each of the trial subjects.

   III. (iii) Adverse events, concomitant medications and intercurrent illnesses are reported in accordance with the protocol on the CRFs.

   IV. (iv) Visits that the subjects fail to make, tests that are not conducted, and examinations that are not performed are clearly reported as such on the CRFs.

   V. (v) All withdrawals and dropouts of enrolled subjects from the trial are reported and explained on the CRFs.

N. Informing the investigator of any CRF entry error, omission, or illegibility. The monitor should ensure that appropriate corrections, additions, or deletions are made, dated, explained (if necessary), and initialled by the investigator or by a member of the investigator's trial staff who is authorized to initial CRF changes for the investigator. This authorization should be documented.

O. Determining whether all adverse events (AEs) are appropriately reported within the time periods required by GCP, the protocol, the IRB/IEC, the sponsor, and the applicable regulatory requirement(s).

P. Determining whether the investigator is maintaining the essential documents (see 8. Essential Documents for the Conduct of a Clinical Trial).

Q. Communicating deviations from the protocol, SOPs, GCP, and the applicable regulatory requirements to the investigator and taking appropriate action designed to prevent recurrence of the detected deviations.

5.18.5 Monitoring Procedures

The monitor(s) should follow the sponsor's established written SOPs as well as those procedures that are specified by the sponsor for monitoring a specific trial.

5.18.6 Monitoring Report

A. The monitor should submit a written report to the sponsor after each trial-site visit or trial-related communication.

B. Reports should include the date, site, name of the monitor, and name of the investigator or other individual(s) contacted.

C. Reports should include a summary of what the monitor reviewed and the monitor's statements concerning the significant findings/facts, deviations and deficiencies, conclusions, actions taken or to be taken and/or actions recommended to secure compliance.

D. The review and follow-up of the monitoring report with the sponsor should be documented by the sponsor's designated representative.

ADDENDUM

E. Reports of on-site and/or centralized monitoring should be provided to the sponsor (including appropriate management and staff responsible for trial and site oversight) in a timely manner for review and follow up. Results of monitoring activities should be documented in sufficient detail to allow verification of compliance with the monitoring plan. Reporting of centralized monitoring activities should be regular and may be independent from site visits.

ADDENDUM

5.18.7 Monitoring Plan

The sponsor should develop a monitoring plan that is tailored to the specific human subject protection and data integrity risks of the trial. The plan should describe the monitoring strategy, the monitoring responsibilities of all the parties involved, the various monitoring methods to be used, and the rationale for their use. The plan should also emphasize the monitoring of critical data and processes. Particular attention should be given to those aspects that are not routine clinical practice and that require additional training. The monitoring plan should reference the applicable policies and procedures.

5.19 Audit

If or when sponsors perform audits, as part of implementing quality assurance, they should consider:

5.19.1 Purpose

The purpose of a sponsor's audit, which is independent of and separate from routine monitoring or quality control functions, should be to evaluate trial conduct and compliance with the protocol, SOPs, GCP, and the applicable regulatory requirements.

5.19.2 Selection and Qualification of Auditors

A. The sponsor should appoint individuals, who are independent of the clinical trials/systems, to conduct audits.

B. The sponsor should ensure that the auditors are qualified by training and experience to conduct audits properly. An auditor's qualifications should be documented.

5.19.3 Auditing Procedures

A. The sponsor should ensure that the auditing of clinical trials/systems is conducted in accordance with the sponsor's written procedures on what to audit, how to audit, the frequency of audits, and the form and content of audit reports.

B. The sponsor's audit plan and procedures for a trial audit should be guided by the importance of the trial to submissions to regulatory authorities, the number of subjects in the trial, the type and complexity of the trial, the level of risks to the trial subjects, and any identified problem(s).

C. The observations and findings of the auditor(s) should be documented.

D. To preserve the independence and value of the audit function, the regulatory authority(ies) should not routinely request the audit reports. Regulatory authority(ies) may seek access to an audit report on a case by case basis when evidence of serious GCP non-compliance exists, or in the course of legal proceedings.

E. When required by applicable law or regulation, the sponsor should provide an audit certificate.

5.20 Noncompliance

5.20.1 Noncompliance with the protocol, SOPs, GCP, and/or applicable regulatory requirement(s) by an investigator/institution, or by member(s) of the sponsor's staff should lead to prompt action by the sponsor to secure compliance.

ADDENDUM

If noncompliance that significantly affects or has the potential to significantly affect human subject protection or reliability of trial results is discovered, the sponsor should perform a root cause analysis and implement appropriate corrective and preventive actions.

5.20.2 If the monitoring and/or auditing identifies serious and/or persistent noncompliance on the part of an investigator/institution, the sponsor should terminate the investiga-tor's/institution's participation in the trial. When an investigator's/institution's parti-cipation is terminated because of noncompliance, the sponsor should notify promptly the regulatory authority(ies).

5.21 Premature Termination or Suspension of a Trial

If a trial is prematurely terminated or suspended, the sponsor should promptly inform the investigators/institutions, and the regulatory authority(ies) of the termination or suspension and the reason(s) for the termination or suspension. The IRB/IEC should also be informed promptly and provided the reason(s) for the termination or suspension by the sponsor or by the investigator/institution, as specified by the applicable regulatory requirement(s).

5.22 Clinical Trial/Study Reports

Whether the trial is completed or prematurely terminated, the sponsor should ensure that the clinical trial reports are prepared and provided to the regulatory agency(ies) as required by the applicable regulatory requirement(s). The sponsor should also ensure that the clinical trial reports in marketing applications meet the standards of the ICH Guideline for Structure and Content of Clinical Study Reports. (NOTE: The ICH Guideline for Structure and Content of Clinical Study Reports specifies that abbreviated study reports may be acceptable in certain cases.)

5.23 Multicentre Trials

For multicentre trials, the sponsor should ensure that:

5.23.1 All investigators conduct the trial in strict compliance with the protocol agreed to by the sponsor and, if required, by the regulatory authority(ies), and given approval/favourable opinion by the IRB/IEC.

5.23.2 The CRFs are designed to capture the required data at all multicentre trial sites. For those investigators who are collecting additional data, supplemental CRFs should also be provided that are designed to capture the additional data.

5.23.3 The responsibilities of coordinating investigator(s) and the other participating investigators are documented prior to the start of the trial.

5.23.4 All investigators are given instructions on following the protocol, on complying with a uniform set of standards for the assessment of clinical and laboratory findings, and on completing the CRFs.

5.23.5 Communication between investigators is facilitated.

6. CLINICAL TRIAL PROTOCOL AND PROTOCOL AMENDMENT(S)

The contents of a trial protocol should generally include the following topics. However, site specific information may be provided on separate protocol page(s), or addressed in a separate agreement, and some of the information listed below may be contained in other protocol referenced documents, such as an Investigator's Brochure.

6.1 General Information

6.1.1 Protocol title, protocol identifying number, and date. Any amendment(s) should also bear the amendment number(s) and date(s).

6.1.2 Name and address of the sponsor and monitor (if other than the sponsor).

6.1.3 Name and title of the person(s) authorized to sign the protocol and the protocol amendment(s) for the sponsor.

6.1.4 Name, title, address, and telephone number(s) of the sponsor's medical expert (or dentist when appropriate) for the trial.

6.1.5 Name and title of the investigator(s) who is (are) responsible for conducting the trial, and the address and telephone number(s) of the trial site(s).

6.1.6 Name, title, address, and telephone number(s) of the qualified physician (or dentist, if applicable), who is responsible for all trial-site related medical (or dental) decisions (if other than investigator).

6.1.7 Name(s) and address(es) of the clinical laboratory(ies) and other medical and/or technical department(s) and/or institutions involved in the trial.

6.2 Background Information

6.2.1 Name and description of the investigational product(s).

6.2.2 A summary of findings from nonclinical studies that potentially have clinical significance and from clinical trials that are relevant to the trial.

6.2.3 Summary of the known and potential risks and benefits, if any, to human subjects.

6.2.4 Description of and justification for the route of administration, dosage, dosage regimen, and treatment period(s).

6.2.5 A statement that the trial will be conducted in compliance with the protocol, GCP and the applicable regulatory requirement(s).

6.2.6 Description of the population to be studied.

6.2.7 References to literature and data that are relevant to the trial, and that provide background for the trial.

6.3 Trial Objectives and Purpose

A detailed description of the objectives and the purpose of the trial.

6.4 Trial Design

The scientific integrity of the trial and the credibility of the data from the trial depend substantially on the trial design. A description of the trial design, should include:

6.4.1 A specific statement of the primary endpoints and the secondary endpoints, if any, to be measured during the trial.

6.4.2 A description of the type/design of trial to be conducted (e.g., double-blind, placebo-controlled, parallel design) and a schematic diagram of trial design, procedures and stages.

6.4.3 A description of the measures taken to minimize/avoid bias, including:

A. Randomization.

B. Blinding.

6.4.4 A description of the trial treatment(s) and the dosage and dosage regimen of the investigational product(s). Also include a description of the dosage form, packaging, and labelling of the investigational product(s).

6.4.5 The expected duration of subject participation, and a description of the sequence and duration of all trial periods, including follow-up, if any.

6.4.6 A description of the "stopping rules" or "discontinuation criteria" for individual subjects, parts of trial and entire trial.

6.4.7 Accountability procedures for the investigational product(s), including the placebo(s) and comparator(s), if any.

6.4.8 Maintenance of trial treatment randomization codes and procedures for breaking codes.

6.4.9 The identification of any data to be recorded directly on the CRFs (i.e., no prior written or electronic record of data), and to be considered to be source data.

6.5 Selection and Withdrawal of Subjects

6.5.1 Subject inclusion criteria.

6.5.2 Subject exclusion criteria.

6.5.3 Subject withdrawal criteria (i.e., terminating investigational product treatment/trial treatment) and procedures specifying:

A. When and how to withdraw subjects from the trial/ investigational product treatment.

B. The type and timing of the data to be collected for withdrawn subjects.

C. Whether and how subjects are to be replaced.

D. The follow-up for subjects withdrawn from investigational product treatment/trial treatment.

6.6 Treatment of Subjects

6.6.1 The treatment(s) to be administered, including the name(s) of all the product(s), the dose(s), the dosing schedule(s), the route/mode(s) of administration, and the treatment period(s), including the follow-up period(s) for subjects for each investigational product treatment/trial treatment group/arm of the trial.

6.6.2 Medication(s)/treatment(s) permitted (including rescue medication) and not permitted before and/or during the trial.

6.6.3 Procedures for monitoring subject compliance.

6.7 Assessment of Efficacy

6.7.1 Specification of the efficacy parameters.

6.7.2 Methods and timing for assessing, recording, and analysing of efficacy parameters.

6.8 Assessment of Safety

6.8.1 Specification of safety parameters.

6.8.2 The methods and timing for assessing, recording, and analysing safety parameters.

6.8.3 Procedures for eliciting reports of and for recording and reporting adverse event and intercurrent illnesses.

6.8.4 The type and duration of the follow-up of subjects after adverse events.

6.9 Statistics

6.9.1 A description of the statistical methods to be employed, including timing of any planned interim analysis(ses).

6.9.2 The number of subjects planned to be enrolled. In multicentre trials, the numbers of enrolled subjects projected for each trial site should be specified. Reason for choice of sample size, including reflections on (or calculations of) the power of the trial and clinical justification.

6.9.3 The level of significance to be used.

6.9.4 Criteria for the termination of the trial.

6.9.5 Procedure for accounting for missing, unused, and spurious data.

6.9.6 Procedures for reporting any deviation(s) from the original statistical plan (any deviation(s) from the original statistical plan should be described and justified in protocol and/or in the final report, as appropriate).

6.9.7 The selection of subjects to be included in the analyses (e.g., all randomized subjects, all dosed subjects, all eligible subjects, evaluable subjects).

6.10 Direct Access to Source Data/Documents

The sponsor should ensure that it is specified in the protocol or other written agreement that the investigator(s)/institution(s) will permit trial-related monitoring, audits, IRB/IEC review, and regulatory inspection(s), providing direct access to source data/documents.

6.11 Quality Control and Quality Assurance

6.12 Ethics

Description of ethical considerations relating to the trial.

6.13 Data Handling and Record Keeping

6.14 Financing and Insurance

Financing and insurance if not addressed in a separate agreement.

6.15 Publication Policy

Publication policy, if not addressed in a separate agreement.

6.16 Supplements

(NOTE: Since the protocol and the clinical trial/study report are closely related, further relevant information can be found in the ICH Guideline for Structure and Content of Clinical Study Reports.)

7. INVESTIGATOR'S BROCHURE

7.1 Introduction

The Investigator's Brochure (IB) is a compilation of the clinical and nonclinical data on the investigational product(s) that are relevant to the study of the product(s) in human subjects. Its purpose is to provide the investigators and others involved in the trial with the information to facilitate their understanding of the rationale for, and their compliance with, many key features of the protocol, such as the dose, dose frequency/interval, methods of administration: and safety monitoring procedures. The IB also provides insight to support the clinical management of the study subjects during the course of the clinical trial. The information should be presented in a concise, simple, objective, balanced, and non-promotional form that enables a clinician, or potential investigator, to understand it and make his/her own unbiased risk-benefit assessment of the appropriateness of the proposed trial. For this reason, a medically qualified person should generally participate in the editing of an IB, but the contents of the IB should be approved by the disciplines that generated the described data.

This guideline delineates the minimum information that should be included in an IB and provides suggestions for its layout. It is expected that the type and extent of information available will vary with the stage of development of the investigational product. If the investigational product is marketed and its pharmacology is widely understood by medical practitioners, an extensive IB may not be necessary. Where permitted by regulatory authorities, a basic product information brochure, package leaflet, or labelling may be an appropriate alternative, provided that it includes current, comprehensive, and detailed information on all aspects of the investigational product that might be of importance to the investigator. If a marketed product is being studied for a new use (i.e., a new indication), an IB specific to that new use should be prepared. The IB should be reviewed at least annually and revised as necessary in compliance with a sponsor's written procedures. More frequent revision may be appropriate depending on the stage of development and the generation of relevant new information. However, in accordance with Good Clinical Practice, relevant new information may be so important that it should be communicated to the investigators, and possibly to the Institutional Review Boards (IRBs)/Independent Ethics Committees (IECs) and/or regulatory authorities before it is included in a revised IB.

Generally, the sponsor is responsible for ensuring that an up-to-date IB is made available to the investigator(s) and the investigators are responsible for providing the up-to-date IB to the responsible IRBs/IECs. In the case of an investigator sponsored trial, the sponsor-investigator should determine whether a brochure is available from the commercial manufacturer. If the investigational product is provided by the sponsor-investigator, then he or she should provide the necessary information to the trial personnel. In cases where preparation of a formal IB is impractical, the sponsor-investigator should provide, as a substitute, an expanded background information section in the trial protocol that contains the minimum current information described in this guideline.

7.2 General Considerations

The IB should include:

7.2.1 Title Page

This should provide the sponsor's name, the identity of each investigational product (i.e., research number, chemical or approved generic name, and trade name(s) where legally permissible and desired by the sponsor), and the release date. It is also suggested that an edition number, and a reference to the number and date of the edition it supersedes, be provided. An example is given in Appendix 1.

7.2.2 Confidentiality Statement

The sponsor may wish to include a statement instructing the investigator/recipients to treat the IB as a confidential document for the sole information and use of the investigator's team and the IRB/IEC.

7.3 Contents of the Investigator's Brochure

The IB should contain the following sections, each with literature references where appropriate:

7.3.1 Table of Contents

An example of the Table of Contents is given in Appendix 2

7.3.2 Summary

A brief summary (preferably not exceeding two pages) should be given, highlighting the significant physical, chemical, pharmaceutical, pharmacological, toxicological, pharmacokinetic, metabolic, and clinical information available that is relevant to the stage of clinical development of the investigational product.

7.3.3 Introduction

A brief introductory statement should be provided that contains the chemical name (and generic and trade name(s) when approved) of the investigational product(s), all active ingredients, the investigational product (s) pharmacological class and its expected position within this class (e.g., advantages), the rationale for performing research with the investigational product(s), and the anticipated prophylactic, therapeutic, or diagnostic indication(s). Finally, the introductory statement should provide the general approach to be followed in evaluating the investigational product.

7.3.4 Physical, Chemical, and Pharmaceutical Properties and Formulation

A description should be provided of the investigational product substance(s) (including the chemical and/or structural formula(e)), and a brief summary should be given of the relevant physical, chemical, and pharmaceutical properties.

To permit appropriate safety measures to be taken in the course of the trial, a description of the formulation(s) to be used, including excipients, should be provided and justified if clinically relevant. Instructions for the storage and handling of the dosage form(s) should also be given.

Any structural similarities to other known compounds should be mentioned.

7.3.5 Nonclinical Studies

Introduction:

The results of all relevant nonclinical pharmacology, toxicology, pharmacokinetic, and investigational product metabolism studies should be provided in summary form. This summary should address the methodology used, the results, and a discussion of the relevance of the findings to the investigated therapeutic and the possible unfavourable and unintended effects in humans.

The information provided may include the following, as appropriate, if known/available:

- Species tested
- Number and sex of animals in each group
- Unit dose (e.g., milligram/kilogram (mg/kg))
- Dose interval
- Route of administration
- Duration of dosing
- Information on systemic distribution
- Duration of post-exposure follow-up
- Results, including the following aspects:
    - Nature and frequency of pharmacological or toxic effects
    - Severity or intensity of pharmacological or toxic effects
    - Time to onset of effects
    - Reversibility of effects
    - Duration of effects
    - Dose response

Tabular format/listings should be used whenever possible to enhance the clarity of the presentation.

The following sections should discuss the most important findings from the studies, including the dose response of observed effects, the relevance to humans, and any aspects to be studied in humans. If applicable, the effective and nontoxic dose findings in the same animal species should be compared (i.e., the therapeutic index should be discussed). The relevance of this information to the proposed human dosing should be addressed. Whenever possible, comparisons should be made in terms of blood/tissue levels rather than on a mg/kg basis.

A. *Nonclinical Pharmacology*

A summary of the pharmacological aspects of the investigational product and, where appropriate, its significant metabolites studied in animals, should be included. Such a summary should incorporate studies that assess potential therapeutic activity (e.g., efficacy models, receptor binding, and specificity) as well as those that assess safety (e.g., special studies to assess pharmacological actions other than the intended therapeutic effect(s)).

B. Pharmacokinetics and Product Metabolism in Animals

A summary of the pharmacokinetics and biological transformation and disposition of the investigational product in all species studied should be given. The discussion of the findings should address the absorption and the local and systemic bioavailability of the investigational product and its metabolites, and their relationship to the pharmacological and toxicological findings in animal species.

C. Toxicology

A summary of the toxicological effects found in relevant studies conducted in different animal species should be described under the following headings where appropriate:

- Single dose
- Repeated dose
- Carcinogenicity
- Special studies (e.g., irritancy and sensitisation)
- Reproductive toxicity
- Genotoxicity (mutagenicity)

7.3.6 Effects in Humans

Introduction:

A thorough discussion of the known effects of the investigational product(s) in humans should be provided, including information on pharmacokinetics, metabolism, pharmacodynamics, dose response, safety, efficacy, and other pharmacological activities. Where possible, a summary of each completed clinical trial should be provided. Information should also be provided regarding results of any use of the investigational product(s) other than from in clinical trials, such as from experience during marketing.

A. Pharmacokinetics and Product Metabolism in Humans

- A summary of information on the pharmacokinetics of the investigational product(s) should be presented, including the following, if available:
- Pharmacokinetics (including metabolism, as appropriate, and absorption, plasma protein binding, distribution, and elimination).
- Bioavailability of the investigational product (absolute, where possible, and/or relative) using a reference dosage form.
- Population subgroups (e.g., gender, age, and impaired organ function).
- Interactions (e.g., product-product interactions and effects of food).
- Other pharmacokinetic data (e.g., results of population studies performed within clinical trial(s).

B. Safety and Efficacy

A summary of information should be provided about the investigational product's/products' (including metabolites, where appropriate) safety, pharmacodynamics, efficacy, and dose response that were obtained from preceding trials in humans (healthy volunteers and/or patients). The implications of this information should be discussed. In cases where a number of clinical trials have been completed, the use of summaries of safety and efficacy across multiple trials by indications in subgroups may provide a clear presentation of the data. Tabular summaries of adverse drug reactions for all the clinical trials (including those for all the studied indications) would be useful. Important differences in adverse drug reaction patterns/incidences across indications or subgroups should be discussed.

The IB should provide a description of the possible risks and adverse drug reactions to be anticipated on the basis of prior experiences with the product under investigation and with related products. A description should also be provided of the precautions or special monitoring to be done as part of the investigational use of the product(s).

C. Marketing Experience

The IB should identify countries where the investigational product has been marketed or approved. Any significant information arising from the marketed use should be summarised (e.g., formulations, dosages, routes of administration, and adverse product reactions). The IB should also identify all the countries where the investigational product did not receive approval/registration for marketing or was withdrawn from marketing/registration.

7.3.7 Summary of Data and Guidance for the Investigator

This section should provide an overall discussion of the nonclinical and clinical data, and should summarise the information from various sources on different aspects of the investigational product(s), wherever possible. In this way, the investigator can be provided with the most informative interpretation of the available data and with an assessment of the implications of the information for future clinical trials.

Where appropriate, the published reports on related products should be discussed. This could help the investigator to anticipate adverse drug reactions or other problems in clinical trials.

The overall aim of this section is to provide the investigator with a clear understanding of the possible risks and adverse reactions, and of the specific tests, observations, and precautions that may be needed for a clinical trial. This understanding should be based on the available physical, chemical, pharmaceutical, pharmacological, toxicological, and clinical information on the investigational product(s). Guidance should also be provided to the clinical investigator on the recognition and treatment of possible overdose and adverse drug reactions that is based on previous human experience and on the pharmacology of the investigational product.

7.4 APPENDIX 1:
TITLE PAGE (Example)
SPONSOR'S NAME
Product:
Research Number:
Name(s): Chemical, Generic (if approved)

Trade Name(s) (if legally permissible and desired by the sponsor)

INVESTIGATOR'S BROCHURE

Edition Number:
Release Date:

Replaces Previous Edition Number:
Date:

7.5 APPENDIX 2:
TABLE OF CONTENTS OF INVESTIGATOR'S BROCHURE (Example)

NB: References on 1. Publications
2. Reports

These references should be found at the end of each chapter
Appendices (if any) 8. ESSENTIAL DOCUMENTS FOR THE CONDUCT OF A CLINICAL TRIAL

8.1 Introduction

Essential Documents are those documents which individually and collectively permit evaluation of the conduct of a trial and the quality of the data produced. These documents serve to demonstrate the compliance of the investigator, sponsor and monitor with the standards of Good Clinical Practice and with all applicable regulatory requirements.

Essential Documents also serve a number of other important purposes. Filing essential documents at the investigator/institution and sponsor sites in a timely manner can greatly assist in the successful management of a trial by the investigator, sponsor and monitor. These documents are also the ones which are usually audited by the sponsor's independent audit function and inspected by the regulatory authority(ies) as part of the process to confirm the validity of the trial conduct and the integrity of data collected.

The minimum list of essential documents which has been developed follows. The various documents are grouped in three sections according to the stage of the trial during which they will normally be generated: 1) before the clinical phase of the trial commences, 2) during the clinical conduct of the trial, and 3) after completion or termination of the trial. A description is given of the purpose of each document, and whether it should be filed in either the investigator/institution or sponsor files, or both. It is acceptable to combine some of the documents, provided the individual elements are readily identifiable.

Trial master files should be established at the beginning of the trial, both at the investigator/institution's site and at the sponsor's office. A final close-out of a trial can only be done when the monitor has reviewed both investigator/institution and sponsor files and confirmed that all necessary documents are in the appropriate files.

Any or all of the documents addressed in this guideline may be subject to, and should be available for, audit by the sponsor's auditor and inspection by the regulatory authority(ies).

ADDENDUM

The sponsor and investigator/institution should maintain a record of the location(s) of their respective essential documents including source documents. The storage system used during the trial and for archiving (irrespective of the type of media used) should provide for document identification, version history, search, and retrieval.

Essential documents for the trial should be supplemented or may be reduced where justified (in advance of trial initiation) based on the importance and relevance of the specific documents to the trial.

The sponsor should ensure that the investigator has control of and continuous access to the CRF data reported to the sponsor. The sponsor should not have exclusive control of those data.

When a copy is used to replace an original document (e.g., source documents, CRF), the copy should fulfill the requirements for certified copies.

The investigator/institution should have control of all essential documents and records generated by the investigator/institution before, during, and after the trial.

8.2 Before the Clinical Phase of the Trial Commences

During this planning stage the following documents should be generated and should be on file before the trial formally starts

	Title of Document	Purpose	Investigator/ Institution	Sponsor
8.2.1	**INVESTIGATOR'S BROCHURE**	To document that relevant and current scientific information about the investigational product has been provided to the investigator	X	X
8.2.2	**SIGNED PROTOCOL AND AMENDMENTS, IF ANY, AND SAMPLE CASE REPORT FORM (CRF)**	To document investigator and sponsor agreement to the protocol/ amendment(s) and CRF	X	X
8.2.3	**INFORMATION GIVEN TO TRIAL SUBJECT- INFORMED CONSENT FORM(including all applicable translations)**	To document the informed consent	X	X
	- ANY OTHER WRITTEN INFORMATION	To document that subjects will be given appropriate written information (content and wording) to support their ability to give fully informed consent	X	X
	- ADVERTISEMENT FOR SUBJECT RECRUITMENT (if used)	To document that recruitment measures are appropriate and not coercive	X	
8.2.4	**FINANCIAL ASPECTS OF THE TRIAL**	To document the financial agreement between the investigator/institution and the sponsor for the trial	X	X

	Title of Document	Purpose	Investigator/ Institution	Sponsor
8.2.5	**INSURANCE STATEMENT(where required)**	To document that compensation to subject(s) for trial-related injury will be available	X	X
8.2.6	**SIGNED AGREEMENT BETWEEN INVOLVED PARTIES, e.g.:** - investigator/institution and sponsor - investigator/institution and CRO - sponsor and CRO - investigator/institution and authority(ies) (where required)	To document agreements	 X X X	 X X (where required) X X
8.2.7	**DATED, DOCUMENTED APPROVAL/FAVOURABLE OPINION OF INSTITUTIONAL REVIEW BOARD (IRB) /INDEPENDENT ETHICS COMMITTEE (IEC) OF THE FOLLOWING:** - protocol and any amendments - CRF (if applicable) - informed consent form(s) - any other written information to be provided to the subject(s) - advertisement for subject recruitment	To document that the trial has been subject toIRB/IEC review and given approval/favourable opinion. To identify the version number and date of the document(s)	X	X

	Title of Document	Purpose	Investigator/ Institution	Sponsor
8.2.8	**INSTITUTIONAL REVIEW BOARD/ INDEPENDENT ETHICS COMMITTEE COMPOSITION**	To document that the IRB/IEC is constituted in agreement with GCP	X	X (where required)
8.2.9	**REGULATORY AUTHORITY(IES) AUTHORISATION/APPROVAL/NOTIFICATION OF PROTOCOL** (where required)	To document appropriate authorisation/ approval/notification by the regulatory authority(ies) has been obtained prior to initiation of the trial in compliance with the applicable regulatory requirement(s)	X (where required)	X (where required)
8.2.10	**CURRICULUM VITAE AND/OR OTHER RELEVANT DOCUMENTS EVIDENCING QUALIFICATIONS OF INVESTIGATOR(S) AND SUB-INVESTIGATOR(S)**	To document qualifications and eligibility to conduct trial and/or provide medical supervision of subjects	X	X
8.2.11	**NORMAL VALUE(S)/ RANGE(S) FOR MEDICAL/ LABORATORY/TECHNICAL PROCEDURE(S) AND/OR TEST(S) INCLUDED IN THE PROTOCOL**	To document normal values and/or ranges of the tests		X

	Title of Document	Purpose	Investigator/ Institution	Sponsor
8.2.12	**MEDICAL/LABORATORY/TECHNICAL PROCEDURES / TESTS** - certification or - accreditation or - established quality control and/or external quality assessment or - other validation (where required)	To document competence of facility to perform required test(s), and support reliability of results	X (where required)	X
8.2.13	**SAMPLE OF LABEL(S) ATTACHED TO INVESTIGATIONAL PRODUCT CONTAINER(S)**	To document compliance with applicable labelling regulations and appropriateness of instructions provided to the subjects		X
8.2.14	**INSTRUCTIONS FOR HANDLING OF INVESTIGATIONAL PRODUCT(S) AND TRIAL-RELATED MATERIALS** (if not included in protocol or Investigator's Brochure)	To document instructions needed to ensure proper storage, packaging, dispensing and disposition of investigational products and trial-related materials	X	X
8.2.15	**SHIPPING RECORDS FOR INVESTIGATIONAL PRODUCT(S) AND TRIAL-RELATED MATERIALS**	To document shipment dates, batch numbers and method of shipment of investigational product(s) and trial-related materials. Allows tracking of product batch, review of shipping conditions, and accountability	X	X

	Title of Document	Purpose	Investigator/ Institution	Sponsor
8.2.16	CERTIFICATE(S) OF ANALYSIS OF INVESTIGATIONAL PRODUCT(S) SHIPPED	To document identity, purity, and strength of investigational product(s) to be used in the trial		X
8.2.17	DECODING PROCEDURES FOR BLINDED TRIALS	To document how, in case of an emergency, identity of blinded investigational product can be revealed without breaking the blind for the remaining subjects' treatment	X	X (third party if applicable)
8.2.18	MASTER RANDOMISATION LIST	To document method for randomisation of trial population		X (third party if applicable)
	Title of Document	**Purpose**	**Investigator/ Institution**	**Sponsor**
8.2.19	PRE-TRIAL MONITORING REPORT	To document that the site is suitable for the trial (may be combined with 8.2.20)	X	
8.2.20	TRIAL INITIATION MONITORING REPORT	To document that trial procedures were reviewed with the investigator and the investigator's trial staff (may be combined with 8.2.19)	X	X

8.3 During the Clinical Conduct of the Trial

In addition to having on file the above documents, the following should be added to the files during the trial as evidence that all new relevant information is documented as it becomes available

	Title of Document	Purpose	Investigator/ Institution	Sponsor
8.3.1	**INVESTIGATOR'S BROCHURE UP-DATES**	To document that investigator is informed in a timely manner of relevant information as it becomes available	X	X
8.3.2	**ANY REVISION TO:** - protocol/ amendment(s) and CRF - informed consent form - any other written information provided to subjects - advertisement for subject recruitment (if used)	To document revisions of these trial related documents that take effect during trial	X	X

	Title of Document	Purpose	Investigator/ Institution	Sponsor
8.3.3	**DATED, DOCUMENTED APPROVAL/FAVOURABLE OPINION OF INSTITUTIONAL REVIEW BOARD (IRB) /INDEPENDENT ETHICS COMMITTEE (IEC) OF THE FOLLOWING:** - protocol amendment(s) - revision(s) of: - informed consent form - any other written information to be provided to the subject - advertisement for subject recruitment (if used) - any other documents given approval/favourable opinion - continuing review of trial (where required)	To document that the amendment(s) and/or revision(s) have been subject to IRB/IEC review and were given approval/favourable opinion. To identify the version number and date of the document(s).	X	X
8.3.4	**REGULATORY AUTHORITY(IES) AUTHORISATIONS/APPROVALS/NOTIFICATIONS WHERE REQUIRED FOR:** - protocol amendment(s) and other documents	To document compliance with applicable regulatory requirements	X (where required)	X
8.3.5	**CURRICULUM VITAE FOR NEW INVESTIGATOR(S) AND/OR SUB-INVESTIGATOR(S)**	(see 8.2.10)	X	X

	Title of Document	Purpose	Investigator/ Institution	Sponsor
8.3.6	**UPDATES TO NORMAL VALUE(S)/ RANGE(S) FOR MEDICAL/ LABORATORY/ TECHNICAL PROCEDURE(S)/ TEST(S) INCLUDED IN THE PROTOCOL**	To document normal values and ranges that are revised during the trial (see 8.2.11)	X	X
8.3.7	**UPDATES OF MEDICAL/LABORATORY/ TECHNICAL PROCEDURES/TESTS** - certification or - accreditation or - established quality control and/or external quality assessment or - other validation (where required)	To document that tests remain adequate throughout the trial period (see 8.2.12)	X (where required)	X
8.3.8	**DOCUMENTATION OF INVESTIGATIONAL PRODUCT(S) AND TRIAL-RELATED MATERIALS SHIPMENT**	(see 8.2.15)	X	X
8.3.9	**CERTIFICATE(S) OF ANALYSIS FOR NEW BATCHES OF INVESTIGATIONAL PRODUCTS**	(see 8.2.16)		X
8.3.10	**MONITORING VISIT REPORTS**	To document site visits by, and findings of, the monitor		X

	Title of Document	Purpose	Investigator/ Institution	Sponsor
8.3.11	**RELEVANT COMMUNICATIONS OTHER THAN SITE VISITS** - letters - meeting notes - notes of telephone calls	To document any agreements or significant discussions regarding trial administration, protocol violations, trial conduct, adverse event (AE) reporting	X	X
8.3.12	**SIGNED INFORMED CONSENT FORMS**	To document that consent is obtained in accordance with GCP and protocol and dated prior to participation of each subject in trial. Also to document direct access permission (see 8.2.3)	X	
8.3.13	**SOURCE DOCUMENTS**	To document the existence of the subject and substantiate integrity of trial data collected. To include original documents related to the trial, to medical treatment, and history of subject	X	
8.3.14	**SIGNED, DATED AND COMPLETED CASE REPORT FORMS (CRF)**	To document that the investigator or authorised member of the investigator's staff confirms the observations recorded	X (copy)	X (original)
8.3.15	**DOCUMENTATION OF CRF CORRECTIONS**	To document all changes/additions or corrections made to CRF after initial data were recorded	X (copy)	X (original)

	Title of Document	Purpose	Investigator/ Institution	Sponsor
8.3.16	**NOTIFICATION BY ORIGINATING INVESTIGATOR TO SPONSOR OF SERIOUS ADVERSE EVENTS AND RELATED REPORTS**	Notification by originating investigator to sponsor of serious adverse events and related reports in accordance with 4.11	X	X
8.3.17	**NOTIFICATION BY SPONSOR AND/ OR INVESTIGATOR, WHERE APPLICABLE, TO REGULATORY AUTHORITY(IES) AND IRB(S)/IEC(S) OF UNEXPECTED SERIOUS ADVERSE DRUG REACTIONS AND OF OTHER SAFETY INFORMATION**	Notification by sponsor and/or investigator, where applicable, to regulatory authorities and IRB(s)/ IEC(s) of unexpected serious adverse drug reactions in accordance with 5.17 and 4.11.1 and of other safety information in accordance with 5.16.2 and 4.11.2	X (where required)	X
8.3.18	**NOTIFICATION BY SPONSOR TO INVESTIGATORS OF SAFETY INFORMATION**	Notification by sponsor to investigators of safety information in accordance with 5.16.2	X	X
8.3.19	**INTERIM OR ANNUAL REPORTS TO IRB/IEC AND AUTHORITY(IES)**	Interim or annual reports provided to IRB/IEC in accordance with 4.10 and to authority(ies) in accordance with 5.17.3	X	X (where required)
8.3.20	**SUBJECT SCREENING LOG**	To document identification of subjects who entered pre-trial screening	X	X (where required)

	Title of Document	Purpose	Investigator/ Institution	Sponsor
8.3.21	**SUBJECT IDENTIFICATION CODE LIST**	To document that investigator/institution keeps a confidential list of names of all subjects allocated to trial numbers on enrolling in the trial. Allows investigator/ institution to reveal identity of any subject	X	
8.3.22	**SUBJECT ENROLMENT LOG**	To document chronological enrolment of subjects by trial number	X	
8.3.23	**INVESTIGATIONAL PRODUCTS ACCOUNTABILITY AT THE SITE**	To document that investigational product(s) have been used according to the protocol	X	X
8.3.24	**SIGNATURE SHEET**	To document signatures and initials of all persons authorised to make entries and/or corrections on CRFs	X	X
8.3.25	**RECORD OF RETAINED BODY FLUIDS/ TISSUE SAMPLES (IF ANY)**	To document location and identification of retained samples if assays need to be repeated	X	X

8.4 After Completion or Termination of the Trial

After completion or termination of the trial, all of the documents identified in Sections 8.2 and 8.3 should be in the file together with the following

	Title of Document	Purpose	Investigator/ Institution	Sponsor
8.4.1	**INVESTIGATIONAL PRODUCT(S) ACCOUNTABILITY AT SITE**	To document that the investigational product(s) have been used according to the protocol. To documents the final accounting of investigational product(s) received at the site, dispensed to subjects, returned by the subjects, and returned to sponsor	X	X
8.4.2	**DOCUMENTATION OF INVESTIGATIONAL PRODUCT DESTRUCTION**	To document destruction of unused investigational products by sponsor or at site	X (if destroyed at site)	X
8.4.3	**COMPLETED SUBJECT IDENTIFICATION CODE LIST**	To permit identification of all subjects enrolled in the trial in case follow-up is required. List should be kept in a confidential manner and for agreed upon time	X	
8.4.4	**AUDIT CERTIFICATE (if available)**	To document that audit was performed		X

	Title of Document	Purpose	Investigator/ Institution	Sponsor
8.4.5	**FINAL TRIAL CLOSE-OUT MONITORING REPORT**	To document that all activities required for trial close-out are completed, and copies of essential documents are held in the appropriate files		X
8.4.6	**TREATMENT ALLOCATION AND DECODING DOCUMENTATION**	Returned to sponsor to document any decoding that may have occurred		X
8.4.7	**FINAL REPORT BY INVESTIGATOR TO IRB/IEC WHERE REQUIRED, AND WHERE APPLICABLE, TO THE REGULATORY AUTHORITY(IES)**	To document completion of the trial	X	
8.4.8	**CLINICAL STUDY REPORT**	To document results and interpretation of trial	X (if applicable)	X

Index

Symbols

A

B

E

F

G

H

I

S

T

U

V

W

ABOUT CENTERWATCH

Since 1994, CenterWatch has been the recognized global leader in providing clinical trials information to a broad and influential spectrum of clinical research professionals ranging from top sponsors and CROs to research sites and niche providers, as well as an engaged population of patients interested in clinical research and volunteering.

Clinical Research News and Analysis

The CenterWatch Monthly

The CenterWatch Monthly has been a leader in reporting and analyzing the trends impacting the clinical research landscape. Every issue provides readers with unparalleled, data-rich market knowledge, including regulatory updates, informative short columns on industry topics and detailed drug pipeline analysis to help you better navigate and anticipate a changing landscape and assist you in gaining a competitive advantage for greater success.

CWWeekly

CWWeekly provides expanded analysis on the week's top business and financial news, informative conversations with clinical research executives and insightful strategies on study conduct, technology and global trial issues.

Research Practitioner

This bimonthly newsletter is a valuable educational and career advancement resource providing diverse and comprehensive articles that go beyond what staff "should do" and teaches them "how to" incorporate critical concepts, regulatory updates and strategies to more effectively manage and execute clinical trials—all while earning valuable nursing contact hours accepted by organizations such as ACRP, CCIP and SoCRA.

White Paper Online Library

A collection of white papers written by industry professionals offering a more detailed look at specific topics of the clinical research industry. Each white paper article investigates and analyzes current trends in the industry and the impact on the research community. White papers are complimentary to access on Centerwatch.com.

Patient Enrollment Support

Clinical Trials Listing Service™

CenterWatch's *Clinical Trials Listing Service*™ is the leading online resource for patients interested in clinical trial participation, having reached more than 25 million potential study volunteers since launching in 1994. Today, with 80,000+ global listings and a range of exclusive outreach efforts designed to maximize traffic to your clinical trial listings, CTLS continues to be a valuable and important addition to any patient enrollment strategy. Sponsors, CROs and research centers can also post trial-specific web ads for additional exposure.

Career and Educational Services

JobWatch

JobWatch (centerwatch.com/jobwatch) is a key clinical research recruitment and career resource for professionals currently involved in the industry or professionals interested in obtaining a career in the life sciences or clinical research field.

JobWatch provides job listings, upcoming industry events, educational programs, company profiles and more. Registered job seekers can also manage resumes, set up email alerts and apply directly for positions online. Employers can review resumes, post and manage current openings and maximize exposure with a variety of recruitment and advertising opportunities online along with utilizing the various distribution channels *JobWatch* offers to reach professionals.

Clinical Research Training Guides

CenterWatch's training guide series offers effective and practical tools for those interested in clinical research as well as seasoned professionals seeking to better understand their roles and improve the management of their clinical trials operations in a safe and ethical manner.

- The CRA's Guide to Monitoring Clinical Research

- The CRC's Guide to Coordinating Clinical Research
- The PI's Guide to Conducting Clinical Research
- Protecting Study Volunteers in Research

Regulatory Compliance

Standard Operating Procedures for Good Clinical Practice by Sites

Developed to help clinical research sites meet the challenge of maintaining rigorous standards in a world of diminishing resources. The template has been expanded to include more procedures to assess study feasibility, recruit subjects and ensure regulatory compliance and is based on the Code of Federal Regulations and GCP guidances.

Standard Operating Procedures for Good Clinical Practice by Sponsors of Clinical Trials: Drugs and Biologics

Developed to assist pharmaceutical and biotechnology companies maintain the quality performance and ethical conduct of clinical trials while adhering to U.S. federal regulations. The template contains 30 procedures addressing all Good Clinical Practice requirements and is based on FDA regulations and ICH guidelines.

Standard Operating Procedures for Good Clinical Practice by Sponsors of Medical Device Clinical Trials

Provides detailed SOPs to address specific requirements for medical device research practices to adhere to a discrete set of FDA regulations and guidance. Organizations that sponsor clinical research on new medical devices must implement procedures that comply with both Good Clinical Practice guidelines and federal regulations.

Benchmark Reports

These data-driven reports are compiled from CenterWatch surveys conducted among clinical research professionals. The *Global Site Relationships and Financial and Operating Practices* reports focus on financial analysis, operating challenges and building relationships between sites/sponsors/CROs. They are recommended for all professionals interested in site relationship data between sponsors and CROs.

- Global Site Relationship Benchmark Report for CROs

- Global Site Relationship Benchmark Report for Sponsors
- Site Financial and Operating Benchmark Report

Management Reports and Resource Guides

- The 21st Century Take on Observational Studies: Using Real-World Evidence in the New Millennium
- Clinical Trials Adverse Even Reporting Guide
- Clinical Trial Agreements - A Guide to Key Words and Phrases
- GCP Qualification Audits Choosing Quality Contractors and Sites
- GCP Questions, FDA Answers
- Regenerative Medicine Steps to Accelerate Development
- The Revised Common Rule: New Requirements for Clinical Trials
- Risk-Based Monitoring of Clinical Trials - New Trends and Best Practices
- Risk Management in Clinical Trials - The New ICH E6 Focus

Business Development

Industry Provider Profile Pages

Industry Provider Profile Pages, located on Centerwatch.com, create visibility for contract service providers to showcase their products and services online to the clinical trials community making it a useful and cost-effective way for providers to generate new business leads, increase exposure and reach a captive and targeted audience. Profile Pages are customizable and can include images and links to video presentations, demos and company documents.

Research Center Profiles

This global directory of research centers provides comprehensive listings of hundreds of investigative sites giving your company the critical information needed to find qualified investigators experienced in conducting clinical trials. *Research Center Profiles* are free to search and have an advanced search for centers based on performance metrics, staff certification and are also categorized by therapeutic area, medical conditions and geographic location.